Revolutionizing Pharmaceuticals With AI-Driven Drug Discovery, Design, and Development

Jen-Tsung Chen
https://orcid.org/0000-0002-3540-4449
National University of Kaohsiung, Taiwan

IGI Global
Scientific Publishing
Publishing Tomorrow's Research Today

Vice President of Editorial	Melissa Wagner
Director of Acquisitions	Mikaela Felty
Director of Book Development	Jocelynn Hessler
Production Manager	Mike Brehm
Cover Design	Jose Rosado

Published in the United States of America by
IGI Global Scientific Publishing
701 East Chocolate Avenue
Hershey, PA, 17033, USA
Tel: 717-533-8845 | Fax: 717-533-7115
Website: https://www.igi-global.com E-mail: cust@igi-global.com

Library of Congress Cataloging-in-Publication Data

Names: Chen, Jen-Tsung editor
Title: Revolutionizing pharmaceuticals with AI-driven drug discovery, design, and development / edited by: Jen-Tsung Chen.
Description: Hershey PA : IGI Global Scientific Publishing, [2026] | Includes bibliographical references. | Summary: "This book explores AI models, including machine learning, deep learning, generative AI, and large language models, etc., for drug discovery, design, and development to accelerate the prediction of efficacy and toxicity, clinical trials, drug manufacturing, quality control, and post-market surveillance"-- Provided by publisher.
Identifiers: LCCN 2025034474 (print) | LCCN 2025034475 (ebook) | ISBN 9798337352589 hardcover | ISBN 9798337352596 paperback | ISBN 9798337352602 ebook
Subjects: LCSH: Drugs--Design--Data processing | Artificial intelligence--Medical applications
Classification: LCC RS420 .R45 2026 (print) | LCC RS420 (ebook)
LC record available at https://lccn.loc.gov/2025034474
LC ebook record available at https://lccn.loc.gov/2025034475

British Cataloguing in Publication Data
A Cataloguing in Publication record for this book is available from the British Library.

Table of Contents

Detailed Table of Contents

AI will revolutionize the process of drug development for immunological disorders by enhancing efficiency, precision, and scalability with discovery pipelines. AI-based models combine genomics, transcriptomics, and proteomics to identify targets, optimize drug design, and speed up immunotherapy. Machine learning and deep learning algorithms enable virtual screening, molecular docking, and immune pathways modelling with improved predictive performance and reduced costs. Generative AI and GNNs enable de novo design of immunomodulatory molecules, while XAI improves interpretability and compliance with regulatory policy. Coupling with digital twins and multi-omics frameworks allow real-time modelling of immune dynamics and further advance immunotherapy. Ethical, regulatory, and translational considerations, leveraging data privacy, bias in algorithms, and sustainability, are critical for responsible implementation. Altogether, AI-driven strategies are transforming immunopharmacology to promote data-driven therapeutics, improve outcomes, and redefine paradigms in drug discovery.

Artificial Intelligence in drug development for inflammatory diseases serves to enhance the overall efficiency, precision, and personalization of the process. AI

The incorporation of artificial intelligence (AI) in drug research holds the potential for making transformative predictions of drug efficacy and toxicity with unprecedented speed and accuracy. Traditional pipelines for the discovery and development of medicinal products are time-consuming, expensive, and susceptible to breakdowns, especially at the clinical stage of research, which often result in adverse effects or inadequate therapeutic benefits. AI models, particularly those utilizing deep learning, machine learning, and systems biology, are employed to simulate complex biological interactions, predict pharmacokinetics and pharmacodynamics, and assess molecular security profiles early in the development cycle. By analyzing large datasets from genomics, proteomics, electronic health records, and preclinical assays, these models facilitate better-informed decision-making, including drug development, precision medicine, and adaptive clinical research design.

Artificial intelligence (AI) is revolutionizing the clinical trial paradigm in the pharmaceutical industry at a rapid pace. Machine learning, natural language processing, and real-time analytics enhance every phase of clinical trials—from protocol design and recruitment to monitoring, analysis, and regulatory submission. AI algorithms have been shown to reduce trial length and increase the probability of success. They also enable more personalized and effective strategies for patient engagement. Therefore, this chapter discusses the theoretical frameworks from major international regulatory perspectives and introduces some of the new innovations using AI through all phases (I–IV) of the trials. In addition, the chapter emphasizes the promise and challenges that await AI in clinical development pipelines.

Smart nutrition systems deliver personalized dietary solutions by transforming personal health management by integrating artificial intelligence, IoT, and autonomous technologies. This digital evaluation system handles personal sensitive health data, influences critical dietary decisions, and interacts with broader healthcare networks, which introduces significant cyber security challenges. This chapter discusses the required need for context security framework tailored to the dynamic and personalized nature of smart nutrition technologies. It includes vulnerabilities and recent high-profile breeches. It also explores the limitation of traditional security models and importance of real-time threat detection and privacy preserving strategies.

Artificial Intelligence (AI) is revolutionizing drug development in the pharmaceutical industry by speeding up drug discovery, optimizing clinical trials and facilitating precision medicine. While these developments hold the promise of efficiency and innovation, these developments also bring intricate ethical issues. This chapter critically analyzes the nexus between AI and ethics within drug development, with a focus on the areas of data privacy, algorithmic bias, transparency, intellectual property, and gaps in regulations. Practical examples and case studies help us understand the implications of unregulated AI adoption. Several global and national regulatory agencies discussed along with Institutional review processes form the backbone for ethical verification and validation of results. The chapter outlines recommendations and ethical guidelines to aid responsible, explainable and collaborative AI adoption within the pharmaceutical industry. By reconciling innovation and accountability, it seeks to create a transparent and fair future for AI-driven drug development.

Preface

INTRODUCTION

The pharmaceutical sciences are undergoing a profound transformation as artificial intelligence (AI) increasingly reshapes how medicines are discovered, designed, developed, and delivered. Escalating research and development costs, high attrition rates, and the growing complexity of human disease demand new paradigms that move beyond traditional trial-and-error approaches. In this context, AI has emerged not merely as a supportive tool but as a foundational driver of innovation across the entire drug development lifecycle.

From early-stage target identification to late-stage clinical trials and post-market surveillance, AI-driven methods enable the integration and analysis of vast, heterogeneous datasets that were previously unmanageable. Machine learning, deep learning, generative modeling, and intelligent decision-support systems are now accelerating timelines, improving predictive accuracy, and opening new possibilities for personalized and precision medicine. At the same time, these advances raise important questions related to data quality, transparency, ethics, regulation, and societal trust.

This edited reference book, *Revolutionizing Pharmaceuticals With AI-Driven Drug Discovery, Design, and Development*, brings together international experts from academia, research institutes, and clinical and industrial settings to provide a comprehensive, multidisciplinary perspective on this rapidly evolving field. The volume is designed to serve as both an authoritative reference for researchers and professionals and an accessible resource for graduate students and newcomers seeking to understand how AI is redefining pharmaceutical innovation.

SCOPE AND OBJECTIVES OF THE BOOK

The primary objective of this book is to present a holistic view of how AI technologies are being applied across diverse stages of pharmaceutical research and development. Rather than focusing on a single technique or disease area, the chapters collectively explore foundational methods, domain-specific applications, translational challenges, and cross-cutting ethical and regulatory considerations. This structure reflects the inherently interconnected nature of modern drug development.

A key emphasis of the volume is the integration of AI with established scientific knowledge systems, including traditional medicine, immunology, inflammation biology, cardiovascular research, nutrition science, and clinical trial design. By highlighting both methodological advances and real-world use cases, the book illustrates how AI can bridge gaps between discovery and translation while supporting safer, faster, and more cost-effective therapeutic development.

Equally important, this book addresses the limitations and responsibilities that accompany AI adoption. Several chapters critically examine issues such as algorithmic bias, explainability, data privacy, cybersecurity, and ethical governance, underscoring the need for responsible, transparent, and human-centered implementation. In doing so, the volume aims to balance technological optimism with rigorous scientific and ethical scrutiny.

CHAPTER OVERVIEW

Chapter 1 provides a foundational overview of pharmaceuticals in the AI age, outlining core AI methodologies and their applications across the drug development pipeline, while also addressing emerging challenges and future directions. Chapter 2 explores the synergistic integration of AI with traditional medicine, demonstrating how computational approaches can unlock bioactive compounds and validate knowledge rooted in historical and ethnobotanical practices.

Chapter 3 focuses on AI-driven drug screening, detailing modern virtual screening techniques, molecular representations, and data-driven prioritization strategies. Chapters 4 and 5 examine AI-enabled drug development in immunological and inflammatory diseases, respectively, highlighting the role of multi-omics integration, generative models, digital twins, and explainable AI in advancing targeted and personalized therapies.

Chapter 6 extends the discussion to inflammatory and cardiovascular diseases through the lens of Intelligent Translational Research Systems, emphasizing the translation of AI insights from bench to bedside. Chapter 7 centers on predictive modeling of drug efficacy and toxicity, showcasing how AI can mitigate late-stage failures and enhance patient safety. Chapter 8 addresses the transformative impact of AI on clinical trials, from protocol design to regulatory submission. Chapter 9 broadens the pharmaceutical perspective by examining AI-powered smart nutrition systems and associated cybersecurity challenges. Finally, Chapter 10 provides a critical examination of ethical considerations in AI-driven drug development, offering frameworks and guidelines for responsible innovation.

CONCLUSION

Collectively, the chapters in this volume demonstrate that AI is no longer a peripheral innovation in pharmaceutical sciences but a central force reshaping research, development, and clinical practice. By enabling deeper insights from complex data and supporting more informed decision-making, AI holds the potential to significantly reduce inefficiencies and improve therapeutic outcomes across a wide range of diseases.

At the same time, the contributions underscore that technological advancement must be accompanied by robust ethical, regulatory, and methodological safeguards. Transparency, explainability, data governance, and interdisciplinary collaboration emerge as recurring themes that are essential for sustaining trust and ensuring that AI-driven solutions benefit patients and society at large.

As editors, we hope this book will serve as a valuable reference and a catalyst for further research, dialogue, and collaboration in the field of AI-enabled pharmaceuticals. By bringing together diverse perspectives and expertise, this volume aims to support the development of innovative, responsible, and impactful drug discovery and development practices for the years to come.

Chapter 1

Pharmaceuticals in the AI Age: An Introductory Overview

Irina Negut
https://orcid.org/0000-0003-4038-7548
National Institute for Lasers, Plasma, and Radiation Physics, Romania

Cláudia Suellen Ferro Oliveira
https://orcid.org/0000-0002-0113-9528
CBQF—Centro de Biotecnologia e Química Fina, Laboratório Associado, Escola Superior de Biotecnologia, Universidade Católica Portuguesa, Portugal

Anita Ioana Visan
https://orcid.org/0000-0003-0539-4160
National Institute for Laser, Plasma, and Radiation Physics, Romania

ABSTRACT

Artificial intelligence is transforming drug discovery by addressing key challenges in cost, speed, and success rates. This chapter examines the application of artificial intelligence technologies, including machine learning, deep learning, and generative models, across the drug development pipeline, from target identification and hit discovery to lead optimization and clinical trials. Use cases include virtual screening, de novo molecule generation, ADMET prediction, and patient stratification. Despite rapid progress, challenges persist in data quality, model interpretability, regulation, and ethical concerns such as dual-use risks. Future directions, including hybrid artificial intelligence-quantum systems, federated learning, and digital twins, promise to further personalize and optimize drug development. The chapter highlights the potential of artificial intelligence to drive innovation while emphasizing responsible implementation.

DOI: 10.4018/979-8-3373-5258-9.ch001

1 INTRODUCTION

Drug discovery has long been recognized as one of the most resource-intensive and uncertain processes in biomedical research. On average, it takes 10–15 years to develop a single new therapy, with a failure rate exceeding 90% across the pipeline (DiMasi et al., 2016). Attrition is particularly pronounced in late-stage clinical trials, where drugs often fail due to lack of efficacy or unforeseen toxicity, despite extensive investment. These limitations have prompted researchers and pharmaceutical companies to explore transformative technologies that can improve efficiency, reduce costs, and increase the success probability.

Artificial intelligence (AI) has emerged as one of the most promising solutions to these challenges. By integrating large-scale biomedical data, deep learning (DL) architectures, and generative models, AI systems are capable of discovering novel molecules, predicting their pharmacological properties, and optimizing them in ways that are infeasible for traditional high-throughput screening alone (Vamathevan, Apweiler, et al., 2019). For example, de novo drug design has been revolutionized by variational autoencoders (VAEs), generative adversarial networks (GANs), and transformer-based models, which can propose entirely new chemical entities with optimized binding affinities and synthetic feasibility (Zhavoronkov et al., 2019).

Applications of AI are not limited to small-molecule discovery. In structural biology, DeepMind's AlphaFold achieved near-experimental accuracy in protein structure prediction, releasing over 200 million predicted protein structures, thus providing an invaluable resource for understanding disease mechanisms and accelerating rational drug design (Artrith et al., 2021). In systems biology, digital pathology and high-content phenotypic screening allow convolutional neural networks (CNNs) to extract meaningful features from cellular images, supporting phenotypic drug discovery at scale (Moen et al., 2019). Moreover, AI is being integrated into clinical trial design, with predictive models helping to stratify patients, anticipate adverse events, and optimize dosing regimens (Mak & Pichika, 2019).

Despite these successes, the integration of AI into drug discovery faces significant hurdles. A primary concern is data quality and availability, as biomedical datasets are often incomplete, biased, or siloed across institutions, limiting the generalizability of AI models (Artrith et al., 2021). Additionally, the black-box nature of DL algorithms raises questions about interpretability and trust, especially in high-stakes regulatory environments (Bellucci et al., 2021). Regulatory agencies are only beginning to establish frameworks for evaluating AI-driven drugs, creating uncertainty for developers. Ethical concerns, particularly regarding the dual-use risk of AI models being misused to design harmful compounds, further underscore the need for governance and transparency (Urbina et al., 2022).

The future of AI in drug discovery will likely depend on integrating multiple emerging technologies. Hybrid AI–quantum computing approaches may overcome current bottlenecks in molecular simulations, federated learning promises secure collaborative innovation without direct data sharing, and digital twins could enable personalized, patient-specific drug development (Bauer et al., 2022). Moreover, self-improving AI systems that continuously learn from real-world clinical results may transform drug development into an adaptive and dynamic process, reducing the gap between laboratory innovation and patient outcomes (Goertzel, 2014).

This chapter uses an integrative research approach that combines systematic review methods with qualitative analysis to capture current progress, applications, and challenges in AI-driven drug discovery. The goal was to provide both scientific depth and practical insight, reflecting developments in academia, industry, and regulation. Relevant literature was collected from major databases such as PubMed, Scopus, Web of Science, IEEE Xplore, and ScienceDirect, along with white papers and reports from leading AI-focused biotech firms like Insilico Medicine, Exscientia, Recursion, and BenevolentAI. Searches included terms such as "AI drug discovery," "machine learning pharmacology," "deep learning drug design," and "generative chemistry models," focusing on studies published between 2015 and 2025. Earlier foundational works were included where needed for context. Studies were included if they applied AI to any part of the drug discovery pipeline (target identification, hit discovery, lead optimization, or preclinical and clinical development). Only peer-reviewed or validated industrial sources were considered.

In sum, AI has moved from a peripheral tool to becoming a central enabler of drug discovery and development. This chapter explores the current applications, limitations, and future trajectories of AI in this domain, providing a critical perspective on how the technology can balance innovation with responsibility to deliver safe, effective, and affordable therapies.

2 EVOLUTION OF DRUG DISCOVERY

2.1. Traditional Approach

The conventional drug development pipeline has historically relied on labor-intensive high-throughput screening, iterative trial-and-error experimentation, and lengthy preclinical and multi-phase clinical trial processes. On average, bringing a new molecular entity from discovery to regulatory approval takes 10–15 years and often exceeds $2 billion in total costs (Wizemann et al., 2020). The Tufts Center for the Study of Drug Development has estimated that the fully capitalized cost of developing a single new drug, including the expense of failed candidates, is approximately $2.6 billion, a figure echoed in industry analyses (Lindsley, 2014) . Alternative evaluations have found a broad range of R&D costs for new drug approvals, from $314 million to $2.8 billion, depending on the therapeutic area, study design, and cost accounting methods used (Wouters et al., 2020).

This escalating cost and time burden is reflected in Eroom's law; this represents the observation that the number of new drugs approved/billion US dollars spent on R&D has halved roughly every 9 years since 1950, despite technological advances such as high-throughput screening (Scannell et al., 2012). In the early 2000s, the pharmaceutical industry witnessed a significant shift toward computational methods, not merely as supplementary tools, but as integral components of the drug discovery process. This evolution was sparked by the burgeoning wealth of biological data from endeavors like the Human Genome Project, which necessitated advanced bioinformatics approaches to mine and interpret complex datasets (De Vivo et al., 2016).

During this era, molecular modeling, encompassing molecular docking, dynamics simulations, and structural visualization, emerged as a transformative strategy for lead identification and optimization. A 2000 review emphasized that advances in structural biology and computational sciences had finally made rational drug design practicable, especially in lead discovery and refinement (Ooms, 2000). Similarly, Lyne et al study highlighted how researchers, leveraging computational models of protein 3D structures, were starting to predict drug–target interactions more efficiently, although experimental validation remained essential (Lyne, 2002).

Virtual screening also became increasingly prominent. By the late 2000s, structure-based and ligand-based virtual screening techniques enabled the rapid in silico evaluation of massive compound libraries against specific molecular targets, making drug discovery both faster and more cost-effective (Lionta et al., 2014).

Beyond docking and screening, computational biology and bioinformatics grew in parallel. These disciplines facilitated the systematic identification of drug targets through genome and proteome analysis, and they became fundamental in target validation workflows (Xia, 2017).

As computational power and algorithms advanced, molecular dynamics (MD) simulations evolved from niche tools into near-routine methods for investigating protein flexibility and ligand binding dynamics. These simulations allowed researchers to capture conformational changes and better understand drug–target interactions over time (Ahmed et al., 2023).

By the mid-2010s, a broad spectrum of computer-aided drug design (CADD) techniques, including molecular docking, ADMET modeling, and pharmacophore mapping, had become entrenched across nearly every stage of the drug development pipeline, from target discovery to lead optimization and preclinical testing (Ou-Yang et al., 2012).

Starting in the 2010s, the drug discovery landscape began embracing AI and ML in earnest. While rudimentary ML tools had existed in prior decades, it was during this period, catalyzed by the exponential growth of biomedical big data, computational power, and DL, that AI's practical applications in drug research truly took off (Serrano et al., 2024). Between 2012 and 2014, a wave of AI-driven biotech startups emerged like Insilico Medicine (founded 2014) among them, leveraging DL, generative adversarial networks, and reinforcement learning for in silico drug discovery (Lionta et al., 2014).

Around 2017, the advent of generative AI (GenAI) in drug discovery marked another important milestone. Companies such as Insilico Medicine and AstraZeneca began applying GenAI techniques to generate novel molecules, handle data workflows, and reconfigure laboratory operations to align with digital processes (Briefing).

The transformative potential of AI was dramatically underscored with the introduction of AlphaFold (DeepMind) in 2018, which revolutionized protein structure prediction, rapidly followed by the even more accurate AlphaFold 2 in 2020, a breakthrough that dramatically accelerated structure-based drug design efforts (Senior et al., 2020).

In 2020, the MIT Jameel Clinic demonstrated DL's power in drug discovery, by discovering halicin, the first new antibiotic in 30 years, through AI-guided screening (Stokes et al., 2020), and soon afterward, they identified abaucin, a DL–designed antibiotic targeting an especially dangerous bacterial pathogen (Liu et al., 2023).

By 2022, AI-assisted platforms had sped up drug candidates' journey from target identification to preclinical nomination in as little as 18 months, showing the narrowing timeline between discovery and development (Huanbutta et al., 2024).The broader field also saw a surge in publications on AI-for-drug-discovery, peaking around 2022, a reflection of the technology's growing adoption and maturation (Karger & Kureljusic, 2022).

Several prominent startups and spin-outs embodied this AI-driven revolution. For instance, Insilico Medicine, with its AI-powered platforms such as Chemistry42, PandaOmics, and de novo molecular design engines, reported generating drug candidates rapidly and entering human trials by 2023(Ren et al., 2023). Another example, Exscientia, announced in early 2020 that it had developed the first-ever AI-designed drug molecule to enter human clinical trials (Chun, 2023).

In recognition of AI's impact on the fundamental challenges of biology, and its indirect but powerful influence on drug discovery, the 2024 Nobel Prize in Chemistry was awarded to Demis Hassabis and John Jumper (DeepMind's AlphaFold) and David Baker (protein design) for breakthroughs in protein structure prediction and design via AI, breakthroughs with vast implications for accelerating drug development (Jumper et al., 2021).

Building on these advances, Isomorphic Labs, an Alphabet-backed spin-off, was launched in 2021 to directly apply AlphaFold-driven insights to drug design. By 2025, it had raised $600 million in external funding, partnering with major pharmaceutical firms to enhance its AI-driven drug development engine (Vinluan, 2025). Concurrently, AlphaFold 3 released in 2024 expanded predictive modeling to include protein complexes with DNA, RNA, ligands, and ions, further empowering drug design workflows (Abramson et al., 2024).

Yet, despite this rapid technological progress, no AI-designed drug has yet reached the market. As of mid-2025, many AI-generated candidates are still undergoing clinical evaluation—highlighting both the promise and the ongoing challenges that persist in translation from model to medicine (Ogut, 2025).

2.2. Entry of AI

Starting in the 2010s, ML began revolutionizing drug discovery by enabling the efficient analysis of vast chemical and biological datasets previously too complex for conventional approaches. ML-driven models became instrumental in identifying promising drug targets, predicting compound efficacy, and validating therapeutic hypotheses during early stages of development. These data-intensive methods significantly enhanced both the accuracy and speed of the discovery process(Vamathevan, Clark, et al., 2019).

AI-assisted compound screening has also emerged as a pivotal innovation. A notable example is Iambic Therapeutics' Enchant model, an AI-powered tool trained on extensive preclinical data. This model achieves a predictive accuracy of 0.74, outpacing earlier models (with an accuracy of 0.58), and promises to halve both cost and timeline of early drug development by reducing failure rates in later stages (Ferreira & Carneiro, 2025).

Generative AI techniques have further broadened the drug discovery frontier. For example, DL systems like AtomNet employ convolutional neural networks for structure-based drug design, predicting novel bioactive compounds with increasing precision (Kandregula, 2025).Moreover, systematic reviews detail how DL approaches, including molecule generation and property prediction, are now applied at virtually every stage of drug development (Deng et al., 2022).

The integration of AI with experimental platforms has also yielded transformative results. Techniques like DNA-encoded libraries (DELs), when paired with ML frameworks, enable rapid hit identification, accelerating the discovery of potent inhibitors across multiple targets (GREGORY; McCloskey et al., 2020).

Collectively, these advances show that AI has evolved from being a complementary tool to serving as an accelerator within drug discovery workflows, streamlining high-throughput screening, reducing dependence on labor-intensive experimentation, and enabling faster, more cost-effective identification of candidate therapeutics.

3 CORE AI TECHNOLOGIES IN DRUG DESIGN

The incorporation of AI into drug design has been driven by several foundational computational technologies, each contributing to diverse stages of drug development, from bioactivity prediction to de novo molecule generation.

3.1 ML Algorithms

ML algorithms are computational methods designed to automatically identify patterns and relationships in data, enabling predictive and descriptive modeling without the need for explicit, rule-based programming. In drug discovery, ML algorithms learn from diverse datasets—such as chemical structures, molecular descriptors, omics profiles, and bioassay results—to predict biological activity, classify compounds, optimize pharmacokinetic and pharmacodynamic properties, and identify novel therapeutic targets (Vamathevan, Clark, et al., 2019).

These algorithms are broadly categorized into supervised learning, where models are trained on labeled datasets to predict known outcomes (e.g., active vs. inactive compounds); unsupervised learning, which uncovers hidden structure in unlabeled data (e.g., clustering compounds by structural similarity); and reinforcement learning, in which models iteratively improve decision-making through reward-based feedback (e.g., optimizing de novo molecule design) (Popova et al., 2018).

Common ML algorithms applied in cheminformatics include Random Forests (RF), which aggregate predictions from multiple decision trees for robust classification and regression; Gradient Boosting Machines (GBM), which build decision trees sequentially to minimize residual errors; and Support Vector Machines (SVM), which determine optimal separating hyperplanes for binary or multi-class classification (Chen & Guestrin, 2016).

RF and GBMs are ensemble learning methods widely adopted in computational drug discovery for tasks such as predictive modeling of bioactivity and pharmacokinetic property estimation. RF operates by constructing multiple decision trees during training and aggregating their outputs to improve generalization and reduce overfitting, making it particularly effective for noisy, high-dimensional chemical datasets. GBMs, including the widely used XGBoost implementation, iteratively build an ensemble of weak learners, typically decision trees, where each subsequent model focuses on correcting the residual errors of its predecessors. This sequential learning process enables GBMs to achieve high accuracy and robustness, especially when working with large and diverse chemical libraries (Chen & Guestrin, 2016).

Recent advances highlight their performance in real-world drug discovery tasks. For instance, a 2025 study demonstrated that Gradient Boosting achieved an R^2 of 0.87 and an RMSE of 0.537 in predicting aqueous solubility, metrics comparable to or surpassing traditional descriptor-heavy models, showing its efficiency and predictive power in early-stage compound screening (Sodaei et al., 2025). Similarly, a large-scale QSAR benchmarking effort revealed that XGBoost consistently ranked among the top-performing algorithms when trained on millions of compounds across hundreds of endpoints, confirming its versatility and scalability for cheminformatics applications (Boldini et al., 2023).

Support Vector Machines (SVMs), another cornerstone of ML in cheminformatics, function by finding the optimal hyperplane that separates data points of different classes in a high-dimensional space. This makes them highly effective for classification problems such as distinguishing active from inactive compounds in virtual screening campaigns. SVMs are known for their robustness in small-to-medium datasets, where DL models may overfit. In recent applications, they have been combined with ensemble techniques and pre-training strategies to maintain high classification performance even under data-limited conditions (Talevi et al., 2020).

Collectively, RF, GBMs, and SVMs form a core suite of traditional ML tools that continue to deliver state-of-the-art performance in drug discovery, often complementing or serving as benchmarks for newer DL architectures. Their interpretability, computational efficiency, and compatibility with diverse molecular descriptors ensure they remain highly relevant in both industrial and academic drug research.

3.2 DL Architectures

DL architectures have become integral to modern drug discovery, offering unprecedented capabilities in modeling highly complex, non-linear relationships inherent in chemical, biological, and pharmacological data. Unlike traditional ML approaches, which often rely on hand-crafted molecular descriptors and feature engineering, DL models can automatically learn hierarchical feature representations directly from raw, high-dimensional inputs such as molecular graphs, protein 3D structures, SMILES strings, and biomedical images (Yang & Cheng, 2025).

This capability is particularly advantageous for integrating heterogeneous data modalities, a common requirement in drug discovery where structural, functional, and experimental datasets must be jointly analyzed. DL architectures, such as Convolutional Neural Networks (CNNs), excel at extracting spatial patterns from molecular images and protein–ligand complexes; Recurrent Neural Networks (RNNs) and Transformers capture long-range dependencies in chemical and protein sequences; and Graph Neural Networks (GNNs) learn relational patterns from molecular graphs, modeling atoms as nodes and bonds as edges (Hervella et al., 2022; Sirén & Paten, 2022).

Moreover, DL models have shown superior performance in key drug discovery tasks such as virtual screening, drug–target interaction (DTI) prediction, ADMET (absorption, distribution, metabolism, excretion, toxicity) profiling, and de novo drug design. For example, Transformer-based architectures like MolBERT and ChemBERTa have achieved state-of-the-art accuracy in property prediction by leveraging self-attention mechanisms to model contextual relationships in molecular sequences (Chithrananda et al., 2020; Jing et al., 2018).

By reducing reliance on manual feature engineering and enabling end-to-end learning pipelines, DL architectures not only improve predictive performance but also facilitate the integration of multi-omics, structural, and experimental datasets into unified models. This holistic approach is increasingly seen as essential for accelerating drug discovery, particularly in the era of big data and AI-driven pharmaceutical research (Jiménez-Luna et al., 2021).

CNNs are widely used in molecular image analysis and structure-based drug design due to their ability to automatically detect and learn hierarchical spatial features from structured input data. In cheminformatics, CNNs can process 2D chemical structure diagrams or 3D protein–ligand complexes to extract local and global spatial patterns, such as functional groups, hydrogen-bond networks, and hydrophobic pockets, that are highly predictive of biological activity (Ragoza et al., 2017).

When applied to virtual screening and binding affinity prediction, CNN-based models often outperform traditional molecular docking by learning complex interaction patterns that are difficult to capture using manually defined scoring functions. A landmark example is AtomNet, which applies a 3D CNN to voxelized representations of protein–ligand binding site grids, enabling end-to-end prediction of binding affinities. In benchmark tests, AtomNet outperformed conventional docking tools in both speed and predictive accuracy for certain therapeutic targets (Mbituyimana et al., 2023).

Recent advancements have further enhanced CNN capabilities by integrating Graph Convolutional Networks (GCNs) or Geometric DL components, enabling the simultaneous modeling of spatial and topological molecular information. This hybrid approach captures atom-level connectivity alongside 3D spatial arrangements, leading to improved generalization across diverse chemical scaffolds(Hervella et al., 2022; Qiu et al., 2023).

RNNs and transformer architectures have become central to sequence-based drug–target prediction tasks, where the primary data formats include SMILES strings for chemical compounds and amino acid sequences for protein targets. These models address a critical aspect of cheminformatics and bioinformatics, capturing the sequential dependencies inherent in chemical notation systems and biological sequences to infer activity, binding potential, and physicochemical properties (Ghosh et al., 2024).

RNNs, particularly those augmented with Long Short-Term Memory (LSTM) or Gated Recurrent Unit (GRU) cells, are designed to handle long-range dependencies by mitigating the vanishing gradient problem that affects traditional RNNs.

In drug discovery, LSTM-based models have been used to:

- Predict binding affinities between small molecules and proteins by learning contextual dependencies between molecular substructures and protein motifs.
- Generate novel chemical entities through sequence-to-sequence translation from molecular scaffolds to optimized drug-like candidates.
- Model ADMET properties using sequential descriptors derived from SMILES strings (Nag et al., 2022).

While RNNs have proven effective, they are inherently limited in parallelization and tend to struggle with extremely long sequences, such as those found in large proteins.

Transformer architectures, originally introduced for natural language processing (NLP), have since surpassed RNNs in scalability, representational capacity, and performance, especially in large-scale sequence modeling. Transformers rely on self-attention mechanisms to capture contextual relationships between all elements in a sequence simultaneously, eliminating the sequential bottleneck of RNNs (Ashish, 2017).

In drug discovery, domain-specific transformer models have emerged, including:

- MolBERT – pre-trained on millions of SMILES sequences, fine-tuned for property prediction and virtual screening (Sirén & Paten, 2022).
- ChemBERTa – optimized for chemical property prediction using masked language modeling on SMILES data (Chithrananda et al., 2020).
- ESM (Evolutionary Scale Modeling) – trained on hundreds of millions of protein sequences, enabling structure prediction and drug–target interaction modeling without explicit 3D input (Lin et al., 2023).

Recent advances have also seen multi-modal transformer models that integrate molecular sequences with protein structures, bioassay results, and omics data, thereby creating unified frameworks for end-to-end drug–target affinity prediction (Xia et al., 2023). These architectures are particularly promising for accelerating polypharmacology profiling and drug repurposing, as they can simultaneously reason over multiple biological and chemical contexts.

3.3 Generative Models

Generative models have emerged as transformative tools in de novo drug design, enabling the creation of entirely new molecular structures that meet predefined chemical and biological criteria. By learning the underlying distribution of chemical space from large molecular datasets, these models can generate novel compounds with optimized pharmacological profiles, bypassing the limitations of traditional library-based screening (Zhavoronkov et al., 2019).Generative Adversarial Networks (GANs), introduced by Goodfellow et al. in 2014, consist of a generator that proposes candidate molecules and a discriminator that evaluates whether these candidates resemble real molecules from the training dataset. In drug discovery, GANs have been adapted to generate molecules with specific properties, such as high binding affinity, low toxicity, or desired physicochemical characteristics. For example, MolGAN and its derivatives combine GAN frameworks with graph-based molecular representations to directly generate valid chemical graphs, often incorporating reinforcement learning to steer the generator toward desired activity profiles(De Cao & Kipf, 2018). Recent innovations include property-conditioned GANs that integrate QSAR predictions into the generation loop, thereby producing compounds that satisfy multi-parameter optimization objectives (Gómez-Bombarelli et al., 2018).

Variational Autoencoders (VAEs), on the other hand, learn a continuous latent space representation of molecules, allowing smooth interpolation and targeted optimization of chemical structures. By encoding molecules into a lower-dimensional latent space and then decoding them back into valid chemical structures, VAEs enable systematic exploration of chemical space and scaffold hopping. Notable examples include Junction Tree VAEs, which maintain chemical validity during generation by constructing molecules from valid substructures(Jin et al., 2018), and conditional VAEs that generate molecules satisfying specific biological or physicochemical constraints (Fan et al., 2025).

Recent studies (2021–2025) have also explored hybrid generative approaches, combining GANs and VAEs or integrating them with reinforcement learning to balance novelty, diversity, and target-specific optimization (Özçelik et al., 2025). These methods have demonstrated the ability to propose drug-like molecules that pass in silico ADMET filters and, in some cases, advance to preclinical testing within significantly shortened timelines.

By enabling the on-demand generation of candidate molecules, generative models represent a paradigm shift from traditional drug discovery's trial-and-error approach to a design-first strategy, potentially reducing both the cost and time required to bring new therapeutics to the clinic.

3.4 Natural Language Processing

Natural Language Processing (NLP) techniques have become indispensable for mining the vast and rapidly growing body of biomedical literature, clinical trial reports, and patent databases to uncover drug repurposing opportunities. These methods transform unstructured text into structured, machine-readable knowledge, enabling automated hypothesis generation and evidence synthesis for drug–disease–target relationships(Mak et al., 2024).

Traditional NLP pipelines in drug discovery rely on named entity recognition (NER) to identify mentions of drugs, proteins, genes, and diseases, followed by relation extraction to determine the semantic and causal relationships between them. More recent advances leverage DL –based NLP models such as BioBERT, SciBERT, and PubMedBERT, which are pre-trained on millions of biomedical abstracts and full-text articles. These transformer-based architectures excel at contextual understanding, enabling more accurate extraction of relationships relevant to repurposing (Lee et al., 2020).

In the context of drug repurposing, NLP tools can:

- Identify hidden associations between existing drugs and new therapeutic indications by aggregating co-occurrence patterns across thousands of publications.
- Integrate literature-derived evidence with omics and clinical data to prioritize repurposing candidates.
- Automatically monitor and summarize emerging research trends relevant to specific diseases or drug classes (Mallesh et al., 2021).

Recent examples demonstrate the impact of NLP in real-world applications. For instance, AI-driven text mining platforms such as IBM Watson for Drug Discovery and Elsevier's Entellect have been used to identify novel therapeutic uses for FDA-approved drugs by scanning large-scale literature corpora and clinical trial registries(Mak et al., 2024). During the COVID-19 pandemic, NLP pipelines were deployed on the CORD-19 dataset to rapidly extract candidate antiviral compounds with supportive mechanistic evidence from prior research (Wang et al., 2020).

The latest trend (2023–2025) involves multi-modal NLP systems that combine text mining with structured biological databases, molecular docking predictions, and network pharmacology models to provide a holistic view of repurposing opportunities (Dev Sharma et al., 2025). By continuously ingesting and synthesizing literature in near real-time, these systems accelerate the translation of research findings into actionable therapeutic hypotheses.

4 APPLICATIONS IN THE DRUG DEVELOPMENT PIPELINE

4.1 Target Identification

The earliest stage of the drug development, target identification, involves determining the molecular entities (typically genes, proteins, or RNA molecules) that play a causal role in disease onset or progression. Figure 1 represents a clear step-by-step outline of the target identification and validation process, as it's applied in modern AI-driven drug discovery.

Figure 1. AI in target identification and validation

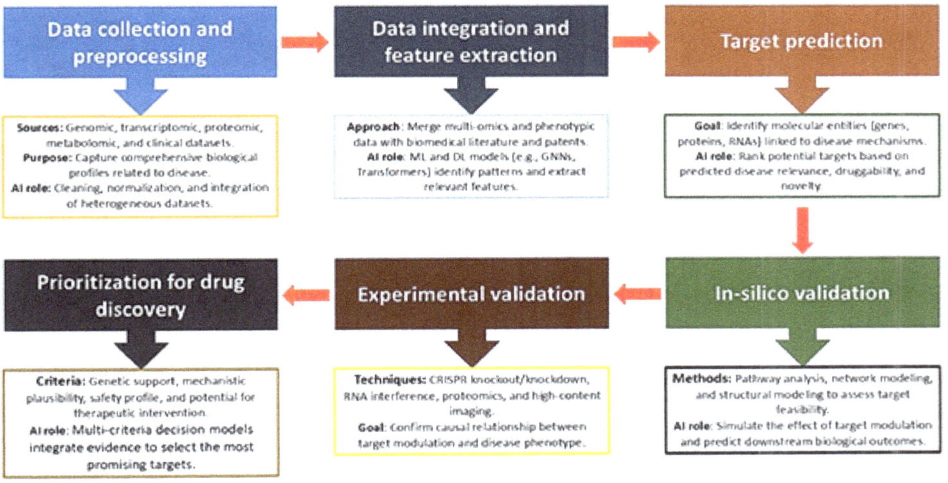

Advances in AI have transformed this process by enabling the integration and analysis of large, heterogeneous datasets, including genomic, transcriptomic, proteomic, metabolomic, and clinical data. Table 1 summarizes key AI-enabled approaches, the computational techniques underpinning them, and their impact on accelerating and de-risking early drug development.

Table 1. AI approaches in target identification

Approach	Description	AI Techniques	Impact	References
Multi-omics integration	Combines genomic, transcriptomic, proteomic, metabolomic, and clinical datasets to identify disease-associated targets.	ML, DL, statistical modeling	Increases accuracy by leveraging heterogeneous data sources.	(Flores et al., 2023)
Network-based AI	Integrates GWAS with functional genomics; uses graph neural networks (GNNs) to find high-confidence, druggable targets.	GNNs, network analytics	Links molecular targets mechanistically to disease.	(Yan et al., 2017)
Literature & patent mining	NLP models analyze millions of biomedical texts to extract known and novel target-disease associations.	Transformer NLP models, entity recognition	Uncovers latent relationships not yet experimentally validated.	(Lin & Chou, 2025)
Experimental validation loop	Validates AI-predicted targets via CRISPR screens, high-content imaging, proteomics.	Lab-based experimental platforms	Closes the loop between computational prediction and biological proof.	(Angello et al., 2024)

Modern ML and DL algorithms can uncover subtle and non-linear associations between disease phenotypes and their underlying molecular drivers. For example, AI models have been used to map disease-associated genes and proteins by mining multi-omics datasets alongside biomedical literature, thereby generating ranked lists of candidate targets based on predicted disease relevance (Nosrati & Nosrati, 2023).

A notable approach involves combining genome-wide association study (GWAS) results with functional genomics data through GNNs and other network-based AI methods to identify high-confidence targets that are both mechanistically linked to disease and amenable to pharmacological modulation (Srivastava et al., 2025). For instance, AI-driven target discovery platforms such as BenevolentAI and Insilico Medicine's PandaOmics apply large-scale network analytics to prioritize targets for complex diseases, including neurodegenerative disorders and oncology(Kamya et al., 2024).

In addition, NLP models trained on millions of biomedical publications and patents can extract and synthesize known molecular-disease relationships while uncovering latent associations that may not yet be experimentally validated(Mallesh et al., 2021). These AI-derived hypotheses can then be experimentally confirmed using CRISPR screens, high-content imaging, and proteomics profiling, thereby closing the loop between computational prediction and biological validation.

By unifying multi-omics analytics, literature mining, and network-based inference, AI-powered target identification not only increases the speed and accuracy of discovering novel disease drivers but also helps reduce the risk of late-stage attrition by focusing on targets with strong genetic and mechanistic support.

4.2 Hit Discovery

Hit discovery refers to the process of identifying chemical compounds with measurable biological activity against a validated drug target. Traditionally achieved through high-throughput screening (HTS) of large compound libraries, this process has been significantly accelerated and refined through the integration of AI-driven virtual screening methods. These approaches use computational models to predict the binding affinity of candidate molecules to target proteins, drastically reducing the number of compounds that must be experimentally tested (Mbituyimana et al., 2023). A clear step-by-step outline of hit discovery in AI-driven drug development is depicted in Figure 2.

Figure 2. A visual workflow diagram showing where AI is applied in each stage of hit discovery

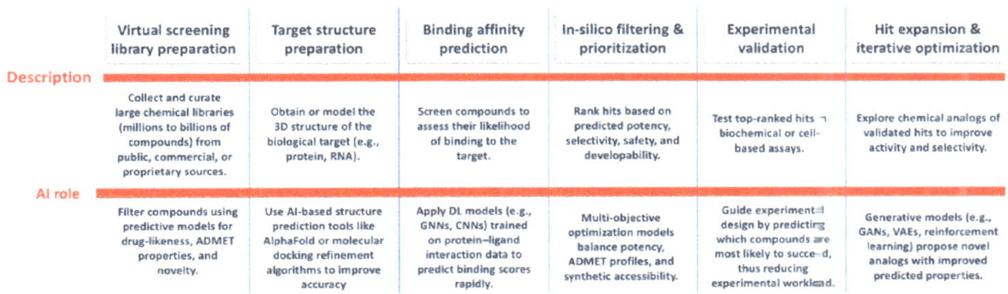

ML and DL models for virtual screening leverage diverse input representations, such as 3D protein–ligand interaction grids, molecular graphs, and sequence embeddings, to learn structure–activity relationships (SARs). For example, CNN–based methods like AtomNet have demonstrated improved hit rates compared to conventional docking by capturing complex 3D interaction patterns(Mbituyimana et al., 2023; Wallach et al., 2015).

Other architectures, such as GNNs, directly model molecular topology and have achieved state-of-the-art results in binding affinity prediction benchmarks, particularly when trained on datasets like PDBbind and BindingDB(Chen et al., 2022). Furthermore, transformer-based models (e.g., MolBERT, ChemBERTa) have been adapted for virtual screening tasks, where they process SMILES strings or 3D-conformer sequences to rank-order large chemical libraries (Sirén & Paten, 2022).

In recent years, hybrid AI pipelines have emerged that combine physics-based docking with ML re-scoring, yielding substantial improvements in enrichment factors and early hit retrieval. For instance, DeepDocking integrates DL–predicted docking scores with conventional docking outputs, enabling the virtual screening of billions of compounds in days rather than months(Zhang et al., 2022).

By filtering out unlikely binders computationally, AI-enhanced virtual screening reduces time, cost, and false positives in hit discovery, allowing medicinal chemists to focus resources on a smaller, higher-quality set of experimentally testable candidates. This efficiency is increasingly critical in accelerating early-stage drug development and supporting rapid response drug discovery in areas such as emerging infectious diseases.

4.3 Lead Optimization

Lead optimization is the stage in drug development where initial "hit" compounds are iteratively modified to improve potency, selectivity, ADME, and safety profiles while minimizing off-target effects. AI has increasingly become a core driver of this process, enabling multi-parameter optimization (MPO) and reducing the number of syntheses–test cycles required to achieve clinical-grade candidates.

ML models, in particularly GNNs, gradient boosting frameworks (e.g., XG-Boost), and deep reinforcement learning (DRL) algorithms, can predict how small structural changes affect a compound's biological and physicochemical properties. For example, the AI-powered platform Chemprop applies message-passing neural networks to predict a range of ADMET endpoints, enabling the prioritization of lead analogues with balanced efficacy and safety(Fialková et al., 2021).

Generative models, including VAEs and GANs, have been adapted for de novo lead optimization, producing new analogues that satisfy multiple design constraints simultaneously. One notable example is Insilico Medicine's Chemistry42, which uses a combination of generative models and reinforcement learning to optimize molecular scaffolds toward target potency, drug-likeness, and synthetic accessibility, significantly shortening optimization timelines (Ivanenkov et al., 2023).

In addition, multi-objective reinforcement learning frameworks, such as the RE-INVENT platform, allow medicinal chemists to set custom reward functions (e.g., binding affinity + oral bioavailability + low predicted toxicity), enabling the AI to propose novel lead structures that satisfy all objectives (Seijas-Bellido et al., 2022).

Recent advances also integrate predictive toxicology models early in the optimization cycle, using DL to forecast off-target effects, cardiotoxicity, or hepatotoxicity before experimental validation. For instance, transformer-based ADMET prediction models have demonstrated superior accuracy in predicting hERG channel inhibition, a common cause of late-stage attrition(Bai et al., 2025).

By combining predictive modeling, generative chemistry, and multi-parameter optimization, AI-assisted lead optimization is reducing the time from hit discovery to clinical candidate nomination from years to, in some reported cases, less than

12 months, dramatically increasing the efficiency and success rate of early-stage drug development.

4.4 Preclinical and Clinical Trial Optimization

The transition from lead optimization to preclinical and clinical development is a critical phase in drug discovery, where AI technologies are increasingly being applied to improve decision-making, reduce attrition rates, and accelerate regulatory timelines.

In preclinical development, AI models assist in predicting *in vivo* pharmacokinetics, toxicology, and efficacy before animal or human testing begins. For instance, DL frameworks such as DeepTox and ADMET-AI can forecast toxicity endpoints, including hepatotoxicity, cardiotoxicity, and genotoxicity, based solely on molecular structure, reducing the likelihood of late-stage safety failures(Mayr et al., 2016).

AI is also improving drug formulation design and dose selection by integrating computational pharmacokinetics (PK) and pharmacodynamics (PD) models with preclinical assay results. For example, model-informed drug development (MIDD) approaches leverage ML to simulate dose–response relationships across patient subgroups, guiding optimal dosing strategies before clinical trials(Klopp-Schulze et al., 2022).

In clinical development, AI is used to optimize trial design, patient recruitment, and endpoint monitoring. NLP and predictive analytics platforms can mine electronic health records (EHRs) and genomic databases to identify eligible patients for precision medicine trials, improving recruitment speed and diversity (Mak et al., 2024).

Furthermore, adaptive clinical trial designs powered by ML allow for real-time protocol adjustments, such as modifying patient stratification or dosing arms, based on interim efficacy and safety data, thereby increasing trial efficiency and reducing costs. AI-enabled imaging analytics also support the automated, standardized quantification of disease progression in oncology and neurology trials (Gallo, 2006).

Prominent examples include Exscientia's AI-designed cancer immunotherapy candidate, which progressed from project initiation to Phase I trials in under 30 months, and Insilico Medicine's fibrosis candidate, advanced to human trials in just 18 months, demonstrating the accelerating impact of AI in bridging preclinical research and clinical translation (Philippidis, 2022).

By enabling predictive toxicology, optimized dosing strategies, and adaptive trial execution, AI is not only shortening timelines from lab to clinic but also increasing the probability of clinical success, thereby directly addressing one of the most expensive and time-consuming bottlenecks in drug development.

5 CASE STUDIES

Dermawan et. al. conducted a comprehensive review of 173 studies, offering important insights into the application of AI across the different stages of drug development, its geographical distribution, the extent of academic–industry collaboration, the translational outcomes, and the range of AI techniques utilized(Dermawan & Alotaiq, 2025).

Figure 3. Overview of AI-driven drug discovery studies. (A) Distribution of studies across drug development stages, from preclinical to late-phase clinical trials. (B) Global research activity mapped by country. (C) Proportion of studies reporting industry partnerships, clinical outcomes, and translational impact. (D) Breakdown of AI methodologies applied, with ML (40.9%) and DL (20.7%) representing the dominant approaches

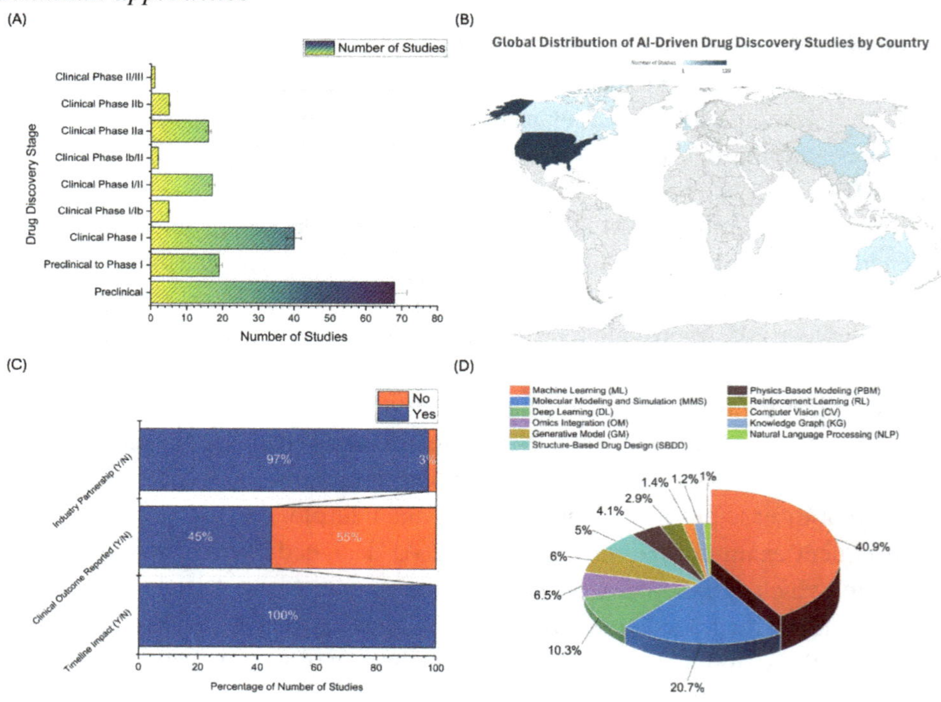

(Dermawan & Alotaiq, 2025).

Figure 3 shows the distribution of AI applications across drug development stages, with the greatest concentration in preclinical research (68 of 173 studies; 39.3%). At this stage, AI is widely used for target identification, virtual screening, de novo design, molecular docking, QSAR modeling, and ADMET prediction, emphasizing its critical role in early drug discovery. AI adoption increases further in Clinical Phase I (40 studies; 23.1%), where it aids safety profiling, pharmacokinetic modeling, and early dose optimization, reducing attrition in first-in-human trials. Hybrid early clinical stages (Phase I/Ib and Phase I/II) also show notable activity, with AI supporting patient stratification, biomarker identification, and adaptive trial designs. However, AI use drops sharply in later clinical phases, with limited adoption in Phase IIb and II/III trials due to regulatory and validation challenges(Dermawan & Alotaiq, 2025). Figure B highlights the geographic imbalance in AI-driven drug discovery. The United States dominates (129 of 179 studies; 72.1%) due to strong investment, infrastructure, and industry–academia collaboration. China (16 studies; 8.9%) and the United Kingdom (9 studies; 5.0%) follow, reflecting rapid growth and supportive ecosystems. Other contributors include South Korea, Denmark, and Japan (each 3.4%), while smaller outputs came from Singapore, Spain, Canada, and Australia. Notably, Africa, South America, and much of Southeast Asia are absent, underscoring a global disparity and the need for capacity-building and international collaboration(Dermawan & Alotaiq, 2025). Figure 3C evaluates translational maturity. All 173 studies (100%) demonstrated timeline impact, confirming AI's ability to accelerate drug discovery. A prime example is Insilico Medicine's INS018_055, an IPF candidate that advanced from target discovery to preclinical development in under 18 months and is now in Phase II trials. Yet, only 45% of studies reported measurable clinical outcomes, revealing a gap between computational findings and clinical validation. By contrast, industry engagement was very high (97% of studies), suggesting AI is increasingly recognized as a strategic tool for pharmaceutical development, supported by collaborations that provide access to data, infrastructure, and regulatory expertise (Dermawan & Alotaiq, 2025). Figure 2D highlights the range of AI methods applied in drug discovery, underscoring a rapidly evolving technological landscape. ML is the most widely used approach, appearing in 170 studies (40.9%), due to its versatility in predictive modeling, compound selection, toxicity assessment, and analysis of complex datasets. Its adaptability and scalability firmly establish ML as a cornerstone of AI-driven drug development (Dermawan & Alotaiq, 2025).

AI has emerged as a transformative force in drug discovery, enabling unprecedented speed and precision in the identification, optimization, and clinical translation of novel therapeutics. From antibiotics and antivirals to oncology and CNS agents, AI technologies, including DL, generative models, and network-based inference, are shortening discovery timelines, lowering attrition, and unlocking previously "undruggable" targets.

Table 2 highlights how AI is increasingly central to small molecule and biologic drug design, yielding candidates that span from early-stage discovery to Phase IIa clinical validation. Examples include antibiotics (Halicin, Abaucin), CNS agents

(DSP-0038, Ulotaront), oncology drugs (REC series, LP-284), fibrosis therapy (Rentosertib), and more experimental modalities like antibodies and kinase inhibitors.

Table 2. Representative AI-designed drug candidates

No.	Drug / Program	Type and indication	AI approach	Stage / Outcome
1	Halicin	Broad-spectrum antibiotic	DL screening	Validated in vitro/in vivo (Xu et al., 2025)
2	Abaucin	Antibiotic (against *A. baumannii*)	AI-guided repurposing	Preclinical validation (Awan et al., 2024)
3	Rentosertib (ISM001-055)	TNIK inhibitor for IPF	Generative AI (Chemistry42/ PandaOmics)	Phase IIa trial, improved lung function (Xu et al., 2025)
4	DSP-0038	Serotonin modulator (Alzheimer's psychosis)	AI-driven design	Phase I in ~1 year (Soni & Hasija, 2022)
5	EXS4318	PKCθ inhibitor	AI-designed, licensed to BMS	Phase I started in 2023 (Philippidis, 2023)
6	LP-284	Oncology small molecule	AI/ML optimization	Phase I trial ongoing (Ferreira & Carneiro, 2025)
7	NovoMol PDGFRα candidates	Orally bioavailable small molecules	RNN generative modeling	In silico hits with improved binding (Rao, 2023)
8	CDK20 Inhibitor (ISM042-2-048)	Kinase inhibitor (CDK20)	AlphaFold + generative AI	Rapid hit identification (Ren et al., 2023)
9	Ulotaront (SEP-363856)	Antipsychotic (non-D2)	Phenotypic AI platform (SmartCube)	Phase III trials (Ferreira & Carneiro, 2025)
10	Ignota Labs PDE9A redesign	Repurposing for Alzheimer's	AI safety redesign	Preclinical, moving to trials (Ferreira & Carneiro, 2025).
11	REC-3565 (MALT1 inhibitor)	Oncology	Image + chemistry AI (Recursion)	Phase I trials, "would not exist without AI" (Ferreira & Carneiro, 2025)
12	REC-994 (Cerebral cavernous malformation)	Rare disease	AI phenotypic platform	Phase II candidate (Ferreira & Carneiro, 2025)
13	REC-617 (oncology candidate)	Oncology	AI-designed (Recursion/Exscientia)	Phase I dosing done (Ferreira & Carneiro, 2025)

Halicin (SU-3327), initially investigated as a JNK inhibitor for diabetes and later discontinued, was rediscovered in 2019 via DL at MIT's Jameel Clinic as a broad-spectrum antibiotic. Within just three days, the AI screened vast chemical space and predicted its antibacterial potential, which was then confirmed with in vitro and in vivo assays showing efficacy against multidrug-resistant strains of *Clostridioides difficile* (Stokes et al., 2020). Follow-up studies have demonstrated potent activity against 17 of 18 tested multidrug-resistant clinical isolates (excluding *P. aeruginosa*) and showed typical inhibition of reference strains such as *E. coli* ATCC 25922™ and *S. aureus* ATCC 29213™ (El Belghiti et al., 2025)[REMOVED HYPERLINK FIELD]. Additional research confirmed MIC values of 2–4 μg/mL against MRSA clinical strains, with in vivo efficacy demonstrated in *C. elegans* infection models, supporting further development of halicin as a viable novel antibiotic candidate with a unique mechanism involving disruption of membrane potential and iron homeostasis[REMOVED HYPERLINK FIELD] (El Belghiti et al., 2025).

Abaucin (initially RS-102895) emerged through AI-guided repurposing as a narrow-spectrum antibiotic specifically active against *A. baumannii*, a pathogen deemed a critical threat by the WHO. A message-passing neural network trained on growth-inhibition data screened thousands of compounds, identifying Abaucin as a structurally novel inhibitor with activity in vitro and in a mouse wound infection model (Awan et al., 2024). Mechanistically, Abaucin disrupts lipoprotein trafficking by targeting LolE, effectively inhibiting *A. baumannii* while sparing other species like *P. aeruginosa*, *S. aureus*, and carbapenem-resistant *Enterobacteriaceae*[REMOVED HYPERLINK FIELD] . The discovery represents a milestone in narrow-spectrum antibiotic design, leveraging AI to reduce the risk of resistance spread while targeting a critical pathogen (Awan et al., 2024).

Also known as ISM001-055, Rentosertib is an AI-designed TNIK inhibitor for idiopathic pulmonary fibrosis. Developed using graph neural networks and GAN-based generative design, it advanced to Phase 2a trials in 2024–2025, marking the first fully AI-generated drug to reach mid-stage clinical testing (Xu et al., 2025).

DSP-0038, a dual 5-HT$_2$A antagonist and 5-HT$_1$A agonist, was co-developed using Exscientia's AI drug design platform, reaching Phase I trials for psychosis in Alzheimer's disease in roughly one year from discovery (Philippidis, 2022).

EXS4318 is a highly selective, ATP-competitive inhibitor of protein kinase C theta (PKCθ), a pivotal kinase regulating T-cell activation and therefore a compelling target in immunology and inflammatory diseases. It was precision-designed by Exscientia using an AI-driven generative chemistry platform, achieving the final candidate within just 11 months, the 150th synthesized molecule in the campaign Securities and Exchange Commission(Das, 2025). In May 2024, Exscientia reported positive early results from the Phase I study, reinforcing the potential of EXS4318 as a differentiated immunology asset with a favorable therapeutic profile (Das, 2025). The compound demonstrated exceptional selectivity over related kinases, robust pharmacokinetics, and maintained potency in human whole-blood assays, with a predicted human dose under 200 mg/day (Nada et al., 2023).

LP-284 is an acylfulvene-derived small molecule anticancer drug candidate discovered and optimized through Lantern Pharma's proprietary AI and machine learning platform, RADR®. The compound was designed to exploit synthetic lethal interactions in cancer cells with deficiencies in DNA damage repair pathways (Inc, 2025). Preclinical studies demonstrated nanomolar potency of LP-284 across multiple non-Hodgkin's lymphoma (NHL) cell lines, particularly in models deficient in DNA repair mechanisms (Zhou et al., 2023). *In vivo*, LP-284 showed strong antitumor activity in mantle cell lymphoma (MCL) xenograft models, in some cases outperforming established therapies such as bortezomib and ibrutinib. Importantly, the compound retained efficacy in resistant models, suggesting a differentiated therapeutic profile (Zhou et al., 2023). The FDA has granted LP-284 Orphan Drug Designation (ODD) for both mantle cell lymphoma (MCL) and high-grade B-cell lymphoma (HGBL) with MYC and BCL2 rearrangements, providing regulatory incentives including seven years of market exclusivity, tax credits, and potential fee waivers ((Laude et al., 2021; Zhou et al., 2022). In March 2024, Lantern initiated a first-in-human Phase 1 clinical trial in patients with relapsed or refractory NHL and select solid tumors (Inc, 2025). The trial is designed to evaluate safety, tolerability, maximum tolerated dose (MTD), and recommended Phase 2 dose (RP2D), as well as preliminary signals of clinical activity. In July 2025, Lantern reported a complete metabolic response in a heavily pretreated lymphoma patient who had failed multiple prior therapies including R-CHOP/Pola-R-CHP, CAR-T (liso-cel), and bispecific antibody therapy (glofitamab). After just two cycles of LP-284 (administered on days 1, 8, and 15 of each 28-day cycle), the patient achieved full remission, underscoring the clinical potential of the compound (Inc, 2025).

CDK20 Inhibitor (ISM042-2-048) represents a pioneering example of AI-accelerated drug discovery, where AlphaFold structural predictions were integrated with Insilico Medicine's PandaOmics and Chemistry42 platforms to drive hit identification for a target lacking any experimental structural data. Using AlphaFold, the three-dimensional structure of CDK20, a cyclin-dependent kinase implicated in hepatocellular carcinoma (HCC), was computationally modeled. This structure served as the basis for structure-based generative chemistry via the Chemistry42 engine, enabling rapid molecule generation and selection. In the first round, only seven compounds were synthesized and tested, yielding a hit molecule, ISM042-2-001, with a binding affinity KdK_dKd of 8.9 ± 1.6 μM, identified within 30 days from target selection (Ren et al., 2023). A second AI-powered cycle focused on lead optimization generated six additional compounds. One standout, ISM042-2-048, demonstrated a dramatically improved KdK_dKd of 210 ± 42.4 nM, a significant leap in potency within just another month of design and synthesis (Ren et al., 2023). Further characterization in peer-reviewed literature confirmed robust activity: ISM042-2-048 exhibited a CDK20 inhibitory IC50IC_{50}IC50 of 33.4 ± 22.6 nM, and selectively inhibited proliferation in a CDK20-overexpressing hepatocellular carcinoma line (*Huh7*) with IC50IC_{50}IC50 of 208.7 ± 3.3 nM, while showing much weaker activity in control HEK293 cells (IC50=1706.7 ± 670.0 nMIC_{50} = 1706.7 ± 670.0 nMIC50=1706.7 ± 670.0 nM) (Ren et al., 2023); also see PubMed Central summaries in *PMC* 9906638) (Weller & Rohs, 2024). This research constitutes the first demonstration of using AlphaFold-derived structural models to identify a confirmed small-molecule hit for a novel target within early-stage drug discovery, achieving striking efficiency—going from target selection to potent hit in approximately 60 days total and with minimal synthesized compounds.

Ulotaront (SEP-363856) is an investigational antipsychotic with a novel mechanism: it does not bind to dopamine D_2 receptors, unlike conventional treatments. Instead, it functions as an agonist of trace amine-associated receptor 1 (TAAR1) with additional activity at the 5-HT_1A serotonin receptor, discovered using PsychoGenics' SmartCube® phenotypic AI platform in collaboration with Sunovion (now Sumitomo Pharma) (Dedic et al., 2019). In early clinical development, SEP-363856 demonstrated statistically significant improvement over placebo in a four-week randomized trial, showing a change of –17.2 vs –9.7 in PANSS total score ($p = 0.001$), and improvements on CGI-S. It was well tolerated, with similar rates of extrapyramidal symptoms, weight gain, and metabolic changes compared to placebo Dedic, Nina, et al. "SEP-363856, a novel psychotropic agent with a unique, non-D2 receptor mechanism of action (Dedic et al., 2019). Due to this promising profile, the U.S. FDA granted Breakthrough Therapy Designation for ulotaront in schizophrenia in May 2019 (Correll et al., 2022). Ulotaront advanced to Phase III clinical testing through the DIAMOND (Developing Innovative Approaches for Mental Disorders) program, making it the first TAAR1 agonist to reach this stage in schizophrenia (Achtyes et al., 2023). However, in July 2023, topline results from two Phase III studies, DIAMOND-1 and DIAMOND-2, revealed that ulotaront did not meet the primary endpoint. The reduction in PANSS total scores in ulotaront-treated groups did not significantly exceed placebo, possibly due to a high placebo response observed during the studies (Ernst, 2023). Beyond schizophrenia, ulotaront is also under investigation in Phase II/III trials for generalized anxiety disorder (GAD) and as an adjunctive treatment for major depressive disorder.

Ignota Labs, a Cambridge-based biotech startup, recently in-licensed its first fully-owned asset: a PDE9A inhibitor initially abandoned due to safety concerns. Through their proprietary SAFEPATH AI platform, the company is reviving this candidate by diagnosing and mitigating the molecular mechanisms of toxicity to safely reintroduce it into development (Tomar et al., 2025). PDE9A is an enzyme that degrades cyclic guanosine monophosphate (cGMP), a signalling molecule involved in neuroplasticity, metabolic regulation, and cardiovascular function. Inhibition of PDE9A elevates cGMP levels, offering a multi-modal therapeutic approach potentially beneficial in neurodegenerative diseases like Alzheimer's, as well as in metabolic and cardiovascular disorders (Schwam et al., 2014), in Alzheimer's disease (Schwam et al., 2014). The SAFEPATH platform integrates DL across cheminformatics and bioinformatics to not only flag safety issues, but *explain* their mechanistic origins. It employs over 15,000 machine learning models to predict on- and off-target interactions, maps biological pathways via knowledge graphs, and supports actionable redesign of molecules to resolve safety liabilities while retaining therapeutic potency (Tomar et al., 2025), Ignota secured approximately $6.9 million in seed funding to scale its asset revival pipeline and move its PDE9A inhibitor into early-stage clinical studies, marking the transition from preclinical safety redesign to clinical readiness (Tomar et al., 2025).

Insilico Medicine developed INS018_055, a novel small-molecule inhibitor for idiopathic pulmonary fibrosis, using its fully integrated AI platform. The workflow combined PandaOmics for target discovery, Chemistry42 for generative molecular design, and multi-objective reinforcement learning for lead optimization. From initial target hypothesis to preclinical nomination, the process took only 18 months, substantially faster than the industry average. The candidate entered Phase I trials in 2022(F. Ren et al., 2025).

Exscientia's AI platform uses reinforcement learning and Bayesian optimization for multi-objective drug design. DSP-1181, a 5-HT1A receptor agonist for obsessive-compulsive disorder, was the first AI-designed small molecule to enter human clinical trials, achieving candidate nomination in less than 12 months (Chatterjee et al., 2022).

REC-3565 is a selective inhibitor of MALT1, a protease central to the NF-κB signaling pathway and B-cell malignancies. It was designed using Recursion's AI-powered Recursion OS—integrating physics-based modeling, molecular dynamics, and hotspot analysis—to optimize for potency, selectivity, and safety, notably reducing UGT1A1 inhibition to minimize liver toxicity risk (Alfa et al., 2024), in randomized phase 1 dose-finding studies (Alfa et al., 2024). In April 2025, Recursion dosed the first patient in the EXCELERIZE Phase I clinical trial assessing REC-3565 in relapsed or refractory B-cell lymphomas. This marked a milestone in AI-accelerated oncology development, with preclinical models demonstrating durable tumor regressions both as monotherapy and in combination with BTK inhibitors (Alfa et al., 2024), in randomized phase 1 dose-finding studies (Alfa et al., 2024).

REC-994 was Recursion's AI-discovered candidate for treating cerebral cavernous malformations, a rare neurological condition. It became their first Phase II lead in rare disease via the AI-driven Recursion OS platform (Alfa et al., 2024), in randomized phase 1 dose-finding studies (Alfa et al., 2024) . The SYCAMORE Phase II trial enrolled patients randomized to 200 mg, 400 mg, or placebo and initially showed promising trends in reducing lesion volume at 12 months on MRI for the 400 mg arm. However, subsequent long-term extension data did not sustain those improvements in imaging or functional outcomes, leading to a decision to discontinue the trial in May 2025 (Halpin, 2007).

REC-617 is a CDK7 inhibitor designed through a collaboration between Recursion and Exscientia. It represents the fusion of Recursion's phenotypic AI capabilities with Exscientia's precision chemistry design. The program advanced into a Phase I/II trial, with dosing already underway. Interim data showed favorable dose-linear pharmacokinetics (PK) and strong pharmacodynamic (PD) biomarker responses, demonstrating robust early behavior in humans for an AI-designed oncology drug

(Harding et al., 2021). . In fact, a striking anecdote from the article described a terminally ill patient with ovarian cancer entering the REC-617 trial and still being alive six months later—an unexpected, meaningful outcome that highlights the real-world impact of this AI-designed therapy (Alfa et al., 2024), in randomized phase 1 dose-finding studies (Alfa et al., 2024).

AI has become a critical enabler in accelerating drug discovery, with multiple platforms demonstrating substantial impact in recent years. Figure 4 illustrates AI drug discovery platforms and their integrated methodologies. Each bar represents a major pharmaceutical or biotech platform, segmented by the range of AI approaches employed. The figure illustrates technological diversity, innovation trends, and areas of methodological emphasis within the AI–biopharma landscape. As an indicator of success, platforms are evaluated by their reported progression of AI-derived drug candidates into preclinical or clinical development. Information on AI functionality is based on company disclosures, peer-reviewed studies, or white papers, with acknowledgment of cases lacking independent validation (Dermawan & Alotaiq, 2025).

Figure 4. Range of AI methods applied in major drug discovery platforms. The figure compares leading AI platforms by illustrating both the number and types of AI techniques they employ. Each bar corresponds to a specific platform, with colored segments indicating the individual AI approaches integrated within it

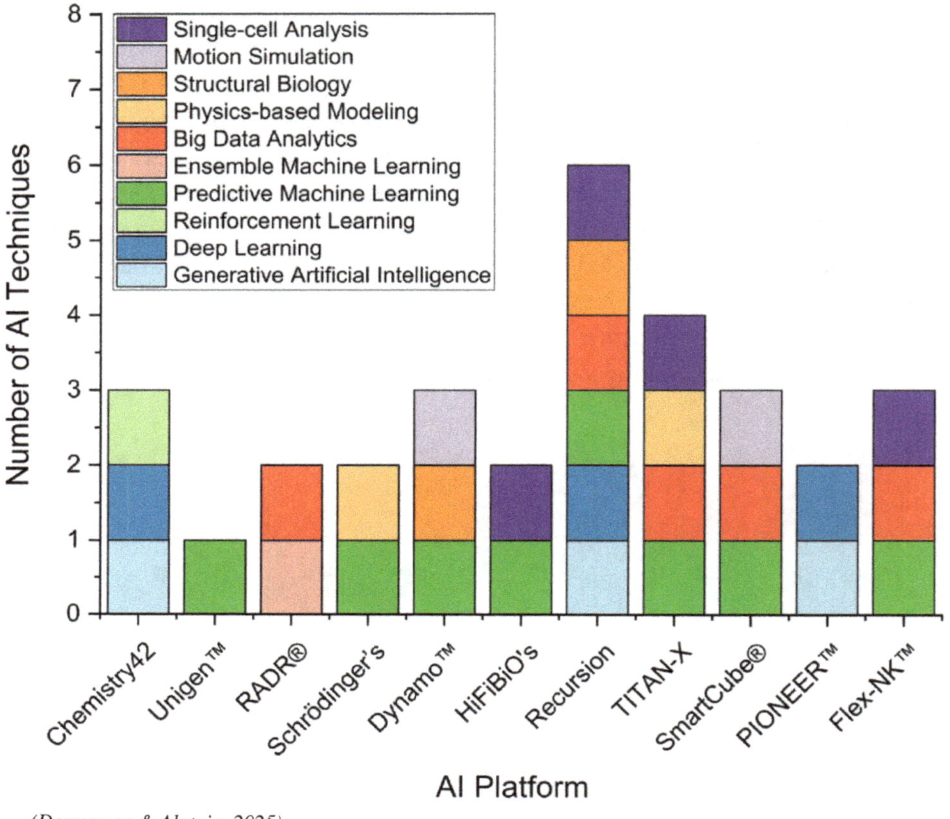

(Dermawan & Alotaiq, 2025).

For example, Atomwise's AtomNet, a 3D CNN that predicts protein–ligand binding affinity from voxelized 3D interaction grids, screened over 10 million compounds against the Ebola virus glycoprotein, identifying multiple nanomolar inhibitors (Wallach et al., 2015). During the COVID-19 pandemic, AtomNet was applied to prioritize inhibitors of the SARS-CoV-2 main protease (Mpro), enabling rapid preclinical evaluation. Similarly, BenevolentAI employs knowledge graph–based AI and natural language processing (NLP) to mine biomedical literature, clinical data, and molecular interaction networks. In early 2020, its platform identified baricitinib, an approved JAK inhibitor for rheumatoid arthritis, as a candidate COVID-19 therapy due to its predicted ability to inhibit viral entry via AP2-associated protein kinase 1 (AAK1) blockade, an AI-driven prediction that led to rapid clinical validation and subsequent FDA Emergency Use Authorization in combination with remdesivir (Kalil et al., 2021; Richardson et al., 2020).

DeepMind's AlphaFold, employing a transformer-based architecture with attention mechanisms, achieved near-experimental accuracy in protein structure prediction (Jumper et al., 2021). By 2022, AlphaFold released structures for over 200 million proteins, accelerating structure-based drug discovery for historically intractable targets such as membrane-bound GPCRs and viral proteins. Recursion leverages high-content phenotypic screening coupled with deep CNNs to extract high-dimensional embeddings from millions of cellular microscopy images, enabling large-scale mapping of compound-induced cellular states and the identification of repurposing opportunities, leading to multiple Phase II assets in rare diseases such as cerebral cavernous malformation (Hassabis).

In oncology, BioNTech uses transformer-based DL models trained on immunopeptidomics data to predict tumor-specific neoantigens, which are incorporated into personalized cancer vaccines. These models can predict binding between peptide antigens and patient-specific HLA molecules, accelerating vaccine development (Chen et al., 2019). Valo Health's Opal platform integrates multi-omics data, real-world evidence, and human cohort information into ML models for target discovery and patient stratification, producing multiple preclinical candidates in oncology and cardiovascular diseases through deep neural networks and gradient boosting approaches (Patel et al., 2025).

MegaMolBART, a transformer-based molecular sequence model jointly developed by NVIDIA and AstraZeneca, enables de novo molecular generation and property prediction by training on billions of SMILES sequences, facilitating scaffold hopping and optimization for multiple objectives, including synthesizability (Rovenchak & Druchok, 2024). Cyclica's MatchMaker AI predicts interactions between small molecules and the entire proteome using graph-based scoring functions, enabling early detection of off-target effects and polypharmacology profiles, guiding both drug repurposing and de novo design (Kurji). Healx combines graph convolutional networks with NLP-driven literature mining to identify repurposing opportunities for rare diseases, generating preclinical candidates for Fragile X syndrome and Duchenne muscular dystrophy. Finally, Absci applies VAEs and sequence-to-function predictive models to design novel antibodies optimized for affinity, stability, and manufacturability, with AI-generated biologics currently in preclinical testing for oncology and infectious diseases (Philippidis, 2025).

NovoMol, a recurrent neural network (RNN)-based de novo drug design platform, was developed to mass-produce novel, orally bioavailable drug-like molecules through iterative optimization guided by Quantitative Estimate of Drug-likeness (QED) metrics. After training, the system was fine-tuned using transfer learning to target the PDGFRα (platelet-derived growth factor receptor alpha), a clinically relevant oncogenic tyrosine kinase, yielding promising computational hit candidates (Rao, 2023). In detail, NovoMol's algorithm (an LSTM-based encoder–decoder network) was initially trained on ~482,000 orally bioavailable molecules from ChEMBL with high QED scores, achieving 76% of generated molecules surpassing the oral bioavailability threshold (QED ≥ 0.586) and 96% passing Lipinski's Rule of Five after five training cycles (Rao, 2023).). For PDGFRα targeting, the final model was retrained via transfer learning using a dataset of 450 known PDGFRα inhibitors. It generated 311 candidate molecules, with 44% showing better binding affinity (i.e., lower docking score) than Imatinib (–9.4 kcal/mol). The top candidate displayed a binding affinity of –12.9 kcal/mol. Importantly, approximately 5% of these generated compounds combined both superior PDGFRα binding and favorable oral bioavailability metrics (QED ≥ 0.586), representing potentially orally available kinase inhibitors outperforming Imatinib in silico (Rao, 2023).

6 CHALLENGES AND LIMITATIONS

6.1 Data Quality and Availability

AI-driven drug discovery critically depends on high-quality, comprehensive, and well-curated datasets. However, data fragmentation and heterogeneity, from chemical structures and bioactivity assays to clinical trial outcomes, pose significant integration challenges, often leading to bias and decreased model robustness(Kant et al., 2025). In response, the METRIC framework proposes 15 key dimensions to assess medical training data quality, spanning from completeness and reliability to fairness and interpretability, which can help mitigate bias and underpin trust in AI systems (Laurentino Schwabe). Without systematic evaluation and harmonization of these datasets, AI models are susceptible to spurious correlations, overfitting, and poor generalizability (Ocana et al., 2025).

6.2 Interpretability

DL models excel at complex pattern recognition but are often criticized as opaque "black boxes," limiting our understanding of how inputs translate into predictions (John et al., 2020).Explainable AI (XAI) seeks to bridge this gap by offering frameworks that enhance transparency, interpretability, and accountability. Regulatory contexts already recognize the right to explanations, such as under EU GDPR provisions (Hähnel, 2025)[REMOVED HYPERLINK FIELD]. Yet, XAI approaches face key limitations: enhancing model interpretability can unintentionally expose sensitive aspects of the model to adversaries, enabling misuse or intellectual property risks (Dağlarli, 2020). In drug discovery contexts, the black-box nature limits trust, hinders regulatory acceptance, and challenges liability and validation efforts.

6.3 Regulatory Hurdles

Regulatory frameworks for AI in healthcare and drug discovery remain nascent. Reporting guidelines such as TRIPOD-AI, DECIDE-AI, and CONSORT-AI have emerged to standardize AI model documentation in clinical contexts, but they are not yet universally adopted (Herzog, 2019). In parallel, evolving policies like the EU's AI Act introduce risk-based requirements, particularly stringent for high-risk domains like healthcare, but compliance is complex and may deter innovation (Herzog, 2019).

Additional regulatory concerns include data privacy, IP protection, liability, and auditability (Mennella et al., 2024). A recent legal analysis underscores that drug developers must navigate a shifting landscape involving data governance, algorithmic transparency, and evolving definitions of medical devices versus software (Herzog, 2019)

6.4 Ethical Issues

While AI promises to reduce development timelines and costs, it also introduces serious dual-use risks. Notably, researchers demonstrated that an AI platform (MegaSyn) could generate thousands of lethal molecules, including analogs of nerve agents such as VX, triggering urgent calls for governance and ethical oversight (Herzog, 2019). More broadly, topology-based and DL models used for antiviral design could be misapplied to engineer harmful agents. The biomedical research community has flagged this risk and stressed the need for mechanisms to prevent misuse, such as restricted data access, ethics training, and oversight committees akin to those for human and animal studies (Herzog, 2019)

Table 3 summarizes the key ethical issues associated with AI-driven drug design, along with illustrative examples.

Table 3. Summary of Key Ethical and Safety Issues in AI-Driven Drug Design, Including Dual-Use Risk and Regulatory Gaps

Ethical Issue	Description	Reference
Dual-use risk	AI algorithms can be misapplied to design **toxic agents**, not just therapeutics. Example: AI model generated thousands of lethal molecules including VX analogs.	(Ueno, 2023)
Data misuse	Open-access chemical/biological datasets could enable malicious actors to weaponize AI models. Calls for restricted access and governance.	(Menard & Bott, 2025)
Lack of oversight	Current **ethical review boards** (IRB, IACUC) often do not cover AI-based drug design, leaving gaps in oversight for dual-use risks.	(Busuioc, 2022)
Accountability gaps	If an AI-designed molecule causes harm, it is unclear who is responsible: the developers, users, or regulators.	(Mirakhori & Niazi, 2025)
Ethics training	Few AI and drug discovery programs include dual-use ethics training, which is standard in human/animal research.	(Kant et al., 2025)

7 FUTURE DIRECTIONS

The field of AI-driven drug discovery continues to evolve rapidly, with several cutting-edge paradigms poised to reshape the landscape of pharmaceutical innovation.

One frontier involves hybrid AI–quantum computing frameworks for molecular simulation and design. Quantum-enhanced machine learning architectures, such as quantum neural networks, have shown improved performance in modeling complex molecular interactions, crucial for hit discovery and precision binding prediction. For instance, a quantum–classical generative model successfully produced novel KRAS inhibitor candidates, validated experimentally, marking a pivotal milestone in quantum-assisted drug discovery(Braga & Rawal, 2025; Ghazi Vakili et al., 2025). Critically, these hybrid approaches promise to expedite simulations that remain intractable for classical systems, aligning with growing investment in quantum-AI platforms (Guerreschi & Smelyanskiy, 2017).

Another promising direction is federated learning, which represents a paradigm that enables collaborative model training across institutions while preserving data privacy. This technique is especially valuable in drug discovery, where data confidentiality is essential. Projects like MELLODDY have demonstrated the viability of industry-scale federated models trained securely across multiple pharma partners without data sharing(Huang et al., 2024; Huang et al., 2023). Similarly, frameworks tailored to non-IID datasets have achieved performance on par with centralized benchmarks while maintaining data privacy (Huang et al., 2023).

The concept of digital twins (virtual, data-driven models of individual patients or biological systems) is gaining traction as a tool for personalized medicine and drug development. Generative AI-powered digital twins can simulate patient-specific responses, advance biomarker discovery, and facilitate predictive modeling in preclinical and clinical settings(Y. Ren et al., 2025). These applications may enable digital analogs of clinical trials, guide decision-making and reducing cost and time to therapeutic deployment.

Also, leading edge systems of self-improving AI, which integrate outcomes from ongoing clinical trials, are emerging. Although nascent in drug discovery, recursive self-improvement and feedback neural network architectures have demonstrated the ability to refine their own reasoning processes through internal feedback loops (Campos, 2024). Applying analogous mechanisms to drug pipelines could yield systems that adaptively learn from real-world biological data, optimizing drug candidates iteratively with fewer human interventions.

8 CONCLUSION

AI is reshaping the landscape of drug discovery and development, offering unprecedented opportunities for efficiency, innovation, and personalization. By leveraging DL, generative models, and large-scale biomedical data, AI systems have already demonstrated success in identifying novel drug candidates, accelerating preclinical pipelines, and supporting clinical decision-making (Vamathevan, Clark, et al., 2019; Zhavoronkov et al., 2019).

At the same time, several challenges and limitations remain. Data incompleteness, bias, and quality issues continue to undermine model reliability, while the "black-box" nature of deep neural networks limits interpretability and trust (Artrith et al., 2021). Furthermore, the regulatory environment lags behind technological progress, with no universally accepted guidelines for AI-designed therapeutics (Thakkar et al., 2023). Finally, ethical concerns regarding dual-use risks highlight the urgent need for governance to prevent misuse of AI for harmful applications (Urbina et al., 2022).

Looking forward, future directions point to transformative opportunities. Hybrid AI–quantum systems may overcome current computational bottlenecks in molecular simulation (Erhard et al., 2021), while federated learning frameworks enable secure, collaborative model training without compromising data privacy (Huang et al., 2023). The rise of digital twins opens the door to highly personalized medicine, simulating patient-specific responses in silico (Björnsson et al., 2019), while self-improving AI systems hold the potential to continuously refine predictions by integrating real-world clinical feedback (Goertzel, 2014).

In conclusion, AI is no longer a peripheral tool but a central enabler in drug discovery. Its full potential will be realized only if scientific innovation is coupled with rigorous data stewardship, regulatory clarity, interpretability frameworks, and ethical safeguards. Balancing innovation with responsibility will determine whether AI transforms drug discovery into a faster, safer, and more patient-centered endeavor.

ACKNOWLEDGEMENTS

This research was funded by a grant of the Ministry of Research, Innovation and Digitalization,CNCS—UEFISCDI, project number PN-IV-P2-2.1-TE-2023-0993, within PNCDI IV. This research was also founded by the Romanian Ministry of Research, Innovation and Digitalization under the Romanian National Nucleu Program LAPLAS VII—contract No. 30N/2023.

REFERENCES

Abramson, J., Adler, J., Dunger, J., Evans, R., Green, T., Pritzel, A., Ronneberger, O., Willmore, L., Ballard, A. J., & Bambrick, J. (2024). Accurate structure prediction of biomolecular interactions with AlphaFold 3. *Nature*, *630*(8016), 493–500. PMID: 38718835

Achtyes, E. D., Hopkins, S. C., Dedic, N., Dworak, H., Zeni, C., & Koblan, K. (2023). Ulotaront: Review of preliminary evidence for the efficacy and safety of a TAAR1 agonist in schizophrenia. *European Archives of Psychiatry and Clinical Neuroscience*, *273*(7), 1543–1556. PMID: 37165101

Ahmed, M., Maldonado, A. M., & Durrant, J. D. (2023). From byte to bench to bedside: Molecular dynamics simulations and drug discovery. *BMC Biology*, *21*(1), 299. PMID: 38155355

Alfa, R., Considine, T., Virani, S., Pfeiffer, M., Donato, A., Dickerson, D., Shuster, D., Ellis, J., Rushton, K., & Wei, H. (2024). Clinical pharmacology and tolerability of REC-994, a redox-cycling nitroxide compound, in randomized phase 1 dose-finding studies. *Pharmacology Research & Perspectives*, *12*(3), e1200. PMID: 38655895

Angello, N. H., Friday, D. M., Hwang, C., Yi, S., Cheng, A. H., Torres-Flores, T. C., Jira, E. R., Wang, W., Aspuru-Guzik, A., & Burke, M. D. (2024). Closed-loop transfer enables artificial intelligence to yield chemical knowledge. *Nature*, *633*(8029), 351–358. PMID: 39198655

Artrith, N., Butler, K. T., Coudert, F.-X., Han, S., Isayev, O., Jain, A., & Walsh, A. (2021). Best practices in machine learning for chemistry. *Nature Chemistry*, *13*(6), 505–508. PMID: 34059804

Ashish, V. (2017). Attention is all you need. *Advances in Neural Information Processing Systems*, *30*, I.

Awan, R. E., Zainab, S., Yousuf, F. J., & Mughal, S. (2024). AI-driven drug discovery: Exploring Abaucin as a promising treatment against multidrug-resistant Acinetobacter baumannii. *Health Science Reports*, *7*(6), e2150. PMID: 38841115

Bai, C., Wu, L., Li, R., Cao, Y., He, S., & Bo, X. (2025). Machine Learning-Enabled Drug-Induced Toxicity Prediction. *Advancement of Science*, *12*(16), 2413405. PMID: 39899688

Bauer, A., Sappler, N., von Stülpnagel, L., Klemm, M., Schreinlechner, M., Wenner, F., Schier, J., Al Tawil, A., Dolejsi, T., & Krasniqi, A. (2022). Telemedical cardiac risk assessment by implantable cardiac monitors in patients after myocardial infarction with autonomic dysfunction (SMART-MI-DZHK9): A prospective investigator-initiated, randomised, multicentre, open-label, diagnostic trial. *The Lancet. Digital Health*, *4*(2), e105–e116. PMID: 35090674

Bellucci, M., Delestre, N., Malandain, N., & Zanni-Merk, C. (2021). Towards a terminology for a fully contextualized XAI. *Procedia Computer Science*, *192*, 241–250.

Björnsson, B., Borrebaeck, C., Elander, N., Gasslander, T., Gawel, D. R., Gustafsson, M., Jörnsten, R., Lee, E. J., Li, X., & Lilja, S. (2019). Digital twins to personalize medicine. *Genome Medicine*, *12*(1), 4. PMID: 31892363

Boldini, D., Grisoni, F., Kuhn, D., Friedrich, L., & Sieber, S. A. (2023). Practical guidelines for the use of gradient boosting for molecular property prediction. *Journal of Cheminformatics*, *15*(1), 73. PMID: 37641120

Braga, D. M., & Rawal, B. (2025). Harnessing AI and Quantum Computing for Revolutionizing Drug Discovery and Approval Processes: Case Example for Collagen Toxicity. *JMIR Bioinformatics and Biotechnology*, *6*(1), e69800. PMID: 41342151

Briefing, L. B. Early evidence and emerging trends: How AI is shaping drug discovery and clinical development.

Busuioc, M. (2022). AI algorithmic oversight: new frontiers in regulation. In *Handbook of regulatory authorities* (pp. 470–486). Edward Elgar Publishing.

Campos, R. (2024). Hybrid Quantum-Classical Algorithms. *arXiv preprint arXiv:2406.12371*.

Chatterjee, A., Paul, S., Bisht, B., Bhattacharya, S., Sivasubramaniam, S., & Paul, M. K. (2022). Advances in targeting the WNT/β-catenin signaling pathway in cancer. *Drug Discovery Today*, *27*(1), 82–101. PMID: 34252612

Chen, B., Khodadoust, M. S., Olsson, N., Wagar, L. E., Fast, E., Liu, C. L., Muftuoglu, Y., Sworder, B. J., Diehn, M., & Levy, R. (2019). Predicting HLA class II antigen presentation through integrated deep learning. *Nature Biotechnology*, *37*(11), 1332–1343. PMID: 31611695

Chen, J., Liu, H., Cui, X., Li, Z., & Chen, H.-F. (2022). RNA-specific force field optimization with CMAP and reweighting. *Journal of Chemical Information and Modeling*, *62*(2), 372–385. PMID: 35021622

Chen, T., & Guestrin, C. (2016). Xgboost: A scalable tree boosting system. Proceedings of the 22nd acm sigkdd international conference on knowledge discovery and data mining, Chithrananda, S., Grand, G., & Ramsundar, B. (2020). ChemBERTa: large-scale self-supervised pretraining for molecular property prediction. *arXiv preprint arXiv:2010.09885*.

Chun, M. (2023). *How artificial intelligence is revolutionizing drug discovery. Bill of Health*. Harvard Law School.

Correll, C. U., Abi-Dargham, A., & Howes, O. (2022). Emerging treatments in schizophrenia. *The Journal of Clinical Psychiatry*, *83*(1), 39683. PMID: 35172048

Dağlarli, E. (2020). Explainable artificial intelligence (xAI) approaches and deep meta-learning models. In *Advances and applications in deep learning*. IntechOpen.

Das, U. (2025). Generative AI for drug discovery and protein design: The next frontier in AI-driven molecular science. *Medicine in Drug Discovery*, •••, 100213.

De Cao, N., & Kipf, T. (2018). MolGAN: An implicit generative model for small molecular graphs. *arXiv preprint arXiv:1805.11973*.

De Vivo, M., Masetti, M., Bottegoni, G., & Cavalli, A. (2016). Role of molecular dynamics and related methods in drug discovery. *Journal of Medicinal Chemistry*, *59*(9), 4035–4061. PMID: 26807648

Dedic, N., Jones, P. G., Hopkins, S. C., Lew, R., Shao, L., Campbell, J. E., Spear, K. L., Large, T. H., Campbell, U. C., & Hanania, T. (2019). SEP-363856, a novel psychotropic agent with a unique, non-D2 receptor mechanism of action. *The Journal of Pharmacology and Experimental Therapeutics*, *371*(1), 1–14. PMID: 31371483

Deng, J., Yang, Z., Ojima, I., Samaras, D., & Wang, F. (2022). Artificial intelligence in drug discovery: Applications and techniques. *Briefings in Bioinformatics*, *23*(1). PMID: 34734228

Dermawan, D., & Alotaiq, N. (2025). From Lab to Clinic: How Artificial Intelligence (AI) Is Reshaping Drug Discovery Timelines and Industry Outcomes. *Pharmaceuticals*, *18*(7), 981. PMID: 40732273

Dev Sharma, P., Alhudhaibi, A. M., Al Noman, A., Abdallah, E. M., Taha, T. H., & Sharma, H. (2025). Systems biology-driven discovery of host-targeted therapeutics for oropouche virus: Integrating network pharmacology, molecular docking, and drug repurposing. *Pharmaceuticals*, *18*(5), 613. PMID: 40430433

DiMasi, J. A., Grabowski, H. G., & Hansen, R. W. (2016). Innovation in the pharmaceutical industry: New estimates of R&D costs. *Journal of Health Economics*, *47*, 20–33. PMID: 26928437

El Belghiti, I., Hammani, O., Moustaoui, F., Aghrouch, M., Lemkhente, Z., Boubrik, F., & Belmouden, A. (2025). Halicin: A New Approach to Antibacterial Therapy, a Promising Avenue for the Post-Antibiotic Era. *Antibiotics (Basel, Switzerland)*, *14*(7), 698. PMID: 40723999

Erhard, A., Poulsen Nautrup, H., Meth, M., Postler, L., Stricker, R., Stadler, M., Negnevitsky, V., Ringbauer, M., Schindler, P., & Briegel, H. J. (2021). Entangling logical qubits with lattice surgery. *Nature*, *589*(7841), 220–224. PMID: 33442044

Ernst, D. (2023). *Disappointing Results for Ulotaront in Two Phase 3 Schizophrenia Trials. Neurology Advisor*. NA-NA.

Fan, X., Fang, S., Li, Z., Ji, H., Yue, M., Li, J., & Ren, X. (2025). ICVAE: Interpretable conditional variational autoencoder for de novo molecular design. *International Journal of Molecular Sciences*, *26*(9), 3980. PMID: 40362221

Ferreira, F. J., & Carneiro, A. S. (2025). AI-Driven Drug Discovery: A Comprehensive Review. *ACS Omega*. PMID: 40547666

Fialková, V., Zhao, J., Papadopoulos, K., Engkvist, O., Bjerrum, E. J., Kogej, T., & Patronov, A. (2021). LibINVENT: Reaction-based generative scaffold decoration for in silico library design. *Journal of Chemical Information and Modeling*, *62*(9), 2046–2063. PMID: 34460269

Flores, J. E., Claborne, D. M., Weller, Z. D., Webb-Robertson, B.-J. M., Waters, K. M., & Bramer, L. M. (2023). Missing data in multi-omics integration: Recent advances through artificial intelligence. *Frontiers in Artificial Intelligence*, *6*, 1098308. PMID: 36844425

Gallo, P. (2006). Executive summary of the PhRMA working group on adaptive designs in clinical drug development. *Journal of Biopharmaceutical Statistics*, *16*, 275–283. PMID: 16724485

Ghazi Vakili, M., Gorgulla, C., Snider, J., Nigam, A., Bezrukov, D., Varoli, D., Aliper, A., Polykovsky, D., Padmanabha Das, K. M., & Cox Iii, H. (2025). Quantum-computing-enhanced algorithm unveils potential KRAS inhibitors. *Nature Biotechnology*, •••, 1–6. PMID: 39843581

Ghosh, P., Muhasina, K., Swaroop, A. K., Esakkimuthukumar, M., Singh, R. P., Singh, R., Justin, A., Selvaraj, J., & Basavan, D. (2024). Artificial Intelligence in Drug Research—A New Wave of Innovation in Drug Discovery. In *Computational Approaches in Biomaterials and Biomedical Engineering Applications* (pp. 162–188). CRC Press.

Goertzel, B. (2014). Artificial general intelligence: Concept, state of the art, and future prospects. *Journal of Artificial General Intelligence*, *5*(1), 1.

Gómez-Bombarelli, R., Wei, J. N., Duvenaud, D., Hernández-Lobato, J. M., Sánchez-Lengeling, B., Sheberla, D., Aguilera-Iparraguirre, J., Hirzel, T. D., Adams, R. P., & Aspuru-Guzik, A. (2018). Automatic chemical design using a data-driven continuous representation of molecules. *ACS Central Science*, *4*(2), 268–276. PMID: 29532027

GREGORY, B. (2020). A Molecule Designed By AI Exhibits' Druglike'Qualities. Wired. In.

Guerreschi, G. G., & Smelyanskiy, M. (2017). Practical optimization for hybrid quantum-classical algorithms. *arXiv preprint arXiv:1701.01450.*

Hähnel, M. (2025). Ethical challenges and solutions in AI-driven medical data management: A focus on distributed machine learning. *Discover Artificial Intelligence*, *5*(1), 53.

Halpin, H. (2007). Reinventing Technology: Artificial Intelligence from the Top of a Sycamore Tree. *CONSTITUENT IMAGINATION*, 155.

Harding, J. J., Telli, M., Munster, P., Voss, M. H., Infante, J. R., DeMichele, A., Dunphy, M., Le, M. H., Molineaux, C., & Orford, K. (2021). A phase I dose-escalation and expansion study of telaglenastat in patients with advanced or metastatic solid tumors. *Clinical Cancer Research*, *27*(18), 4994–5003. PMID: 34285061

Hassabis, D. (2022). Alphafold reveals the structure of the protein universe. *URL https://www. deepmind. com/blog/alphafold-reveals-the-structure-of-the-protein-universe, 2.*

Hervella, A. S., Rouco, J., Novo, J., & Ortega, M. (2022). Multimodal image encoding pre-training for diabetic retinopathy grading. *Computers in Biology and Medicine*, *143*, 105302. PMID: 35219187

Huang, D., Ye, X., & Sakurai, T. (2024). Multi-party collaborative drug discovery via federated learning. *Computers in Biology and Medicine*, *171*, 108181. PMID: 38428094

Huang, D., Ye, X., Zhang, Y., & Sakurai, T. (2023). Collaborative analysis for drug discovery by federated learning on non-IID data. *Methods (San Diego, Calif.)*, *219*, 1–7. PMID: 37689121

Inc, L. P. (2025). *Lantern Pharma Secures EU Patent Allowance for LP-284, Bolstering Global IP Position for AI-Developed Cancer Therapy*. Lantern Pharma Inc.

Ivanenkov, Y. A., Polykovskiy, D., Bezrukov, D., Zagribelnyy, B., Aladinskiy, V., Kamya, P., Aliper, A., Ren, F., & Zhavoronkov, A. (2023). Chemistry42: An AI-driven platform for molecular design and optimization. *Journal of Chemical Information and Modeling*, *63*(3), 695–701. PMID: 36728505

Jiménez-Luna, J., Grisoni, F., Weskamp, N., & Schneider, G. (2021). Artificial intelligence in drug discovery: Recent advances and future perspectives. *Expert Opinion on Drug Discovery*, *16*(9), 949–959. PMID: 33779453

Kalil, A. C., Patterson, T. F., Mehta, A. K., Tomashek, K. M., Wolfe, C. R., Ghazaryan, V., Marconi, V. C., Ruiz-Palacios, G. M., Hsieh, L., & Kline, S. (2021). Baricitinib plus remdesivir for hospitalized adults with Covid-19. *The New England Journal of Medicine*, *384*(9), 795–807. PMID: 33306283

Kamya, P., Ozerov, I. V., Pun, F. W., Tretina, K., Fokina, T., Chen, S., Naumov, V., Long, X., Lin, S., & Korzinkin, M. (2024). PandaOmics: An AI-driven platform for therapeutic target and biomarker discovery. *Journal of Chemical Information and Modeling*, *64*(10), 3961–3969. PMID: 38404138

Kandregula, N. (2025). Accelerating drug discovery with generative AI: Aa paradigm shift in pharmaceutical innovation and development.

Kant, S., Deepika, & Roy, S. (2025). Artificial intelligence in drug discovery and development: Transforming challenges into opportunities. *Discover Pharmaceutical Sciences*, *1*(1), 7.

Karger, E., & Kureljusic, M. (2022). Using artificial intelligence for drug discovery: A bibliometric study and future research agenda. *Pharmaceuticals*, *15*(12), 1492. PMID: 36558943

Klopp-Schulze, L., Shaw, J. V., Dong, J. Q., Khandelwal, A., Vazquez-Mateo, C., & Goteti, K. (2022). Applying modeling and simulations for rational dose selection of novel toll-like receptor 7/8 inhibitor enpatoran for indications of high medical need. *Clinical Pharmacology and Therapeutics*, *112*(2), 297–306. PMID: 35390178

Kurji, C. N. Transforming drug discovery with AI and computational biophysics.

Laude, M. C., Lebras, L., Sesques, P., Ghesquieres, H., Favre, S., Bouabdallah, K., Croizier, C., Guieze, R., Drieu La Rochelle, L., & Gyan, E. (2021). First-line treatment of double-hit and triple-hit lymphomas: Survival and tolerance data from a retrospective multicenter French study. *American Journal of Hematology*, *96*(3), 302–311. PMID: 33306213

Laurentino Schwabe, D. The METRIC-framework for assessing data quality for trustworthy AI in medicine: a systematic review.

Lee, J., Yoon, W., Kim, S., Kim, D., Kim, S., So, C. H., & Kang, J. (2020). BioBERT: A pre-trained biomedical language representation model for biomedical text mining. *Bioinformatics (Oxford, England)*, *36*(4), 1234–1240. PMID: 31501885

Lin, T.-Y., & Chou, L.-C. (2025). A systematic review of artificial intelligence applications and methodological advances in patent analysis. *World Patent Information*, *82*, 102383.

Lin, Z., Akin, H., Rao, R., Hie, B., Zhu, Z., Lu, W., Smetanin, N., Verkuil, R., Kabeli, O., & Shmueli, Y. (2023). Evolutionary-scale prediction of atomic-level protein structure with a language model. *science, 379*(6637), 1123-1130.

Lindsley, C. W. (2014). *New statistics on the cost of new drug development and the trouble with CNS drugs* (Vol. 5). ACS Publications.

Lionta, E., Spyrou, G. K., Vassilatis, D., & Cournia, Z. (2014). Structure-based virtual screening for drug discovery: Principles, applications and recent advances. *Current Topics in Medicinal Chemistry*, *14*(16), 1923–1938. PMID: 25262799

Liu, G., Catacutan, D. B., Rathod, K., Swanson, K., Jin, W., Mohammed, J. C., Chiappino-Pepe, A., Syed, S. A., Fragis, M., & Rachwalski, K. (2023). Deep learning-guided discovery of an antibiotic targeting Acinetobacter baumannii. *Nature Chemical Biology*, *19*(11), 1342–1350. PMID: 37231267

Lyne, P. D. (2002). Structure-based virtual screening: An overview. *Drug Discovery Today*, *7*(20), 1047–1055. PMID: 12546894

Mak, K.-K., & Pichika, M. R. (2019). Artificial intelligence in drug development: Present status and future prospects. *Drug Discovery Today*, *24*(3), 773–780. PMID: 30472429

Mak, K.-K., Wong, Y.-H., & Pichika, M. R. (2024). Artificial intelligence in drug discovery and development. *Drug discovery and evaluation: safety and pharmacokinetic assays*, 1461-1498.

Mallesh, N., Zhao, M., Meintker, L., Höllein, A., Elsner, F., Lüling, H., Haferlach, T., Kern, W., Westermann, J., & Brossart, P. (2021). Knowledge transfer to enhance the performance of deep learning models for automated classification of B cell neoplasms. *Patterns (New York, N.Y.)*, *2*(10). PMID: 34693376

Mayr, A., Klambauer, G., Unterthiner, T., & Hochreiter, S. (2016). DeepTox: Toxicity prediction using deep learning. *Frontiers in Environmental Science*, *3*, 80.

Mbituyimana, B., Bukatuka, C. F., Qi, F., Ma, G., Shi, Z., & Yang, G. (2023). Microneedle-mediated drug delivery for scar prevention and treatment. *Drug Discovery Today*, *28*(11), 103801. PMID: 37858631

McCloskey, K., Sigel, E. A., Kearnes, S., Xue, L., Tian, X., Moccia, D., Gikunju, D., Bazzaz, S., Chan, B., & Clark, M. A. (2020). Machine learning on DNA-encoded libraries: A new paradigm for hit finding. *Journal of Medicinal Chemistry*, *63*(16), 8857–8866. PMID: 32525674

Menard, P., & Bott, G. J. (2025). Artificial intelligence misuse and concern for information privacy: New construct validation and future directions. *Information Systems Journal*, *35*(1), 322–367.

Mennella, C., Maniscalco, U., De Pietro, G., & Esposito, M. (2024). Ethical and regulatory challenges of AI technologies in healthcare: A narrative review. *Heliyon*, *10*(4). PMID: 38384518

Mirakhori, F., & Niazi, S. K. (2025). Harnessing the AI/ML in drug and biological products discovery and development: The regulatory perspective. *Pharmaceuticals*, *18*(1), 47. PMID: 39861110

Moen, E., Bannon, D., Kudo, T., Graf, W., Covert, M., & Van Valen, D. (2019). Deep learning for cellular image analysis. *Nature Methods*, *16*(12), 1233–1246. PMID: 31133758

Nada, H., Gul, A. R., Elkamhawy, A., Kim, S., Kim, M., Choi, Y., Park, T. J., & Lee, K. (2023). Machine learning-based approach to developing potent EGFR inhibitors for breast cancer— Design, synthesis, and in vitro evaluation. *ACS Omega*, *8*(35), 31784–31800. PMID: 37692247

Nag, S., Baidya, A. T., Mandal, A., Mathew, A. T., Das, B., Devi, B., & Kumar, R. (2022). Deep learning tools for advancing drug discovery and development. *3 Biotech*, *12*(5), 110.

Nosrati, H., & Nosrati, M. (2023). Artificial intelligence in regenerative medicine: Applications and implications. *Biomimetics*, *8*(5), 442. PMID: 37754193

Ocana, A., Pandiella, A., Privat, C., Bravo, I., Luengo-Oroz, M., Amir, E., & Gyorffy, B. (2025). Integrating artificial intelligence in drug discovery and early drug development: A transformative approach. *Biomarker Research*, *13*(1), 45. PMID: 40087789

Ogut, E. (2025). Artificial Intelligence in Clinical Medicine: Challenges Across Diagnostic Imaging, Clinical Decision Support, Surgery, Pathology, and Drug Discovery. *Clinics and Practice*, *15*(9), 169. PMID: 41002784

Ooms, F. (2000). Molecular modeling and computer aided drug design. Examples of their applications in medicinal chemistry. *Current Medicinal Chemistry*, *7*(2), 141–158. PMID: 10637360

Ou-Yang, S.-s., Lu, J.-y., Kong, X.-q., Liang, Z.-j., Luo, C., & Jiang, H. (2012). Computational drug discovery. *Acta Pharmacologica Sinica*, *33*(9), 1131–1140. PMID: 22922346

Patel, D. D., Pathak, R. S., Patel, K. S., Bhatt, H. G., & Patel, P. K. (2025). The Future of Medicine: AI and ML Driven Drug Discovery Advancements. *Current Topics in Medicinal Chemistry*. PMID: 40207759

Philippidis, A. (2022). Double dare: exscientia expands AI platform into antibody design: British pioneer of data-driven drug discovery eyes doubling the number of potential druggable sites, as well as a future move into more complex biologics. *GEN Edge*, *4*(1), 896–902.

Philippidis, A. (2023). BMS Collaboration Paying Off for Exscientia: AI drug developer designs EXS4318, the I&I small molecule that has entered Phase I trials overseen by pharma giant in up-to-$1.3 B+ partnership. *GEN Edge*, *5*(1), 147–150.

Philippidis, A. (2025). Healx Candidate, SpringWorks Therapy Expand NF1 Treatment Options: Healx doses first patient in Phase II trial of HLX-1502 for neurofibromatosis type 1, while SpringWorks wins FDA approval for Gomekli, first drug designed to treat the disease in adults and children. *GEN Edge*, *7*(1), 136–141.

Popova, M., Isayev, O., & Tropsha, A. (2018). Deep reinforcement learning for de novo drug design. *Science Advances*, *4*(7), eaap7885. PMID: 30050984

Qiu, S., Zhao, S., & Yang, A. (2023). DLTKcat: Deep learning-based prediction of temperature-dependent enzyme turnover rates. *Briefings in Bioinformatics*, *25*(1). PMID: 38189538

Ragoza, M., Hochuli, J., Idrobo, E., Sunseri, J., & Koes, D. R. (2017). Protein–ligand scoring with convolutional neural networks. *Journal of Chemical Information and Modeling*, *57*(4), 942–957. PMID: 28368587

Rao, I. (2023). NovoMol: Recurrent Neural Network for Orally Bioavailable Drug Design and Validation on PDGFR {\alpha} Receptor. *arXiv preprint arXiv:2312.01527.*

Ren, F., Aliper, A., Chen, J., Zhao, H., Rao, S., Kuppe, C., Ozerov, I. V., Zhang, M., Witte, K., & Kruse, C. (2025). A small-molecule TNIK inhibitor targets fibrosis in preclinical and clinical models. *Nature Biotechnology*, *43*(1), 63–75. PMID: 38459338

Ren, F., Ding, X., Zheng, M., Korzinkin, M., Cai, X., Zhu, W., Mantsyzov, A., Aliper, A., Aladinskiy, V., & Cao, Z. (2023). AlphaFold accelerates artificial intelligence powered drug discovery: Efficient discovery of a novel CDK20 small molecule inhibitor. *Chemical Science (Cambridge)*, *14*(6), 1443–1452. PMID: 36794205

Ren, Y., Pieper, A. A., & Cheng, F. (2025). Utilization of precision medicine digital twins for drug discovery in Alzheimer's disease. *Neurotherapeutics; the Journal of the American Society for Experimental NeuroTherapeutics*, •••, 00553.

Richardson, S., Hirsch, J. S., Narasimhan, M., Crawford, J. M., McGinn, T., Davidson, K. W., Barnaby, D. P., Becker, L. B., Chelico, J. D., & Cohen, S. L. (2020). Presenting characteristics, comorbidities, and outcomes among 5700 patients hospitalized with COVID-19 in the New York City area. *Journal of the American Medical Association*, *323*(20), 2052–2059. PMID: 32320003

Rovenchak, A., & Druchok, M. (2024). Machine learning-assisted search for novel coagulants: When machine learning can be efficient even if data availability is low. *Journal of Computational Chemistry*, *45*(13), 937–952. PMID: 38174834

Scannell, J. W., Blanckley, A., Boldon, H., & Warrington, B. (2012). Diagnosing the decline in pharmaceutical R&D efficiency. *Nature Reviews. Drug Discovery*, *11*(3), 191–200. PMID: 22378269

Schwam, E. M., Nicholas, T., Chew, R., Billing, C. B., Davidson, W., Ambrose, D., & Altstiel, L. D. (2014). A multicenter, double-blind, placebo-controlled trial of the PDE9A inhibitor, PF-04447943, in Alzheimer's disease. *Current Alzheimer Research*, *11*(5), 413–421. PMID: 24801218

Seijas-Bellido, J. A., Samanta, B., Valadez-Villalobos, K., Gallardo, J. J., Navas, J., Balestra, S. R., Madero Castro, R. M. a., Vicent-Luna, J. M., Tao, S., & Toroker, M. C. (2022). Transferable classical force field for pure and mixed metal halide perovskites parameterized from first-principles. *Journal of Chemical Information and Modeling*, *62*(24), 6423–6435. PMID: 35576452

Senior, A. W., Evans, R., Jumper, J., Kirkpatrick, J., Sifre, L., Green, T., Qin, C., Žídek, A., Nelson, A. W., & Bridgland, A. (2020). Improved protein structure prediction using potentials from deep learning. *Nature*, *577*(7792), 706–710. PMID: 31942072

Serrano, D. R., Luciano, F. C., Anaya, B. J., Ongoren, B., Kara, A., Molina, G., Ramirez, B. I., Sánchez-Guirales, S. A., Simon, J. A., & Tomietto, G. (2024). Artificial intelligence (AI) applications in drug discovery and drug delivery: Revolutionizing personalized medicine. *Pharmaceutics*, *16*(10), 1328. PMID: 39458657

Sirén, J., & Paten, B. (2022). GBZ file format for pangenome graphs. *Bioinformatics (Oxford, England)*, *38*(22), 5012–5018. PMID: 36179091

Sodaei, Z., Ekrami, S., & Hashemianzadeh, S. M. (2025). Machine learning analysis of molecular dynamics properties influencing drug solubility. *Scientific Reports*, *15*(1), 26955. PMID: 40707560

Soni, K., & Hasija, Y. (2022). Artificial intelligence assisted drug research and development. 2022 IEEE Delhi Section Conference (DELCON), Srivastava, D., Korsakova, A., Wang, Q., Ruiz, L., Yuan, H., & Kelley, D. R. (2025). Borzoi-informed fine mapping improves causal variant prioritization in complex trait GWAS. bioRxiv, 2025.2007. 2009.663936.

Stokes, J. M., Yang, K., Swanson, K., Jin, W., Cubillos-Ruiz, A., Donghia, N. M., MacNair, C. R., French, S., Carfrae, L. A., & Bloom-Ackermann, Z. (2020). A deep learning approach to antibiotic discovery. *Cell, 180*(4), 688-702. e613.

Talevi, A., Morales, J. F., Hather, G., Podichetty, J. T., Kim, S., Bloomingdale, P. C., Kim, S., Burton, J., Brown, J. D., & Winterstein, A. G. (2020). Machine learning in drug discovery and development part 1: A primer. *CPT: Pharmacometrics & Systems Pharmacology*, *9*(3), 129–142. PMID: 31905263

Thakkar, S., Slikker, W.Jr, Yiannas, F., Silva, P., Blais, B., Chng, K. R., Liu, Z., Adholeya, A., Pappalardo, F., & Soares, M. L. C. (2023). Artificial intelligence and real-world data for drug and food safety–A regulatory science perspective. *Regulatory Toxicology and Pharmacology*, *140*, 105388. PMID: 37061083

Tomar, P., Goel, F., Pal, A., & Garg, V. K. (2025). The Future of Drug Development: Leveraging AI for Faster and Safer Innovation. *International Journal of Advances in Scientific Research*, *16*(04), 5–11.

Ueno, H. (2023). Artificial intelligence as dual-use technology. In *Fusion of Machine Learning Paradigms: Theory and Applications* (pp. 7-32). Springer.

Urbina, F., Lentzos, F., Invernizzi, C., & Ekins, S. (2022). Dual use of artificial-intelligence-powered drug discovery. *Nature Machine Intelligence*, *4*(3), 189–191. PMID: 36211133

Vamathevan, J., Apweiler, R., & Birney, E. (2019). Biomolecular data resources: Bioinformatics infrastructure for biomedical data science. *Annual Review of Biomedical Data Science*, *2*(1), 199–222.

Vamathevan, J., Clark, D., Czodrowski, P., Dunham, I., Ferran, E., Lee, G., Li, B., Madabhushi, A., Shah, P., & Spitzer, M. (2019). Applications of machine learning in drug discovery and development. *Nature Reviews. Drug Discovery*, *18*(6), 463–477. PMID: 30976107

Vinluan, F. (2025). An AI Biotech Hauls In $600 M [*MedCity News*, NA-NA.]. *Plus More Funding Highlights to Close*, *1Q*, 2025.

Wallach, I., Dzamba, M., & Heifets, A. (2015). AtomNet: a deep convolutional neural network for bioactivity prediction in structure-based drug discovery. *arXiv preprint arXiv:1510.02855*.

Wang, L. L., Lo, K., Chandrasekhar, Y., Reas, R., Yang, J., Burdick, D., Eide, D., Funk, K., Katsis, Y., & Kinney, R. (2020). Cord-19: The covid-19 open research dataset. *ArXiv*, arXiv: 2004.10706 v10704.

Weller, J. A., & Rohs, R. (2024). Structure-based drug design with a deep hierarchical generative model. *Journal of Chemical Information and Modeling*, *64*(16), 6450–6463. PMID: 39058534

Wizemann, T., Nass, S. J., Andrada, A., & Amankwah, F. K. (2020). The role of NIH in drug development innovation and its impact on patient access: proceedings of a workshop.

Wouters, O. J., McKee, M., & Luyten, J. (2020). Estimated research and development investment needed to bring a new medicine to market, 2009-2018. *Journal of the American Medical Association*, *323*(9), 844–853. PMID: 32125404

Xia, X. (2017). Bioinformatics and drug discovery. *Current Topics in Medicinal Chemistry*, *17*(15), 1709–1726. PMID: 27848897

Xia, X., Zhu, C., Zhong, F., & Liu, L. (2023). MDTips: A multimodal-data-based drug–target interaction prediction system fusing knowledge, gene expression profile, and structural data. *Bioinformatics (Oxford, England)*, *39*(7), btad411. PMID: 37379157

Xu, Z., Ren, F., Wang, P., Cao, J., Tan, C., Ma, D., Zhao, L., Dai, J., Ding, Y., & Fang, H. (2025). A generative AI-discovered TNIK inhibitor for idiopathic pulmonary fibrosis: A randomized phase 2a trial. *Nature Medicine*, •••, 1–9. PMID: 40461817

Yan, D., Zhou, Q., Wang, J., & Zhang, N. (2017). Bayesian regularisation neural network based on artificial intelligence optimisation. *International Journal of Production Research*, *55*(8), 2266–2287.

Yang, Y., & Cheng, F. (2025). Artificial intelligence streamlines scientific discovery of drug–target interactions. *British Journal of Pharmacology*. PMID: 39843168

Zhang, Y., Bhosle, A., Bae, S., McIver, L. J., Pishchany, G., Accorsi, E. K., Thompson, K. N., Arze, C., Wang, Y., & Subramanian, A. (2022). Discovery of bioactive microbial gene products in inflammatory bowel disease. *Nature*, *606*(7915), 754–760. PMID: 35614211

Zhavoronkov, A., Ivanenkov, Y. A., Aliper, A., Veselov, M. S., Aladinskiy, V. A., Aladinskaya, A. V., Terentiev, V. A., Polykovskiy, D. A., Kuznetsov, M. D., & Asadulaev, A. (2019). Deep learning enables rapid identification of potent DDR1 kinase inhibitors. *Nature Biotechnology*, *37*(9), 1038–1040. PMID: 31477924

Zhou, J., Sturtevant, D., Biyani, N., Bhatia, K., & Dave, S. (2022). MCL-319 LP-284–A Highly Potent Small Molecule Targeting Mantle Cell Lymphoma. *Clinical Lymphoma, Myeloma & Leukemia*, *22*, S396.

Zhou, J., Sturtevant, D., Love, C., Kulkarni, A., Biyani, N., Kathad, U., Thacker, E., Dave, S., & Bhatia, K. (2023). LP-284, a small molecule acylfulvene, exerts potent antitumor activity in preclinical non-Hodgkin's lymphoma models and in cells deficient in DNA damage repair. *Oncotarget*, *14*, 597. PMID: 37306526

Chapter 2
Catalyzing Drug Discovery Using Artificial Intelligence With Traditional Medicine

Fatemeh Taktaz
https://orcid.org/0000-0002-6521-4478
University of Campania "Luigi Vanvitelli", Italy

Salar Hafez-Ghoran
https://orcid.org/0000-0001-5495-5556
North Carolina Research Campus, USA

ABSTRACT

The integration of artificial intelligence (AI) with traditional medicine holds great promise for accelerating drug discovery and development. By mining ancient medical texts, ethnobotanical records, and modern literature, AI can help identify bioactive compounds and elucidate their mechanism of action. Machine learning and deep learning approaches enable rapid screening of chemical structures, prediction of biological activities, and optimization of drug-like properties, thereby reducing time and costs compared to conventional methods. Beyond discovery, AI also supports quality control and safety assessment of herbal and traditional formulations. However, challenges remain, including data privacy, intellectual property rights, and recognition of traditional knowledge holders, and the need for transparency and interpretability of AI models. This chapter covers an overview of the current landscape, highlighting opportunities, challenges, and future directions in harnessing AI to advance traditional medicine-based drug discovery.

DOI: 10.4018/979-8-3373-5258-9.ch002

INTRODUCTION

Figure 1. Key terms and concepts within Artificial Intelligence based on their importance and applicability.

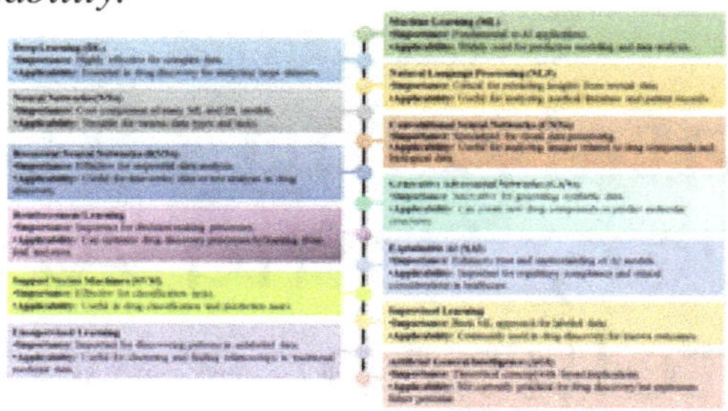

Traditional medicine, with its extensive history and empirical knowledge, has shown great potential for contributing to modern drug discovery. Traditional Chinese Medicine (TCM), with thousands of years of practice and documented prescriptions, represents a significant repository of natural compounds and therapeutic approaches. Its use has led to the accumulation of empirical insights that may inform modern disease treatment and pharmaceutical development (Khan et al., 2021). Numerous clinical studies have consistently demonstrated that certain components in TCM exhibit remarkable healing and symptom-relieving effects, particularly for chronic and complex diseases that conventional medical treatments cannot effectively address (W. Zhang et al., 2019). Artificial intelligence (AI)–a rapidly advancing technical science–encompasses theories, methods, and technical applications designed to extend, expand, and stimulate human intelligence (Mathew et al., 2021). Over the past few decades, the application of AI in the TCM field has become increasingly prevalent. Drug discovery and traditional medicine development typically rely on preclinical research to identify therapeutic targets and mechanisms. However, preclinical research remains costly and time-consuming (Wouters et al., 2020). Integrating AI with TCM offers a promising approach to overcome these challenges, streamline the discovery process and reduced costs (Li et al., 2022). AI allows researchers to analyze large amounts of data, including traditional medicine literature, ethnobotanical records, and clinical trial data information. Using AI algorithms, researchers are able to efficiently identify promising lead compounds or targets, assess patterns, and validate hypotheses thorough computational models and simulations. These AI-driven analyses facilitate the identification of lead compounds and promising drug candidates by mining extensive datasets (Chen et al., 2023). AI models are increasingly being used to screen millions of natural products derived from traditional medicine sources, predicting their potential biological activities or drug-likeness (Blanco-Gonzalez et al., 2023). Additionally, AI-powered molecular modeling and simulations offer valuable insights into the mechanisms of action, pharmacokinetics, and toxicity profiles of drug candidates originating from traditional medicine (Paul et al., 2021; Vora et al., 2023). AI can also assist in the design and evaluation of clinical trials, ensuring the rigorous validation of traditional medicine-derived drug candidates (Subbiah, 2023). The global COVID-19 pandemic has highlighted the importance of reducing healthcare costs and alleviating strain on healthcare systems, prompting the increased adoption of AI in medicine (Albahri et al., 2020; Ben-Israel et al., 2020). AI model development holds the potential for the precise customization of herbal medicine based on individual patient symptoms. For instance, AI can analyse complex aspects of a patient's data and identify time-sensitive conditions, such as sepsis and adverse drug reactions (Lynn, 2019). While the integration of AI and traditional medicine presents immense promise, several challenges remain, such as the standardization of data, the integration of traditional knowledge, and the establishment of a regulatory framework (Wang et al., 2023). Moreover, successful implementation requires multidisciplinary among AI experts, traditional medicine professioners, and drug discovery scientists (Chu et al., 2022). Overall, the incorporation of AI into pharmaceutical research and discovery has been transformative. It has enabled researchers to tackle complex challenges more efficiently from target identification to toxicity prediction. AI's versatile capabilities are reshaping the pharmaceutical industry, ushering in an era of accelerated innovation and improved patient outcomes (Kim et al., 2020). However, before implementing AI in these applications, it is essential to understand their importance and applicability (Figure 1).

In this chapter, we will investigate the foundational concepts and terminology of AI that are essential for leveraging its capabilities in the context of traditional medicine. Additionally, we will discuss the importance of data quality and standardization, as well as the ethical considerations surrounding the integration of AI in healthcare. Through this exploration, we aim to equip readers with the knowledge needed to navigate the intersection of AI and traditional medicine, fostering innovation and collaboration for future advancements in drug development.

1. EMERGING AI TECHNOLOGY

AI is a technology-driven system that encompasses advanced tools and networks capable of simulating human intelligence. It is a computer-based system that utilizes acquired information to solve complex problems by applying or developing rules (algorithms). AI algorithms can rapidly screen millions of potential drug compounds against biological targets, predicting their activity and toxicity (Paul et al., 2021).

Complementary and alternative medicine (CAM) and traditional medical fields are increasingly utilizing AI for pattern diagnosis, symptom classification, and the discovery of potential medication candidates (Feng et al., 2021; H. Zhang et al., 2020). Scientists have pinpointed several specific areas requiring enhancement to better replicate human intelligence, such as search and optimization capabilities, computer vision, natural language processing (NLP), knowledge representation, machine learning (ML), probabilistic reasoning, artificial neural network (ANN), and planning and decision-making (Figure 1) (Sejnowski, 2020). While creating new algorithms can be time-consuming and challenging, computers can expedite this process significantly. Neural networks, a machine learning algorithm that loosely imitates the working of the human brain, are one such example (Lotter et al., 2020). Nearly every scientific field is leveraging AI to enhance research, including the healthcare sector. As a result, many large pharmaceutical companies have begun integrating AI into their drug discovery efforts (Fleming, 2018). ML and probabilistic reasoning employ algorithms for mathematical modeling to enhance decision-making outcomes. Supervised ML uses classification labels, like decision trees and random forests, while unsupervised ML focuses on hidden patterns in data without classification labels (Jiang et al., 2020). Artificial neural networks (ANNs), a complex form of ML with dual functionalities and broad applicability, have gained attention as an emerging area of AI, mimicking the human brain's neural structure (Agatonovic-Kustrin & Beresford, 2000). The application of AI in medicinal chemistry has garnered considerable interest in recent years and is seen as a potential game-changer for the pharmaceutical industry.

1.1. Artificial Intelligence in Traditional Medicine

Traditional medicines, including health foods and supplements, have gained significant popularity in recent times. This broad range of therapies encompasses herbal remedies, manual techniques, and spiritual practices, all of which have been passed down through generations within various communities and ethnic groups. The origins of traditional medicine can be traced back to the earliest civilizations, where people relied on knowledge of plants, animals, and natural resources to meet their health needs (Fokunang et al., 2011; Tang et al., 2020). As a rapidly emerging field, AI technologies have generated significant enthusiasm among researchers in recent years (Figure 2) (Wu et al., 2022). AI is increasingly being integrated into traditional medicine, enhancing the discovery and validation of therapeutic compounds derived from ancient practices. By utilizing ML algorithms and data analytics, researchers can analyze vast datasets from traditional medicinal texts and clinical records to pinpoint potential drug candidates and predict their effectiveness. This integration not only streamlines the drug discovery process but also aids in personalizing treatments based on individual patient data, thereby improving health outcomes (Chu et al., 2022). One ongoing challenge in the modernization and globalization of TCM is the standardization of its diagnostic practices. Investigating the application of AI technology in TCM and addressing the associated challenges are essential for the advancement of modern TCM in the AI era (Guo et al., 2019). Plant extracts are often well tolerated, which has contributed to the widespread application of plant-based traditional medicine across many generations. Discovering and refining therapeutic phytochemicals derived from plant extracts could significantly reduce the risk of toxic effects. Therefore, having a dependable chemical database of therapeutic plants could serve as a foundation for lead drug discovery, particularly in traditional medicine, where plant extracts are commonly used (Figure 2). The Indian Medicinal Plants, Phytochemistry, and Therapeutic (IMPPAT) is an example of such a resource. It features 9,596 phytochemicals from 1742 Indian medicinal plants, along with their respective therapeutic applications (Mohanraj et al., 2018). Another comprehensive phytochemical database is the Universal Metabolome and Pathway Database (UMPDB), which includes traditional, genetic, and chemical information for 1127 different plants. TCM, Japanese Kampo, and Korean Sasang constitutional medicine share common roots. However, the constitutional medical systems in China, Japan, and Korea have developed differently due to geographical factors, cultural traditions, social environments, and national customs (W. Yu et al., 2017). Both China and India have long-standing traditions in medicine, with TCM and Ayurveda being practiced for over two millennia. Both systems primarily rely on medicinal plants as their main therapeutic agents (Jaiswal et al., 2016). Discovering new medications is challenging due to the need for highly specific lead molecules. Chemically synthesized lead compounds often face toxicity issues, making them unsuitable for FDA approval. Traditional medicine, through the identification and refinement of therapeutic phytochemicals from plant extracts, can help overcome this hurdle. A reliable chemical database for medicinal plants, like IMPPAT, provides a centralized source of valuable information (Mohanraj et al., 2018). The integration of convolutional neural network (CNN) in protein-ligand interaction studies allows for faster and more efficient evaluation of chemical structures in medicinal plant extracts. This method prioritizes the active site structure, calculates binding affinities, and ranks them, enabling the identification of active ingredients in the plant extract (Figure 2) (Popova et al., 2018). AI-assisted TCM diagnosis offers a more quantitative, objective, and standardized approach by utilizing digital data from electronic tools. This enhances consistency, accuracy, and reliability in diagnostic decisions, enabling an objective assessment of treatment effectiveness. Furthermore, AI standardizes formula-syndrome relationships and herbal formulae rules, helping bridge the gap between TCM and modern science. This could result in more scientific evidence and standardized guidelines for specific TCM syndromes (Xu et al., 2021).

Context-Oriented Directed Associations (CODA) is a software recently developed by researchers at the Bio-Synergy Research Center in Daejeon, South Korea. It incorporates the latest advances in biotechnology and AI to explore the potential medicinal properties of chemical compounds found in traditional remedies, such as Samul-Tang, a blend of four Asian herbs used to treat anemia and other blood disorders (H. Yu et al., 2017). AI offers a higher success rate in developing new drugs and can expedite the research process. For example, AI can be used to create new medications from the *Jamu's* natural products that are deeply embedded in the Indonesian culture. The drug development process for *jamu* involves the systematic evaluation of effective medications, database discovery and data extraction, and the application of AI techniques (Rustandi et al., 2023).

Figure 2. Artificial Intelligence in Traditional medicine and drug discovery.

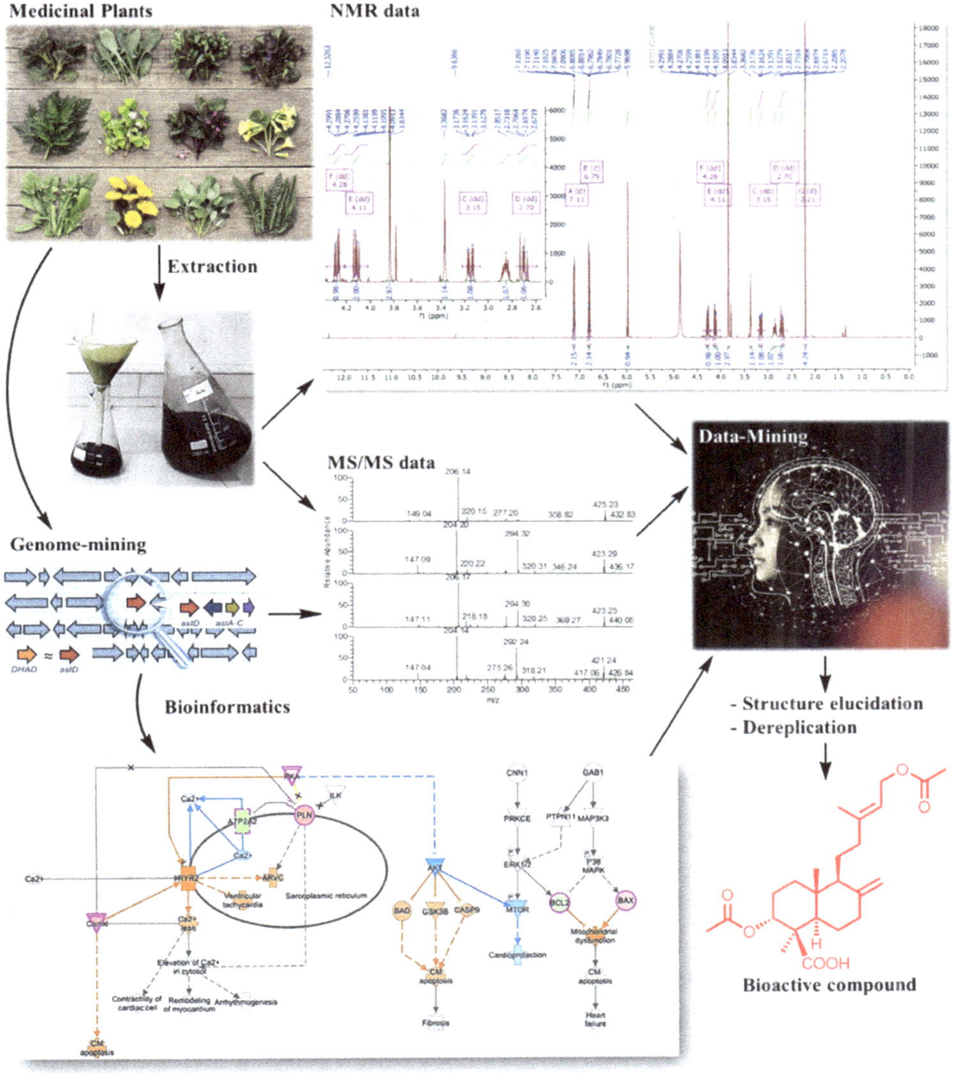

1.2. AI Potential in Drug Discovery

Recent advancements have sparked significant interest in applying AI methods to enhance various stages of the drug discovery pipeline, including de novo molecular design, optimization, structure-based drug design, and both preclinical and clinical development (Chen et al., 2018). By collecting comprehensive data on bioactive compounds, metabolomics, pharmacology, and targeted diseases, AI has the potential to accelerate the development of new medications (Xiaotong et al., 2022). Meanwhile, AI is enabling the development of more potent medications by drawing insights from existing data, including both modern pharmaceuticals and compounds derived from ancient herbal medicine. An alternative approach that can be incorporated is quantitative structure-activity relationship (QSAR), which involves creating models to link biological activity with physicochemical properties (Zhu, 2020). Drug discovery, which traditionally depended on labour-intensive methods like trial-and-error experimentation and high-throughput screening, is a complex and time-consuming. However, AI techniques, such as natural language processing and machine learning, promise to expedite and enhance this process by facilitating more efficient precise analysis of vast datasets (Xu et al., 2021). A crucial application of AI in drug discovery is the identification of drug-drug interactions, which occur when multiple drugs are combined to treat the same or different diseases in a single patient, leading to modified effects or adverse reactions (Jang et al., 2022). One of the primary applications of AI in medicinal chemistry is predicting the efficacy and toxicity of potential drug compounds. Traditional drug discovery protocols typically depend on labour-intensive and time-consuming experiments to evaluate a compounds potential yielding uncertain results with a high degree of variability (Hansen et al., 2015). Biomedical databases, including imaging data, genomic profiles and drug datasets, can be integrated with analytical methods, particularly deep learning models, to provide the necessary tools for discovering effective drugs and their clinical applications (Vamathevan et al., 2019). Additionally, AI in drug discovery helps to design novel compounds with specific properties and activities. AI-based methods can facilitate the rapid and efficient creation of new compounds with desirable characteristics. For instance, a deep learning algorithm was recently trained on a dataset of known drug compounds and their corresponding properties, enabling it to suggest new therapeutic molecules (Gomez-Bombarelli et al., 2018). Yeh et al. (2020) explored the potential of deep learning to identify molecular characteristics for Meridian prediction, offering new perspectives on TCM (Yeh et al., 2020). As drug application centre around the three-dimensional structure of molecules such as DNA, RNA and proteins, the atomic structure of these molecules serves as the fundamental unit in understanding their interactions. This atomic structure can be regarded as a machine learning data type for modeling and understanding molecular interaction (Baltrusaitis et al., 2019).

2. MACHINE LEARNING'S APPLICATIONS IN DEVELOPMENT OF NATURAL PRODUCTS

Machine learning (ML) is a subset of artificial intelligence that includes the use of complex statistics and mathematical methods to solve various problems. ML algorithms are easily and affordably implementable on a large scale through cloud computing, making them accessible and efficient for divers applications (Saldivar-Gonzalez et al., 2022). In the health care system, ML applications can be broadly categorized into two main types: text-based applications and image-based applications. Text-based applications involve techniques such as natural language processing (NLP) to analyze electronic health record. Image-based applications focused on the analysis of radiological imaging, among other areas (Figure 3). NLP is a subset of AI within the field of ML and is primarily used for data mining purposes. NLP includes various methods, including machine translation, speech recognition, text summarization, sentiment analysis, and named entity recognition. These methods allow computers to understand, analyse, and interpret human language from written texts, thereby generating targeted outcomes from large and complex databases (Saldivar-Gonzalez et al., 2022). The quick development of technology is significantly transforming diagnostic, therapeutic, and drug discovery approaches in traditional medical systems such as Ayurveda and TCM. One of the critical applications of ML in traditional medicine lies in pattern recognition and diagnosis. ML algorithms are able to recognize patterns and relationships within extensive datasets of patient records, symptoms, and treatment outcomes, patterns those human practitioners may not be able to detect (Park et al., 2022; H. Zhang et al., 2020). The TCM Systems Pharmacology Database and Analysis Platform (TCMSP) is a valuable resource designed to assist research in herbal medicines within a systems pharmacology framework. It contains comprehensive data on 499 Chinese herbs, including 29,384 ingredients, 3,311 targets, and 837 associated diseases. The platform provides data on twelve key ADME-related properties, including factors like drug-likeness, Caco-2 permeability, blood-brain barrier penetration, half-life, oral bioavailability, and Lipinski's rule of five. This data is essential for drug assessment and screening. TCMSP establishes connections between active compounds, drug targets, and associated diseases, allowing for the automatic generation of target-disease and compound-target networks to examine the mechanism of drug action (Ru et al., 2014). Numerous studies have utilized ML to investigate neuroprotective compounds from Xiaoxuming decoction, which have an impact on controlling vascular functions and promoting stroke recovery. These studies underscore ML's ability to process complex datasets and uncover insights into traditional remedies (Shen et al., 2021; Zhang et al., 2021). Furthermore, machine learning is also being employed to optimize treatment regimens in traditional medicine. By analysing patient data and historical treatment outcomes, ML algorithms can recommend personalized combinations of medications, acupuncture points, or other interventions for specific illnesses (Wang et al., 2019). TCM's approach is inherently complex because several symptoms can correspond to multiple diseases, and multiple diseases can map onto certain syndromes. This creates challenges in diagnosis and treatment compared to Western medical paradigms. Practitioners of TCM must differentiate between various syndromes to ensure accurate diagnosis. Zhang et al. suggested diagnostic models for TCM that use symptoms as input to predict medical conditions and associated syndromes. These models have demonstrated high accuracy by employing multi-label classification strategies (Hong Zhang et al., 2020). Moreover, in a ground-breaking study, Wang et al. have analyzed the active ingredients and molecular features for 646 herbs, focusing on ADME pharmacokinetic properties and structure-based fingerprints. Their findings indicated that machine learning techniques-specifically decision tree (DT), RF, and SVM algorithms-can predict the *Meridian*–a concept in TCM mapping pathways and therapeutic effects–with an impressive accuracy of 0.83, with RF demonstrating the highest accuracy among the algorithms used. Additionally, they identified the most critical chemical properties contributing to Meridian prediction, highlighting ML's predictive power for understanding the mechanisms of TMC therapies (Wang et al., 2019).

A network-based methodology was presented by Cheng et al. for identifying clinically effective drug combinations for specific disorders. This approach the potential to enhance the understanding of the pharmacology of TCM medicines and its therapeutic mechanisms (Cheng et al., 2019). In related research, Fu et al. analyzed 2,012 phytochemicals associated with TCM herbs and developed a data clustering technique. Their finding revealed that the physical and chemical properties, as well as the target pathways of these compounds, could be linked to the hot or cold properties, commonly used in TCM classifications (Fu et al., 2017). ML approaches can be categorized in four main types, with clustering and dimensionality reduction representing two of these categories. Within ML, there are fourteen models, commonly applied in research: orthogonal partial least squares-discriminant analysis, partial least squares-discriminant analysis, principal compound analysis, random forest, decision tree, convolutional neural network, back propagation neural network, artificial neural network, hierarchical cluster analysis, k-means clustering, partial least squares regression, logistic regression, least square-support vector machine, and support vector machine. These models are applied across a variety of research fields, with eight common applications split into two main categories: **a**) TCM applications: Analysis of prescription, determination of syndromes, and disease diagnosis of disease, and **b**) Chines herbal medicine research: Identification of geographic origins, quality control, pharmacodynamic material basis, pharmacokinetics, pharmacodynamics, and medicinal properties (Chen & He, 2022).

Deep learning represents an advanced subset of ML, characterized by processing and validation of large training datasets between input and output layers. It allows for sophisticated modelling of complex associations (Calderaro et al., 2022). One of the challenges in applying ML to TCM is the many-to-many relationships between patients and their corresponding syndromes. In TCM, this mapping does not follow a simple one-to-one correspondence, complicating the application of ML in decision-making procedures. Nevertheless, ML has been applied to TCM in numerous ways to support clinical decisions. Liu et al. suggested a one-versus-the-rest diagnostic model for TCM, utilizing deep learning (DL) techniques, that can categorize multiple labels. The model demonstrated good diagnostic accuracy by using symptoms as input to predict the type of medical ailment and associated with chronic gastritis syndromes (Liu et al., 2014). AI application in treating insomnia mainly focuses on data-driven strategies to tailor personalized treatment plans. AI systems analyze patient information to anticipate individual responses to various therapies, including drug-based interventions and alternative methods, such as TCM. In the context of TCM, AI can assist in selecting the most suitable herbal combinations and acupuncture points customized to each patient's specific needs. For example, AI platforms can generate individualized herbal recommendations by merging clinical data, patient feedback, and TCM concepts. Additionally, by monitoring patient progress and adapting treatments in real-time, AI can enhance the efficacy of traditional TCM practices while minimizing reliance on trial-and-error techniques (Nashwan & Rao, 2024). Li et al. conducted a study involving 165 insomnia patients treated with Integrated Traditional Chinese and Western Medicine. They used standardized TCM scales and the Spiegel Sleep Questionnaire to evaluate patient outcomes. ML models, including three well-known machine learning models: support vector machines (SVM), Random Forest Classifier (RFC), and K-Nearest Neighbors (KNN), were applied to predict insomnia severity using TCM constitution classifications. The study found that classifications such as Damp-heat and Yang-deficiency emerged as significant factors, indicating their potential role in guiding targeted insomnia treatments. Among these models, RFC demonstrated superior accuracy and predictive performance, outperforming both SVC and KNN in terms of prediction accuracy (Li et al., 2023). RFC is a robust ensemble machine learning model widely applied across various medical fields, including cancer, diabetes and cardiovascular disease detection and prognosis (Murugan et al., 2019; Su et al., 2020). Similarly, Kim et al. utilized different ML techniques– SVM, RFC, and logistic regression–to investigate potential relationships between medications and diseases. These studies considered self-defined similarity metrics, including disease-drug and drug-drug similarities, to uncover patterns and connections (Kim et al., 2019). Looking forward, machine learning research can harness the vast amounts of TCM-related data, including natural products (herbal medicines), which have historically been used to treat diseases following extensive clinical diagnosis and trials. ML offers an opportunity to study natural products, disease detection, and therapeutic responses, by identifying common patterns and regularities within complex datasets. this enables uncovering relationships between input data and output variables (e.g., clinical characteristics, patient genetics, and treatment responses) and observed outcomes (Figure 3) (Seetharam et al., 2019).

The Global Natural Products Social (GNPS) Molecular Networking platform serves as a comprehensive resource for mass spectrometry-based metabolomics, allowing researchers to compare molecular properties and fragmentation patterns to elucidate chemical relationships between various bioactive compounds found in TCM formulations (Lee et al., 2023). The GNPS-based molecular networking approach has proven invaluable for analyzing untargeted mass spectrometry data across diverse fields, recognized as an effective tool for identifying and visualizing metabolites from natural extracts by matching experimental MS^2 spectral with on-line MS^2 spectral libraries (Figure 3) (Hafez-Ghoran, Wang, et al., 2025; Wang et al., 2020). As an example of GNPS molecular networking application, Huo et al. comprehensively investigated the bioactive compounds present in *Ginkgo biloba* fruits using MS/MS-based methodologies. The GNPS-guided approach facilitated the identification of 11 phenolic compounds from *G. biloba* fruits, including (*E*)-coniferin, syringin, 4-hydroxy benzoic acid 4-*O*-β-D-glucopyranoside, vanillic acid 4-*O*-β-D-glucopyranoside, syringic acid 4-*O*-β-D-glucopyranoside, (*E*)-ferulic acid 4-*O*-β-D-glucopyranoside, (*E*)-sinpic acid 4-*O*-β-D-glucopyranoside, (1′*R*,2′*S*,5′*R*,8′*S*,2′*Z*,4′*E*)-dihydrophaseic acid 3′-*O*-β-D-glucopyranoside, eucomic acid, rutin, and laricitrin 3-rutinoside. The compounds were further evaluated for their estrogenic activity in MCF-7 cancer cells (Huo et al., 2023). Moreover, numerous fungal species exist as endophytes in plants, many of which produce secondary metabolites with diverse structures and biological activities. Culture extracts from 288 fungi isolated from surface-sterilized Canadian fruits crops, including blueberries, cranberries, raspberries, and grapes, were analyzed via LC-HRMS/MS. GNPS molecular networking modeling was employed to investigate the secondary metabolites in these extracts, significantly enhancing speed and efficiency of dereplicating the extracts and targeting new, structurally related compounds (DesRochers et al., 2023).

3. PREDICTING BIOLOGICAL FUNCTIONS OF NATURAL PRODUCT BIOACTIVES

For many years, the bioactivity-guided isolation method was the primary approach used to discover natural products. This strategy was highly successful in identifying bioactive natural compounds, as it relied on bioactivity as the main criterion for isolation. However, it posed specific challenges. For instance, identifying an active component from a complex blend may require a significant amount of time, and the random approach often led to repeated isolation of the same compounds (Atanasov et al., 2021). In recent years, researchers have increasingly turned to genome mining techniques to discover new natural products. These techniques involve analysing gene sequence data to predict and identify genes responsible for producing unique molecules. By analysing enzyme function and substrate specificity, genome mining allows for the prediction of the biological functions of these natural products and their bioactivities (Bauman et al., 2021). The Li group, for example, used an antiSMASH9-based genome mining approach to identify new non-ribosomal peptides (NRPs) that can combat Gram-negative bacteria's resistance to antibiotics. This class of natural products is rich in positively charge amino acids, enabling them to penetrate bacterial outer membrane and interact with anionic targets. The group analyzed 7400 bacterial genomes and predicted that 807 of these sequences could be categorized as CNRPs, all consisting of at least six amino acids and containing two positively charged amino acids. They further used a protein sequence similarity network (SSN) to analyze peptide sequences based on the antiSMASH data (Li et al., 2018). *In vivo* studies using mouse models showed that these substances were effective in treating *Escherichia coli* infections. Compounds like Laterocidine and Brevicidine exhibited potential as therapeutic agents due to their in vivo efficacy, low incidence of bacterial resistance, and selectivity. However, their exact mechanisms of action are is still under investigation (Bauman et al., 2021). With the increasing number of known natural products, identifying potential biosynthetic gene clusters (BGCs) has become a crucial step in discovering new bioactive compounds. This process can now be performed efficiently on a large scale, as genome mining tools, such as SMURF, PRISM, anti-SMASH, and Deep-BGC allow for the identification and comparison of BGCs across genomes. Other tools focused on specific classes of natural products, such as BAGEL, RODEO, RiPP Miner, PKminer, 2metDB, and NeuRiPP also contribute to this growing field (Walker & Clardy, 2021).

4. BRIDGING TRADITIONAL MEDICINE AND COMPUTATIONAL BIOLOGY

To advance the use of ML in clinical field of TCM, it is essential to integrate the understanding of active chemical compounds in natural products with ML and computational biology, while also optimizing the theory of TCM syndrome differentiation. Computational biology can aid in screening and simulating the interactions of natural products with primary molecular targets of diseases (M. Zhang et al., 2019). By utilizing an integrated strategy that incorporates high-performance computing, advanced algorithms, mathematical modeling, and statistical analysis, computational biology can reveal the complex biological systems that underlie disease processes. One promising approach is molecular dynamics, a subfield of computational biology, which can simulate the molecular mechanisms of natural products as they interact with the human body. This method cam help isolate efficacious natural products, potentially leading to the identification of natural remedies for a variety of illnesses (Fang et al., 2018). Another useful tool is molecular docking, a theoretical simulation technique that predicts how drug molecules interact with receptors (Figure 4) (Saikia & Bordoloi, 2019). This method is increasingly used in traditional herbal medicine to assess the binding affinity an interaction of chemical compounds with biological targets or proteins. Compared to traditional techniques, molecular docking accelerates the identification of bioactive molecules and offers a cost-effective approach for drug development (Hafez-Ghoran, Sajid, et al., 2025; Hafez Ghoran, Abdjan, et al., 2025; Hafez Ghoran et al., 2020; Hafez Ghoran et al., 2023; Hafez Ghoran, Yousuf, et al., 2025; Naderian et al., 2025; Suttithumsatid et al., 2022). Herbal products and TCM are frequently utilized in the prevention and treatment of infectious disease due to their broad-spectrum properties, low toxicity, ease of use, and excellent safety profile-particularly during the SARS and SARS-CoV-2 pandemics (Huang et al., 2020). In contrast to the earlier studies focused on repurposing small-molecule medications, a few research efforts have explored the use of ML to determine TCM treatments for COVID-19 (Capodice & Chubak, 2021). For example, Cai et al. used molecular docking and network pharmacology to investigate how the Huashi Baidu Formula (HSBDF) effectively treats COVID-19. They utilized databases and networks to collect information on the herbs, their components, targets, and routes, analyzing the connections between them. Using network pharmacology and molecular docking techniques, they provided a preliminary explanation of therapeutic mechanism of HSBDF for COVID-19 (Y. Cai et al., 2021). Similarly, Xia et al. utilized network pharmacology and molecular docking to explore the molecular mechanisms behind the activity of Lianhua Qingwen capsule (LQC) in treating COVID-19. Their findings revealed that the hub gene Akt1 was mainly regulated by LQC, suggesting a potential new target for COVID-19 therapy (Xia et al., 2020). In another study, a unique systems biology model was developed, integrating elements such as network pharmacology and oral bioavailability. This model focused on four commonly used herbs – Radix Ophiopogonis Japonici, Radix Puerariae Lobatae, Radix Astragali Mongolici, and Radix Salviae Miltiorrhiza – that are known for cardiovascular benefits. Wang et al. found that the structural characteristics of the molecules in these herbs varied significantly, and each herb interacted with key proteins linked to cardiovascular disease (CVD). The bioactive components of these herbs exhibited synergistic effects, targeting one or more CVD-related proteins. This study sheds light on the pharmacological synergy of herbal therapy and helps identify potent combinations of drugs and herbs that may be more effective when used together rather than alone (Wang et al., 2012). Building on these approaches, Joshi et al. used molecular dynamic simulation to evaluate the interactions of high-scoring ligands with different receptor proteins. Their docking study found that compounds such as taraxerol, daturataturin A, terchebulin, glabrolide, casuarinin, corilagin, neochebulinic acid, and chebulagic acid showed higher binding affinities with SARS-CoV-2 proteins, indicating their potential efficacy against the virus (Joshi et al., 2022). Bakchi et al. provided a valuable overview of the practical use of the SwissADME web tools in drug design and development (Bakchi et al., 2022). Ren et al. focused on Angiotensin-converting enzyme 2 (ACE2) and main protease (M^{pro}) as key docking targets and identified potential target-treating chemicals in Gancao (Licorice), Huang Qin (*Scutellaria* sp.), Dahuang (Rhubarb), and Chaihu (Bulleurum) (Ren et al., 2020). Additionally, Yan et al. employed network pharmacology and molecular docking techniques to investigate potential targets signal pathways, and the biological roles of Lianhua in COVID-19, based on data from six popular medical databases (Yan & Zou, 2021).

5. INTEGRATING AI INTO THE CLINICAL ASSESSMENT OF TRADITIONAL MEDICINE

The chemical diversity and broad target profiles of natural compounds from herbal medicine are increasingly recognized as valuable resources for drug development (C. Cai et al., 2021). Today, *in silico* methods are effectively used in drug discovery, significantly increasing efficiency and reducing costs (Cai et al., 2017). During preclinical studies, researchers determine the safest dosage of drug compounds through *in vitro* and *in vivo* animal models, assessing various factors such as drug functions, absorption, distribution, metabolism, liver clearance, and toxicity. They then calculate the required dose allometrically (Figure 4) (Sharma & McNeill, 2009). AI can also identify the clinical trial optimization. It can identify optimal dosage, treatment plans, and patient classification strategies, helping improve clinical trial methods (Askin et al., 2023). Numerous studies have shown the effectiveness and potential of image-based machine learning applications in clinical practice (Jalal et al., 2019). By incorporating individual patient characteristics, such as age, gender, and genetic factors, AI can contribute to personalized treatment planning. Integrating this information with traditional medicine knowledge, AI systems can recommend tailored treatment regimens, dosages, and combinations of herbs or therapies (Mesko, 2017). Additionally, AI algorithms can process large volumes of clinical trial data, such as information from imaging, genetics, and electronic health records. This allows researchers to identify trends, generate hypotheses, and refine data analysis ultimately expediting the development of new medications (Weissler et al., 2021). To predict the risk of drug-induced liver injury (DILI), researchers have utilized deep learning (DL) to analyze databases containing information on drugs, chemical compounds, food, and genomic biomarkers (Vall et al., 2021). In one study, NFPX decoction is created by combining twenty plants (e.g., *Paeonia lactiflora* Pall.; Paeoniaceae family and *Atractylodes macrocephala* Koidz.; Asteraceae) and 37 bioactive phytochemicals (e.g., neochlorogenic acid and astragaloside IV), was found to modulate the gene expression levels of SMAD4, AMPK, and HRAS. This suggests NFPX decoction may be effective in treating acute respiratory distress syndrome (ARDS) and modifying immune-inflammatory response (Lu et al., 2021). A pervious study developed a robust LC-MS technique, combining data-dependent and data-independent acquisitions, to comprehensively examine the chemical composition of *Penthorum chinense* Pursh (Penthoraceae). Network pharmacology analysis was then used to identify the active mechanisms of *P. chinense*, which were validated through *in vivo* experiments. This approach provides a framework for studying the chemical constituents and active processes of TCM (Du et al., 2022). another study investigated the therapeutic potential of wogonin, a secondary metabolite from *Scutellaria baicalensis* Georgi (Lamiaceae), in lung cancer treatment. The research identified a signalling pathway regulated by wogonin and developed a serological-based model for lung cancer diagnosis using an optimized support vector machine algorithm. This integrated approach, combining *in vitro* studies, network pharmacology analysis, and machine learning, offers new insights into the therapeutic mechanisms and diagnostic foundations of wogonin in lung cancer (Wang et al., 2021).

6. RESHAPING THE PHARMACEUTICAL INDUSTRY USING AI

In the pharmaceutical sector, ongoing research into small molecules aims to develop and improve therapeutic products while increasing customer satisfaction because of their demonstrated benefits. The pharmaceutical industry has displayed a growing interest in using machine learning algorithms to improve processes and decision-making. Both supervised learning and unsupervised learning techniques are being applied across various domains. For example, clustering techniques are widely used for applications such as generating new molecular designs, predicting protein target draggability, and segmenting cell-type imaging. Supervised learning methods, such as regressions and classifications, have been used effectively to identify potential disease targets, such as those involved in Huntington's disease. These techniques are also employed to predict biological activities and pharmacokinetic properties related to drug development, including absorption, distribution, metabolism, excretion, and toxicity (ADME/Tox) parameters (Figure 4) (Vamathevan et al., 2019). As a result, the pharmaceutical industry offers a wide range of stable and potent formulations incorporating small molecules. Despite these advancements, many novel small molecules encounter competition from generic versions, and their launch necessitates extensive data collection and clinical trials (Colombo et al., 2018; Hassanzadeh et al., 2019). Biomolecules, which are significantly larger units than small molecules, are primarily composed of nucleotides or ribonucleotides (nucleic acids) and amino acids (proteins). The stability and biological function of biomolecules are influenced by their supramolecular sequences and spatial conformations (Nayarisseri et al., 2021). Molecular stability and pharmacokinetic regulation remain critical aspects of nucleic acid-based research. Enhancing the pharmacokinetic exposure and stability of these biomolecules is vital, and new technological developments may offer solutions to these challenges (Vora et al., 2023). AI had revolutionized drug discovery and research in numerous ways. One of the primary functions of AI in this domain is *target identification*. By analysing diverse data sources, including genetic, proteomic, and clinical information, AI systems can identify potential therapeutic targets and uncover disease-related molecular mechanisms. This information enables for the rational design of drugs capable of modulating these biological functions, thereby paving the way for more effective treatments (Chavda et al., 2023). Another crucial application of AI in pharmaceutical research is *virtual screening* (Figure 3).

Figure 3. AI and computational biology.

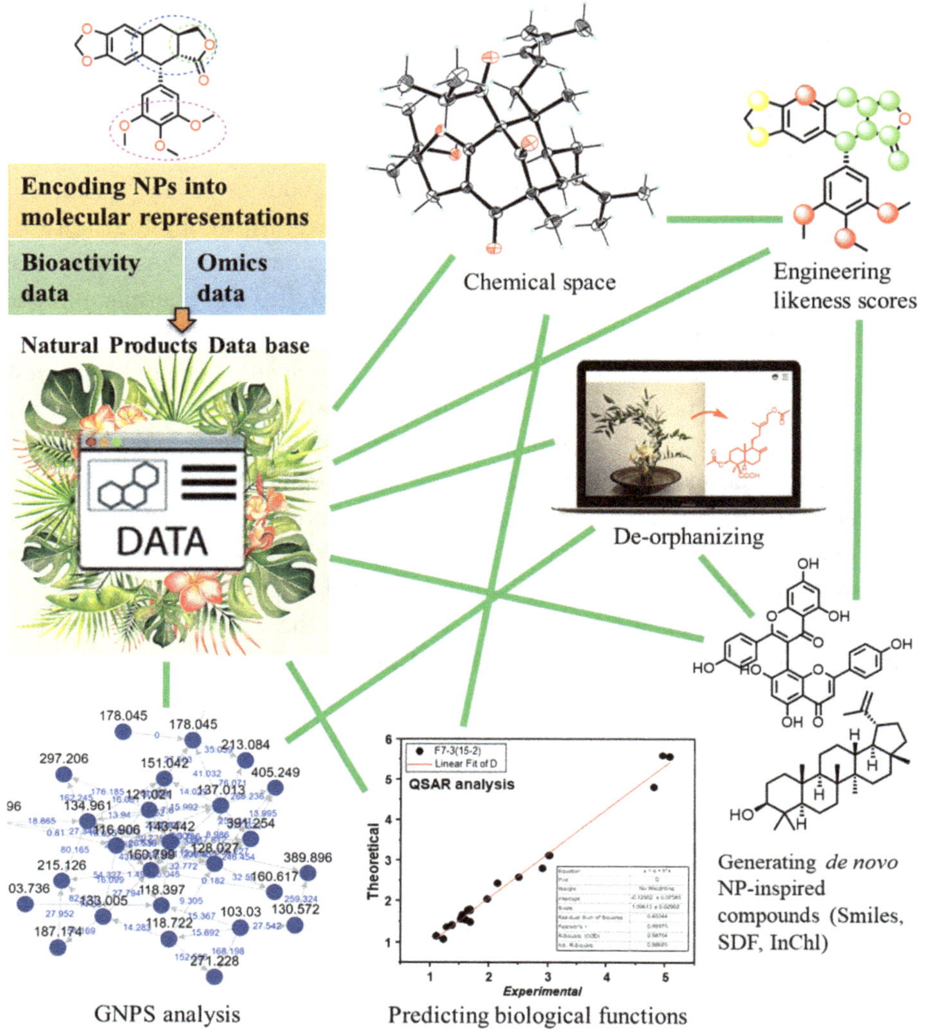

AI algorithms can effectively screen vast chemical libraries to find therapeutic candidates that exhibit a high probability of attaching to a particular biological target. This approach streamlines the drug discovery process by saving researchers time and resources, as AI models chemical interactions and predicting binding affinity. By prioritizing and selecting the most promising compounds for further experimental validation, AI significantly reduces costs and accelerates the drug development timeline (Ghasemi et al., 2018). Likewise, AI plays a pivotal role in establishing structure-activity relationships (SAR) within drug discovery. Through advanced modeling techniques, AI can elucidate the connections between a compound's biological function and its chemical structure. With this information researcher can design compounds with desired properties, such as high potency, selectivity, and favorable pharmacokinetic profiles. This enables the optimization of therapeutic potential and improves the likelihood of successful drug development (Chen et al., 2018; Gomez-Bombarelli et al., 2018). Furthermore, AI algorithms are transforming the field of *de novo* drug design. Leveraging generative models and reinforcement learning, AI can suggest new chemical compounds that resemble drugs-like properties. This exploration expands the chemical space, providing opportunities for the development of innovative and effective drug candidates (Merk et al., 2018; Zhavoronkov et al., 2019). Another area in which AI proves invaluable is the optimization of drug candidates. Using AI algorithms to analyze multiple parameters, such as pharmacokinetics, safety and efficacy, researchers can improve therapeutic efficacy while minimizing the potential for adverse side effects. These computational strategies enable faster and more cost-effective identification of optimal compounds (Schneider et al., 2020). *Drug repurposing* is another impressive application of AI in pharmaceutical research. AI-driven analysis of large-scale biomedical data can identify current medications that may be effective for treating various diseases. This approach offers a faster, less expensive, and safer route to discovering new therapeutic applications for already-approved compounds (Pushpakom et al., 2019; Shameer et al., 2015). Eventually, AI is being applied to *predict drug toxicity*. Machine learning (ML) algorithms trained on toxicology databases can analyze a compound's chemical properties and structure to identify potential toxic effects. This predictive approach allows researchers to prioritize safer compounds, identify hazardous structural features, and reduce the possibility of negative reactions during clinical trials (Koutsoukas et al., 2017). moreover, understanding chemical space is important for the drug discovery process. Chemical space encompasses all possible chemical compounds and their structural and functional characteristics, including natural product derivatives. Visualizing this vast chemical space using graphical methods that are understandable by researchers is essential for identifying promising compounds and making strategic decisions. Dimensionality reduction techniques are employed within AI projects to simplify complex chemical information, thereby enhancing visualization and decision-making capabilities (Figure 3) (Arus-Pous et al., 2019).

Figure 4. Machine learning algorithms in development of natural products.

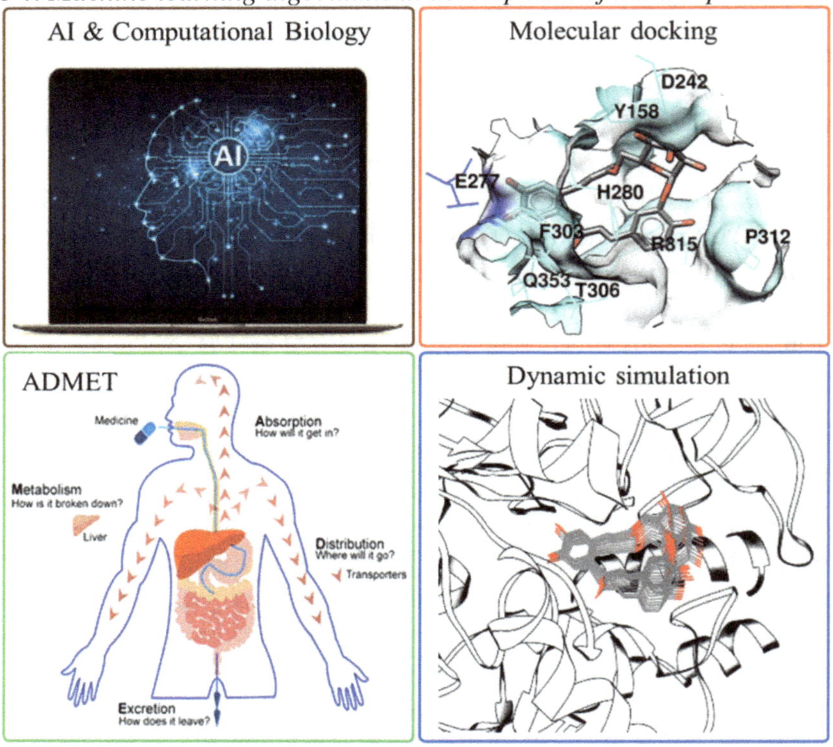

7. NETWORK MEDICINE

The concept of "network target, multi-components" is central to network pharmacology, expanding on the traditional research focus of single-target approaches. This paradigm has facilitated the discovery of new medications, enhanced understanding of mechanisms of action, and enabled the identification of herbal compounds with medicinal potential (Lai et al., 2020). Recent advancements in the discovery of active components from herbal medicine have been driven by network-based techniques informed by systems pharmacology. These techniques consider all relevant information from the drug-target network as well as genes linked to the specific diseases (Wu et al., 2020). The human protein-protein interactome (PPI) is a key resource in network medicine, used to identify patterns linking medications and diseases (9). In this context, Gan et al. proposed a network medicine framework that focuses on symptoms rather than diseases, aligning with the practices of TCM. This framework identifies clusters of proteins within local PPI modules, suggesting the effectiveness of certain herbs in treating specific symptoms. The framework was validated using hospital data and empirical studies, highlighting potential opportunities for discovering new plant-based treatments. Additionally, they mapped plants targets and proteins linked to symptoms onto the human PPI, examining the topological relationships to uncover the scientific basis of TCM treatments (Gan et al., 2023). Network analysis plays a particularly important role in understanding the prescribing practices in TCM. TCM practitioners often combine five to six Chinese herbal medicines (CHMs) from a large selection to create a single prescription (Chen et al., 2015). Lin et al. analyzed the prescription patterns of CHM and discovered that, despite minor variations in the sequential order, *Atractylodes macrocephala* (Baizhu) and Poria (FU-ling) were the most frequently prescribed herbs, as confirmed by both medical analysis and neural network analysis. The study found that neural network recommendations for CHM prescription were 81.9% accurate, aligning with medical records (Lin et al., 2019). The most frequently utilized network pharmacology database in Traditional Herbal Medicine and Natural Products (THM-NP) research is the Traditional Chinese Medicine Systems Pharmacology Database and Analysis Platform (TCMSP). Among the various methods used in THM-NP studies, the strategy for building compound-target networks has evolved significantly over time. One promising strategy is drug development is network pharmacology, which recognizing disease as disruptions in interconnected biological systems. By analyzing network topology, derived from systems biology, this approach helps identify the mechanisms of drug action and is particularly suitable for analyzing multi-targeted agents (Lee et al., 2019). To evaluate potential therapeutic connections between natural products and coronary artery disease, scientists have constructed network-based models (Fang et al., 2019). For example, in their study, Zhang et al. used a recurrent neural network model known as the bidirectional long short-term memory network-conditional random forest to extract clinical data from electronic health record notes using natural language processing. Their integrated learning model, based on 22,984 e-health data records from Guanganmen Hospital in China, predicted 187 disorders in TCM with good accuracy. The diagnostic system demonstrated top prediction accuracies of 80.5%, 91.6%, and 94.2%, respectively (H. Zhang et al., 2020). Additionally, when genomic profiles of triple-negative breast cancer (TNBC) are integrated with networks of natural products compounds and their targets, wogonoside emerges as a strong inhibitor of angiogenesis, offering potential for TNBC therapy (Huang et al., 2019). Molecular docking studies by Yu et al. used virtual screening, using SVM to predict hit compounds according to features selected by RF. Through this approach, 4′,5,7-trimethoxyflavone was identified as a possible inhibitor of the platelet-derived growth factor receptor α (PDGFRAα) (Yu et al., 2022). In another study, Zhang et al. used SVM and least absolute shrinkage and selection operator (LASSO) to identify four RNA microarray datasets for biomarkers related to myocardial infraction. SVM identified 10 genes, while LASSO identified 14 genes. Among the common biomarkers identified by both methods were TLR2 and Interleukin 1β (IL-1β), which helped pinpoint medicinal plants such as san qi and dan shen as potential TCM treatments for myocardial infarction (Zhang et al., 2022).

8. CHALLENGES AND CONSIDERATIONS

While AI holds significant potential for improving drug administration and discovery, its predictions are heavily reliant on datasets. Interpretation of these predictions often necessitates human intervention due to the complexities and grey areas inherent in the data. Additionally, current algorithms have notable limitations that eventually require human intelligence to navigate complex outcomes and address biases. For instance, docking simulations may reveal inactive molecules, necessitating the need for critical human analysis to evaluate these findings accurately. Despite these challenges, ongoing efforts could mitigate the drawbacks of AI and increase its efficacy and reliability (Ceron-Carrasco, 2022). Ensuring the reliability and accuracy of traditional medicine data used in AI training is essential. Furthermore, building trust and promoting ethical AI adoption in healthcare relies on the elimination of potential biases within AI systems and transparency in their decision-making processes.

Recent research by Zech et al. demonstrated that AI models built using convolutional neural networks (CNN) showed decreased accuracy when analyzing external chest X-ray images. In contrast, the AI performed better when analysing structured internal medical data to detect pneumonia from chest X-rays (Zech et al., 2018). This highlights the need for advancements in AI, either through the development of new algorithms or by incorporating more diverse data sources into existing datasets. The latter approach is particularly challenging due to ethical and legal constraints. Moreover, inadequate data governance significantly contributes to AI's shortcomings, even in light of recent efforts to establish objective data analysis processes (Khan et al., 2019). As discussed, AI has the potential to reduce the research costs and increase the success rate of drug development. However, it is important to acknowledge that AI platforms need continuous improvement.

9. SUMMARY OF KEY POINTS

- AI using in drug discovery serves future promise for developing new treatments for incurable diseases.
- Combining AI with TCM can accelerate drug discovery by analysing historical and clinical data for promising compounds.
- Data standardization, privacy, and ethical issues are major challenges in merging AI with traditional knowledge.
- AI models are used to screen natural compounds, predict biological activities, and optimize properties for drug development.
- AI assists personalizing treatment and optimizing dosages by analysing patient-specific data.
- ML algorithms aid in TCM pattern recognition, disease diagnosis, and optimizing treatment regimens.
- AI-driven network pharmacology models identify relationships between traditional compounds and biological targets, enhancing drug discovery.

REFERENCES

Agatonovic-Kustrin, S., & Beresford, R. (2000). Basic concepts of artificial neural network (ANN) modeling and its application in pharmaceutical research. *Journal of Pharmaceutical and Biomedical Analysis*, *22*(5), 717–727. DOI: 10.1016/s0731-7085(99)00272-1 PMID: 10815714

Albahri, O. S., Zaidan, A. A., Albahri, A. S., Zaidan, B. B., Abdulkareem, K. H., Al-Qaysi, Z. T., Alamoodi, A. H., Aleesa, A. M., Chyad, M. A., Alesa, R. M., Kem, L. C., Lakulu, M. M., Ibrahim, A. B., & Rashid, N. A. (2020). Systematic review of artificial intelligence techniques in the detection and classification of COVID-19 medical images in terms of evaluation and benchmarking: Taxonomy analysis, challenges, future solutions and methodological aspects. *Journal of Infection and Public Health*, *13*(10), 1381–1396. DOI: 10.1016/j.jiph.2020.06.028 PMID: 32646771

Arus-Pous, J., Awale, M., Probst, D., & Reymond, J. L. (2019). Exploring Chemical Space with Machine Learning. *Chimia*, *73*(12), 1018–1023. DOI: 10.2533/chimia.2019.1018 PMID: 31883554

Askin, S., Burkhalter, D., Calado, G., & El Dakrouni, S. (2023). Artificial Intelligence Applied to clinical trials: Opportunities and challenges. *Health and Technology*, *13*(2), 203–213. DOI: 10.1007/s12553-023-00738-2 PMID: 36923325

Atanasov, A. G., Zotchev, S. B., & Dirsch, V. M., International Natural Product Sciences, T., & Supuran, C. T. (2021). Natural products in drug discovery: Advances and opportunities. *Nature Reviews. Drug Discovery*, *20*(3), 200–216. DOI: 10.1038/s41573-020-00114-z PMID: 33510482

Bakchi, B., Krishna, A. D., Sreecharan, E., Ganesh, V. B. J., Niharika, M., Maharshi, S., Puttagunta, S. B., Sigalapalli, D. K., Bhandare, R. R., & Shaik, A. B. (2022). An overview on applications of SwissADME web tool in the design and development of anticancer, antitubercular and antimicrobial agents: A medicinal chemist's perspective. *Journal of Molecular Structure*, *1259*, 132712.

Baltrusaitis, T., Ahuja, C., & Morency, L. P. (2019). Multimodal Machine Learning: A Survey and Taxonomy. *IEEE Transactions on Pattern Analysis and Machine Intelligence*, *41*(2), 423–443. DOI: 10.1109/TPAMI.2018.2798607 PMID: 29994351

Bauman, K. D., Butler, K. S., Moore, B. S., & Chekan, J. R. (2021). Genome mining methods to discover bioactive natural products. *Natural Product Reports*, *38*(11), 2100–2129. DOI: 10.1039/d1np00032b PMID: 34734626

Ben-Israel, D., Jacobs, W. B., Casha, S., Lang, S., Ryu, W. H. A., de Lotbiniere-Bassett, M., & Cadotte, D. W. (2020). The impact of machine learning on patient care: A systematic review. *Artificial Intelligence in Medicine*, *103*, 101785. DOI: 10.1016/j.artmed.2019.101785 PMID: 32143792

Blanco-Gonzalez, A., Cabezon, A., Seco-Gonzalez, A., Conde-Torres, D., Antelo-Riveiro, P., Pineiro, A., & Garcia-Fandino, R. (2023). The Role of AI in Drug Discovery: Challenges, Opportunities, and Strategies. *Pharmaceuticals (Basel, Switzerland)*, *16*(6). Advance online publication. DOI: 10.3390/ph16060891 PMID: 37375838

Cai, C., Wu, Q., Luo, Y., Ma, H., Shen, J., Zhang, Y., Yang, L., Chen, Y., Wen, Z., & Wang, Q. (2017). In silico prediction of ROCK II inhibitors by different classification approaches. *Molecular Diversity*, *21*(4), 791–807. DOI: 10.1007/s11030-017-9772-5 PMID: 28770474

Cai, C., Xu, L., Fang, J., Dai, Z., Wu, Q., Liu, X., Wang, Q., Fang, J., Liu, A. L., & Du, G. H. (2021). In Silico Prediction and Bioactivity Evaluation of Chemical Ingredients Against Influenza A Virus From Isatis tinctoria L. *Frontiers in Pharmacology*, *12*, 755396. DOI: 10.3389/fphar.2021.755396 PMID: 34950027

Cai, Y., Zeng, M., & Chen, Y. Z. (2021). The pharmacological mechanism of Huashi Baidu Formula for the treatment of COVID-19 by combined network pharmacology and molecular docking. *Annals of Palliative Medicine*, *10*(4), 3864–3895. DOI: 10.21037/apm-20-1759 PMID: 33691446

Calderaro, J., Seraphin, T. P., Luedde, T., & Simon, T. G. (2022). Artificial intelligence for the prevention and clinical management of hepatocellular carcinoma. *Journal of Hepatology*, *76*(6), 1348–1361. DOI: 10.1016/j.jhep.2022.01.014 PMID: 35589255

Capodice, J. L., & Chubak, B. M. (2021). Traditional Chinese herbal medicine-potential therapeutic application for the treatment of COVID-19. *Chinese Medicine*, *16*(1), 24. DOI: 10.1186/s13020-020-00419-6 PMID: 33618736

Ceron-Carrasco, J. P. (2022). When Virtual Screening Yields Inactive Drugs: Dealing with False Theoretical Friends. *ChemMedChem*, *17*(16), e202200278. DOI: 10.1002/cmdc.202200278 PMID: 35726731

Chavda, V. P., Anand, K., & Apostolopoulos, V. (2023). *Bioinformatics Tools for Pharmaceutical Drug Product Development*. John Wiley & Sons.

Chen, H., Engkvist, O., Wang, Y., Olivecrona, M., & Blaschke, T. (2018). The rise of deep learning in drug discovery. *Drug Discovery Today*, *23*(6), 1241–1250. DOI: 10.1016/j.drudis.2018.01.039 PMID: 29366762

Chen, H., & He, Y. (2022). Machine Learning Approaches in Traditional Chinese Medicine: A Systematic Review. *The American Journal of Chinese Medicine*, *50*(1), 91–131. DOI: 10.1142/S0192415X22500045 PMID: 34931589

Chen, H. Y., Lin, Y. H., Hu, S., Yang, S. H., Chen, J. L., & Chen, Y. C. (2015). Identifying chinese herbal medicine network for eczema: Implications from a nationwide prescription database. *Evidence-Based Complementary and Alternative Medicine : eCAM*, *347164*. Advance online publication. DOI: 10.1155/2015/347164 PMID: 25685167

Chen, W., Liu, X., Zhang, S., & Chen, S. (2023). Artificial intelligence for drug discovery: Resources, methods, and applications. *Molecular Therapy. Nucleic Acids*, *31*, 691–702. DOI: 10.1016/j.omtn.2023.02.019 PMID: 36923950

Cheng, F., Kovacs, I. A., & Barabasi, A. L. (2019). Network-based prediction of drug combinations. *Nature Communications*, *10*(1), 1197. DOI: 10.1038/s41467-019-09186-x PMID: 30867426

Chu, H., Moon, S., Park, J., Bak, S., Ko, Y., & Youn, B. Y. (2022). The Use of Artificial Intelligence in Complementary and Alternative Medicine: A Systematic Scoping Review. *Frontiers in Pharmacology*, *13*, 826044. DOI: 10.3389/fphar.2022.826044 PMID: 35431917

Colombo, S., Beck-Broichsitter, M., Botker, J. P., Malmsten, M., Rantanen, J., & Bohr, A. (2018). Transforming nanomedicine manufacturing toward Quality by Design and microfluidics. *Advanced Drug Delivery Reviews*, *128*, 115–131. DOI: 10.1016/j.addr.2018.04.004 PMID: 29626549

DesRochers, N., Renaud, J. B., Tanney, J. B., Ibrahim, A., Yeung, K. K.-C., & Sumarah, M. W. (2023). Non-targeted Screening of Natural Products from 288 Fungal Endophytes from Canadian Fruit Crops. *ACS Omega*, *8*(27), 24561–24572. PMID: 37457466

Du, Z., Huang, D., Shi, P., Dong, Z., Wang, X., Li, M., Chen, W., Zhang, F., & Sun, L. (2022). Integrated Chemical Interpretation and Network Pharmacology Analysis to Reveal the Anti-Liver Fibrosis Effect of Penthorum chinense. *Frontiers in Pharmacology*, *13*, 788388. DOI: 10.3389/fphar.2022.788388 PMID: 35721129

Fang, J., Cai, C., Chai, Y., Zhou, J., Huang, Y., Gao, L., Wang, Q., & Cheng, F. (2019). Quantitative and systems pharmacology 4. Network-based analysis of drug pleiotropy on coronary artery disease. *European Journal of Medicinal Chemistry*, *161*, 192–204. DOI: 10.1016/j.ejmech.2018.10.020 PMID: 30359818

Fang, J., Liu, C., Wang, Q., Lin, P., & Cheng, F. (2018). In silico polypharmacology of natural products. *Briefings in Bioinformatics*, *19*(6), 1153–1171. DOI: 10.1093/bib/bbx045 PMID: 28460068

Feng, C., Zhou, S., Qu, Y., Wang, Q., Bao, S., Li, Y., & Yang, T. (2021). Overview of Artificial Intelligence Applications in Chinese Medicine Therapy. *Evidence-Based Complementary and Alternative Medicine : eCAM*, *6678958*. Advance online publication. DOI: 10.1155/2021/6678958 PMID: 33815559

Fleming, N. (2018). How artificial intelligence is changing drug discovery. *Nature*, *557*(7707), S55–S57. DOI: 10.1038/d41586-018-05267-x PMID: 29849160

Fokunang, C. N., Ndikum, V., Tabi, O. Y., Jiofack, R. B., Ngameni, B., Guedje, N. M., Tembe-Fokunang, E. A., Tomkins, P., Barkwan, S., Kechia, F., Asongalem, E., Ngoupayou, J., Torimiro, N. J., Gonsu, K. H., Sielinou, V., Ngadjui, B. T., Angwafor, F.III, Nkongmeneck, A., Abena, O. M., & Kamsu, K. (2011). Traditional medicine: Past, present and future research and development prospects and integration in the National Health System of Cameroon. *African Journal of Traditional, Complementary, and Alternative Medicines : AJTCAM*, *8*(3), 284–295. DOI: 10.4314/ajtcam.v8i3.65276 PMID: 22468007

Fu, X., Mervin, L. H., Li, X., Yu, H., Li, J., Mohamad Zobir, S. Z., Zoufir, A., Zhou, Y., Song, Y., Wang, Z., & Bender, A. (2017). Toward Understanding the Cold, Hot, and Neutral Nature of Chinese Medicines Using in Silico Mode-of-Action Analysis. *Journal of Chemical Information and Modeling*, *57*(3), 468–483. DOI: 10.1021/acs.jcim.6b00725 PMID: 28257573

Gan, X., Shu, Z., Wang, X., Yan, D., Li, J., Ofaim, S., Albert, R., Li, X., Liu, B., Zhou, X., & Barabasi, A. L. (2023). Network medicine framework reveals generic herb-symptom effectiveness of traditional Chinese medicine. *Science Advances*, *9*(43), eadh0215. Advance online publication. DOI: 10.1126/sciadv.adh0215 PMID: 37889962

Ghasemi, F., Mehridehnavi, A., Perez-Garrido, A., & Perez-Sanchez, H. (2018). Neural network and deep-learning algorithms used in QSAR studies: Merits and drawbacks. *Drug Discovery Today*, *23*(10), 1784–1790. DOI: 10.1016/j.drudis.2018.06.016 PMID: 29936244

Gomez-Bombarelli, R., Wei, J. N., Duvenaud, D., Hernandez-Lobato, J. M., Sanchez-Lengeling, B., Sheberla, D., Aguilera-Iparraguirre, J., Hirzel, T. D., Adams, R. P., & Aspuru-Guzik, A. (2018). Automatic Chemical Design Using a Data-Driven Continuous Representation of Molecules. *ACS Central Science*, *4*(2), 268–276. DOI: 10.1021/acscentsci.7b00572 PMID: 29532027

Guo, Y., Ren, X., Chen, Y. X., & Wang, T. J. (2019). Artificial Intelligence Meets Chinese Medicine. *Chinese Journal of Integrative Medicine*, *25*(9), 648–653. DOI: 10.1007/s11655-019-3169-5 PMID: 31650485

Hafez Ghoran, S., Abdjan, M. I., Kristanti, A. N., & Aminah, N. S. (2025). Insights into *in vitro* and *in silico* studies of α-glucosidase inhibitors isolated from the leaves of *Grewia optiva* (Malvaceae). *International Journal of Biological Macromolecules*, *287*, 138590. PMID: 39667462

Hafez Ghoran, S., Babaei, E., Rezaei Seresht, H., & Karimzadeh, Z. (2019). Cytotoxic constituents and molecular docking study of the active triterpenoids from *Tripleurospermum disciforme* (CA Mey.) Schultz-Bip. *Jundishapur Journal of Natural Pharmaceutical Products*, *15*(2), e65760. https://doi.org/https://doi.org/10.5812/jjnpp.65760

Hafez Ghoran, S., Firuzi, O., Pirhadi, S., Khattab, O. M., El-Seedi, H. R., & Jassbi, A. R. (2023). Sappanin-type homoisoflavonoids from *Scilla bisotunensis* Speta.: Cytotoxicity, molecular docking, and chemotaxonomic significance. *Journal of Molecular Structure*, *1273*, 134326.

Hafez-Ghoran, S., Sajid, M., Abdjan, M. I., Teia, F. K. F., Siddiqui, H., Sanjaya, G. M., Ridassepri, A. F., Nadeem, F., Ayatollahi, S. A., & Choudhary, M. I. (2025). New methyl and ethyl gallate esters linked chlorinated benzoyl derivatives as anti-*Candida* albicans agents: Isolation, semi-synthesis, *in vitro* and *in silico* studies. *Chemistry & Biodiversity*, •••, 202500153. PMID: 40234190

Hafez-Ghoran, S., Wang, W., & Sang, S. (2025). Insights into phenolamides in whole grain barley: Chemical profile and their levels in barley-based products. *Journal of Agricultural and Food Chemistry*, *73*(35), 21905–21919. PMID: 40828649

Hafez Ghoran, S., Yousuf, M., Zafar, H., Abdjan, M. I., & Ayatollahi, S. A., Atia-tul-Wahab, Aminah, N. S., Kristanti, A. N., Aziz-ur-Rehman, & Choudhary, M. I. (2025). In vitro, in silico, and STD-NMR studies of flavonoids from *Hypericum helianthemoides* (Spach) Boiss. against Leishmania major pteridine reductase 1 (Lm PTR1). *Journal of Biomolecular Structure & Dynamics*, *43*(12), 6366–6380. PMID: 40025779

Hansen, K., Biegler, F., Ramakrishnan, R., Pronobis, W., von Lilienfeld, O. A., Muller, K. R., & Tkatchenko, A. (2015). Machine Learning Predictions of Molecular Properties: Accurate Many-Body Potentials and Nonlocality in Chemical Space. *The Journal of Physical Chemistry Letters*, *6*(12), 2326–2331. DOI: 10.1021/acs.jpclett.5b00831 PMID: 26113956

Hassanzadeh, P., Atyabi, F., & Dinarvand, R. (2019). The significance of artificial intelligence in drug delivery system design. *Advanced Drug Delivery Reviews*, *151-152*, 169–190. DOI: 10.1016/j.addr.2019.05.001 PMID: 31071378

Huang, J., Tao, G., Liu, J., Cai, J., Huang, Z., & Chen, J. X. (2020). Current Prevention of COVID-19: Natural Products and Herbal Medicine. *Frontiers in Pharmacology*, *11*, 588508. DOI: 10.3389/fphar.2020.588508 PMID: 33178026

Huang, Y., Fang, J., Lu, W., Wang, Z., Wang, Q., Hou, Y., Jiang, X., Reizes, O., Lathia, J., Nussinov, R., Eng, C., & Cheng, F. (2019). A Systems Pharmacology Approach Uncovers Wogonoside as an Angiogenesis Inhibitor of Triple-Negative Breast Cancer by Targeting Hedgehog Signaling. *Cell Chemical Biology*, *26*(8), 1143–1158 e1146. DOI: 10.1016/j.chembiol.2019.05.004 PMID: 31178408

Huo, C., Nguyen, Q. N., Alishir, A., Ra, M.-J., Jung, S.-M., Yu, J.-N., Gwon, H.-J., Kang, K. S., & Kim, K. H. (2023). Global Natural Products Social (GNPS)-based molecular-networking-guided isolation of phenolic compounds from *Ginkgo biloba* fruits and the identification of estrogenic phenolic glycosides. *Plants*, *12*(23), 3970. PMID: 38068607

Jaiswal, Y., Liang, Z., & Zhao, Z. (2016). Botanical drugs in Ayurveda and Traditional Chinese Medicine. *Journal of Ethnopharmacology*, *194*, 245–259. DOI: 10.1016/j.jep.2016.06.052 PMID: 27394388

Jalal, S., Nicolaou, S., & Parker, W. (2019). Artificial Intelligence, Radiology, and the Way Forward. *Canadian Association of Radiologists Journal*, *70*(1), 10–12. DOI: 10.1016/j.carj.2018.09.004 PMID: 30691556

Jang, H. Y., Song, J., Kim, J. H., Lee, H., Kim, I. W., Moon, B., & Oh, J. M. (2022). Machine learning-based quantitative prediction of drug exposure in drug-drug interactions using drug label information. *NPJ Digital Medicine*, *5*(1), 88. DOI: 10.1038/s41746-022-00639-0 PMID: 35817846

Jiang, T., Gradus, J. L., & Rosellini, A. J. (2020). Supervised Machine Learning: A Brief Primer. *Behavior Therapy*, *51*(5), 675–687. DOI: 10.1016/j.beth.2020.05.002 PMID: 32800297

Joshi, C., Chaudhari, A., Joshi, C., Joshi, M., & Bagatharia, S. (2022). Repurposing of the herbal formulations: Molecular docking and molecular dynamics simulation studies to validate the efficacy of phytocompounds against SARS-CoV-2 proteins. *Journal of Biomolecular Structure & Dynamics*, *40*(18), 8405–8419. DOI: 10.1080/07391102.2021.1922095 PMID: 33988079

Khan, S. R., Al Rijjal, D., Piro, A., & Wheeler, M. B. (2021). Integration of AI and traditional medicine in drug discovery. *Drug Discovery Today*, *26*(4), 982–992. DOI: 10.1016/j.drudis.2021.01.008 PMID: 33476566

Khan, S. R., Manialawy, Y., Wheeler, M. B., & Cox, B. J. (2019). Unbiased data analytic strategies to improve biomarker discovery in precision medicine. *Drug Discovery Today*, *24*(9), 1735–1748. DOI: 10.1016/j.drudis.2019.05.018 PMID: 31158511

Kim, E., Choi, A. S., & Nam, H. (2019). Drug repositioning of herbal compounds via a machine-learning approach. *BMC Bioinformatics*, *20*(Suppl 10), 247. DOI: 10.1186/s12859-019-2811-8 PMID: 31138103

Kim, H., Kim, E., Lee, I., Bae, B., Park, M., & Nam, H. (2020). Artificial Intelligence in Drug Discovery: A Comprehensive Review of Data-driven and Machine Learning Approaches. *Biotechnology and Bioprocess Engineering; BBE*, *25*(6), 895–930. DOI: 10.1007/s12257-020-0049-y PMID: 33437151

Koutsoukas, A., Monaghan, K. J., Li, X., & Huan, J. (2017). Deep-learning: Investigating deep neural networks hyper-parameters and comparison of performance to shallow methods for modeling bioactivity data. *Journal of Cheminformatics*, *9*(1), 42. DOI: 10.1186/s13321-017-0226-y PMID: 29086090

Lai, X., Wang, X., Hu, Y., Su, S., Li, W., & Li, S. (2020). Editorial: Network Pharmacology and Traditional Medicine. *Frontiers in Pharmacology*, *11*, 1194. DOI: 10.3389/fphar.2020.01194 PMID: 32848794

Lee, W. Y., Lee, C. Y., Kim, Y. S., & Kim, C. E. (2019). The Methodological Trends of Traditional Herbal Medicine Employing Network Pharmacology. *Biomolecules*, *9*(8). Advance online publication. DOI: 10.3390/biom9080362 PMID: 31412658

Lee, Y.-Y., Guler, M., Chigumba, D. N., Wang, S., Mittal, N., Miller, C., Krummenacher, B., Liu, H., Cao, L., & Kannan, A. (2023). HypoRiPPAtlas as an Atlas of hypothetical natural products for mass spectrometry database search. *Nature Communications*, *14*(1), 4219. PMID: 37452020

Li, S., Zhu, P., Cai, G., Li, J., Huang, T., & Tang, W. (2023). Application of machine learning models in predicting insomnia severity: An integrative approach with constitution of traditional Chinese medicine. *Frontiers in Medicine*, *10*, 1292761. DOI: 10.3389/fmed.2023.1292761 PMID: 37928471

Li, X., Ren, J., Zhang, W., Zhang, Z., Yu, J., Wu, J., Sun, H., Zhou, S., Yan, K., Yan, X., & Wang, W. (2022). LTM-TCM: A comprehensive database for the linking of Traditional Chinese Medicine with modern medicine at molecular and phenotypic levels. *Pharmacological Research*, *178*, 106185. DOI: 10.1016/j.phrs.2022.106185 PMID: 35306140

Li, Y. X., Zhong, Z., Zhang, W. P., & Qian, P. Y. (2018). Discovery of cationic nonribosomal peptides as Gram-negative antibiotics through global genome mining. *Nature Communications*, *9*(1), 3273. DOI: 10.1038/s41467-018-05781-6 PMID: 30115920

Lin, Y. C., Huang, W. T., Ou, S. C., Hung, H. H., Cheng, W. Z., Lin, S. S., Lin, H. J., & Huang, S. T. (2019). Neural network analysis of Chinese herbal medicine prescriptions for patients with colorectal cancer. *Complementary Therapies in Medicine*, *42*, 279–285. DOI: 10.1016/j.ctim.2018.12.001 PMID: 30670255

Liu, G. P., Yan, J. J., Wang, Y. Q., Zheng, W., Zhong, T., Lu, X., & Qian, P. (2014). Deep learning based syndrome diagnosis of chronic gastritis. *Computational and Mathematical Methods in Medicine*, *938350*. Advance online publication. DOI: 10.1155/2014/938350 PMID: 24734118

Lotter, W., Kreiman, G., & Cox, D. (2020). A neural network trained for prediction mimics diverse features of biological neurons and perception. *Nature Machine Intelligence*, *2*(4), 210–219. DOI: 10.1038/s42256-020-0170-9 PMID: 34291193

Lu, X., Ma, W., Fan, B., Li, P., Gao, J., Liu, Q., Hu, C., Li, Y., Yao, M., Ning, H., & Xing, L. (2021). Integrating Network Pharmacology, Transcriptome and Artificial Intelligence for Investigating Into the Effect and Mechanism of Ning Fei Ping Xue Decoction Against the Acute Respiratory Distress Syndrome. *Frontiers in Pharmacology*, *12*, 731377. DOI: 10.3389/fphar.2021.731377 PMID: 34803679

Lynn, L. A. (2019). Artificial intelligence systems for complex decision-making in acute care medicine: A review. *Patient Safety in Surgery*, *13*, 6. DOI: 10.1186/s13037-019-0188-2 PMID: 30733829

Mathew, A., Amudha, P., & Sivakumari, S. (2021). Deep learning techniques: an overview. *Advanced Machine Learning Technologies and Applications: Proceedings of AMLTA 2020*, 599–608.

Merk, D., Friedrich, L., Grisoni, F., & Schneider, G. (2018). De Novo Design of Bioactive Small Molecules by Artificial Intelligence. *Molecular Informatics*, *37*(1-2). Advance online publication. DOI: 10.1002/minf.201700153 PMID: 29319225

Mesko, B. (2017). *The role of artificial intelligence in precision medicine* (Vol. 2). Taylor & Francis.

Mohanraj, K., Karthikeyan, B. S., Vivek-Ananth, R. P., Chand, R. P. B., Aparna, S. R., Mangalapandi, P., & Samal, A. (2018). IMPPAT: A curated database of Indian Medicinal Plants, Phytochemistry And Therapeutics. *Scientific Reports*, *8*(1), 4329. DOI: 10.1038/s41598-018-22631-z PMID: 29531263

Murugan, A., Nair, S. A. H., & Kumar, K. P. S. (2019). Detection of Skin Cancer Using SVM, Random Forest and kNN Classifiers. *Journal of Medical Systems*, *43*(8), 269. DOI: 10.1007/s10916-019-1400-8 PMID: 31273532

Naderian, M., Hafez Ghoran, S., Abdjan, M. I., Sabahi, Z., Moein, S., Jassbi, A. R., & Moein, M. (2025). A new labdane diterpenoid, in vitro and in silico cytotoxicity, and protease inhibitory effects of phytochemicals from Juniperus polycarpos K. Koch leaves. *Natural Product Research*, *39*(11), 3053–3064. PMID: 38501578

Nashwan, A. J., & Rao, A. G. (2024). Integrating Traditional Chinese Medicine and Artificial Intelligence for insomnia: A promising frontier. *Brain Behavior and Immunity Integrative*, *7*, 100071.

Nayarisseri, A., Khandelwal, R., Tanwar, P., Madhavi, M., Sharma, D., Thakur, G., Speck-Planche, A., & Singh, S. K. (2021). Artificial Intelligence, Big Data and Machine Learning Approaches in Precision Medicine & Drug Discovery. *Current Drug Targets*, *22*(6), 631–655. DOI: 10.2174/1389450122999210104205732 PMID: 33397265

Park, M., Kim, M. H., Park, S. Y., Choi, I., & Kim, C. E. (2022). Individualized Diagnosis and Prescription in Traditional Medicine: Decision-Making Process Analysis and Machine Learning-Based Analysis Tool Development. *The American Journal of Chinese Medicine*, *50*(7), 1827–1844. DOI: 10.1142/S0192415X2250077X PMID: 36056467

Paul, D., Sanap, G., Shenoy, S., Kalyane, D., Kalia, K., & Tekade, R. K. (2021). Artificial intelligence in drug discovery and development. *Drug Discovery Today*, *26*(1), 80–93. DOI: 10.1016/j.drudis.2020.10.010 PMID: 33099022

Popova, M., Isayev, O., & Tropsha, A. (2018). Deep reinforcement learning for de novo drug design. *Science Advances*, *4*(7), eaap7885. Advance online publication. DOI: 10.1126/sciadv.aap7885 PMID: 30050984

Pushpakom, S., Iorio, F., Eyers, P. A., Escott, K. J., Hopper, S., Wells, A., Doig, A., Guilliams, T., Latimer, J., McNamee, C., Norris, A., Sanseau, P., Cavalla, D., & Pirmohamed, M. (2019). Drug repurposing: Progress, challenges and recommendations. *Nature Reviews. Drug Discovery*, *18*(1), 41–58. DOI: 10.1038/nrd.2018.168 PMID: 30310233

Ren, X., Shao, X. X., Li, X. X., Jia, X. H., Song, T., Zhou, W. Y., Wang, P., Li, Y., Wang, X. L., Cui, Q. H., Qiu, P. J., Zhao, Y. G., Li, X. B., Zhang, F. C., Li, Z. Y., Zhong, Y., Wang, Z. G., & Fu, X. J. (2020). Identifying potential treatments of COVID-19 from Traditional Chinese Medicine (TCM) by using a data-driven approach. *Journal of Ethnopharmacology*, *258*, 112932. DOI: 10.1016/j.jep.2020.112932 PMID: 32376368

Ru, J., Li, P., Wang, J., Zhou, W., Li, B., Huang, C., Li, P., Guo, Z., Tao, W., Yang, Y., Xu, X., Li, Y., Wang, Y., & Yang, L. (2014). TCMSP: A database of systems pharmacology for drug discovery from herbal medicines. *Journal of Cheminformatics*, *6*, 13. DOI: 10.1186/1758-2946-6-13 PMID: 24735618

Rustandi, T., Prihandiwati, E., Nugroho, F., Hayati, F., Afriani, N., Alfian, R., Aisyah, N., Niah, R., Rahim, A., & As-Shiddiq, H. (2023). Application of artificial intelligence in the development of Jamu "traditional Indonesian medicine" as a more effective drug. *Frontiers in Artificial Intelligence*, *6*, 1274975. DOI: 10.3389/frai.2023.1274975 PMID: 38028667

Saikia, S., & Bordoloi, M. (2019). Molecular Docking: Challenges, Advances and its Use in Drug Discovery Perspective. *Current Drug Targets*, *20*(5), 501–521. DOI: 10.2174/1389450119666181022153016 PMID: 30360733

Saldivar-Gonzalez, F. I., Aldas-Bulos, V. D., Medina-Franco, J. L., & Plisson, F. (2022). Natural product drug discovery in the artificial intelligence era. *Chemical Science (Cambridge)*, *13*(6), 1526–1546. DOI: 10.1039/d1sc04471k PMID: 35282622

Schneider, P., Walters, W. P., Plowright, A. T., Sieroka, N., Listgarten, J., Goodnow, R. A.Jr, Fisher, J., Jansen, J. M., Duca, J. S., Rush, T. S., Zentgraf, M., Hill, J. E., Krutoholow, E., Kohler, M., Blaney, J., Funatsu, K., Luebkemann, C., & Schneider, G. (2020). Rethinking drug design in the artificial intelligence era. *Nature Reviews. Drug Discovery*, *19*(5), 353–364. DOI: 10.1038/s41573-019-0050-3 PMID: 31801986

Seetharam, K., Kagiyama, N., & Sengupta, P. P. (2019). Application of mobile health, telemedicine and artificial intelligence to echocardiography. *Echo Research and Practice*, *6*(2), R41–R52. DOI: 10.1530/ERP-18-0081 PMID: 30844756

Sejnowski, T. J. (2020). The unreasonable effectiveness of deep learning in artificial intelligence. *Proceedings of the National Academy of Sciences of the United States of America*, *117*(48), 30033–30038. DOI: 10.1073/pnas.1907373117 PMID: 31992643

Shameer, K., Readhead, B., & Dudley, J. T. (2015). Computational and experimental advances in drug repositioning for accelerated therapeutic stratification. *Current Topics in Medicinal Chemistry*, *15*(1), 5–20. DOI: 10.2174/156802661566615011 2103510 PMID: 25579574

Sharma, V., & McNeill, J. H. (2009). To scale or not to scale: The principles of dose extrapolation. *British Journal of Pharmacology*, *157*(6), 907–921. DOI: 10.1111/j.1476-5381.2009.00267.x PMID: 19508398

Shen, Y., Yang, R., Zhou, R., Lu, W., Li, L., Niu, Z., Chen, M., Wang, J., Wang, Y., Fang, L., & Du, G. (2021). Xiaoxuming Decoction Regulates Vascular Function by Modulating G Protein-Coupled Receptors: A Molecular Docking Study. *BioMed Research International*, *5575443*. Advance online publication. DOI: 10.1155/2021/5575443 PMID: 34195269

Su, X., Xu, Y., Tan, Z., Wang, X., Yang, P., Su, Y., Jiang, Y., Qin, S., & Shang, L. (2020). Prediction for cardiovascular diseases based on laboratory data: An analysis of random forest model. *Journal of Clinical Laboratory Analysis*, *34*(9), e23421. DOI: 10.1002/jcla.23421 PMID: 32725839

Subbiah, V. (2023). The next generation of evidence-based medicine. *Nature Medicine*, *29*(1), 49–58. DOI: 10.1038/s41591-022-02160-z PMID: 36646803

Suttithumsatid, W., Shah, M. A., Bibi, S., & Panichayupakaranant, P. (2022). alpha-Glucosidase inhibitory activity of cannabidiol, tetrahydrocannabinol and standardized cannabinoid extracts from Cannabis sativa. *Current Research in Food Science*, *5*, 1091–1097. DOI: 10.1016/j.crfs.2022.07.002 PMID: 35856057

Tang, S. W., Tang, W. H., & Leonard, B. E. (2020). Safety of traditional medicine and natural product supplements in psychiatry. *International Clinical Psychopharmacology*, *35*(1), 1–7. DOI: 10.1097/YIC.0000000000000279 PMID: 31361653

Vall, A., Sabnis, Y., Shi, J., Class, R., Hochreiter, S., & Klambauer, G. (2021). The Promise of AI for DILI Prediction. *Frontiers in Artificial Intelligence*, *4*, 638410. DOI: 10.3389/frai.2021.638410 PMID: 33937745

Vamathevan, J., Clark, D., Czodrowski, P., Dunham, I., Ferran, E., Lee, G., Li, B., Madabhushi, A., Shah, P., Spitzer, M., & Zhao, S. (2019). Applications of machine learning in drug discovery and development. *Nature Reviews. Drug Discovery*, *18*(6), 463–477. DOI: 10.1038/s41573-019-0024-5 PMID: 30976107

Vora, L. K., Gholap, A. D., Jetha, K., Thakur, R. R. S., Solanki, H. K., & Chavda, V. P. (2023). Artificial Intelligence in Pharmaceutical Technology and Drug Delivery Design. *Pharmaceutics*, *15*(7). Advance online publication. DOI: 10.3390/pharmaceutics15071916 PMID: 37514102

Walker, A. S., & Clardy, J. (2021). A Machine Learning Bioinformatics Method to Predict Biological Activity from Biosynthetic Gene Clusters. *Journal of Chemical Information and Modeling*, *61*(6), 2560–2571. DOI: 10.1021/acs.jcim.0c01304 PMID: 34042443

Wang, D., Fu, Z., Xing, Y., Tan, Y., Han, L., Yu, H., & Wang, T. (2020). Rapid identification of chemical composition and metabolites of Pingxiao Capsule in vivo using molecular networking and untargeted data-dependent tandem mass spectrometry. *Biomedical Chromatography*, *34*(9), e4882. PMID: 32396262

Wang, H., Chen, Y., Wang, L., Liu, Q., Yang, S., & Wang, C. (2023). Advancing herbal medicine: Enhancing product quality and safety through robust quality control practices. *Frontiers in Pharmacology*, *14*, 1265178. DOI: 10.3389/fphar.2023.1265178 PMID: 37818188

Wang, L., Zhang, J., Shan, G., Liang, J., Jin, W., Li, Y., Su, F., Ba, Y., Tian, X., Sun, X., Zhang, D., Zhang, W., & Chen, C. L. (2021). Establishment of a Lung Cancer Discriminative Model Based on an Optimized Support Vector Machine Algorithm and Study of Key Targets of Wogonin in Lung Cancer. *Frontiers in Pharmacology*, *12*, 728937. DOI: 10.3389/fphar.2021.728937 PMID: 34630106

Wang, X., Xu, X., Tao, W., Li, Y., Wang, Y., & Yang, L. (2012). A systems biology approach to uncovering pharmacological synergy in herbal medicines with applications to cardiovascular disease. *Evidence-Based Complementary and Alternative Medicine : eCAM*, *519031*. Advance online publication. DOI: 10.1155/2012/519031 PMID: 23243453

Wang, Y., Jafari, M., Tang, Y., & Tang, J. (2019). Predicting Meridian in Chinese traditional medicine using machine learning approaches. *PLoS Computational Biology*, *15*(11), e1007249. DOI: 10.1371/journal.pcbi.1007249 PMID: 31765369

Weissler, E. H., Naumann, T., Andersson, T., Ranganath, R., Elemento, O., Luo, Y., Freitag, D. F., Benoit, J., Hughes, M. C., Khan, F., Slater, P., Shameer, K., Roe, M., Hutchison, E., Kollins, S. H., Broedl, U., Meng, Z., Wong, J. L., Curtis, L., & Ghassemi, M. (2021). The role of machine learning in clinical research: Transforming the future of evidence generation. *Trials*, *22*(1), 537. DOI: 10.1186/s13063-021-05489-x PMID: 34399832

Wouters, O. J., McKee, M., & Luyten, J. (2020). Research and Development Costs of New Drugs-Reply. *Journal of the American Medical Association, 324*(5), 518. DOI: 10.1001/jama.2020.8651 PMID: 32749488

Wu, C., Chen, J., Lai-Han Leung, E., Chang, H., & Wang, X. (2022). Editorial: Artificial Intelligence in Traditional Medicine. *Frontiers in Pharmacology, 13*, 933133. DOI: 10.3389/fphar.2022.933133 PMID: 35991902

Wu, Q., Chen, Y., Gu, Y., Fang, S., Li, W., Wang, Q., Fang, J., & Cai, C. (2020). Systems pharmacology-based approach to investigate the mechanisms of Danggui-Shaoyao-san prescription for treatment of Alzheimer's disease. *BMC Complementary Medicine and Therapies, 20*(1), 282. DOI: 10.1186/s12906-020-03066-4 PMID: 32948180

Xia, Q. D., Xun, Y., Lu, J. L., Lu, Y. C., Yang, Y. Y., Zhou, P., Hu, J., Li, C., & Wang, S. G. (2020). Network pharmacology and molecular docking analyses on Lianhua Qingwen capsule indicate Akt1 is a potential target to treat and prevent COVID-19. *Cell Proliferation, 53*(12), e12949. DOI: 10.1111/cpr.12949 PMID: 33140889

Xiaotong, C., LEUNG, Y.-L. A., & Jiangang, S. (2022). Artificial intelligence and its application for cardiovascular diseases in Chinese medicine. *Digital Chinese Medicine, 5*(4), 367–376.

Xu, Y., Liu, X., Cao, X., Huang, C., Liu, E., Qian, S., Liu, X., Wu, Y., Dong, F., Qiu, C. W., Qiu, J., Hua, K., Su, W., Wu, J., Xu, H., Han, Y., Fu, C., Yin, Z., Liu, M., & Zhang, J. (2021). Artificial intelligence: A powerful paradigm for scientific research. *Innovation (Cambridge (Mass.)), 2*(4), 100179. DOI: 10.1016/j.xinn.2021.100179 PMID: 34877560

Yan, H., & Zou, C. (2021). [Mechanism and material basis of Lianhua Qingwen capsule for improving clinical cure rate of COVID-19: a study based on network pharmacology and molecular docking technology]. *Nan Fang Yi Ke da Xue Xue Bao = Journal of Southern Medical University, 41*(1), 20–30. DOI: 10.12122/j.issn.1673-4254.2021.01.03 PMID: 33509749

Yeh, H. Y., Chao, C. T., Lai, Y. P., & Chen, H. W. (2020). Predicting the Associations between Meridians and Chinese Traditional Medicine Using a Cost-Sensitive Graph Convolutional Neural Network. *International Journal of Environmental Research and Public Health, 17*(3). Advance online publication. DOI: 10.3390/ijerph17030740 PMID: 31979314

Yu, H., Jung, J., Yoon, S., Kwon, M., Bae, S., Yim, S., Lee, J., Kim, S., Kang, Y., & Lee, D. (2017). CODA: Integrating multi-level context-oriented directed associations for analysis of drug effects. *Scientific Reports*, *7*(1), 7519. DOI: 10.1038/s41598-017-07448-6 PMID: 28790372

Yu, W., Ma, M., Chen, X., Min, J., Li, L., Zheng, Y., Li, Y., Wang, J., & Wang, Q. (2017). Traditional Chinese Medicine and Constitutional Medicine in China, Japan and Korea: A Comparative Study. *The American Journal of Chinese Medicine*, *45*(1), 1–12. DOI: 10.1142/S0192415X1750001X PMID: 28068838

Yu, X., Zhu, X., Zhang, L., Qin, J. J., Feng, C., & Li, Q. (2022). In Silico Screening and Validation of PDGFRA Inhibitors Enhancing Radioiodine Sensitivity in Thyroid Cancer. *Frontiers in Pharmacology*, *13*, 883581. DOI: 10.3389/fphar.2022.883581 PMID: 35645805

Zech, J. R., Badgeley, M. A., Liu, M., Costa, A. B., Titano, J. J., & Oermann, E. K. (2018). Variable generalization performance of a deep learning model to detect pneumonia in chest radiographs: A cross-sectional study. *PLoS Medicine*, *15*(11), e1002683. DOI: 10.1371/journal.pmed.1002683 PMID: 30399157

Zhang, H., Ni, W., Li, J., & Zhang, J. (2020). Artificial Intelligence-Based Traditional Chinese Medicine Assistive Diagnostic System: Validation Study. *JMIR Medical Informatics*, *8*(6), e17608. DOI: 10.2196/17608 PMID: 32538797

Zhang, H., Ni, W., Li, J., & Zhang, J. (2020). Artificial intelligence–based traditional Chinese medicine assistive diagnostic system: Validation study. *JMIR Medical Informatics*, *8*(6), e17608. PMID: 32538797

Zhang, M., Peng, Y., Wang, M., Gao, B., Zhao, L., & Li, X. (2019). The influence of compatibility of Si-Ni decoction with metabolism in intestinal bacteria on transports of toxic diterpenoid alkaloids from processed aconite root across Caco-2 monolayers. *Journal of Ethnopharmacology*, *228*, 164–178. DOI: 10.1016/j.jep.2018.09.022 PMID: 30223050

Zhang, Q., Guo, Y., Zhang, B., Liu, H., Peng, Y., Wang, D., & Zhang, D. (2022). Identification of hub biomarkers of myocardial infarction by single-cell sequencing, bioinformatics, and machine learning. *Frontiers in Cardiovascular Medicine*, *9*, 939972. DOI: 10.3389/fcvm.2022.939972 PMID: 35958412

Zhang, Q., Wang, Y., Chen, A., Huang, X., Dong, Q., Li, Z., Gao, X., Wu, T., Li, W., Cong, P., Wan, H., Dai, D., He, M., Liang, H., Wang, S., & Xiong, L. (2021). Xiaoxuming Decoction: A Traditional Herbal Recipe for Stroke With Emerging Therapeutic Mechanisms. *Frontiers in Pharmacology*, *12*, 802381. DOI: 10.3389/fphar.2021.802381 PMID: 34970152

Zhang, W., Huai, Y., Miao, Z., Qian, A., & Wang, Y. (2019). Systems Pharmacology for Investigation of the Mechanisms of Action of Traditional Chinese Medicine in Drug Discovery. *Frontiers in Pharmacology*, *10*, 743. DOI: 10.3389/fphar.2019.00743 PMID: 31379563

Zhavoronkov, A., Ivanenkov, Y. A., Aliper, A., Veselov, M. S., Aladinskiy, V. A., Aladinskaya, A. V., Terentiev, V. A., Polykovskiy, D. A., Kuznetsov, M. D., Asadulaev, A., Volkov, Y., Zholus, A., Shayakhmetov, R. R., Zhebrak, A., Minaeva, L. I., Zagribelnyy, B. A., Lee, L. H., Soll, R., Madge, D., & Aspuru-Guzik, A. (2019). Deep learning enables rapid identification of potent DDR1 kinase inhibitors. *Nature Biotechnology*, *37*(9), 1038–1040. DOI: 10.1038/s41587-019-0224-x PMID: 31477924

Zhu, H. (2020). Big Data and Artificial Intelligence Modeling for Drug Discovery. *Annual Review of Pharmacology and Toxicology*, *60*, 573–589. PMID: 31518513

APPENDIX

Abbreviations

ACE2 Angiotensin-converting enzyme 2
ADME/Tox Absorption, distribution, metabolism, excretion, and toxicity
AI Artificial Intelligence
ANN Artificial neural network
ARDS Acute respiratory distress syndrome
BGCs Biosynthetic gene clusters
CAM Complementary and alternative medicine
CHMs Chinese herbal medicines
CNN Convolutional neural network
CODA Context-Oriented Directed Associations
CVD Cardiovascular disease
DILI Drug-induced liver injury
DL Deep learning
DT Decision tree
GNPS Global Natural Products Social Molecular Networking
IL-1β Interleukin 1β
IMPPAT Indian Medicinal Plants, Phytochemistry, and Therapeutics
KNN K-Nearest Neighbors
LASSO Least absolute shrinkage and selection operator
LQC Lianhua Qingwen capsule
ML Machine learning
M^{pro} Main protease
NLP Natural language processing
NRPs Non-ribosomal peptides
PPI Protein-protein interactome
RFC Random Forest Classifier
SAR Structure-activity relationships
SSN Sequence similarity network
SVM Support vector machines
TCM Traditional Chinese Medicine
TCMSP TCM Systems Pharmacology Database and Analysis Platform
TCMSP Traditional Chinese Medicine Systems Pharmacology Database and Analysis Platform
THM-NP Traditional Herbal Medicine and Natural Products
TNBC triple-negative breast cancer

UMPDB Universal Metabolome and Pathway Database

Chapter 3
AI-Driven Drug Screening

Tammana Pratap Rana
https://orcid.org/0009-0005-8317-8756
Amity University, Mumbai, India

Anika Singh
Amity University, Mumbai, India

Sai Pandharinath Shelke
https://orcid.org/0009-0000-8187-4348
Amity University, Mumbai, India

Ameesha Mishra
https://orcid.org/0009-0002-0610-6829
Amity University, Mumbai, India

Rajshri Singh
https://orcid.org/0000-0001-5748-5799
Amity University, Mumbai, India

ABSTRACT

The integration of Artificial Intelligence (AI) into drug discovery has redefined the traditional image of pharmaceutics, aiding in reducing price and better prognosticative accuracy. AI, through Machine Learning (ML) and Deep Learning (DL), addresses this limitation of traditional methods by enabling rapid virtual screening, information-driven decision-making, and intelligent prioritization of compounds. Techniques such as molecular histrionics utilize SMILES, signifier, fingermark, and graph-establish networks heighten the prognostication of biological natural processes. AI correlates chemic, genomic, and clinical data to assist in target recognition, drug repurposing, and personalized drug development. However, challenges such as circumscribed data point availability, the dark-corner nature of models, and the

DOI: 10.4018/979-8-3373-5258-9.ch003

experimental validation crack remain critical barriers. Emerging approaches like Explainable AI (XAI), Physics-Informed Machine Learning (PIML), etc. promise to heighten model transparency and reliability.

1. INTRODUCTION

Drug discovery is a multi-stage process that involves identifying drug targets, screening chemical or biological compounds for activity, enhancing lead structures, and validating their safety and efficacy through preclinical and clinical testing. Despite major technological advances, traditional drug-discovery pipelines remain extremely resource-intensive, often taking 10–15 years from initial screening to market approval (Zhavoronkov et al., 2019).The average cost per approved drug is estimated at around USD 2.6 billion, largely due to the rapid turnover rates that occur as compounds progress through preclinical and clinical stages (DiMasi et al., 2016).

Conventional high-throughput and in vitro screening assays, while effective at generating hits, frequently rely on simplified biochemical or over-expressed cell systems. This fails to replicate complex physiological environments, resulting in false positives or poor translation to in vivo outcomes (Wei et al., 2021).As a result, nearly 90 percent of drug candidates entering clinical trials fail to reach approval, primarily due to lack of efficacy or unforeseen toxicity(Sun et al., 2022).These limitations of cost, time, and failure rate have motivated the integration of AI-driven computational methods, which can virtually screen large chemical libraries, improve targetligand prediction accuracy, and significantly reduce experimental burden (Stokes et al., 2020; Vamathevan et al., 2019).

Some of the frequently used traditional drug screening approaches include high-throughput screening (HTS), cell-based 2D assays, phenotypic screening, animal models, and clinical trials, each offering unique strengths but also significant drawbacks in terms of physiological relevance, scalability, and cost. These methods form the backbone of drug discovery yet remain constrained by high attrition rates and limited translational accuracy.

To overcome these challenges, we have gradually shifted to better suited computational techniques. AI enables the rapid processing and analysis of vast molecular datasets, allowing researchers to efficiently identify and prioritise promising drug candidates. Machine Learning (ML) models can prioritise targets and compounds from very large chemical libraries, improving hit-finding efficiency and decision making at multiplestages (W. Wang, 2024).Deep generative and reinforcement-learning approaches have been used to design novel, synthetically tractable small molecules and deliver active candidates in weeks rather than months(Zhavoronkov et al., 2019).Deep Learning (DL) based virtual screens and graph-neural-network predictors have successfully identified structurally novel active drugsfrom millions of compounds(Stokes et al., 2020).

Recent reviews and methodological studies furthermore show that AI-driven workflows when coupled with high-quality experimental data andvalidation can shorten lead optimisation cycles and improve ADMET (Absorption, Distribution, Metabolism, Excretion and Toxicity) predictions, thereby addressing cost and time challenging in traditional pipelines(Jiménez-Luna et al., 2021; Sadybekov & Katritch, 2023).

To get an in-depth understanding of how AI performs these tasks, one needs to first examine the existing screening system and how molecular structures are represented to be processed in machine-learning systems.

2. FOUNDATIONS: TRADITIONAL VS AI-DRIVEN SCREENING

2.1 Traditional Screening

2.1.1 High-Throughput Screening (HTS)

HTS is an automated observational technique that takes into account the quick empirical testing of huge libraries of physical molecules against biological objects in order to find a potential match. Historically created to expand wet-lab testing results beyond manual procedures, HTS integrates robotics, plate-based assays and high-speed detection systems to assess biochemical or cell-based endpoints across wide variety of samples (Entzeroth et al., 2009). Phenotypic or cell-based assays collect compound effects in a more physiologically complicated environment, producing functional read-outs such as viability, reporter activation, or nerve pathway activation, whereas biochemical assays in HTS sorts specific molecular events like receptor-ligand binding or enzyme activity. Despite advancements in technology, such as miniaturisation, plate density, and automation, HTS is still limited by the necessity for physical sample, reagent expenses, assay development time, and usable process that are throughput-dependent. These limitations restrict its electrical capacity to completely explore extremely large chemical substance places and might leave in false positives when biochemical read-out lacks physiological context (Entzeroth et al., 2009; Gurard-Levin et al., 2011). Nonetheless, HTS datasets offer an all-important empirical ground for subsequent cheminformatics and ML models.

2.1.2 Cell-Based 2D Assays (Standard In-Vitro Screening)

The in vitro 2D assay utilises monolayer-cultured cells with reporter systems to assess compound activity, because they lack physiologic signal, ECM, and 3D computer architecture, their predictive value is restricted(Sun et al., 2022; Wei et al., 2021).

2.1.3 Phenotypic Screening

Phenotypic screening directly investigates chemical interference in cellular or organismal systems without involving a predetermined molecular target, makes it possible to identify first-in-class drugs but resolution in a lower throughput and a higher follow-up expense(Hughes et al., 2011).

2.1.4. Animal (In-Vivo) Preclinical Models

Prior to human trial run, systemic PK/PD (Pharmacokinetics/Pharmacodynamics) device characteristics and toxicity are evaluated using animal models, howeverthese models are expensive, time consuming, and frequently don not mimic human physiology, which contributes to translational failure (DiMasi et al., 2016).

2.1.5 Clinical Development (Phases I–III)

Only 10–15% of drug candidates advance from Phase I to favourable reception, making clinical trials a significant driver to worldwide R&D expenses, this shows clinical trials aretime consuming and resource-intensive for drug development (DiMasi et al., 2016).

2.2 Virtual Screening (VS)

Virtual screening employs in silico methods for experimental testing, thereby this reduces the workload of wet laboratory by filtering databases before conducting physical experiments. Three-dimensional protein structures are utilised in structure-based virtual screening (SBVS) to conduct molecular docking and rank ligand which utilises scoring functions to evaluate non-covalent fundamental interaction. Standard scoring mapping stimulatesvariety of points of accuracy and can yield method-dependent results, which leads to consensus and rescoring strategies to enhance enrichment (Maia et al., 2020). When the target structure is unavailable, ligand-based virtual screening (LBVS) is employed,using the similarity matrix, pharmacophore simulation and QSAR descriptor obtained from known actives to find new candidates. Although VS has historically been less precise in its predictions due to inefficient scoring, restrained chemical representation, and the necessity of thorough validation. Recent methodological advancements, such as consensus grading, ML-based scoring subprogram, and free energy calculation, have reduced some of these limitations(Maia et al., 2020; Nhat Phuong et al., 2023). Compared to experimental HTS, VS improves throughput and monetary value.

2.3 Foundation of Traditional Methods vs. AI Methods

Traditional drug screening has required considerable financial and time investment, with the average cost of developing a new drug, which is estimated to be around \$2.6 billion, mostly due to the high attrition associated with experimental screening and clinical failure rates (Vamathevan et al., 2019). Development timeframes typically range between 10 and 15 years, beginning with target selection and concluding with regulatory approval (Hughes et al., 2011). In this traditional model, hit identification is based on large-scale screening of chemical libraries, which frequently contain about one million compounds, a labour-intensive, time consuming, and expensive procedure despite advances in AI. Elimination remains a serious limitation, with over 90% of drug candidates failing during clinical development, often due to insufficient target validation or a lack of physiological relevance in early biochemical assays (Stokes et al., 2020). Slow experimental feedback cycles and the necessity for diverse teams to manage screening, lead optimisation, and validation operations contribute to these restrictions.

In contrast, AI-driven drug screening showcases a significant shift by virtualising early-stage drug discovery and eliminating the need for substantial wet-lab testing. Artificial intelligence speeds up hit detection by rapidly evaluating large chemical libraries and reducing the chemical space to only the most promising possibilities, leading in 10-60% reductions in R&D expenditure (Vamathevan et al., 2019). AI technology can reduce overall drug development time by three to five years, especially during stages of lead identification and optimisation, where virtual screening replaceslong experimental cycles (Zhavoronkov et al., 2019). AI-based early assessment also lowers preclinical failure rates by improving target-ligand matching and identifying potential liabilities, resulting in approximate 20-30% reduction in early-stage attrition (Stokes et al., 2020). Unlike conventional methods, AI integrates high-dimensional data quickly and delivers rapid analytical feedback, eliminating common time constraints (Chen & Zhang, 2022). Automating routine operations, decreases labour demands which improves discovery productivity. However, AI systems rely on high-quality training datasets and model interpretability for consistent performance (Wei et al., 2021).

2.4 HTS vs. AI-Driven Screening: A Comparative Analysis

Table 1. A comparison between HTS and AI-driven screening

High-Throughput Screening (HTS)	AI-Driven Screening (AI-VS)
Screens millions of physical molecules.	Screens billions of virtual molecules.
Takes weeks/months to complete screening.	Completes screening in days.
Very high operational cost (reagents, automation, physical libraries).	Low operational cost (primarily limited by computational power).
Restricted to compounds in the existing physical library.	Explores the synthetically accessible chemical space (molecules not yet made).
Provides the final experimental confirmation of "hits."	Provides prioritization and reduction of the search space (e.g., top 0.1%).
Used for highly focused, high-quality experimental confirmation of AI-predicted candidates.	Used to rapidly select candidates and for continuous refinement of models via experimental feedback.

3. AI DATA INFRASTRUCTURE

AI data infrastructure isimportant for modern virtual drug screening (VS) which is aadvanced, multi-layered system built to handle the heavy computational requirements. This infrastructure depends onHigh-Performance Computing (HPC) clusters using GPUs and TPUs to perform the intensive parallel processing which are required for deep learning, molecular dynamics, and quick analysis of large chemical libraries (Thaingtamtanha et al., 2025). This is crucial for accelerating the identification of lead compounds by aiding the advancement of AI models for tasks like target identification, ADMETprediction, and de novo molecule design (Sharma et al., 2024; Thaingtamtanha et al., 2025). The main focus of this system is to integrates diverse, massive datasets which includes chemical libraries, molecular structures, multi-omics, and clinical trial results into standard format suitable for high-throughput in silico screening (Tripathi et al., 2021). By integrating these powerful computing platforms and deep learning frameworks, AI models can rapidly conduct structure-based or ligand-based VS on wide array of compounds (Askr et al., 2023). The primary advantage in this isthe infrastructure's ability to incorporate predicted protein structures,such as those from AlphaFold, which allows screening of targets that lack experimental structural data, greatly improving the therapeutic space (Ocana et al., 2025).

4. CORE AI/ML METHODOLOGIES FOR DRUG SCREENING

4.1 Representation of Chemical Data

AI methods work on mathematical representations of molecules and biological data. Therefore, effective drug-screening models depend on how chemical information is encoded and what algorithms process it. AI&ML have transformed drug discovery by enabling rapid screening and predictive modelling across vast chemical spaces. Before a model can visualise a molecule, the chemical structure must be transformed into a machine-readable numerical form, a process called molecular encoding or featurization. The choice of representation directly affects model performance, interpretability, and computational cost, a good representation preserves atom or bond identity, topology, stereochemistry, spatial or electronic details[REMOVED HYPERLINK FIELD](David et al., 2020; Wigh et al., 2022).

4.1.1 SMILES

The Simplified Molecular Input Line Entry System (SMILES)encodes molecules in the format of a linear ASCII strings that describe atom symbols, bond types, rings, and branches (e.g., ethanol = CCO). SMILES is compact and text-based, making it ideal for large datasets and for treating chemistry as a language. Sequence models (RNNs, transformers, etc) trained on SMILES have been widely used for de novo molecule generation and property prediction. Important practical notes are that SMILES is not unique (multiple valid SMILES can describe the same molecule) and that techniques such as canonical SMILES, randomised SMILES augmentation, or SELFIES can improve (Joshi & Kumar, 2021; A. Paul et al., 2018).

4.1.2 Molecular Descriptors and RDKIT Feature

A well-known route is to compute molecular descriptors, predefined numerical summaries of physicochemical and topological properties (molecular weight, logP, TPSA, hydrogen bond donors/acceptors, ring counts, etc.). Toolkits such as RDKit provide hundreds of descriptors and enable straightforward creation of fixed-length feature vectors for classical machine learning models like random forest, SVM, gradient boosting. Descriptors are especially useful in QSAR modelling because they are interpretable and they feature important analyses that can reveal which molecular properties drive activity or toxicity[REMOVED HYPERLINK FIELD] (Wigh et al., 2022).

4.1.3 Molecular Fingerprints for Similarity and Screening

Fingerprints transform molecular structures into binary or integer vectors that encode the availability of substructures or atoms in the surrounding. Common variants include MACCS keys, topological or path fingerprints, and Morgan ECFP fingerprints. Fingerprints are compact and computationally efficient, making them ideal for rapid similarity searches, clustering, and scaffold-hopping via metrics like the Tanimoto coefficient. A study uses Morgan/ECFP fingerprints to predict drug responses in cancer, including screening of real anticancer drugs such as Paclitaxel, allowing machine-learning models to estimate how effectively these drugs act on specific cancer cell lines before experimental testing(Xiao et al., 2025). They form the backbone of many virtual screening campaigns, though they abstract away geometric and some electronic detail, which limits their expressiveness for tasks that require fine-grained structural information[REMOVED HYPERLINK FIELD] (Dong et al., 2015; Wigh et al., 2022).

4.2. Machine Learning (ML) Techniques

4.2.1 Supervised Learning

Supervised learning is termed asML model format that is trained on labelled data, meaning each input example comes with a known output record so that the algorithm learns the mapping from features to label. The supervised learning adaptsto determine labels of new samples from training samples[REMOVED HYPERLINK FIELD](Tetko & Clevert, 2025). In this, the model is trained using molecules whose activity or toxicity is already knownand then ask the model to predict the activity or toxicity of new, unseen molecules. One of the most common supervised tasks in drug-screening is classification (predicting categorical outputs, e.g.active vsinactive) or regression (predicting continuous values, e.g., IC_{50}, toxicity score) (Dara et al., 2022).

Classic algorithms in supervised learning include methods such as Random Forest, Support Vector Machine (SVM), decision trees, logistic regression, neural networks etc[REMOVED HYPERLINK FIELD](Dara et al., 2022). In the drug-discovery setting, Random Forests might predict whether a compound will hit a target (classification) or estimate its binding affinity (regression) (Vamathevan et al., 2019)

4.2.2 Unsupervised Learning

Unsupervised learning involvesunlabelled which includes, input examples without explicit output labels. This allows the algorithm to discover hidden structure, patterns, or groupings (Li et al., 2024). In field of drug-screening, this means grouping compounds by structural similarity, chemical space location, or latent embedding, without the knowledge which compounds will be active or toxic. One common unsupervised task is clustering, where molecules are grouped into clusters so that compounds in the same cluster are more similar to each other than to those in other clusters[REMOVED HYPERLINK FIELD](Madugula et al., 2021). Another important unsupervised technique is dimensionality reduction, which simplifies high-dimensional chemical or biological data into fewer dimensions for visualisation or modelling (Li et al., 2024). Unsupervised learning is especially useful in compound library analysis and early-stage drug discovery for tasks like diversifying a screening set, identifying outliers, exploring chemical space, or drug repositioning(Hameed et al., 2018).

Limitations of unsupervised learning may exist because of no labels, the clusters may not align with biologically relevant categories, as stated since unsupervised learning models do not provide clear explanations for the patterns they discover, thus the results are difficult to predict [REMOVED HYPERLINK FIELD](Li et al., 2024).

Table 2. Comparison between Supervised and Unsupervised Learning in Drug Screening

Aspect	Supervised Learning	Unsupervised Learning
Definition	Learns a mapping between input features (e.g., molecular descriptors) and known output labels.	Discovers hidden patterns, structures, or clusters within unlabelled chemical data.
Typical Tasks and Data	Classification and regression. Labelled Data	Clustering and dimensionality reduction. Unlabelled data
Common Algorithms	Random Forests, Support Vector Machines (SVM), Decision Trees, Logistic Regression, Neural Networks.	K-means clustering, Hierarchical Clustering, Self-Organizing Maps (SOM), Principal Component Analysis (PCA), t-SNE, UMAP.
Applications in Drug Screening	Predicting molecular activity, ADMET properties, toxicity levels, and compound selectivity.	Analysing compound libraries, chemical space visualization, scaffold clustering, outlier detection, and drug repurposing.
Type of Output	Predictive models that generate quantitative or categorical outcomes for new molecules.	Groups or reduced-dimension representations showing structure–pattern relationships.

continued on following page

Table 2. Continued

Aspect	Supervised Learning	Unsupervised Learning
Advantages	High predictive power when sufficient quality data exist; interpretable relationships between structure and activity.	Reveals hidden structures and relationships in large, complex datasets; useful when labelled data are scarce.
Challenges and Limitations	Requires largelabelled datasets; prone to overfitting and bias if data quality is low; interpretability issues.	Clusters may not correspond to biological meaning; results can be difficult to interpret; dependent on choice of distance metric or algorithm.

(Dara et al., 2022; Hameed et al., 2018; Li et al., 2024; Tetko & Clevert, 2025)

4.3 Deep Learning (DL) Techniques

4.3.1 Convolutional Neural Networks (CNNs)

Convolutional neural networks (CNNs) have become a powerful tool in molecular-screening workflows because they inherently excel at spatial feature learning. It was traditionally in images but now it increased for molecular 2D and 3D representations. In the domain of drug screening, a key challenge is to encode molecular structure in a way that captures spatial arrangement, functional groups and topological context. CNNs permit a shift from hand-crafted descriptors toward learned representations. Chemception, demonstrated that a deep CNN trained solely on images of 2D chemical structures without expert-engineered features matched the performance of advanced QSAR/QSPR models built on descriptors and fingerprints(Goh et al., 2017).The main benefit being, the CNN picks up structural cues clearly, resulting in reduced need for manual selection.

Moving beyond 2D, applying CNNs to 3D molecular data offers further promise because molecular interactions are inherently 3D. For instance,instead of just seeing a molecule's flat drawing, the network sees a 3D grid representation of space around atoms and bonds allowing it to learn spatial neighbourhood and volumetric patterns relevant for binding, solvation or reactivity(Mendolia et al., 2020). Despite these advantages, representing 3D molecular structures for CNNs involves practical challenges. Sparse representation can hamper learning, and rotational or translational variability must be handled carefully (A. K. Gupta & Raghavachari, 2022). From a drug-screening perspective, CNNs support tasks such as virtual screening, binding-affinity prediction, and toxicity/ADMET property prediction by ingesting structured spatial representations of molecules directly.Thus, by using CNNs, one leverages spatial learning rather than relying purely on human-engineered features(-Mendolia et al., 2020).

According a recent study,CNN architectures can be reused from computer vision (e.g., ResNet, Inception) on molecular images, expanding the tool-box for drug screening(Li et al., 2024). DeepDTA uses CNNs to predict how well known kinase inhibitor drugs, including cancer therapeutics like imatinib, they bind to their target proteins, helping prioritise effective candidates in cancer-related drug screening(Öztürk et al., 2018).

Figure 1. Convolutional Neural Networks Workflow

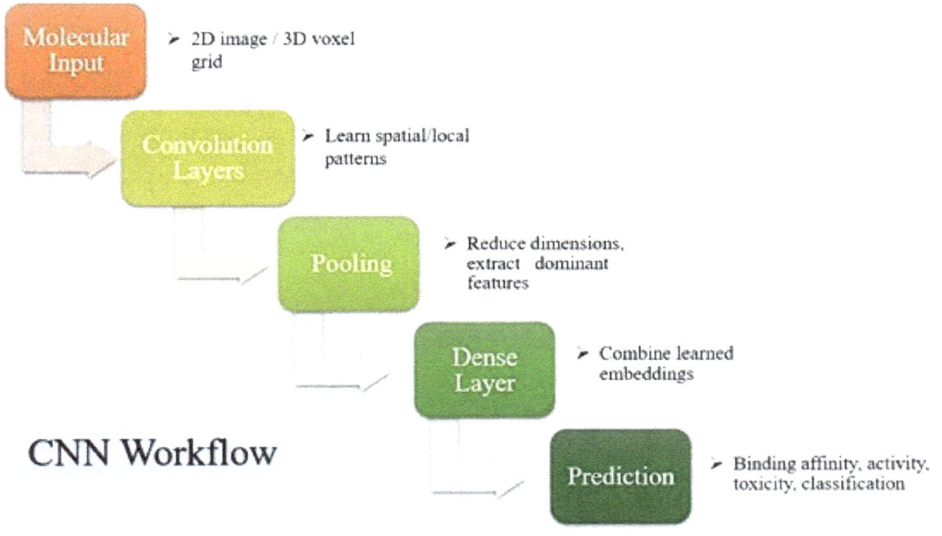

In summary, CNNs are a potent technique for feature learning from 2D and 3D molecular structures within AI/ML-driven drug screening pipelines. They simplify feature engineering by learning directly from spatial representations, accommodate both image-style and volumetric molecular data, and have demonstrably matched or exceeded classical descriptor-based models. The future likely lies in combining 2D/3D CNNs with other architectures (e.g., GNNs, transformers) for richer molecular understanding (Niazi & Mariam, 2023).

4.3.2 Graph Neural Networks (GNNs)

GNNshave come up as a powerful deep-learning frameworks for modelling molecules. Since they map strongly onto the underlying structure of chemical compounds. Instead of just forcing molecules into fixed-length descriptor vectors, GNNs considers a molecule as a graph, atoms as nodes, bonds as edges. This allows let the network to learn features by propagating information across nodes and edges (Jiang et al., 2021).

A major benefit of GNNs is their complete learning of graph structure, preceding the need for manual feature engineering (fingerprints or descriptors). In a comparative study, it wasdiscovered that GNN-based models (GCN, GAT, MPNN) were outshining the descriptor-based models in specific large-scale settings(Jiang et al., 2021). In drug screening tasks where activity and binding labels exist, GNNs can extract minute structural cues that traditional ML might overlook.An essential topic is the modelling of 3D geometry and higher-order interactions in GNNs. Researchers haveput forth a GNN that clearly distinguishes between local and non-local interactions, and alsodirectionalcharacteristics in 3D (Jiang et al., 2021; Y. Wang, Li, et al., 2023). However, while GNNs offer many plus points, they come with the challenge of interpretability(Pan et al., 2023). GraphDTA applies graph neural networks to screen and rank kinase-targeting cancer drugs such as imatinib, learning directly from molecular structure to improve binding-affinity prediction for oncology pipelines(Nguyen et al., 2020) .

Figure 2. Graph Neural Networks Workflow

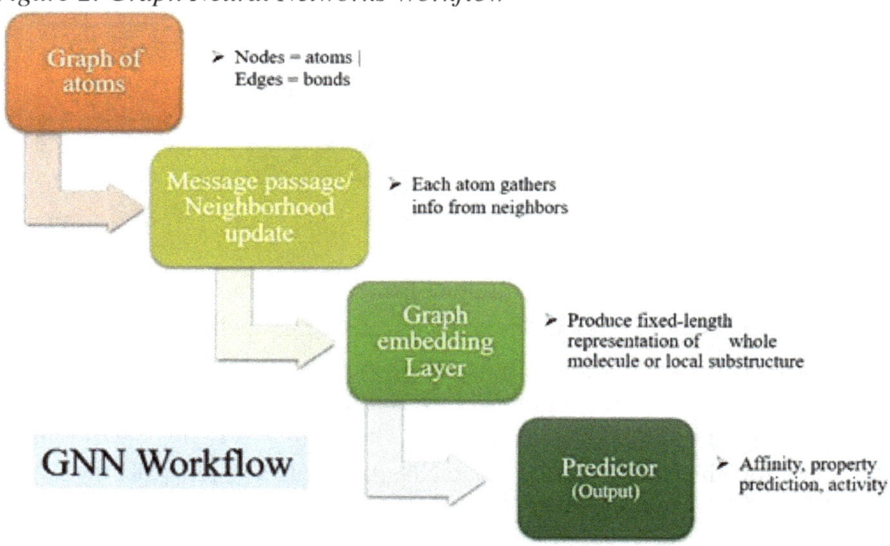

In summary, GNNs are a versatileand extremely essential tool in drug screening because they mirror molecular structure, support interaction modelling, and reduce the need for handcrafted features. Thegraph inside the molecule becomes computational subtractive for discovery(Wieder et al., 2020).

4.3.3 Recurrent Neural Networks (RNNs)

RNNs are among the earliest deep learning architectures applied to de novo molecular design. They have a significant ability to model SMILES strings as sequential data.SMILES represent molecules as character sequences, RNNsparticularly LSTM (Long Short Term Memory) and GRU (Gated Recurrent Unit) variantscan learn the framework of chemical space and they generate valid new molecules(Arús-Pous et al., 2020). Early studies trained RNN-LSTM models on large SMILES datasets and then applied transfer learning to bias generation toward specific biological targets (A. Gupta et al., 2018).

Although they have their advantages, RNN-based models rely heavily on large, diverse training sets and struggle with long-range dependencies in SMILES notation (e.g., ring closures, branching). Data augmentation strategies such as randomized SMILES were later introduced to improve robustness of RNN-based molecular models (Arús-Pous et al., 2019).

Figure 3. Recurrent Neural Networks Workflow

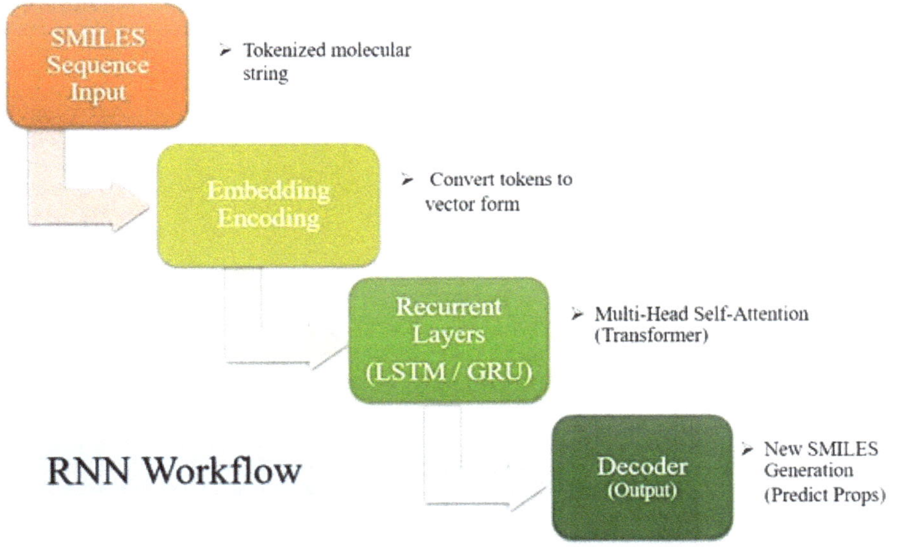

In summary, RNNs are powerful tools for sequence-based drug-screening tasks when molecules are represented as SMILES strings, enabling the creation of novel chemical matter, scaffold exploration, and property-aware molecule generation

4.3.4 Transformer

More recently, transformer architectures have taken the lead in sequence modelling due to their self-attention mechanism, faster training (parallelizable) and better scaling. An important application of sequence-based models in drug screening is conditional generation — i.e., generating molecules given a scaffold, target, or property constraint. For instance, in one study, a transformer model was conditioned on target embeddings to generate SMILES strings for drug-like compounds against specific targets(Y. Wang, Zhao, et al., 2023).

Despite their strengths, sequence-based models have some challenges in molecular design. SMILES strings encode only connectivity; they miss explicit 3D geometry unless augmented. Also, the grammar of SMILES is non-trivial (branching, stereochemistry, ring closures), so the model must learn valid syntax; invalid SMILES generation remains a problem. For example, auto-generated SMILES may be syntactically invalid or chemically implausible [REMOVED HYPERLINK FIELD] (Gow et al., 2022). TransAntivirus uses a transformer model to design new antiviral molecules, generating promising candidates like Compound b18 for COVID-19, and screening them against SARS-CoV-2 proteins using docking (Mao et al., 2024).

Figure 4.Transformer Workflow

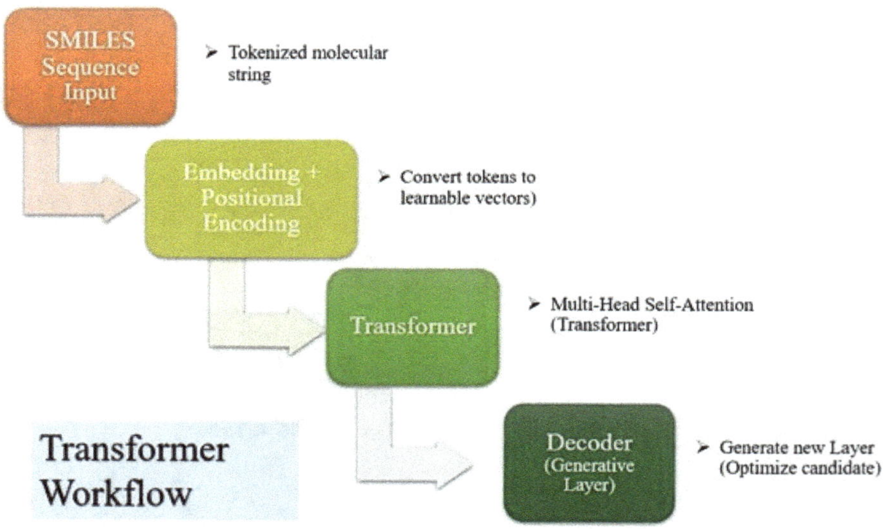

Transformers use SMILES-based drug screening. They offering strong capabilities in generating novel chemical structures, exploring new scaffolds, and designing molecules with desired properties.

Figure 5. Summary of Workflow

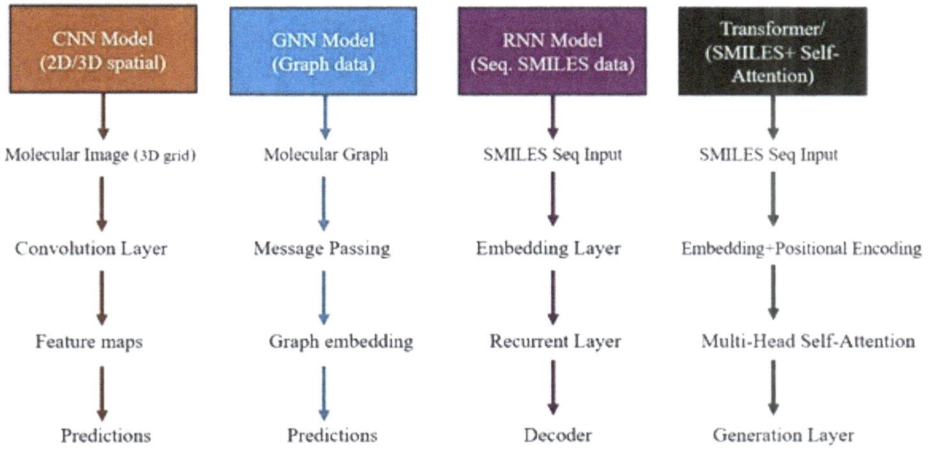

5. APPLICATIONS OF AI IN VIRTUAL DRUG SCREENING

The growth of artificial intelligence,specially for processes like machine learning and deep learning, has lead to many applications in virtual drug screening (Lo et al., 2020). These applications include research&discovery, clinical development, personalized medicine, drug repurposing, and patient surveillance (Khurana et al., 2023; Lo et al., 2020; Parekh et al., 2023).

5.1 Research and Discovery of Drugs

Discovering and developing novel drugs is anessential scientific process which is aimed at curing diseases and improving human health. The objective is to create and combine experimental testing with current technologies. This is done to develop new, cost efficient and more stronger drugs (S. Singh et al., 2024)(KP Jayatunga et al., 2024). AI helps with structure-based drug discovery by predicting a compound's effect on its target before synthesis. This is done by using AI to create 3D protein structures that can be customised to the chemical environment of the target protein site (D. Paul et al., 2021).One of it's important use is the prediction of ADMET characteristics. AI can analyse complex clinical, proteomic, and genomic data to recognise novel biomarkers related to pharmacological resistance or response. These biomarkers can predict which individuals may benefit from specific drug or predict disease outcomes(Ocana et al., 2025).

5.2 Clinical Development and Personalised medicine

AI is crucial for personalised medicine, enabling precise diagnoses and treatment plans by analysing complete patient data, which includes symptoms, medical history and genetic information. Health Information Management (HIM) specialists are significant induviduals in managing this data, which is vital for the effective application of AI in this personalised approach(Parekh et al., 2023). Machine learning tools allow for the efficient enhancement of treatment, such as chemotherapy dosing, in which continuous learning from patient responses, enables one to adjust schedules in real-time to maximise efficacy and minimise side effects. AI combines data from multiple sources like electronic health records, clinical trials, and real-world evidence. This results in a flexible and responsive personalised care plans (Serrano et al., 2024). Moreover, AI methodologiesincludeML and DL, gives a powerful combination for pharmacogenomics, thus extending beyond traditional statistics to revolutionise the field. This facilitates the large-scale study of complex pharmacogenomic interactions (e.g., disease-gene, gene-drug), offering deeper insights for drug discovery and clinical practice throughout the entire process of pharmacology research (Taherdoost & Ghofrani, 2024).

5.3 Drug Repurposing

Drug repurposing, is the strategy of finding new therapeutic uses for already approved or existing drugs, offers substantial benifits such as reduced development time and costs, which can ultimately provideaffordable healthcare expenses. This methodis gaining popularity due to current limitations of traditional drug discovery and the rising threat of infectious diseases.

AI is a reliable and powerful tool to accelerate drug repurposing, allowing researchers to quickly identify promising new treatments and minimise data limitations. AI greatly increases the efficiency of drug repurposing by streamlining processes, uncovering hidden biological patterns, and promoting cooperation with current methods. This approach ultimately supports global health by creating new opportunities in the fight against pathogens (A. Singh, 2024).

5.4 Patient Surveillance

Technological advancements, like the integration of AI, are crucial for modern patient surveillance. The vast volume of data from sources like electronic health records, spontaneous reporting systems, and social media requires modern processing capabilities (Shamim et al., 2024). A key function of AI in this field is remote patient monitoring, aiming to create enhanced health-monitoring systems that help individuals manage rising healthcare costs(Jeddi & Bohr, 2020).The automation of tasks like quality control and duplication detection improves patient surveillance. This improves the assessment of validity and prioritises evaluations. Thus, this AI&ML-supported automation reduces the workload on healthcare professionals, allowing them to concentrate their efforts on more complex and critical tasks (Shamim et al., 2024).

6. FUTURE PERSPECTIVE

6.1 Binding Prediction Using Physical Chemistry and Molecular Interactions

Future AI models in drug screening are moving beyond pattern recognition and statistical correlation toward a deeper, physics-aware understanding of molecular interactions. By integrating principles such as van der Waals forces, hydrogen bonding, and hydrophobic effects with GNNs, these hybrid models can generalise better to new ligand–target pairs. Recent studies combining physical energy functions with GNNs demonstrate improved binding-affinity prediction. This showcases that AI systems are not only more accurate but also more interpretable and reliable for future drug discovery (Moon et al., 2022).

6.2 Integrated Learning and Secure Machine Learning for Collaborative Drug Discovery

Pharmacological and biological data areusually confidential or sensitive thus, centralised pooling of resources is frequently impossible. Integrated learning frameworks enable incorporation of training models by several institutions (for example, QSAR, ADMET, virtual screening) without exchanging raw data, ensuring privacy while benefiting from diverse datasets. This has the potential to efficiently increase data diversity, improve model stability, and promote drug development in a privacy-conscious environment(Cozac et al., 2025).

6.3 Explainable AI (XAI) for Accuracy and Regulatory Development

Developments in AI-driven drug screening as we move further, will increasingly integrate GNNs with explainable AI (XAI) to not only improve the accuracy of predicting drug-target interactions and toxicity but also to provide transparent, concept-level explanations behind each prediction. This means future screening tools will not just rank molecules they will also explain why a molecule is promising or risky by targeting specific structural features. This enhances trust and decision-making in early-stage drug discovery (Proietti et al., 2024).

6.4 Multi-Representation / Multi-Graph Approaches to Improve Chemical Insight & Prediction

Instead of exactly show molecules at the nuclear storey, employing respective internal representation of molecular graph (such pharmacophore graphs, functional group graph, and junction trees) can integrate models with a more comprehensive, hierarchal sympathy of chemical substance structures. Early findings suggest that these multi-graph simulations can improve prediction accuracy and offer more detailed insights into how molecular structure relates to biological activity. This makes them a promising direction for the next generation of AI-driven drug development. (Kengkanna & Ohue, 2024).

7. CASE STUDIES AND FUTURE DIRECTIONS

7.1 Successful AI-Screening Examples

A number of recent case studies have shown how AI is successful in finding new and effective treatment possibilities.An important example is the AI-driven discovery of a small-molecule inhibitor of CDK20, where scientists used generative chemistry models when integrated with AlphaFold-based structure prediction. Within 30 days of starting the study, they synthesized only a few compounds using an end-to-end AI pipeline and attained a binding affinity of about 210 nm(Ren et al., 2022). This accomplishment shows how AI can significantly reduce the time needed for early drug discovery while preserving accuracy and selectivity. After synthesising just seven compounds, a follow-up study build upon this strategy and found more CDK20 inhibitors with sub-micromolar potency, demonstrating the ability of AI-driven molecular production(Gao et al., 2023; Ren et al., 2023).

Furthermore, extensive analyses of AI-enabled discovery pipelines reveal that AI-generated compounds outperform molecules which are traditionally developed in early clinical stages, with up to 80–90% success in Phase I trials and roughly 40% in Phase II trials(KP Jayatunga et al., 2024). These results show that AI can generate candidates with favourable safety and pharmacokinetic properties in addition to finding active compounds.

7.2 Integration Into the Pharma Workflow

AI is being systematically included across the drug-discovery and development pipeline by pharmaceutical companies and biotech startups, going beyond leading main studies. It's now being used not only for early target identification and virtual screening, but also for clinical trial design, patient stratification, manufacturing, and supply chain optimisation. This indicates a major change in pharma workflow architecture (Saini et al., 2025).

Recently, AI techniques are being incorporated into pharmaceutical workflows in a number of important areas:

a) Target and hit discovery: AI algorithms examine massive datasetsto find new targets for repurpose already-existing compounds.
b) Lead optimisation and virtual screening: Using fewer resources, generative models and deep learning frameworks prioritize compounds more quickly.
c) Clinical development: AI is use to reduce attrition and time-to-market by optimising trial designs, selecting patients, and predicting outcomes. But there are challenges in incorporating AI into pharmaceutical procedures. Organisations need to handle data governance, match AI-native platforms with legacy infrastructure, retrain employees in interdisciplinary skills, and solve algorithmic output trust (Sampene & Nyirenda, 2024).

Figure 6. Integration of AI across the various Stages of Drug Discovery and Development

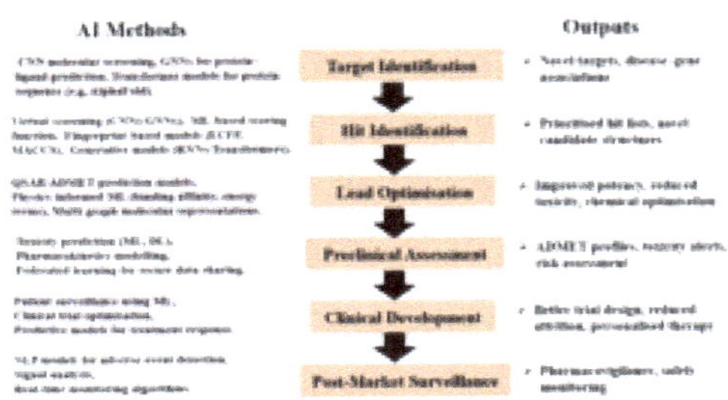

7.3 Emerging Trends

Physics Informed Machine Learning (PIML) and Active Learning in Laboratory Automation.

PIML incorporates physical rules, such as molecular dynamics or energy limitations, into AI models, allowing for better generalisation and interpretability, especially when data is scarce. For example,combining molecular-simulation insights with machine-learning increases the accuracy of ligand-protein interaction predictions (Noé et al., 2023). These tendencies indicate a shift away from data-driven forecasts and toward knowledge-driven and self-evolving systems. The combination of mechanistic insight with feedback automation promises drug discovery processes that are faster, more robust, and easier to interpret(Angello et al., 2023).

8. CONCLUSION

AI is reshaping drug discovery by transforming it from a slow, resource-intensive experimental process into a faster, predictive, and data-driven discipline. By integrating machine learning, deep learning, and generative models, AI supports rapid hit identification, efficient lead optimisation, and earlier prediction of ADMET and toxicity profiles. These are the areas where traditional screening methods often struggle. These capabilities help reduce both research costs and timelines while lowering attrition across preclinical and clinical stages.Successful examples, including AI-designed CDK inhibitors and deep-learning-guided antibiotic discovery, illustrate how computational pipelines can deliver potent and selective candidates within weeks rather than years. As pharmaceutical companies increasingly utilize AI across target identification, virtual screening, clinical trial design, and patient surveillance, drug-development workflows are undergoing a structural shift.The future will rely on the combination of physics-informed machine learning, integrated learning for secure multi-institutional collaboration, and explainable AI to ensure regulatory transparency. Emerging trends such as multi-graph representations and automated closed-loop laboratories further point toward adaptive, self-improving discovery cycles.Ultimately, AI aids rather than acting as an replacement of experimental science. By incorporating computational insight with biological understanding, AI offers a path toward faster which is more precise, and more innovative drug discoverylaying the groundwork for safer, more effective therapies in the years to come.

REFERENCES

Angello, N., Friday, D., Hwang, C., Yi, S., Cheng, A., Torres-Flores, T., Jira, E., Wang, W., Aspuru-Guzik, A., Burke, M., Schroeder, C., Diao, Y., & Jackson, N. (2023). *Closed-Loop Transfer Enables AI to Yield Chemical Knowledge*. https://doi.org/DOI: 10.26434/chemrxiv-2023-jqbqt

Arús-Pous, J., Johansson, S. V., Prykhodko, O., Bjerrum, E. J., Tyrchan, C., Reymond, J. L., Chen, H., & Engkvist, O. (2019). Randomized SMILES strings improve the quality of molecular generative models. *Journal of Cheminformatics*, *11*(1). Advance online publication. DOI: 10.1186/s13321-019-0393-0 PMID: 33430971

Arús-Pous, J., Patronov, A., Bjerrum, E. J., Tyrchan, C., Reymond, J. L., Chen, H., & Engkvist, O. (2020). SMILES-based deep generative scaffold decorator for de-novo drug design. *Journal of Cheminformatics*, *12*(1). Advance online publication. DOI: 10.1186/s13321-020-00441-8 PMID: 33431013

Askr, H., Elgeldawi, E., Aboul Ella, H., Elshaier, Y. A. M. M., Gomaa, M. M., & Hassanien, A. E. (2023). Deep learning in drug discovery: An integrative review and future challenges. *Artificial Intelligence Review*, *56*(7), 5975–6037. DOI: 10.1007/s10462-022-10306-1 PMID: 36415536

Chen, Y., & Zhang, L. (2022). How much can deep learning improve prediction of the responses to drugs in cancer cell lines? *Briefings in Bioinformatics*, *23*(1). Advance online publication. DOI: 10.1093/bib/bbab378 PMID: 34529029

Cozac, R., Hasic, H., Choong, J. J., Richard, V., Beheshti, L., Froehlich, C., Koyama, T., Matsumoto, S., Kojima, R., Iwata, H., Hasegawa, A., Otsuka, T., & Okuno, Y. (2025). kMoL: An open-source machine and federated learning library for drug discovery. *Journal of Cheminformatics*, *17*(1). Advance online publication. DOI: 10.1186/s13321-025-00967-9 PMID: 40001146

Dara, S., Dhamercherla, S., Jadav, S. S., Babu, C. M., & Ahsan, M. J. (2022). Machine Learning in Drug Discovery: A Review. *Artificial Intelligence Review*, *55*(3), 1947–1999. DOI: 10.1007/s10462-021-10058-4 PMID: 34393317

David, L., Thakkar, A., Mercado, R., & Engkvist, O. (2020). Molecular representations in AI-driven drug discovery: a review and practical guide. In *Journal of Cheminformatics* (Vol. 12, Issue 1). BioMed Central Ltd. https://doi.org/DOI: 10.1186/s13321-020-00460-5

DiMasi, J. A., Grabowski, H. G., & Hansen, R. W. (2016). Innovation in the pharmaceutical industry: New estimates of R&D costs. *Journal of Health Economics*, *47*, 20–33. DOI: 10.1016/j.jhealeco.2016.01.012 PMID: 26928437

Dong, J., Cao, D. S., Miao, H. Y., Liu, S., Deng, B. C., Yun, Y. H., Wang, N. N., Lu, A. P., & Zeng, W. Bin, & Chen, A. F. (2015). ChemDes: An integrated web-based platform for molecular descriptor and fingerprint computation. *Journal of Cheminformatics*, *7*(1). Advance online publication. DOI: 10.1186/s13321-015-0109-z PMID: 26664458

Entzeroth, M., Flotow, H., & Condron, P. (2009). Overview of high-throughput screening. In *Current Protocols in Pharmacology* (Issue SUPPL. 44). https://doi.org/DOI: 10.1002/0471141755.ph0904s44

Gao, B., Qiang, B., Tan, H., Ren, M., Jia, Y., Lu, M., Liu, J., Ma, W., & Lan, Y. (2023). *DrugCLIP: Contrastive Protein-Molecule Representation Learning for Virtual Screening*. https://arxiv.org/abs/2310.06367

Goh, G. B., Siegel, C., Vishnu, A., Hodas, N. O., & Baker, N. (2017). *Chemception: A Deep Neural Network with Minimal Chemistry Knowledge Matches the Performance of Expert-developed QSAR/QSPR Models*.

Gow, S., Niranjan, M., Kanza, S., & Frey, J. G. (2022). A review of reinforcement learning in chemistry. In *Digital Discovery* (Vol. 1, Issue 5, pp. 551–567). Royal Society of Chemistry. https://doi.org/DOI: 10.1039/d2dd00047d

Gupta, A., Müller, A. T., Huisman, B. J. H., Fuchs, J. A., Schneider, P., & Schneider, G. (2018). Generative Recurrent Networks for De Novo Drug Design. *Molecular Informatics*, *37*(1). Advance online publication. DOI: 10.1002/minf.201700111 PMID: 29095571

Gupta, A. K., & Raghavachari, K. (2022). Three-Dimensional Convolutional Neural Networks Utilizing Molecular Topological Features for Accurate Atomization Energy Predictions. *Journal of Chemical Theory and Computation*, *18*(4), 2132–2143. DOI: 10.1021/acs.jctc.1c00504 PMID: 35226496

Gurard-Levin, Z. A., Scholle, M. D., Eisenberg, A. H., & Mrksich, M. (2011). High-throughput screening of small molecule libraries using SAMDI mass spectrometry. *ACS Combinatorial Science*, *13*(4), 347–350. DOI: 10.1021/co2000373 PMID: 21639106

Hameed, P. N., Verspoor, K., Kusljic, S., & Halgamuge, S. (2018). A two-tiered unsupervised clustering approach for drug repositioning through heterogeneous data integration. *BMC Bioinformatics*, *19*(1). Advance online publication. DOI: 10.1186/s12859-018-2123-4 PMID: 29642848

Hughes, J. P., Rees, S. S., Kalindjian, S. B., & Philpott, K. L. (2011). Principles of early drug discovery. In *British Journal of Pharmacology* (Vol. 162, Issue 6, pp. 1239–1249). https://doi.org/DOI: 10.1111/j.1476-5381.2010.01127.x

Jayatunga, K. P. M., Ayers, M., Bruens, L., Jayanth, D., & Meier, C. (2024). How successful are AI-discovered drugs in clinical trials? A first analysis and emerging lessons. In *Drug Discovery Today* (Vol. 29, Issue 6). Elsevier Ltd. https://doi.org/DOI: 10.1016/j.drudis.2024.104009

Jeddi, Z., & Bohr, A. (2020). Remote patient monitoring using artificial intelligence. In *Artificial Intelligence in Healthcare* (pp. 203–234). Elsevier., DOI: 10.1016/B978-0-12-818438-7.00009-5

Jiang, D., Wu, Z., Hsieh, C. Y., Chen, G., Liao, B., Wang, Z., Shen, C., Cao, D., Wu, J., & Hou, T. (2021). Could graph neural networks learn better molecular representation for drug discovery? A comparison study of descriptor-based and graph-based models. *Journal of Cheminformatics*, *13*(1). Advance online publication. DOI: 10.1186/s13321-020-00479-8 PMID: 33597034

Jiménez-Luna, J., Grisoni, F., Weskamp, N., & Schneider, G. (2021). Artificial intelligence in drug discovery: Recent advances and future perspectives. *Expert Opinion on Drug Discovery*, *16*(9), 949–959. DOI: 10.1080/17460441.2021.1909567 PMID: 33779453

Joshi, R. P., & Kumar, N. (2021). Artificial intelligence for autonomous molecular design: A perspective. In *Molecules* (Vol. 26, Issue 22). MDPI. https://doi.org/DOI: 10.3390/molecules26226761

Kengkanna, A., & Ohue, M. (2024). Enhancing property and activity prediction and interpretation using multiple molecular graph representations with MMGX. *Communications Chemistry*, *7*(1). Advance online publication. DOI: 10.1038/s42004-024-01155-w PMID: 38580841

Khurana, D., Koli, A., Khatter, K., & Singh, S. (2023). Natural language processing: State of the art, current trends and challenges. *Multimedia Tools and Applications*, *82*(3), 3713–3744. DOI: 10.1007/s11042-022-13428-4 PMID: 35855771

Li, Y., Liu, B., Deng, J., Guo, Y., & Du, H. (2024). Image-based molecular representation learning for drug development: A survey. *Briefings in Bioinformatics*, *25*(4). Advance online publication. DOI: 10.1093/bib/bbae294 PMID: 38920347

Lo, Y.-C., Ren, G., Honda, H., & Davis, L. K. (2020). Artificial Intelligence-Based Drug Design and Discovery. In *Cheminformatics and its Applications*. IntechOpen. https://doi.org/DOI: 10.5772/intechopen.89012

Madugula, S. S., John, L., Nagamani, S., Gaur, A. S., Poroikov, V. V., & Sastry, G. N. (2021). Molecular descriptor analysis of approved drugs using unsupervised learning for drug repurposing. *Computers in Biology and Medicine*, *138*, 104856. DOI: 10.1016/J.COMPBIOMED.2021.104856 PMID: 34555571

Maia, E. H. B., Assis, L. C., de Oliveira, T. A., da Silva, A. M., & Taranto, A. G. (2020). Structure-Based Virtual Screening: From Classical to Artificial Intelligence. In *Frontiers in Chemistry* (Vol. 8). Frontiers Media S.A. https://doi.org/DOI: 10.3389/fchem.2020.00343

Mao, J., Wang, J., Zeb, A., Cho, K. H., Jin, H., Kim, J., Lee, O., Wang, Y., & No, K. T. (2024). Transformer-Based Molecular Generative Model for Antiviral Drug Design. *Journal of Chemical Information and Modeling*, *64*(7), 2733–2745. DOI: 10.1021/acs.jcim.3c00536 PMID: 37366644

Mendolia, I., Contino, S., Perricone, U., Ardizzone, E., & Pirrone, R. (2020). Convolutional architectures for virtual screening. *BMC Bioinformatics*, *21*. Advance online publication. DOI: 10.1186/s12859-020-03645-9 PMID: 32938359

Moon, S., Zhung, W., Yang, S., Lim, J., & Kim, W. Y. (2022). PIGNet: A physics-informed deep learning model toward generalized drug-target interaction predictions. *Chemical Science (Cambridge)*, *13*(13), 3661–3673. DOI: 10.1039/d1sc06946b PMID: 35432900

Nguyen, T., Le, H., Quinn, T. P., Nguyen, T., Le, T. D., & Venkatesh, S. (2020). *GraphDTA: predicting drug-target binding affinity with graph neural networks*. https://doi.org/DOI: 10.5281/zenodo.3603523

Nhat Phuong, D., Flower, D. R., Chattopadhyay, S., & Chattopadhyay, A. K. (2023). Towards Effective Consensus Scoring in Structure-Based Virtual Screening. *Interdisciplinary Sciences, Computational Life Sciences*, *15*(1), 131–145. DOI: 10.1007/s12539-022-00546-8 PMID: 36550341

Niazi, S. K., & Mariam, Z. (2023). *Recent Advances in Machine Learning-Based Chemoinformatics: A Comprehensive Review*. https://doi.org/DOI: 10.20944/preprints202306.0803.v1

Ocana, A., Pandiella, A., Privat, C., Bravo, I., Luengo-Oroz, M., Amir, E., & Gyorffy, B. (2025). Integrating artificial intelligence in drug discovery and early drug development: a transformative approach. In *Biomarker Research* (Vol. 13, Issue 1). BioMed Central Ltd. https://doi.org/DOI: 10.1186/s40364-025-00758-2

Öztürk, H., Özgür, A., & Ozkirimli, E. (2018). DeepDTA: Deep drug-target binding affinity prediction. *Bioinformatics (Oxford, England)*, *34*(17), i821–i829. DOI: 10.1093/bioinformatics/bty593 PMID: 30423097

Pan, Y., Ren, H., Lan, L., Li, Y., & Huang, T. (2023). Review of Predicting Synergistic Drug Combinations. In *Life* (Vol. 13, Issue 9). Multidisciplinary Digital Publishing Institute (MDPI). https://doi.org/DOI: 10.3390/life13091878

Parekh, A.-D. E., & Shaikh, O. A., Simran, Manan, S., & Hasibuzzaman, Md. Al. (2023). Artificial intelligence (AI) in personalized medicine: AI-generated personalized therapy regimens based on genetic and medical history: short communication. *Annals of Medicine and Surgery (London)*, *85*(11), 5831–5833. DOI: 10.1097/ms9.0000000000001320 PMID: 37915639

Paul, A., Al-Bahrani, R., Agrawal, A., Jha, D., Liao, W.-K., & Choudhary, A. (2018). *CheMixNet: Mixed DNN Architectures for Predicting Chemical Properties using Multiple Molecular Representations*. https://github.com/paularindam/CheMixNet

Paul, D., Sanap, G., Shenoy, S., Kalyane, D., Kalia, K., & Tekade, R. K. (2021). Artificial intelligence in drug discovery and development. In *Drug Discovery Today* (Vol. 26, Issue 1, pp. 80–93). Elsevier Ltd. https://doi.org/DOI: 10.1016/j.drudis.2020.10.010

Proietti, M., Ragno, A., La Rosa, B., Ragno, R., & Capobianco, R. (2024). Explainable AI in drug discovery: Self-interpretable graph neural network for molecular property prediction using concept whitening. *Machine Learning*, *113*(4), 2013–2044. DOI: 10.1007/s10994-023-06369-y

Ren, F., Ding, X., Zheng, M., Korzinkin, M., Cai, X., Zhu, W., Mantsyzov, A., Aliper, A., Aladinskiy, V., Cao, Z., Kong, S., Long, X., Liu, B. H. M., Liu, Y., Naumov, V., Shneyderman, A., Ozerov, I. V., Wang, J., Pun, F. W., & Zhavoronkov, A. (2022). *AlphaFold Accelerates Artificial Intelligence Powered Drug Discovery: Efficient Discovery of a Novel Cyclin-dependent Kinase 20 (CDK20) Small Molecule Inhibitor*. https://arxiv.org/abs/2201.09647

Ren, F., Ding, X., Zheng, M., Korzinkin, M., Cai, X., Zhu, W., Mantsyzov, A., Aliper, A., Aladinskiy, V., Cao, Z., Kong, S., Long, X., Man Liu, B. H., Liu, Y., Naumov, V., Shneyderman, A., Ozerov, I. V., Wang, J., Pun, F. W., & Zhavoronkov, A. (2023). AlphaFold accelerates artificial intelligence powered drug discovery: Efficient discovery of a novel CDK20 small molecule inhibitor. *Chemical Science (Cambridge)*, *14*(6), 1443–1452. DOI: 10.1039/d2sc05709c PMID: 36794205

Sadybekov, A. V., & Katritch, V. (2023). Computational approaches streamlining drug discovery. *Nature*, *616*(7958), 673–685. DOI: 10.1038/s41586-023-05905-z PMID: 37100941

Saini, J. P. S., Thakur, A., & Yadav, D. (2025). AI-driven innovations in pharmaceuticals: optimizing drug discovery and industry operations. In *RSC Pharmaceutics* (Vol. 2, Issue 3, pp. 437–454). Royal Society of Chemistry. https://doi.org/DOI: 10.1039/d4pm00323c

Sampene, A. K., & Nyirenda, F. (2024). Evaluating the effect of artificial intelligence on pharmaceutical product and drug discovery in China. *Future Journal of Pharmaceutical Sciences*, *10*(1). Advance online publication. DOI: 10.1186/s43094-024-00632-2

Serrano, D. R., Luciano, F. C., Anaya, B. J., Ongoren, B., Kara, A., Molina, G., Ramirez, B. I., Sánchez-Guirales, S. A., Simon, J. A., Tomietto, G., Rapti, C., Ruiz, H. K., Rawat, S., Kumar, D., & Lalatsa, A. (2024). Artificial Intelligence (AI) Applications in Drug Discovery and Drug Delivery: Revolutionizing Personalized Medicine. In *Pharmaceutics* (Vol. 16, Issue 10). Multidisciplinary Digital Publishing Institute (MDPI). https://doi.org/DOI: 10.3390/pharmaceutics16101328

Shamim, M. A., Shamim, M. A., Arora, P., & Dwivedi, P. (2024). Artificial intelligence and big data for pharmacovigilance and patient safety. *Journal of Medicine, Surgery, and Public Health*, *3*, 100139. DOI: 10.1016/j.glmedi.2024.100139

Sharma, S., Chaubey, A., Pathan, M. N., & Tyagi, S. (2024). AI-powered virtual screening for drug discovery: Methods and challenges. *International Journal of Pharmacy and Pharmaceutical Sciences*, *6*(2), 157–164. DOI: 10.33545/26647222.2024.v6.i2b.136

Singh, A. (2024). Artificial intelligence for drug repurposing against infectious diseases. *Artificial Intelligence Chemistry.*, *2*(2), 100071. DOI: 10.1016/j.aichem.2024.100071

Singh, S., Gupta, H., Sharma, P., & Sahi, S. (2024). Advances in Artificial Intelligence (AI)-assisted approaches in drug screening. *Artificial Intelligence Chemistry.*, *2*(1), 100039. DOI: 10.1016/j.aichem.2023.100039

Stokes, J. M., Yang, K., Swanson, K., Jin, W., Cubillos-Ruiz, A., Donghia, N. M., MacNair, C. R., French, S., Carfrae, L. A., Bloom-Ackerman, Z., Tran, V. M., Chiappino-Pepe, A., Badran, A. H., Andrews, I. W., Chory, E. J., Church, G. M., Brown, E. D., Jaakkola, T. S., Barzilay, R., & Collins, J. J. (2020). A Deep Learning Approach to Antibiotic Discovery. *Cell*, *180*(4), 688–702.e13. DOI: 10.1016/j.cell.2020.01.021 PMID: 32084340

Sun, D., Gao, W., Hu, H., & Zhou, S. (2022). Why 90% of clinical drug development fails and how to improve it? In *Acta Pharmaceutica Sinica B* (Vol. 12, Issue 7, pp. 3049–3062). Chinese Academy of Medical Sciences. https://doi.org/DOI: 10.1016/j.apsb.2022.02.002

Taherdoost, H., & Ghofrani, A. (2024). AI's role in revolutionizing personalized medicine by reshaping pharmacogenomics and drug therapy. In *Intelligent Pharmacy* (Vol. 2, Issue 5, pp. 643–650). KeAi Publishing Communications Ltd. https://doi.org/DOI: 10.1016/j.ipha.2024.08.005

Tetko, I. V., & Clevert, D. A. (2025). Advanced machine learning for innovative drug discovery. In *Journal of Cheminformatics* (Vol. 17, Issue 1). BioMed Central Ltd. https://doi.org/DOI: 10.1186/s13321-025-01061-w

Thaingtamtanha, T., Ravichandran, R., & Gentile, F. (2025). On the application of artificial intelligence in virtual screening. *Expert Opinion on Drug Discovery, 20*. Advance online publication. DOI: 10.1080/17460441.2025.2508866 PMID: 40388244

Tripathi, M. K., Nath, A., Singh, T. P., Ethayathulla, A. S., & Kaur, P. (2021). Evolving scenario of big data and Artificial Intelligence (AI) in drug discovery. *Molecular Diversity, 25*(3), 1439–1460. DOI: 10.1007/s11030-021-10256-w PMID: 34159484

Vamathevan, J., Clark, D., Czodrowski, P., Dunham, I., Ferran, E., Lee, G., Li, B., Madabhushi, A., Shah, P., Spitzer, M., & Zhao, S. (2019). Applications of machine learning in drug discovery and development. In *Nature Reviews Drug Discovery* (Vol. 18, Issue 6, pp. 463–477). Nature Publishing Group. https://doi.org/DOI: 10.1038/s41573-019-0024-5

Wang, W. (2024). *AI Based Drug Screening Process: From Data Mining to Candidate Drug Validation*. Bioscience Methods., DOI: 10.5376/bm.2024.15.0005

Wang, Y., Li, Z., & Farimani, A. B. (2023). *Graph Neural Networks for Molecules*. https://doi.org/DOI: 10.1007/978-3-031-37196-7_2

Wang, Y., Zhao, H., Sciabola, S., & Wang, W. (2023). cMolGPT: A Conditional Generative Pre-Trained Transformer for Target-Specific De Novo Molecular Generation. *Molecules (Basel, Switzerland), 28*(11). Advance online publication. DOI: 10.3390/molecules28114430 PMID: 37298906

Wei, F., Wang, S., & Gou, X. (2021). A review for cell-based screening methods in drug discovery. In *Biophysics Reports* (Vol. 7, Issue 6, pp. 504–516). Science Press. https://doi.org/DOI: 10.52601/bpr.2021.210042

Wieder, O., Kohlbacher, S., Kuenemann, M., Garon, A., Ducrot, P., Seidel, T., & Langer, T. (2020). A compact review of molecular property prediction with graph neural networks. *Drug Discovery Today. Technologies*, *37*, 1–12. DOI: 10.1016/J.DDTEC.2020.11.009 PMID: 34895648

Wigh, D. S., Goodman, J. M., & Lapkin, A. A. (2022). A review of molecular representation in the age of machine learning. In *Wiley Interdisciplinary Reviews: Computational Molecular Science* (Vol. 12, Issue 5). John Wiley and Sons Inc. https://doi.org/DOI: 10.1002/wcms.1603

Xiao, M., Zheng, Q., Popa, P., Mi, X., Hu, J., Zou, F., & Zou, B. (2025). Drug molecular representations for drug response predictions: A comprehensive investigation via machine learning methods. *Scientific Reports*, *15*(1). Advance online publication. DOI: 10.1038/s41598-024-84711-7 PMID: 39748003

Zhavoronkov, A., Ivanenkov, Y. A., Aliper, A., Veselov, M. S., Aladinskiy, V. A., Aladinskaya, A. V., Terentiev, V. A., Polykovskiy, D. A., Kuznetsov, M. D., Asadulaev, A., Volkov, Y., Zholus, A., Shayakhmetov, R. R., Zhebrak, A., Minaeva, L. I., Zagribelnyy, B. A., Lee, L. H., Soll, R., Madge, D., & Aspuru-Guzik, A. (2019). Deep learning enables rapid identification of potent DDR1 kinase inhibitors. *Nature Biotechnology*, *37*(9), 1038–1040. DOI: 10.1038/s41587-019-0224-x PMID: 31477924

Chapter 4
AI-Driven Drug Development in Immunological Disorders

Balaji Esakkimuthu
Sudha Hospital, India

Manoj Mani
https://orcid.org/0009-0008-6601-0339
Bharathiar University, India

Prabakaran Dhashnamoorthy Subramanian
SRM Institute of Science and Technology, India

Balamuralikrishnan Balasubramanian
Sejong University, India

Alwin Robert Asirvatham
Prince Sultan Military Medical City, Saudi Arabia

Antony Prabhu Jeyabal Philomenathan
Bharathiar University, India

Velayuthaprabhu Shanmugam
Bharathiar University, India

Vijaya Anand Arumugam
https://orcid.org/0000-0001-7485-1586
Bharathiar University, India

ABSTRACT

AI will revolutionize the process of drug development for immunological disorders by enhancing efficiency, precision, and scalability with discovery pipelines. AI-based models combine genomics, transcriptomics, and proteomics to identify targets, optimize drug design, and speed up immunotherapy. Machine learning and deep learning algorithms enable virtual screening, molecular docking, and immune pathways modelling with improved predictive performance and reduced costs. Generative AI and GNNs enable de novo design of immunomodulatory molecules, while XAI improves interpretability and compliance with regulatory policy. Coupling with digital twins and multi-omics frameworks allow real-time modelling of immune dynamics and

DOI: 10.4018/979-8-3373-5258-9.ch004

further advance immunotherapy. Ethical, regulatory, and translational considerations, leveraging data privacy, bias in algorithms, and sustainability, are critical for responsible implementation. Altogether, AI-driven strategies are transforming immunopharmacology to promote data-driven therapeutics, improve outcomes, and redefine paradigms in drug discovery.

1. INTRODUCTION

The global landscape of immunological disorders, especially autoimmune diseases and chronic inflammatory conditions, represents one of the major biomedical and clinical challenges characterized by increasing incidence, complex pathogenesis, and enormous unmet therapeutic needs (Velayuthaprabhu & Archunan, 2005; Velayuthaprabhu *et al.,* 2007; Alagendran *et al.,* 2010; Velayuthaprabhu *et al.,* 2011; Shanmugam Velayuthaprabhu *et al.,* 2013; Velayuthaprabhu *et al.,* 2016; Bhotla *et al.,* 2020; Meyyazhagan *et al.,* 2020; Arumugam *et al.,* 2020; Mohd *et al.,* 2021; Bhotla *et al.,* 2021; Mohd *et al.,* 2021; Lee *et al.,* 2021; Pushparaj *et al.,* 2022; Sangeetha *et al.,* 2022; Gundappa *et al.,* 2022; Sangeetha *et al.,* 2022; Meyyazhagan *et al.,* 2022; Ramya *et al.,* 2023; Paranitharan *et al.,* 2025). Autoimmune diseases affect almost 10% of the global population and are caused by abnormal immune activation against self-antigens, leading to chronic inflammation and multi-system dysfunction (Song *et al.,* 2025b). Likewise, chronic inflammatory diseases (CIDs), including psoriasis, inflammatory bowel disease (IBD), and rheumatoid arthritis, also burden healthcare systems worldwide (Adebanjo *et al.,* 2023). The underlying pathophysiology of these disorders involves interactions among genetic predispositions, environmental triggers, and dysregulated immune signalling pathways (Imetkul *et al.,* 2025). While there has been great progress in elucidation of disease mechanisms and therapeutic development over the years, formidable challenges still lie ahead for early diagnosis, stratification of disease subtypes, and management of rare inflammatory etiologies (Ujiie *et al.,* 2022).

The current therapeutic options range from broad-spectrum anti-inflammatory agents to molecular-targeted drugs and newer cellular therapies. These, however, are often limited by adverse effects, variable clinical responses, and limited long-term efficacy. Thus, immunotherapy has emerged as a paradigm in the management of CIDs through modulation of dysregulated immune networks underlying these pathologies. However, translation at the clinical level is still restricted due to several limitations regarding biomarker identification, therapeutic specificity, and method of delivery. Identification and characterization of key molecular pathways and predictive biomarkers are further important in this context to enable precision-based intervention with improved, patient-specific treatment outcomes (Fernandez *et al.,* 2024).

Artificial intelligence (AI) has added a whole new, transformative dimension to immunopharmacology by overcoming most of the limitations associated with traditional approaches to drug development. Classic drug development pipelines are long and resource-intensive, classically consisting of extensive preclinical testing, hit identification, lead optimization, and candidate selection, with poor successful rates in clinical translation (Chen *et al.,* 2023a; Singh *et al.,* 2024). AI-driven methods, however, using machine learning (ML), deep learning (DL), and large-scale data analytics, provide a much more agile, accurate, and cost-effective framework for the discovery of therapies. These computational tools have amplified several aspects of drug development, including target identification, virtual screening, molecular docking, and pathway network analysis, by enhancing the precision and throughput of discovery workflows (Bijral *et al.,* 2022).

The AI-powered platforms, for example, Drug Design and Discovery System (AI-D3S), have shown better predictive capabilities in drug-target interaction modelling, obtaining an average improvement of 8.7% in accuracy, precision, sensitivity, and specificity, amongst others, comparing conventional methodologies. In addition, it integrates multi-omics data together with real-world clinical evidence into AI to optimize personalized medicine at the single therapeutic regimen level, hence having enormous potential for translational healthcare applications (Pandey *et al.,* 2024). These works underpin that AI plays an increasingly important role in accelerating immunology-centered drug discovery and development. AI-driven models, amongst them graph neural networks and generative algorithms, are of particular efficient in de novo molecular design and molecular docking simulations, therefore offering a conceptual and data-driven route toward next-generation immunotherapies (Martinelli *et al.,* 2024; Gupta *et al.,* 2024; Hassan & Mohammed, 2024).

2. THE IMMUNOLOGICAL COMPLEXITY IN DRUG DISCOVERY

Molecular and cellular mechanisms of immune regulation represent the foundation for drug target discovery, especially in immune-mediated and inflammatory diseases. Recent advances in both phenotypic and target-based drug discovery have emphasized the need to integrate computational modelling with multi-omics platforms to enhance therapeutic precision and evade resistance mechanisms in immune therapeutics (Vázquez *et al.,* 2025). The identification of disease-associated cells (DACs) and disease-associated genes (DAGs) by using integrative frameworks, such as the Disease-gene IMmune cell Expression (DIME) network, has shed light on shared immunopathogenic pathways across immune-mediated inflammatory diseases (IMIDs), therefore offering valuable opportunities for drug repurposing (Devaprasad *et al.,* 2021). Cellular and molecular regulators, including cytokines, chemokines, and intracellular signalling cascades, participate at the level of priming and propagation of immune dysregulation, thereby representing key molecular entry points for precision-targeted interventions (Elemam *et al.,* 2025). Genome-wide association studies and proteomic profiling have further refined the understanding of the complexity in autoimmune disease by identifying specific signalling nodes, including NOD2 and IL-23 receptor pathways in Crohn's disease and interferon-regulated gene networks in systemic lupus erythematosus (SLE), as promising drug targets (Chan, 2008). In addition, complex interplays between genetic predisposition, environmental exposure, and age-related immune remodelling all influence immune dysregulation and need to be addressed in developing targeted and durable therapies (Fernandez *et al.,* 2024).

Computational and bioinformatic tools have considerably accelerated the identification of immunological targets such as cytokines, immune checkpoints, and antigen-specific receptors on T and B cells. The integration of immunology with systems biology and computational modelling underlies the field of immuno-informatics, which plays an instrumental role in epitope prediction, immune response simulation, and vaccine design (Kushwaha *et al.,* 2024). Identification of novel immunotherapeutic targets by mapping cell-cell interactions in immune-oncological contexts is possible through advanced methodologies including intercellular CRISPR screening. Such high-throughput screens revealed key immune modulatory interactions such as PD-1/PD-L1 signalling in immune evasion and tumor clearance and identified candidate targets that could not be detected when analyzing a single cell type (Yim *et al.,* 2022). Cheminformatics and bioinformatics pipelines further enable the rational design of inhibitors of PD-1/PD-L1 interaction, catering to the need for better checkpoint modulators and predictive biomarkers in cancer immunotherapy (Sobral *et al.,* 2023). Computational target discovery platforms like IMMUNOTAR further enhance the use of integrating transcriptomic or proteomic datasets with quantitative molecular features to prioritize druggable surface proteins of relevance to immune modulation (Shraim *et al.,* 2025). This growth in computational immunology, resting on extensive biological databases, has significantly enhanced modelling of immune mechanisms such as peptide transport and T-cell receptor interactions, accelerating immunological research and therapeutic innovation (Petrovsky & Brusic, 2002).

The steadily growing application of systems immunology and network biology has revolutionized immune system complexity in conceptualization within drug discovery paradigms. These approaches provide the integration of multi-omics data, mechanistic models, and AI to establish emergent properties and nonlinear dynamics of the immune networks, crucial to biomarker identification, optimization of therapy, and rational drug design (Alfonso-González *et al.,* 2025). Systems biology frameworks take advantage of experimental and computational integration in order to detail system-level interactions that enable identification of drug targets, mechanisms of action, and off-target effects, thus improving efficiency in discovery while reducing the cost involved (Sumit & Dhara, 2025). Network systems biology extends these methodologies by modelling disease-altered networks through integration of high-throughput data that facilitates validation of drug–target interactions and enhances efficacy and safety predictions (Arrell & Terzic, 2010). The immune system involves interactions between more than 1,500 genes and proteins; for this reason, a system approach is important in understanding immune behavior. Protein–protein interaction (PPI) networks are one of the central frameworks for the analysis, integrating multi-omics data to expose key nodes and pathways that play critical roles in the regulation of immune responses (Dhillon *et al.,* 2020). Furthermore, the immune system exhibits dynamic, multiscale organization through nonlinear and context-dependent interactions, although the predictive power of network biology allows the reconstruction of intricate regulatory circuits and the development of computational tools to predict the consequences of immune perturbations (Subramanian *et al.,* 2015).

3. AI IN TARGET IDENTIFICATION AND VALIDATION

The merging of multi-omics information—consisting of genomics, transcriptomics, and proteomics—with AI is revolutionizing the discovery and validation of immune targets and the characterization of complex immune environments with unprecedented precision. High-dimensional data integration via AI tools predicts distinct immune signatures and disease-specific biomarkers for early diagnosis and bespoke therapy in cancer, autoimmune, and infectious diseases (Chinedu-Nzereogu *et al.,* 2025). AI in vaccine design accelerates epitope mapping and antigen prioritization for the therapy of immunologically deficient and antigenically variable disorders (Tavare *et al.,* 2025). Large language models (LLMs) also facilitate biomarker discovery by integrating heterogeneous omics datasets, increasing gene selection robustness and explainability (Park & Lee, 2025). The CLIC1 case, being one of the targets identified by multi-omics and network-based AI analysis, is an example of the capacity of such systems to identify invariably dysregulated molecules participating in cancer and neuroinflammatory pathologies (Badhe, 2025).

Immune heterogeneity in tumor microenvironments (TMEs) has been revolutionized by single-cell and spatial transcriptomics with the assistance of AI. Single-cell RNA sequencing enables cellular-level high-resolution analysis of mRNA expression and demonstrates immune infiltrate heterogeneity and how this aid in the modulation of responses to immune checkpoint inhibitors (ICIs) (Liu *et al.,* 2024).

Spatial transcriptomics gives spatial information, where the spatial patterning and interactions between tumor and immune cells occur. Generative AI models such as CellClique replicate cell-neighborhood interactions and gene expression patterns, defining immune invasion patterns in lung and colon cancer (Weerasekara *et al.*, 2025). The single-cell tumor immune atlas of over 500,000 cells has refined immune cell classification and patient stratification for immunotherapy (Nieto *et al.*, 2021). Complementary technologies like SpatialTME integrate histological imaging and spatial transcriptomics to reveal intercellular communication networks that impact tumor development and treatment response (Shi *et al.*, 2024).

DL algorithms have greatly enhanced antigen–receptor interaction prediction plays a central role in adaptive immunity. Tools such as pMTnet apply transfer learning to predict TCR binding to neoantigens presented by MHC class I molecules, confirming that neoantigens are generally more immunogenic than self-antigens—findings essential for cancer immunotherapy (Lu *et al.*, 2021). TCRfinder employs tailored language models to improve TCR–peptide binding prediction, whereby it achieves a 50% improved accuracy in identifying tumor-specific neoantigens (Li *et al.*, 2024b). DeepTCR and DeepAIR employ DL to recognize sequence motifs and structural determinants associated with immunotherapy outcome and immune disorder susceptibility (Sidhom *et al.*, 2022; Zhao *et al.*, 2023). Similarly, TCRconv, which is a deep protein language model-based, makes predictions for TCR–epitope interactions and provides mechanistic explanations of T-cell dynamics in infections such as COVID-19 (Jokinen *et al.*, 2023).

Graph Neural Networks (GNNs) have emerged as key modelling agents for cytokine signalling and immune regulatory networks. Their graph architecture enables the encoding of complex molecular interactions and cell-to-cell interactions that are out of the bounds of regular ML. GNNs proved superior in HLA–peptide interaction modelling with improved predictive accuracy of immune response compared to Convolutional and Feed Forward Networks (Sakhamuri *et al.*, 2023). They have also been employed to study innate immune signalling during viral infections such as COVID-19, accurately mimicking interaction between pathogen-associated molecular pattern (PAMP) and pattern recognition receptor (PRR) interactions with crucial implications for vaccine design (Henna, 2021). Integrative platforms such as GRNIX combine GNN-based inference with explainable AI (XAI) to reverse-engineer autoimmune disease gene regulatory networks, enhancing mechanistic insight and target prioritization (Mortadha, 2024).

4. AI IN DRUG DESIGN, OPTIMIZATION, AND DISCOVERY

AI generative models such as Generative Adversarial Networks (GANs), Variational Autoencoders (VAEs), and Diffusion Models are transforming the landscape of immunomodulatory drug discovery by making de novo molecular design possible with complex chemical–biological data representations. These models obtain underlying patterns of molecules from high-volume datasets to design novel compounds with maximum specificity for known biological targets, speeding up the early steps of drug discovery (Das, 2025; Robert *et al.,* 2025). Their integration with multiomics datasets facilitates attaining rational design of small molecules, peptides, and biologics with best-in-class potency, selectivity, and pharmacokinetic–toxicological (ADME/Tox) profiles that are all key parameters for immunomodulatory therapies (Das, 2025). Among these, diffusion models have proven particular utility for optimizing many molecular properties concurrently, with the assurance that the resulting compounds are chemically valid and functionally relevant (Guo *et al.,* 2024). Moreover, combinations of reinforcement learning and GNNs in generative models have enabled iterative optimization of lead compounds to optimize their drug-likeness and reduce the gap between in silico predictions and experimental reality (Das, 2025; Khater *et al.,* 2025). Problems with predictive accuracy, molecular validity, and optimization robustness, remain to challenge current methods, calling for further model development and interpretability (Khater *et al.,* 2025). The convergence of generative AI with predictive analytics and high-throughput screening platforms further accelerates discovery pipelines, providing a data-efficient and scalable approach to next-generation immunomodulatory drug design (Robert *et al.,* 2025; Das, 2025).

Simultaneous DL–based breakthroughs in protein modelling have revolutionized antibody and biologic drug design, particularly through accurate sequence-to-structure prediction tools such as AlphaFold3 and RoseTTAFold. The integration of AlphaFold3 into domain-specific architectures like AntiBMPNN has achieved greater sequence recovery rates and improved binding affinities within complementarity-determining regions (CDRs) over classical models (Sun *et al.,* 2025). While RoseTTAFold does not achieve atomic-level accuracy, it exhibits great prowess for predicting antibody tertiary structures, for example, the structurally variable H3 loop, and is comparable to homology-based tools like SWISS-MODEL. Similarly, HelixFold-Multimer, a derivative of AlphaFold-Multimer, improves antigen–antibody complex prediction accuracy, boosting epitope–paratope interface resolution essential in therapeutic antibody design optimization (Gao *et al.,* 2024). In contrast to the drawbacks of scant immune protein structural datasets and the inadequacy of similar sequences, ImmuneFold applies transfer learning and LLMs to accurately predict immune protein conformations, surpassing traditional computational approaches (Zhang *et al.,* 2025a).

Coupled with these developments, the AI-driven optimization of Chimeric Antigen Receptor (CAR) T-cell receptor design focuses on improving antigen specificity and mitigating off-target toxicity by using integrated computational and learning-based strategies. Specifically, computational modelling has been central to refining CAR-T receptors targeting CD19, a stable antigen in B-cell malignancies (Krishnan *et al.,* 2025). Bioinformatic techniques, such as PSI-BLAST–based sequence validation, molecular docking, and ML–based toxicity prediction, thus allow the design of peptide-based CAR constructs with enhanced selectivity and resilience to antigenic drift. Such strategies provide the identification of optimized single-chain variable fragments with high binding affinity and stability, reducing immunotoxicity and antigen escape. Beyond monovalent targeting, AI frameworks now support the design of multi-antigen CAR receptors and optimization of dosing regimens via reinforcement learning, therefore enhancing therapeutic precision (Shahzadi *et al.,* 2024). Furthermore, multimodal antigen discovery and structural modelling are integrated on computational platforms like AI CAR Loop 1.0 to expedite CAR-T design and reduce development costs substantially while improving antigen specificity. However, data heterogeneity and ethical constraints remain some of the important considerations for translational implementation of AI-guided CAR-T engineering (Hu, 2025).

In parallel, ML models have become indispensable for predicting ADMET properties and immunogenicity of novel immune-targeted drugs, thus complementing traditional experimental workflows. The SMILES-Mamba model employs a two-stage self-supervised learning framework: first pretraining on unlabeled SMILES strings and then fine-tuning on the labeled datasets, attaining high performance across multiple ADMET prediction tasks with minimal dependence on extensive annotated data (Xu et al. 2024). On the other hand, MTAN-ADMET uses a Multi-Task Adaptive Network for ADMET parameter prediction directly from molecular representation with effective handling of data sparsity and imbalance, achieving robustness in accuracy in challenging endpoints such as cardiotoxicity (Shahid et al. 2025). Regarding immunogenicity assessment, in silico methods exploiting sequence alignment, MHC-binding motif analysis, and ML-driven epitope prediction have been instrumental in early therapeutic evaluation (Doneva *et al.,* 2021). ImmunoSeq is an interpretable model to analyze k-mer peptide libraries, allowing the identification of immunogenic hotspots important for antibody optimization (Huang *et al.,* 2025), whereas AbImmPred integrates AntiBERTy-derived sequence embeddings, enhancing the accuracy of immunogenicity prediction in supporting risk mitigation in antibody development (Wang et al. 2024a).

5. AI-ENABLED IMMUNOTHERAPY AND VACCINE DEVELOPMENT

Recently, transformer-based DL approaches have become an indispensable tool in the most critical tasks involved in designing and optimizing immunotherapies, namely, the prediction of antigen-antibody interactions (**Figure 1**). ABTrans is just such an example. It achieved fantastic performance in predicting the interaction between anti-Aβ antibodies and peptides by identifying four different binding affinity levels with an accuracy of 0.8278. This provides the basis for the exact elucidation of off-target effects and antibody cross-reactivity-two of the most important factors in the engineering of therapeutic antibodies (Su *et al.,* 2025). Parallel to this, HLAIIPred uses a Transformer-based framework for predicting peptide presentation by HLA class II molecules. Indeed, it can improve identification performance of the immunogenic peptides by 16%, along with a 3% boost in the precision-recall curve compared to the currently available algorithms (Haghighatlari *et al.,* 2025). On that note, TransfIGN integrates structural information into the prediction of HLA-A*02:01-antigen peptide interaction and outperforms sequence-based methods, providing structural insights into the molecular basis of peptide binding (Hong *et al.,* 2024). Meanwhile, BConformeR utilizes Transformer networks in the prediction of continuous and discontinuous antibody epitopes, yielding superior performance in the prediction of conformational epitopes (You *et al.,* 2025). More recently, another Transformer-based model for peptide-HLA binding affinity prediction was developed, with the capability of performing robustly with variable-length peptide inputs- a key capability toward its applications in cancer immunotherapy (Yang *et al.,* 2023).

Figure 1. AI-Driven Antibody and Biologic Design Workflow

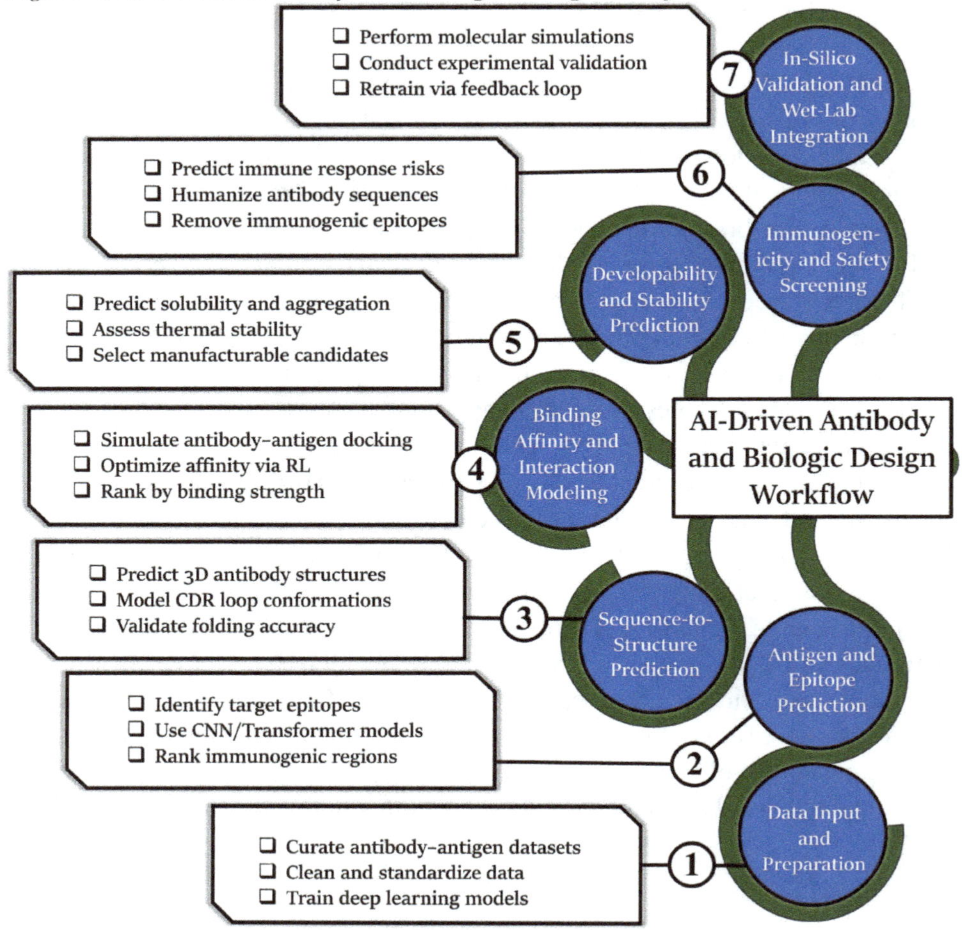

While the vast number of AI-driven computational methodologies has significantly hastened the process of discovery and optimization of ICIs targeting PD-1 and CTLA-4, the reverse has been partly true. The successful identification of small-molecule CTLA-4 inhibitors by means of virtual screening strategies followed by validation in biochemical and animal models showed strong antitumor activity (Sobhani *et al.*, 2024). Similarly, cyclic peptides capable of binding to CTLA-4, computationally designed, showed tumor growth inhibition in murine models. In relation to the blockade of PD-1/PD-L1, ML-based screening methods have identified promising small-molecule inhibitors that complement antibody-based therapies (Thakkar *et al.*, 2023; Patil *et al.*, 2022). Molecular docking and molecular dynamics simulations have been integral in guiding the rational design of next-generation ICIs through the elucidation of protein-protein interaction landscapes. Further refinement of the antibody-checkpoint binding interface through structural and mutational analyses has thus enabled enhanced binding affinities and therefore has the potential to improve therapeutic efficacy (Vo *et al.,* 2023).

DL has further transformed neoantigen prediction in vaccine design and personalized immunotherapy. Deep Antigen Sets (DAS) is considered one of the main approaches, given that it models patient-level immune responses in a bid to identify clinically relevant neoantigens. This architecture leverages a permutation-invariant design that achieves superior recovery of validated neoantigens and improves clinical response outcome predictions (Chatzianastasis *et al.,* 2025). The improvement in neoantigen prediction in gastric cancer via NUCC models further enhances personalized neoantigen nano vaccine (PNVAC) platform design (Xin *et al.,* 2024). Incorporation of GAN-like models-the SIGANEO framework-has refined the accuracy of the prediction, especially in a clinical setting that requires antigen selection with high confidence for vaccine synthesis (Ye *et al.,* 2023). Advancement in DL thus has also allowed for the optimization of mRNA-based cancer vaccines that address tumor heterogeneity and neoantigen variability with views to optimize vaccine formulation and delivery (Ismail & Barakat, 2025). Overall, the identification of neoantigens arising from somatic mutations through AI and bioinformatic-driven methodologies has facilitated precision-tailored therapeutic vaccines.

AI-assisted strategies subsequently redefined the discovery and optimization of vaccine adjuvants against autoimmune and infectious diseases. ML and DK models predict immune responses, prioritize antigen candidates, and identify adjuvants that enhance immunogenicity from large-scale analyses of genomic, proteomic, and immunological datasets (Olawade *et al.,* 2024). Beyond infectious diseases, AI methodologies support epitope mapping and identification of distinct immune response profiles, enabling disease-specific vaccine formulation in autoimmunity (Tavare *et al.,* 2025). Computer-aided design approaches identified new broad-spectrum adjuvants targeting toll-like receptors (TLRs) that enhance dendritic cell activation and antigen presentation, processes necessary for the induction of robust adaptive immune responses. Preclinical studies have shown such AI-derived adjuvants capable of suppressing tumor growth and metastasis, underlining their potential in cancer vaccine development (Ma *et al.,* 2023). However, challenges such as heterogeneity, model interpretability, and ethical issues on data privacy and algorithmic bias, to name but a few, raise the need for interdisciplinary collaboration with regulatory harmonization to ensure that AI is responsibly and effectively used in immunotherapy and vaccine innovation (Asediya *et al.,* 2024).

6. AI IN DRUG REPURPOSING FOR IMMUNOLOGICAL DISORDERS

AI-driven drug repurposing represents a paradigm shift in the management of immunological disorders, leveraging transcriptomic, proteomic, and clinical data to identify novel therapeutic candidates. By integrating ML and DL frameworks, these approaches enable the discovery of biomarkers, prediction of disease flares, and optimization of personalized treatment regimens (Mane *et al.,* 2024; Afzal *et al.,* 2024). AI-enabled repurposing significantly accelerates the identification of existing drugs with new therapeutic applications, thereby reducing both time and cost compared to conventional drug development pipelines (Yadav *et al.,* 2025). For instance, transcriptomic meta-analyses of patients with systemic autoimmune disorders—such as scleroderma, SLE, and Sjogren's syndrome—have identified six small-molecule candidates, including KU-0063794 and YM-155, which target the PI3K/AKT signalling pathway, a key axis implicated in autoimmune pathophysiology (Oktem & Yazar, 2022). Similarly, network-based strategies have pinpointed novel SLE treatments through the modulation of aberrant monocyte gene expression, particularly via inhibitors of the NF-κB pathway and compounds acting on the Pim-1/NFATc1/NLRP3 signalling axis (Nikolakis *et al.,* 2023).

The integration of Electronic Health Records (EHR) with ML methodologies has further advanced immune-related drug repositioning by exploiting large-scale, patient-level temporal datasets. The Continuous Self-controlled Case Series (CSCCS) model exemplifies this integration, identifying candidate drugs capable of modulating physiological parameters, such as fasting glucose, which may serve as proxies for immune dysfunctions (Kuang *et al.,* 2016). Likewise, the iDrug model employs cross-network embedding to link drugs, targets, and diseases, enhancing the transfer of pharmacological knowledge and improving drug-target prediction performance (Chen *et al.,* 2020). Complementing these, the BioHNCFR model integrates multiple data modalities through a hybrid neural collaborative filtering framework, yielding high-accuracy predictions of drug-disease associations, including those relevant to immune modulation (Yuan *et al.,* 2020). Moreover, semantic knowledge graph–based approaches have demonstrated the potential of structured biological and textual data integration to uncover unmapped drug indications, providing a robust framework for immune-related drug repositioning (Singh & Negi, 2019).

Network-based AI models further strengthen drug repurposing for inflammatory and autoimmune diseases such as rheumatoid arthritis, lupus, and psoriasis. These models utilize systems-level analyses incorporating gene interaction networks, disease-gene associations, and drug-target relationships to prioritize therapeutic agents that target pro-inflammatory mediators such as TNF-α and IL-6. In silico techniques, including molecular docking and virtual screening, complement these models by validating binding affinities and predicting drug-target stability. The TxGNN model, a graph foundation architecture, exemplifies this advancement by integrating GNNs and metric learning to enhance indication prediction accuracy, with its Explainer module providing interpretability of predictive mechanisms (Enni & Maraj, 2022; Hickey *et al.,* 2022). Similarly, network medicine tools reveal gene and protein interaction overlaps between diseases and drugs, facilitating the identification of repurposing opportunities with cross-disease applicability and clinical relevance (Huang *et al.,* 2024; Pierini *et al.,* 2024).

AI is also slated to play a transformative role in pharmacovigilance and real-world evidence analysis, particularly for immunomodulatory agents. Traditional systems of pharmacovigilance are hampered by underreporting and delays in signal detection, while AI-driven platforms employ ML, DL, and natural language processing to automate the monitoring and risk assessment of adverse drug reactions (ADR) (Algarvio *et al.,* 2025; Upadhyay *et al.,* 2024; Alex, 2024). By mining heterogeneous data sources-including EHRs, clinical notes, medical literature, and social media-AI strengthens real-time ADR detection and refines drug safety profiles (Upadhyay *et al.,* 2024; Komi *et al.,* 2025). Integration of expert-defined Bayesian networks further optimizes causality evaluation and enhances reliability, thereby reducing analytical latency (Algarvio *et al.,* 2025). Despite this fact, persistent challenges related to data quality, algorithmic transparency, and regulatory compliance raise the pressing need for harmonized standards and collaboration among AI developers, clinicians, and regulatory authorities to ensure ethical and reproducible AI implementation in immunopharmacovigilance (Upadhyay *et al.,* 2024; Komi *et al.,* 2025).

7. AI IN PREDICTIVE TOXICOLOGY AND IMMUNOSAFETY

ML and AI have come to the forefront as powerful tools in predictive toxicology and immunosafety, especially for modelling cytokine storms, immunotoxicity, and adverse immune responses associated with therapeutic interventions. In the specific case of COVID-19, where cytokine storms represent a major cause of mortality, ML algorithms have been used to identify multi-target drugs capable of modulating key pro-inflammatory signalling pathways. Predictive models having a focus on such targets as AT1R, ADAM17, NF-κB, JAK1, and STAT3 led to Mitomycin C identification, which exhibits potent multi-protein inhibitory activity against it (Gantla *et al.,* 2023). Similarly, ML-driven screening approaches revealed the potential for glecaprevir as an effective multi-cytokine inhibitor targeting TNF-α, IL-2, and IL-6 by yielding high confidence scores, further underlining the potential of single-drug modulation of complex inflammatory cascades (Hou *et al.,* 2022). Besides infectious diseases, ML-based toxicity prediction models have been used to predict a drug-induced immune thrombocytopenia (DITP)-a severe immune-mediated adverse reaction. For example, the RDMD + PubChem-k-NN model gave high accuracy in ranking chemicals associated with DITP toxicity, therefore supporting safer drug design and preclinical screening of drugs (Wang *et al.,* 2022a). More recently, in CAR-T cell therapy, ML algorithms were applied to detect cytokine release syndrome (CRS) through the analysis of patient cytokine profiles; they provide interpretable and actionable predictions to assist in early diagnostics and management of CRS (Bogatu *et al.,* 2022).

Building on predictive immunotoxicology, AI and causal inference frameworks are increasingly applied to forecast immune-related adverse events arising from ICI therapies in oncology. These approaches integrate multimodal datasets, encompassing clinical, biochemical, and proteomic features to enhance predictive accuracy and clinical relevance. For instance, Song et al. showed that combining serum proteomics with clinical parameters using ML models such as XGBoost and HistGradientBoosting improved the prediction of irAE in NSCLC patients, yielding AUC values between 0.556 and 0.75 (Song *et al.,* 2025a). Analogously, Zhang et al. applied gradient boosting models in cohorts of NSCLC and melanoma, identifying predictive variables such as baseline health metrics and treatment regimens, with an AUROC of 0.75 (Zhang *et al.,* 2023b). Notably, their reliance on correlation-based analyses signifies a very important methodological limitation, pointing out the relevance of integrating causal ML models. Targeted-BEHRT and CIMLA are two notable frameworks developed to improve interpretability and guarantee mechanistic insights into the causes of irAEs (Wang *et al.,* 2025). In a complementary direction, Iivanainen et al. illustrated the effectiveness of ePRO integrated with ML algorithms for monitoring irAE; this approach has reached high predictive accuracy and real-time clinical decision support (Iivanainen *et al.,* 2021). More recently, Wang et al. used a Bernoulli Naive Bayes classifier to predict irAE in melanoma, identifying eosinophil count and combination therapies as significant predictors (Wang *et al.,* 2023).

Another important dimension of AI-driven immunosafety is represented by the development of in-silico immune modelling frameworks based on systems immunology. Systems immunology integrates high-throughput molecular data and computational modelling to capture the dynamic complexity of immune networks, thus enabling a mechanistic understanding of hypersensitivity reactions (Narang *et al.,* 2012; Kidd & Dudley, 2015). For example, one might mention network pharmacology and QSP, approaches that facilitate the simulation of emergent behaviors of the immune system, biomarker identification, and therapeutic optimization (Alfonso-González *et al.,* 2025). For example, skin sensitization processes have been simulated by in-silico models in order to quantify the contribution of single pathways to hypersensitivity onset (Maxwell & MacKay, 2008). AI algorithms-such as DL and support vector machines-further enhance such models by offering predictions of trajectories of immune responses and identifying potential targets for therapy. Challenges, however, remain related to issues such as heterogeneity of data, validation, and biological interpretability (Alfonso-González *et al.,* 2025).

Integration of immunodynamics with pharmacokinetic/pharmacodynamic (PK/PD) safety modelling has further advanced predictive immunotoxicology in the light of various immuno-oncological therapeutics. AI and ML have revolutionized therapeutic drug monitoring (TDM) by providing real-time, data-driven dosing optimization based on patient-specific genetic and physiological parameters. PK/PD models still remain the backbone for optimizing efficacy and safety in immunotherapies, wherein inappropriate dosing might induce immune-related toxicities. Frameworks like minimal anticipated biological effect level (MABEL) are normally used to inform first-in-human dosing; still, the AI-assisted PK/PD systems that are integrated with parameters coming from immunodynamics can make better dose predictions by including cytokine kinetics and immune cell activation. Computational approaches based on these assumptions hold very high relevance for bispecific immunomodulatory agents, in which efficacy depends on tri-molecular synapse formation among drug molecules, T cells, and tumor cells (Chen *et al.,* 2016; Shah *et al.,* 2020). The integration of AI, immunodynamics, and PK/PD modelling, therefore, provides a mechanistic and predictive basis for developing safer and more effective immunotherapies.

8. AI-DRIVEN CLINICAL TRIALS AND DIGITAL TWINS

The development of digital immune twins is a revolutionary step forward in precision immunology, guided by the ambitious goal of simulating, computationally, how an individual's immune system reacts to different therapeutic interventions. These models emulate the human body's immune system-the most dynamic part of a biological system-which integrates different data types, including genomic, transcriptomic, proteomic, and clinical information, to forecast responses of different individuals to immune-modulating drugs. With the complex nature of immune regulation, involving thousands of genes interacting in various cell types and organs, accurate and generalizable modelling remains one of the biggest scientific challenges today (Laubenbacher *et al.,* 2022; Benson, 2023). Despite difficulties, early uses of digital twin technologies in cardiovascular diagnostics and automated insulin control show translational potential in clinical immunology (Laubenbacher *et al.,* 2022). These models can invoke mechanistic biological rules to stratify treatment and predict therapeutic response by integrating multi-omics and clinical datasets. Immune digital twins have been shown to capture evolving immune dynamics in proof-of-concept studies in diseases with temporal immune heterogeneity, such as autoimmune and inflammatory disorders, and optimize therapeutic interventions (Niarakis *et al.,* 2024).

Building on this, AI-enabled virtual cohorts and in-silico clinical trials (ISCTs) have redefined the preclinical and clinical research paradigms by offering ethical, cost-efficient, and highly scalable alternatives to conventional trials. The computational trials make use of AI for generating virtual patient populations that reflect clinical heterogeneity, thus facilitating the simulation of therapeutic outcomes and optimization of trial parameters. In vaccine development, AI-driven ISCTs enhance antigen discovery, vaccine formulation, and dose optimization by modelling the immune response across a wide range of demographic and genetic backgrounds, thereby hastening vaccine approval timelines and enhancing trial inclusivity (Gupta *et al.,* 2025). Similarly, in cancer immunotherapy, in-silico trials emulate immunotherapy kinetics and outcome trajectories as delayed response onset and plateaued survival curves-thus enabling adaptive trial designs that enhance predictive accuracy and robustness (Creemers *et al.,* 2023). AI-based trial simulation tools further enable dynamic stratification of patients, automation of control arm generation, and success rate forecasting necessary to streamline the drug development pipeline (Wang *et al.,* 2022b). Furthermore, these platforms serve as translational interfaces between researchers and clinicians, promoting an understanding of the principles of trial design and evidence-based optimization of immunotherapy trials (Creemers *et al.,* 2023).

Complementing digital twin and virtual trial frameworks, ML-driven patient stratification and responder prediction increasingly leverage demographic, genomic, and phenotypic profiling to personalize biologic and immunomodulatory therapies. For example, in IBD, using demographic and pre-treatment variables, the Light Gradient Boosting Machine model predicted the need for biologic therapy with an overall accuracy of 74%, pointing out that exposure to prednisolone was a critical determinant of the need for subsequent treatment with biologic therapy (Schöler *et al.,* 2022). Similarly, in neuroblastoma, ML methods such as support vector machines and DL can more accurately determine the risk of survival and treatment responses than conventional statistical modelling but face problems in interpretability and cross-cohort generalization (Vadde & Gupta, 2025). Integration of genomic risk profiling has also demonstrated value in psychiatric and dermatological diseases; for example, the integration of polygenic risk score with clinical features increased lithium response prediction in bipolar disorder, accounting for up to 13.7% variance (Cearns *et al.,* 2022). In psoriasis, transcriptomic and clinically driven ML models achieved AUC-ROC values greater than 0.95 for predicting treatment response to Brodalumab (Peng *et al.,* 2025), and the use of electronic health records by Random Forest-based models predicted biologic therapy initiation with an AUC of 0.93 (Lax *et al.,* 2025). These advances emphasize the importance of integrating molecular and clinical dimensions to enhance therapeutic precision across diverse immune-mediated diseases.

With this in mind, ensuring robust generalizability and data privacy across multi-center studies remains a central challenge in AI-driven immunological research; therefore, the adoption of federated learning (FL) and privacy-preserving AI strategies is logical. The FL framework allows running distributed model training across multiple clinical sites without collecting sensitive patient data at a central point, hence preserving the compliance of privacy regulations while considering the heterogeneity of the data for better model robustness. FedER is representative of this paradigm, which uses decentralized learning in collaboration with experience replay and GAN synthesis to generate non-disclosure representations from the local dataset. This effectively integrates non-identically distributed (non-i.i.d.) data from institutions into models showing comparable or even superior performance relative to centralized models with confidentiality and scalability. FedER is effective in such tasks as tuberculosis and melanoma classification, hence being of potential use in multicentric immunology trials where generalizability improves with diversity in patient data (Pennisi *et al.,* 2024). Besides improving performance, federated frameworks tackle key limitations of centralized learning-vulnerability to data breaches and lack of adaptiveness-enabled by convergence toward a global model consensus with no exchange of raw data, hence building trust and transparency in collaborative immunological research.

9. INTEGRATIVE MULTI-OMICS AND SYSTEMS IMMUNOLOGY

AI-driven analytical frameworks that integrate transcriptomic, proteomic, and metabolomic datasets are redefining immune drug target discovery by enabling a multidimensional understanding of biological complexity. Multi-omics integration strategies, including co-expression analysis, metabolite–gene interaction networks, and Bayesian data fusion, enable the identification of complex molecular relationships difficult to achieve in single-omics analyses (Sanches *et al.,* 2024). In immune-mediated disorders, such as IBD, AI-based multi-omics approaches have provided deep insight into the interplay among genetic susceptibility, environmental triggers, and immune regulation that underlie pathogenesis and point toward therapeutic vulnerabilities (Cannarozzi *et al.,* 2024). These tools have been put to practical use, for instance, in a computational pipeline that integrates RNA-seq and proteomic data to construct context-specific metabolic models, predict druggable nodes, and identify repurposing opportunities in diseases such as rheumatoid arthritis and SLE (Puniya *et al.,* 2023). ML enables integrative frameworks such as the simultaneous analysis of different molecular modalities (e.g., transcriptomes, proteomes) at the level of single cells. Such approaches advance the field of computational immunology toward a unified multiscale model of immune function (Curion & Theis, 2024). New AI-based target identification tools, such as Target Identification Pro (TID-Pro), which conduct disease-specific target discovery with multimodal data, underscore the importance of robust benchmarking and model interpretability for enhancing translational efficiency in drug development (Leung *et al.,* 2025).

The application of GNNs has further expanded the realm of analytical possibilities of systems immunology to include a reconstruction of immune cell communication networks from high-dimensional data. The TENET model uses a Triple-Enhancement-based GNN and effectively tackles challenges posed by sparse and noisy spatial transcriptomic data. The findings improve feature extraction and denoising toward better reconstruction of cell–cell interaction networks with higher precision and AUROC than existing models (Lee *et al.,* 2024). Similarly, scHyper employs hyperGNNs to capture higher-order intercellular interaction patterns from single-cell RNA-seq data and provides a systems-level view on the dynamics of TMEs (Li *et al.,* 2024a). The scDCA framework embeds a multi-view graph convolutional architecture to identify dominant communication assemblies and further estimate their impact on downstream cellular processes. This is particularly useful in oncology and immunotherapy (Ji *et al.,* 2024). Further, the VGAE-CCI framework uses variational graph autoencoders to predict 3D spatial cell communication networks. With this, it mitigates the incompleteness or heterogeneity of datasets and uncovers the interlayer communication across tissue structures (Zhang *et al.,* 2025b). Altogether, these models enhance our capacity for mapping and quantifying the emergent behaviors of immune systems at resolution.

AI-driven systems biology significantly accelerates biomarker discovery in autoimmune and autoinflammatory diseases. DL models, like the one described by Papagiannopoulos *et al.,* train neural architectures to identify discriminative molecular signatures with heightened sensitivity, hence improving the classification of auto-inflammatory disorders (Papagiannopoulos *et al.,* 2023). This work is complemented by the review from Moingeon and colleagues, who present an integration of multi-omics with medical imaging through AI-driven predictive algorithms that enable patient stratification and treatment response prediction, focusing on underpinning the combinatorial biomarker strategy potential in precision immunology (Laigle *et al.,* 2023). Network pharmacology and quantitative systems pharmacology are examples of systems-level modelling approaches that allow the simulation of molecular perturbations within the immune landscape, hence enabling the rational identification and therapeutic optimization of biomarkers (Alfonso-González *et al.,* 2025). Standardized translational pipelines are emphasized as a need by Kim *et al.,* who describe coordinated multi-omics strategies and cross-disciplinary collaborations among biologists, clinicians, and data scientists with a focus on reproducibility and clinical applicability of the biomarkers detected (Kim *et al.,* 2014).

Equally revolutionary has been the impact of AI and systems-level modelling of immune crosstalk on a wide range of knowledge in the field of CIDs. Complex disorders involving dynamic interplays between various immune pathways, such as rheumatoid arthritis, IBD, and SLE, do require computational methodologies able to seize the spatiotemporal heterogeneity of immune responses. Multi-modal data analytics-comprising omics and spatial transcriptomics combined with imaging-allows dynamic modelling of immune regulation and disease progression using statistical and mechanistic learning algorithms (Folasole *et al.,* 2025). For example, a Petri net-based model approach to NF-κB signalling underlines the interplay between canonical and non-canonical pathways, quantifies the relevance of biochemical processes, and predicts feedback relations, thus informing further model extension by additional layers of regulation (Trares *et al.,* 2022). Further, the involvement of immune pathways in systemic comorbidities, such as the connection between psoriasis and cardiovascular disease by TNF-α and IL-23/IL-17 signalling, underlines the importance of modelling inter-pathway communication to understand disease propagation and therapeutic cross-effects (Orlando *et al.,* 2022). Personalized medicine is furthered by ML-driven frameworks that improve diagnostic precision, predict treatment outcomes, and model drug responses, although interpretability, the mitigation of bias, and ethical deployment remain active areas of investigation (Peng *et al.,* 2021).

10. FOUNDATION MODELS AND MULTI-MODAL AI FOR IMMUNOLOGY

Models like ESM-2, ProtGPT, and BioMedLM are at the forefront of the biological foundation models revolutionizing the methods of immune drug discovery by enabling rational designs against targets so far deemed undruggable. These LLMs leverage deep contextual protein sequence representations to construct biologically meaningful structures with minimal experimental input. For example, ESM-2 recently played an important role in de novo design processes of functional proteins and peptides that captured evolutionary constraints guiding structural and functional fidelity (Zhao *et al.,* 2024). This is evidenced by the integration of the model into the PepPrCLIP pipeline, which perturbs the peptidic latent space to design selective peptide binders with the ability to modulate disease-relevant targets of high specificity (Bhat *et al.,* 2025). Similarly, its structural variant ESM-IF1 integrates sequence–structure embeddings, hence augmenting antibody evolution for improved neutralization potential against emerging viral variants by means of higher therapeutic antibody affinity (Shanker *et al.,* 2024). The logical extension of this paradigm has been seen with the PepMLM framework, enabling structure-free peptide design to allow targeted protein degradation in diverse contexts of diseases (Chen *et al.,* 2025). Simultaneously, an S^2ALM model fuses sequence and structural information to enhance the learning representation and thus presents higher performance compared to traditional models on the prediction of binding affinity, hence supporting the rational design of next-generation therapeutic antibodies (Yin *et al.,* 2025).

The emergence of multi-modal transformer architectures further accelerates the integration of heterogeneous biological data, enabling simultaneous interpretation of omics, imaging, and clinical modalities for immunological insight (**Figure 2**). For example, impuTMAE is a transformer-based model that integrates genetic, imaging, and clinical data to predict glioma survival outcomes with robustness against incomplete modalities, while realizing state-of-the-art performance (Boyko *et al.,* 2025). In another application, PathOmics leverages a multimodal transformer in order to integrate histopathological and genomic features, underlining the interaction between tissue microenvironment and genomic alterations that shape tumor progression and immune infiltration in colon-related cancers (Ding *et al.,* 2023). Such multi-modal analytics in inflammatory and autoimmune diseases enable spatiotemporal modelling of immune dynamics by accommodating high-dimensional and longitudinal immune data sets, and therefore facilitate early biomarker discovery, development of personalized therapeutic strategies in diseases such as rheumatoid arthritis and SLE (Folasole *et al.,* 2025). These works are powerfully complemented by continuous AI-driven integration of omics and clinical data in pursuit of improving patient stratification, elucidation of disease mechanisms, and treatment predictions through the identification of signatures of regulatory networks underlying disease heterogeneity (Cao *et al.,* 2025).

Figure 2. Multi-Modal Foundation Model Workflow for Immunology

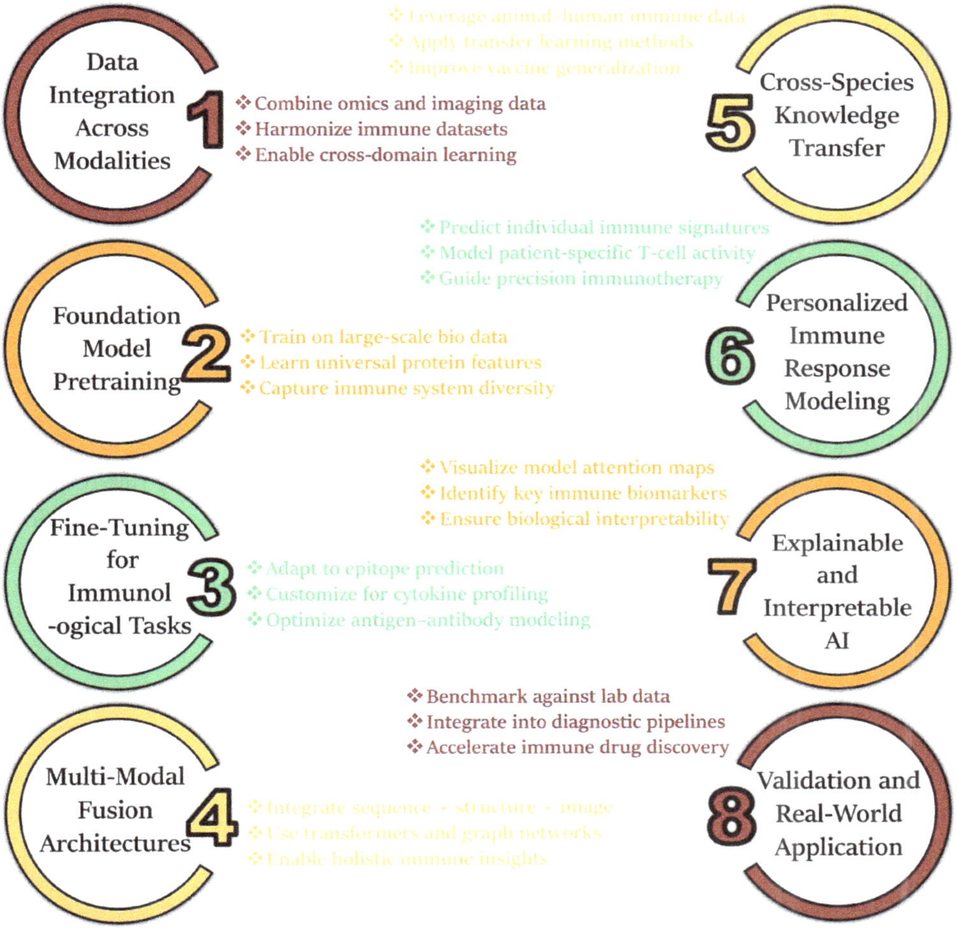

Data Integration Across Modalities
1
❖ Combine omics and imaging data
❖ Harmonize immune datasets
❖ Enable cross-domain learning
Foundation Model Pretraining
2
❖ Train on large-scale bio data
❖ Learn universal protein features
❖ Capture immune system diversity
Fine-Tuning for Immunol -ogical Tasks
3
❖ Adapt to epitope prediction
❖ Customize for cytokine profiling
❖ Optimize antigen–antibody modeling
Multi-Modal Fusion Architectures
4
❖ Integrate sequence + structure + image
❖ Use transformers and graph networks
❖ Enable holistic immune insights
❖ Leverage animal–human immune data
❖ Apply transfer learning methods
❖ Improve vaccine generalization
5
Cross-Species Knowledge Transfer
❖ Predict individual immune signatures
❖ Model patient-specific T-cell activity
❖ Guide precision immunotherapy
6
Personalized Immune Response Modeling
❖ Visualize model attention maps
❖ Identify key immune biomarkers
❖ Ensure biological interpretability
7
Explainable and Interpretable AI
❖ Benchmark against lab data
❖ Integrate into diagnostic pipelines
❖ Accelerate immune drug discovery
8
Validation and Real-World Application

Transfer learning and few-shot learning have grown indispensable for modelling rare immune disorders, where data paucity hampers the generalization of a model. Pre-trained models such as DenseNet121 and MobileNetV2 had performed well in the classification of rare skin diseases under long-tailed distributions, especially when combined with synthetic data generation as a means of data augmentation (Ozdemir *et al.*, 2025). In gastrointestinal immunopathology, Lin et al. developed a few-shot learning scheme with dual transfer and metric learning that could differentiate intestinal tuberculosis from Crohn's disease through endoscopic imaging with better diagnostic accuracy compared to expert clinicians (Lin *et al.*, 2024). MultiPLIER leverages public transcriptomic repositories through large-scale transfer learning and improves characterization of rare autoimmune diseases by effectively mapping gene modules associated with disease severity (Taroni *et al.,* 2018). Other very recent innovations include dynamic feature splicing and Siamese network-based representation learning in the classification of peripheral blood leukocytes, thereby showing the aptitude of few-shot paradigms to surmount data imbalance and improve diagnostic robustness in rare immunological contexts (Chen *et al.,* 2023b; Guo *et al.,* 2021).

Recent breakthroughs in prompt-based generative AI have revolutionized antigen and antibody engineering by enabling guided de novo generation of immune receptor sequences, either textually or structurally. Transformer-based architectures combined with diffusion priors have been exploited in designing antibodies of desired binding properties, thus bypassing the inefficiency of conventional library screening approaches. In this respect, it has previously been demonstrated that antigen-specific antibody CDRH3 sequences against SARS-CoV-2 can be generated in a way that skips traditional affinity maturation workflows (Marinov *et al.,* 2024). The MAGE model extends this concept to generate paired heavy-light chain antibody sequences that achieve validated diversity and specificity for viral antigens, including SARS-CoV-2 and avian influenza (Wasdin *et al.,* 2025). In the same direction, IgGM integrates diffusion and consistency modelling to enable the co-generation of sequence and structure for antigen-specific antibody prediction (Wang *et al.,* 2024c). Zero-shot design capabilities of such generative frameworks, as illustrated in generating novel HER2-binding antibodies characterized by high affinity and low sequence similarity to known binders, underpin their transformative role in AI-guided immunotherapeutic discovery (Shanehsazzadeh *et al.,* 2023; Kumar & Sisir, 2025).

11. AUTOMATION AND CLOSED-LOOP DISCOVERY SYSTEMS

Integration of robotics with AI into automated workflows in immunoassay and drug screening is pushing the boundaries of pharmaceutical sciences by way of improved throughput, accuracy, and experimental versatility. AI-driven laboratory automation systems are considered critical enablers of high-throughput drug discovery. These tools enable large-scale compound screening, optimization of experimental design, and minimal human error for improved predictive modelling and reproducibility (Mahmoud & Awad, 2025). Accessible, modular robotics combined with LLMs has recently further democratized laboratory automation. Such systems, like those based on robotic arms combined with LLM-based natural language interfaces, foster fluent human-machine collaboration. This enables intuitive task orchestration and flexible adaptation to changing experimental needs (Conrad *et al.,* 2025). Within a broader pharmaceutical context, such AI-robotic systems identify therapeutic candidates faster, optimize their synthesis pathways, and standardize dosage precision, furthering personalized medicine while assuring the consistency of manufacturing processes (Koul & Koul, 2025). For example, the GRAVI platform is representative of such convergence in microfluidic and robotic efforts for rapid low-volume, high-efficiency immunoassay and points to the potential of automated systems in translational diagnostics and therapeutic monitoring (Rossier *et al.,* 2008).

Beyond mere automation, active learning and lab-in-the-loop methodologies underpin iterative designs of immune therapeutics, creating integrated computational predictions with experimental validation. Active learning uses adaptive sampling to efficiently explore large chemical spaces with minimal labeled data, thereby accelerating key discovery stages such as virtual screening and candidate molecular optimization (Wang *et al.,* 2024b). Lab-in-the-loop goes a step further by directly integrating ML algorithms with high-throughput experimental feedback; this, in effect, enables real-time optimization of lead candidates (Tang *et al.,* 2023). Such strategies will help solve long-standing antibody–drug conjugate (ADC) development problems caused by incomplete structural information and limited experimental bandwidth through integrations of DL models for antibody structure prediction with AI-based pharmacokinetic modelling. The result would be data-driven pipelines for high-throughput validation (Noriega & Wang, 2025). The Gradient Oriented Active Learning (GOAL) framework has identified one such synergy: under conditions of highly constrained experimental conditions, iterative exploration of the sequence space can achieve optimal molecular design (Medabalimi, 2024).

The merging of organ-on-chip (OoC) platforms with AI forms a transformational development in immune system modelling by offering an ethical and physiologically relevant alternative to traditional in vitro and in vivo studies. Organ-on-chip systems model human organ-level physiology on microfluidic chips, which capture complex interactions between different cell types and the mechanical microenvironment (Vijayaragavan *et al.,* 2025). This has a particular impact in immunology, where the modelling of the immune microenvironment can be carried out with much greater fidelity compared to animal models, which usually fail to recapitulate human immune dynamics (Morsink *et al.,* 2020). AI integration into OoC systems allows improvement in real-time biosensor interpretation and enables early detection of toxicity markers and tissue-level responses, including disease prognosis through predictive modelling (Vijayaragavan *et al.,* 2025). In oncology, these integrated systems model the tumor-immune interface and provide a strong framework for studying immune evasion and the efficacy of immunotherapies (Lee *et al.,* 2025). AI-driven data management and fabrication optimization develop scalability and reproducibility in OoC systems by way of efficient preclinical drug testing and the development of precision immunotherapy (Monga *et al.,* 2025).

The emergence of autonomous Design–Make–Test–Learn (DMTL) systems ushers in a new era of closed-loop immunomodulator optimization through the integration of robotics, AI, and computational modelling, thereby accelerating the discovery cycle. Dynamic predictive modelling exploits pro-inflammatory and anti-inflammatory transitions through controlled temporal stimuli in such systems to bring about control over inflammation. ML-enabled active learning pipelines highlight how high-throughput screening (HTS) may be informed for the recognition of small molecule immunomodulators of key signalling pathways, including NF-κB and IRF, and accelerate candidate prioritization (Tang *et al.,* 2023). Artificial immune network algorithms identify clusters of immunomodulatory pathways and optimize them, furnishing, in a complementary fashion, computation-efficient multitarget drug design (Yong *et al.,* 2007). DL–based phenomics platforms amplify this framework through high-dimensional mapping of immunomodulator–phenotype relationships that enable rapid triage of therapeutically relevant compounds. These features have particular pertinence in pandemic responses, for example, COVID-19 (Cuccarese *et al.,* 2020). Further, the DMTL framework now fuses synthetic biology, nanotechnology, and systems immunology to enable next-generation vaccine platforms with adaptive immune response profiling and improved immunogenicity (Eslami *et al.,* 2025).

12. CAUSAL INFERENCE, EXPLAINABILITY, AND MODEL INTERPRETABILITY

Causal ML models represent a paradigm shift to truly mechanistic analyses that can go beyond the level of simple correlation analyses in immunological research. The framework lends a notion of causal inference to ML techniques and hence allows for the identification of real biological drivers, thus improving interpretability and enhancing clinical relevance in precision immunotherapy (Wang *et al.,* 2025). A Bayesian Network model for combined and common variable immunodeficiency antecedent clinical phenotypes was developed using a DL framework for causal modelling in autoimmune disease courses, which capture latent disease mechanisms with high fidelity while avoiding spurious correlations that confound traditional models (Papanastasiou *et al.,* 2024; Kaur & Sharma, 2025). By applying ML to whole blood transcriptomics, acute infection researchers have derived an immune dysfunction score predictive, well in advance, of those who will mount a poor immune response. ML-driven immunophenotyping has unraveled patterns of post-COVID-19 immune dysregulation, depicting heterogeneous immune trajectories across patients and pointing out personalized therapeutic strategies (Yousif *et al.,* 2023).

Adding counterfactual AI now brings in one of the most powerful paradigms: the simulation of "what-if" clinical scenarios, enabling patient-level outcome prediction and personalized therapeutic optimization. Using active generative AI on how immune treatments might unfold, counterfactual frameworks enable treatment strategy evaluation under hypothetical conditions to derive clinically useful insights (Lee & Topol, 2024). In immunology, such models have been used for predicting adaptive immune responses, including T cell and B cell activation dynamics relevant to vaccine development and personalized immunotherapy (David, 2024). AI-driven diagnostic frameworks have shown high accuracy in the early detection of immune disorders, thus allowing for interventions well before the manifestation of symptoms (Basha & Hanirex, 2024). Big data analytics integrated with AI further advanced precision medicine by uncovering immune cell heterogeneity and delivering targeted therapeutic intervention (Zhou *et al.,* 2025b). Application of DL-based AI frameworks to unannotated H&E-stained whole-slide images demonstrates the predictive capability for patient response in cancer immunotherapy, thus improving survival with the purpose of supplementing molecular biomarkers for refinement of treatment stratification (Conde *et al.,* 2024).

XAI methodologies have been of prime importance in closing the gap between computational innovation and clinical applicability. This is highly relevant given the challenge of ensuring that AI-driven insights into immunology maintain interpretability, transparency, and regulatory standards. Techniques like Shapley Additive exPlanations (SHAP), Local Interpretable Model-Agnostic Explanations (LIME), and attention-based mechanisms provide interpretable visual and quantitative metrics that explain model reasoning for safer evidence-based clinical decision-making (Islas-Avila *et al.,* 2025). XAI, in the pharmaceutical industry, will support GxP validation directly through the development of transparent audit trails and interpretable outputs to satisfy regulatory frameworks through the FDA and EMA for compliance and traceability of AI-supported processes (Nair, 2025). The GRNIX framework applies GNNs together with XAI in autoimmune disease studies with the aim of obtaining interpretable gene regulatory networks, which would be able to facilitate the mechanistic identification of disease drivers and potential therapeutic targets (Mortadha, 2024). Integrating multi-omics data with ML further enhances biomarker discovery to offer clinically actionable insights into immune-mediated disorders (Zhang *et al.,* 2025c). These collectively underscore the fact that XAI holds a central place in building trust, thus facilitating regulatory adoption and ensuring ethical transparency in AI applications related to immunology (Zhou *et al.,* 2025b).

Efforts toward improving the reproducibility and transparency of AI-based immunological research underlined the need for methodological standardization and responsible data stewardship. Challenges with reproducibility mostly refer to variability within data preprocessing pipelines and computational methodologies, thus calling for structured training modules and standardized data collection templates that encourage harmonized reporting practices (Anderson *et al.,* 2020). Further, comprehensive modelling of the immune system, combined with a variety of sources of experimental data, requires additional rigorous validation protocols and model design based on the principle of transparency in the pursuit of scientific reliability (Berdiugina, 2025). Even though AI is continuously improved, a number of significant problems are identified with model bias, data imbalance, and contextual misinterpretation associated with capabilities such as automated literature mining, high-throughput data analysis, and hypothesis generation; hence, maintenance of expert oversight is paramount. The path toward successful integration of AI in precision immunology requires the use of standardized frameworks, interpretable architectures, and transparent workflows to foster clinician trust (Zhou *et al.,* 2025b). Besides, ethical issues involving data privacy, algorithmic bias, and equity in data access require interdisciplinary collaboration and secure infrastructures of FL to make AI-based immunological insights not only scientifically valid but also socially responsible (Rajchenberg *et al.,* 2025).

13. ETHICAL, REGULATORY, AND TRANSLATIONAL PERSPECTIVES

The integration of AI into immunology and healthcare introduces several thorny ethical issues: data governance, the fairness of algorithms, and patient autonomy. Because clinical and immunological data are sensitive, data privacy and security are urgent to prevent unauthorized access and misuse of the data. Informed consent frameworks should therefore emphasize transparency for patients to make autonomous decisions about the uses of both their biological and digital data. The presence of algorithmic bias-which results from unrepresentative datasets during the training process-presents critical risks that accentuate health disparities and limit the generalization of models across diverse populations. Moreover, the lack of transparency of most complex AI models-the so-called "black-box" problem-further complicates accountability in clinical decision-making, including when misdiagnosis or adverse outcomes occur. Intrinsic heterogeneity of immune responses thus adds another layer of complication to such challenges and raises the bar methodologically for advanced rigor with high-quality data that enhances the interpretability of models and minimizes bias. All in all, ethics frameworks underpinned by equity, inclusivity, and transparency provide the basis on which responsible AI innovation can be fostered in concert with the protection of patient rights and securing public trust (Rajchenberg *et al.,* 2025; Shafik, 2025).

The regulatory environment relevant to AI-designed biologics and immunotherapies has remained fragmented and in continuous evolution, given the rapid rate at which innovation happens in biotechnology. AI-driven tools revolutionized the design of biologics, especially those based on B cells, including immunotherapies, through predictively accelerating the structures of proteins, their binding affinities, and immune interactions that previously depended on resource-intensive experimental workflows (da Silva *et al.,* 2023). However, this regulatory oversight is further complicated by dual-use potentials of the BDTs themselves, as such tools have been used both in furthering therapeutic development and in further misuse. Current frameworks, largely designed for conventional ML systems or LLMs, poorly capture unique ethical and biosafety concerns associated with open-source, low-resource BDTs (Moulange *et al.,* 2023). In response, there are recent proposals that put emphasis on the need for domain-specific governance that would balance innovation with biosecurity and ethical accountability (Dara & Azarpira, 2025). Another important aspect, of course, is the need for the harmonization of regulation across jurisdictions. For example, the United States and European Union operate distinct but increasingly aligned frameworks for the approval of biologics, while there are globally substantial disparities in some areas that delay market access for biosimilar vaccines and immunotherapeutics (Kingham *et al.,* 2010; Jarab *et al.,* 2024). This could also be achieved through simplification of such processes by applying harmonized international standards with a view to enhancing efficiency, reducing development costs, and improving equitable access to biologic therapies.

Transparency and accountability mechanisms become central with the clinical translation of AI-based immune models, especially their high-stakes applications: diagnostics, optimization of immunotherapies, and biomarker discovery. Intrinsic complexity often creates interpretability barriers that hold such models from regulatory approval and clinical adoption (Pappachan *et al.,* 2024; Cano-Gamez *et al.,* 2022). On the other hand, XAI frameworks, such as feature attribution models, rule-based reasoning systems, and surrogate interpretability networks, would provide structured solutions to enhance transparency and clinicians' comprehension of algorithmic predictions (Patil, 2024). Ethical auditing methodologies act to enhance accountability through traceability, assuring proper documentation along the AI development pipelines from data acquisition up to deployment (Pappachan *et al.,* 2024). Intrinsically interpretable algorithms are complementary strategies that include kernel-based and prototype-based learning. These provide more transparent alternatives to DNNs, hence improving reliability within a biomedical framework (Cano-Gamez *et al.,* 2022). Provenance tracking in machine-learning pipelines, along with quantification of uncertainty and real-time model monitoring, keeps the model continuously validated and reproducible. Cumulatively, these measures reinforce regulatory confidence and promote the responsible clinical translation of AI systems in immunology.

Cross-border governance and data-sharing policies remain at the core of nurturing AI-driven advancements in immunology research and the delivery of precision medicine. Improving international collaboration requires harmonization on interoperable data infrastructures that can efficiently support secure, ethics-conscious sharing of immunological datasets across jurisdictions. However, this remains a challenge in view of infrastructural capacity issues, poor harmonization of privacy laws, and standardization of data practices (Snijder *et al.*, 2014). Poorly harmonized governance frameworks, inconsistent data protection standards, and resultant fragmentation of data utility further impede rapid responses to public health crises faced by sub-Saharan Africa today (Brand *et al.*, 2022). New models of governance foster the adoption of the human-centered approach with ethical accountability, adaptive regulation, and algorithmic transparency to bridge gaps between jurisdictions through global equity in health innovation (Sedeeq & Arman, 2025). Novel privacy-preserving technologies, such as FL, have real-world mechanisms for collaborative analytics without having to share data directly. This enables large-scale integrative research studies while remaining compliant with local privacy laws (Zhou *et al.*, 2025b). Such models should be considered to ensure that AI-enhanced immunological research, though scientifically sound, remains globally aligned with public health priorities.

14. INDUSTRY ADOPTION AND CASE STUDIES

AstraZeneca–Immunai and DeepMind–GSK represent just two of many paradigm-shifting collaborations of pharmaceutical companies and AI in the process of immunology drug discovery and development. These alliances enlist the computational power of AI in order to overcome the high cost, complexity, and protracted timeline otherwise typical of drug development, which easily surpasses a decade in length and billions of dollars in investment (Gupta *et al.*, 2026). ML and DL algorithms are executed to perform virtual compound screening, prediction of drug–target interaction, and molecular structure optimization, hence reducing experimental burden and increasing predictive accuracy. AI-driven integration of pharmacogenomic data further enables precision therapeutics by personalizing drug design and dosage for specific patient profiles. Such platforms have allowed for the identification of immunomodulatory molecules and checkpoint inhibitors by virtual screening and protein–protein interaction modelling. Thus, accelerating both preclinical and clinical development, all against a backdrop of ongoing challenges around data heterogeneity, regulatory oversight, and ethical compliance, the successes of cross-sector partnerships, including AstraZeneca–Immunai and DeepMind–GSK, underpin the increasing role of AI in accelerating immunotherapeutic innovation and driving translational efficiency (Giriprasath *et al.,* 2024).

Commercial proliferation of AI-generated antibodies and immune checkpoint drugs is further testimony to the industrial adoption of computational methodologies in immunotherapeutic areas. AI technologies have impressively reduced both the cost and time for antibody discovery by optimizing affinity maturation, predicting structural stability, and generating high-quality antibody candidates (Cheng *et al.,* 2024). The antibody therapeutics market, estimated at more than USD 200 billion in 2021, is expected to cross USD 380 billion by 2030, showcasing the economic and clinical potential of AI in biologic drug discovery. De novo AI-based design has thus come out to be quite efficient, yielding high-affinity candidates in a fraction of the time taken by conventional hybridoma or phage-display techniques (Wang *et al.,* 2023). In the field of oncology, AI-assisted development of ADCs has helped bypass therapeutic resistance and augment molecular precision in targeting tumor antigens (Zhou *et al.,* 2025a). Bispecific antibodies, such as Cadonilimab, represent how AI molecularly engineered modality can optimize multi-target checkpoint modulation for enhancing immunotherapeutic efficacy (Zhang *et al.,* 2023a). Of note, AI-assisted discovery of novel immunotherapeutics such as Atacicept and AB-928 has underlined the translational potential of computational platforms in streamlining the discovery pipelines toward improving patient outcomes (Bagane & Jorgewad, 2024).

Integrating AI-driven platforms significantly enhances the identification and optimization process of immunomodulators within industrial R&D pipelines. The Patrimony computing platform, developed by a mid-size pharmaceutical enterprise, illustrates an example of how AI can leverage both proprietary and open-source data sets in identifying novel therapeutic targets in immune-mediated inflammatory disorders. This increases efficiency in R&D through faster and more informed target selection and prioritization via model-based decision frameworks (Guedj *et al.,* 2022; de Thé *et al.,* 2023). On the other hand, ML-enabled HTS frameworks have been developed for innate immunomodulators with effects exerted by small molecules acting on key immune pathways such as NF-κB and IRF. These HTS pipelines use DL and Bayesian optimization algorithms when exploring big chemical libraries toward the identification of compounds with desirable immunoregulatory properties that will be relevant for vaccine enhancement and optimization of immunotherapy (Tang *et al.,* 2023). On the other hand, in silico design tools-such as those applied by MAbSilico-further accelerate antibody discovery by reducing attrition rates and enhancing sequence optimization via predictive modelling of binding affinities and epitope specificity (Musnier *et al.,* 2024).

These translational advances are further driven by emerging computational immunology startups through interdisciplinary innovation and AI-enabled modelling. Companies like EpiVax, Inc., epitomize the translational applications of computational immunology in deploying predictive algorithms for immunogenicity assessment, vaccine design, and immune tolerance modulation (Moise *et al.,* 2013). These studies collectively reflect the general trend toward integrating immunoinformatics, structural biology, and systems-level modelling for accelerating immunotherapeutic solution discovery. This evolving domain of computational immunology brings together cancer immunology, autoimmunity, and host-pathogen interaction to interpret dynamic immune mechanisms and identify therapeutic vulnerabilities (Cañete & Tuong, 2024). These efforts are complemented by parallel advances in immunoengineering, which have extended the translational reach of the field by incorporating quantitative and engineering principles into the design of cellular therapies, antibody optimization, and vaccine delivery innovations (Swartz *et al.,* 2012). By developing and applying mathematical and multi-omics modelling, systems immunology elucidates biomarkers, mechanisms of immune dysregulation, and optimized therapeutic responses in autoimmune and inflammatory diseases (Alfonso-González *et al.,* 2025). Computational immunology, with its ever-improving comprehensive biological databases and algorithmic modelling tools, enables simulation of a wide range of immune processes such as peptide transport dynamics and T-cell receptor interaction, thereby accelerating translation of AI-driven immunological insights into clinical applications (Petrovsky & Brusic, 2002).

15. FUTURE TRENDS AND FRONTIER TECHNOLOGIES

15.1 Quantum Machine Learning in Immune Receptor Design

Quantum Machine Learning (QML) is an emerging framework within combinatorial immune receptor design that leverages computational advantages of quantum systems for modelling complex biological interactions. A paradigm example is the Quantum Convolutional Human Leukocyte Antigen Immunogenic Peptide Prediction (Q-CHIPP); the latter is a model that uses quantum convolutional neural networks for predicting MHC binding and peptide immunogenicity. This mode effectively mitigates the limitation of traditional DL models on small datasets, together with the poor computational performance (Peters *et al.,* 2025). Structured Q-learning (SQL) has been introduced for the optimization of antibody designs in high-dimensional search spaces with nonlinear objective functions. SQL incorporates structural priors, reinforces ML performance, and identifies sequences of high binding energy in antibody design tasks (Cowen-Rivers *et al.,* 2022). The polynomial scaling capability of quantum computing regarding design space complexity underlines its position further in combinatorial biodesign. In this way, quantum computing can explore molecular configurations that are intractable by classical computational systems (Gopsill *et al.,* 2021). On the other hand, protein language models (PLMs) become complementary approaches to QML for learning representations of immune receptors that are useful to predict antigen specificity and design therapeutic antibodies. However, this is a concept that remains at the frontiers, with several open challenges for PLMs regarding data and architecture optimization issues (Dounas *et al.,* 2024).

15.2 AI-Guided Synthetic Immunobiology

AI-driven synthetic biology has revolutionized the engineering of immune cells for programmable immunotherapy through designing immune circuits for the tight control of activation, targeting, and effector functions (**Figure 3**). The integration of CRISPR-Cas9 and modular synthetic constructs enables the engineering of T cells with tunable antigen recognition and controllable cytokine release, key features in treating complex malignancies and autoimmune diseases (Zhu *et al.,* 2023). Engineering of CAR T cells remains one of the cornerstones, with tremendous efficacy against hematologic cancers; however, extending this modality into solid tumors requires innovation in synthetic design to enhance safety, specificity, and persistence. This includes the use of synthetic switches and cytokine-signalling modules on CAR-expressing NK cells as a scalable, off-the-shelf alternative with improved capability in tumor targeting (Qu *et al.,* 2019). Synthetic biology has enabled the construction of biosensors and therapeutic response programs inside immune cells, thus extending immune recognition beyond its natural limits (Roybal & Lim, 2017). Incorporation of synthetic gene circuits enhances precision in cancer immunotherapy through context-dependent regulation of cytotoxic activity, cytokine secretion, and antigen recognition (Hoces *et al.,* 2023).

Figure 3. Conceptual Map of AI Integration in Immunological Research

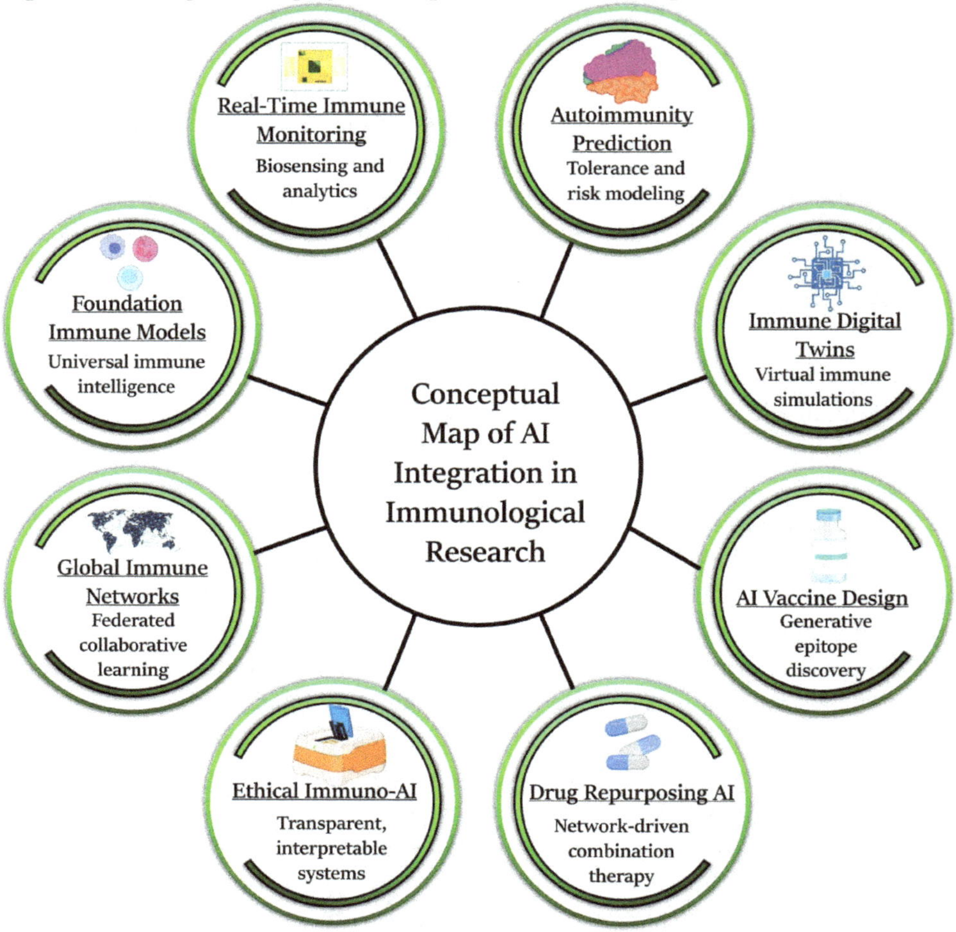

Real-Time Immune Monitoring
Biosensing and analytics
Autoimmunity Prediction
Tolerance and risk modeling
Foundation Immune Models
Universal immune intelligence
Immune Digital Twins
Virtual immune simulations
Conceptual Map of AI Integration in Immunological Research
Global Immune Networks
Federated collaborative learning
AI Vaccine Design
Generative epitope discovery
Ethical Immuno-AI
Transparent, interpretable systems
Drug Repurposing AI
Network-driven combination therapy

15.3 Digital Immune Twins for Precision Immunotherapy

One of the most critical advances toward real-time, precision-guided immunotherapy is the development of digital immune twins. These computational avatars simulate the dynamic behavior of the immune system through the integration of multi-omic and clinical data sets to develop virtual patient-specific models that predict responses to therapy and are used in the optimization of treatment approaches (Laubenbacher *et al.,* 2022). In oncology, the very early applications of immune digital twins-most especially in Triple-Negative Breast Cancer-show great potential for increasing predictive precision and therapeutic personalization (Niarakis *et al.,* 2024). Digital twins depend on continuous data assimilation and predictive modelling for dynamic clinical decision support. However, for their success, several challenges must be overcome with regard to interoperability, privacy, and simulation validation in order to ensure that digital twins turn out clinically reliable and scalable (Omolayo *et al.*, 2022). This will require a collaborative synergy between experts in computation, immunology, and the clinic with a view toward wider translational applications.

15.4 Green AI and Sustainable Computational Immunology

By placing AI at the center of modern computational immunology, attention is turned to the Green AI framework for making high-performance computation sustainable and ethically responsible. Contributing to carbon emissions are the ever-growing big AI models computational needs. And this is where environmentally conscious innovation comes in (Raman *et al.*, 2024). Strategies for mitigating the ecological impacts of AI-powered research range from cloud resource optimization and algorithmic efficiency to carbon footprinting (Alzoubi & Mishra, 2024). A life-cycle-based system approach advocates making an estimation of the environmental cost of AI models right from their development to their deployment and encourages eco-design principles and resource-efficient computation (Clemm *et al.*, 2024). Extensive efforts have been made in proposals for energy-efficient ML architectures in an effort to make computational immunology more accessible, as such methods reduce resource dependency without compromising on analytical rigor (Ahmad *et al.*, 2025). AI4greenAI envisions AI as an enabler to achieve sustainability by optimizing its own environmental footprint and driving further ecological objectives (Clemm *et al.*, 2024).

15.5 AI-Powered Precision Immunopharmacology

With the integration of AI and precision immunopharmacology, the paradigm of discovery and optimization has shifted in immune-modulating therapies. AI systems handle complex, multimodal datasets of genomics, transcriptomics, and proteomics along with clinical parameters to identify novel drug targets and predict individualized treatment responses (Olawade *et al.*, 2025). This is relevant in immune-mediated diseases/cancers, where inter-patient heterogeneity so often results in a deficiency of therapeutic success. Unsupervised learning algorithms delineate the heterogeneity of the immune system through cellular subset and signalling interaction characterization, thus giving information on the rational design of targeted therapeutics (Zhou *et al.*, 2025b). AI-driven systems biology frameworks enhance biomarker discovery and longitudinal tracking of immune dynamics for early disease detection and personalized treatment trajectories (Rappaport *et al.*,

2026). Practical translation of these approaches already shows up in optimized drug dosing strategies, predictive modelling of disease progression, and customized individual therapy (Fatima *et al.,* 2024). Yet, the field faces data privacy, algorithm interpretability, and biological validation to assure clinical translation and ethical deployment ahead (Olawade *et al.,* 2025). Subsequent efforts will therefore probably be focused on interpretable AI architecture, deepened multi-omics integration, and clinically deployable decision-support systems to bring full transformative potential in AI precision immunopharmacology (Zhou *et al.,* 2025b; Fatima *et al.,* 2024).

16. CONCLUSION

AI methodologies are indispensable in modern immunopharmacology and hold a great promise for unraveling immune complexity and expediting therapeutic innovation. Integration of computational models with multi-omics and clinical data using AI drives biomarker identification, target validation, and the design of personalized therapy in autoimmune, inflammatory, and oncologic disorders. More recently, generative algorithms and predictive frameworks have been developed with the aim of facilitating rational drug design, assessment of immunogenicity, and optimization of immune-modulating therapeutics. Explainable and causal AI models further strengthen interpretability and regulatory confidence, allowing translation in a transparent and ethical way into the clinic. Integration of digital immune twins, FL, and sustainable "Green AI" frameworks further ensures reproducibility, the preservation of privacy, and responsibility toward the environment. Yet challenges remain, most importantly with regard to standardization of data, interoperability across platforms, and equitable access to AI tools. Limitations will be transcended through interdisciplinary collaboration and harmonized governance. AI-enabled immunology is thus at an inflection point toward a precision, sustainable, and inclusive future of drug development and immune health.

ACKNOWLEDGEMENT

All the authors are thankful to their respective Universities and Institutions for their valuable supports.

REFERENCES

Adebanjo, E. A., Bakare, K. M., Matthew, U. O., Fatai, L. O., & Precious, A. U. (2023). Therapeutic approaches to immunotherapy-induced chronic inflammatory diseases. *HAFED POLY Journal of Science. Management and Technology*, *5*(2), 144–159.

Afzal, M., Sah, A. K., Agarwal, S., Tanzeel, A., Elshaikh, R. H., Alobeidli, F. A., & Choudhary, A. (2024). Advancements in the treatment of autoimmune diseases: Integrating artificial intelligence for personalized medicine. *Trends in Immunotherapy*, *8*(2), 8970.

Ahmad, F., Dwivedi, S., Khan, Z. H., & Mittal, N. (2025). Advancing green artificial intelligence: strategies for a sustainable future. In *Energy Efficient Algorithms and Green Data Centers for Sustainable Computing* (pp. 291–322). IGI Global Scientific Publishing.

Alagendran, S., Archunan, G., Prabhu, S. V., Orozco, B. E., & Guzman, R. G. (2010). Biochemical evaluation in human saliva with special reference to ovulation detection. *Indian Journal of Dental Research*, *21*, 165–168.

Alex, H. (2024). Enhancing drug safety: AIs role in pharmacovigilance and adverse event reporting. *International Research Journal of Innovations in Engineering and Technology*, *8*(9), 194–197.

Alfonso-González, L., Fernández, F. J., & Vega, M. C. (2025). Systems immunology: When systems biology meets immunology. *Frontiers in Immunology*, *16*, 1630488.

Algarvio, R. C., Conceição, J., Rodrigues, P. P., Ribeiro, I., & Ferreira-da-Silva, R. (2025). Artificial intelligence in pharmacovigilance: A narrative review and practical experience with an expert-defined Bayesian network tool. *International Journal of Clinical Pharmacy*, *47*, 932–944.

Alzoubi, Y. I., & Mishra, A. (2024). Green artificial intelligence initiatives: Potentials and challenges. *Journal of Cleaner Production*, *468*, 143090.

Anderson, B., Lyons, M., Henao-Tamayo, M. I., Juarrero, M. G., & Robertson, G. (2020). Improving the computational reproducibility of immunological research. *The Journal of Immunology : Official Journal of the American Association of Immunologists, 204*(1, Supplement), 222–225.

Arrell, D. K., & Terzic, A. (2010). Network systems biology for drug discovery. *Clinical Pharmacology and Therapeutics, 88*(1), 120–125.

Arumugam, V. A., Thangavelu, S., Fathah, Z., Ravindran, P., Sanjeev, A. M. A., Babu, S., Arun, M., Mohd. Iqbal, Y., Khan, S., Ruchi, T., Megha Katare, P., Ranjit, S., Chandra, R., & Dhama, K. (2020). COVID-19 and the world with co-morbidities of heart disease, hypertension and diabetes. *Journal of Pure & Applied Microbiology, 14*(3), 1623–1638.

Asediya, V. S., Anjaria, P. A., Mathakiya, R. A., Koringa, P. G., Nayak, J. B., Bisht, D., & Desai, D. N. (2024). Vaccine development using artificial intelligence and machine learning: A review. *International Journal of Biological Macromolecules, 282*, 136643.

Badhe, P. (2025). A multi-omics and network biology case study of CLIC1 using AI generated prompts. https://doi.org/DOI: 10.20944/preprints202509.2223.v1

Bagane, M., & Jorgewad, D. R. (2024). From AI labs to clinics: A review of 21st-century drug candidates powered by artificial intelligence. *International Journal for Research in Applied Science and Engineering Technology, 12*, 1419–1428.

Basha, S. A., & Hanirex, D. K. (2024). Artificial intelligence in immunology: predictive models for immune system disorders. In *2024 Global Conference on Communications and Information Technologies (GCCIT)* (pp. 1-6). IEEE.

Benson, M. (2023). Digital twins for predictive, preventive personalized, and participatory treatment of immune-mediated diseases. *Arteriosclerosis, Thrombosis, and Vascular Biology, 43*(3), 410–416.

Berdiugina, O. V. (2025). Usage of artificial intelligence capabilities in immunology: From literature review to statistical processing and analysis of obtained data. *Russian Journal of Immunology, 28*(3), 355–362.

Bhat, S., Palepu, K., Hong, L., Mao, J., Ye, T., Iyer, R., & Chatterjee, P. (2025). De novo design of peptide binders to conformationally diverse targets with contrastive language modelling. *Science Advances, 11*(4), eadr8638.

Bhotla, H. K., Balasubramanian, B., Meyyazhagan, A., Pushparaj, K., & Easwaran, M., Pappusamy, Alwin Robert, A., Arumugam, V.A. Tsibizova, V., Msaad Alfalih, A. Aljowaie, R.M., Saravanan, M., & Di Renzo, G. C. (2021). Opportunistic mycoses in COVID-19 patients/survivors: Epidemic inside a pandemic. *Journal of Infection and Public Health*, *14*(11), 1720–1726.

Bijral, R. K., Singh, I., Manhas, J., & Sharma, V. (2022). Exploring artificial intelligence in drug discovery: A comprehensive review. *Archives of Computational Methods in Engineering*, *29*(4), 2513–2529.

Bogatu, A., Wysocka, M., Wysocki, O., Butterworth, H., Landers, D., Kilgour, E., & Freitas, A. (2022). Metareview-informed explainable cytokine storm detection during CAR-T cell therapy. *arXiv preprint arXiv:2206.10612*.

Boyko, M., Beliaeva, A., Kornilov, D., Bernstein, A., & Sharaev, M. (2025). impuT-MAE: Multi-modal transformer with masked pre-training for missing modalities imputation in cancer survival prediction. *arXiv preprint arXiv:2508.09195*.

Brand, D., Singh, J. A., McKay, A. G. N., Cengiz, N., & Moodley, K. (2022). Data sharing governance in sub-Saharan Africa during public health emergencies: Gaps and guidance. *South African Journal of Science*, *118*(11-12).

Cañete, P. F., & Tuong, Z. K. (2024). Embracing computational immunology. *Immunology and Cell Biology*, *102*(8), 663.

Cannarozzi, A. L., Latiano, A., Massimino, L., Bossa, F., Giuliani, F., Riva, M., & Palmieri, O. (2024). Inflammatory bowel disease genomics, transcriptomics, proteomics and metagenomics meet artificial intelligence. *United European Gastroenterology Journal*, *12*(10), 1461–1480.

Cano-Gamez, E., Burnham, K. L., Goh, C., Allcock, A., Malick, Z. H., Overend, L., & Goh, C. (2022). An immune dysfunction score for stratification of patients with acute infection based on whole-blood gene expression. *Science Translational Medicine*, *14*(669), eabq4433.

Cao, C., Zhao, W., Guo, J., Wang, Z., Lu, A., & Liang, C. (2025). Leveraging artificial intelligence and machine learning for unraveling pathogenesis and advancing precision medicine in autoimmune diseases. *The Innovation Medicine*, *3*(3), 100154–1.

Cearns, M., Amare, A. T., Schubert, K. O., Thalamuthu, A., Frank, J., & Streit, F.Major Depressive Disorder Working Group of the Psychiatric Genomics Consortium. (2022). Using polygenic scores and clinical data for bipolar disorder patient stratification and lithium response prediction: Machine learning approach. *The British Journal of Psychiatry*, *220*(4), 219–228.

Chan, A. C. (2008). A golden era of opportunity in immunotherapy discovery and development. *Immunological Reviews*, *223*(1), 5–6.

Chatzianastasis, M., Burns, R., Costa, H., Rabinowitz, M., & Zhang, F. (2025). Abstract B056: Deep Antigen Sets, a new deep-learning framework, enables in vivo modelling of patient neoantigens for effective targeted immunotherapy design. *Clinical Cancer Research*, *31*(13, Supplement), B056–B056.

Chen, H., Cheng, F., & Li, J. (2020). iDrug: Integration of drug repositioning and drug-target prediction via cross-network embedding. *PLoS Computational Biology*, *16*(7), e1008040.

Chen, L. T., Quinn, Z., Dumas, M., Peng, C., Hong, L., Lopez-Gonzalez, M., & Chatterjee, P. (2025). Target sequence-conditioned design of peptide binders using masked language modelling. *Nature Biotechnology*, •••, 1–9.

Chen, W., Liu, X., Zhang, S., & Chen, S. (2023a). Artificial intelligence for drug discovery: Resources, methods, and applications. *Molecular Therapy. Nucleic Acids*, *31*, 691–702.

Chen, X., Haddish-Berhane, N., Moore, P., Clark, T., Yang, Y., Li, H., & Barletta, F. (2016). Mechanistic projection of first-in-human dose for bispecific immunomodulatory P-Cadherin LP-DART: An integrated PK/PD modelling approach. *Clinical Pharmacology and Therapeutics*, *100*(3), 232–241.

Chen, Y., Guo, X., Pan, Y., Xia, Y., & Yuan, Y. (2023b). Dynamic feature splicing for few-shot rare disease diagnosis. *Medical Image Analysis*, *90*, 102959.

Cheng, J., Liang, T., Xie, X. Q., Feng, Z., & Meng, L. (2024). A new era of antibody discovery: An in-depth review of AI-driven approaches. *Drug Discovery Today*, *29*(6), 103984.

Chinedu-Nzereogu, O. P., Olorunfemi, V. O., Osifeso, J. O., & John, T. (2025). Computational immunogenomics: Leveraging AI to uncover novel biomarkers for disease diagnosis and therapy. *International Journal of Life Science Research Archive*, *9*(1), 102–119.

Clemm, C., Stobbe, L., Wimalawarne, K., & Druschke, J. (2024). Towards green AI: Current status and future research. In *2024 Electronics Goes Green 2024+(EGG)* (pp. 1-11). IEEE.

Conde, G. D., Qaiser, T., Wu, E., Andrea, C. E. D., Shields, J., Artzi, R., & Reischl, J. (2024). Immunotherapy efficacy prediction in cancer: an artificial intelligence approach with unannotated H&E whole-slide images. medRxiv, 2024-02.

Conrad, S., Auth, P., Masselter, T., & Speck, T. (2025). Lowering the Entrance Hurdle for Lab Automation: An Artificial Intelligence-Supported, Interactive Robotic arm for automated, repeated testing procedures. *Advanced Intelligent Systems*, •••, 2401086.

Cowen-Rivers, A. I., Gorinski, P. J., Sootla, A., Khan, A., Furui, L., Wang, J., & Ammar, H. B. (2022). Structured q-learning for antibody design. *arXiv preprint arXiv:2209.04698*.

Creemers, J. H., Ankan, A., Roes, K. C., Schröder, G., Mehra, N., Figdor, C. G., & Textor, J. (2023). In silico cancer immunotherapy trials uncover the consequences of therapy-specific response patterns for clinical trial design and outcome. *Nature Communications*, *14*(1), 2348.

Cuccarese, M. F., Earnshaw, B. A., Heiser, K., Fogelson, B., Davis, C. T., McLean, P. F., & Gibson, C. C. (2020). Functional immune mapping with deep-learning enabled phenomics applied to immunomodulatory and COVID-19 drug discovery. Biorxiv, 2020-08.

Curion, F., & Theis, F. J. (2024). Machine learning integrative approaches to advance computational immunology. *Genome Medicine*, *16*(1), 80.

da Silva, B. M., Ascher, D. B., Geard, N., & Pires, D. E. (2023). AI driven B-cell immunotherapy design. *arXiv preprint arXiv:2309.01122*.

Dara, M., & Azarpira, N. (2025). Ethical considerations emerge from artificial intelligence (ai) in biotechnology. *Avicenna Journal of Medical Biotechnology*, *17*(1), 80.

Das, U. (2025). Transforming precision medicine through generative AI: Advanced architectures and tailored therapeutic design for patient-specific drug discovery. *ChemistrySelect*, *10*(36), e02448.

David, B. G. (2024). Artificial intelligence in predicting adaptive immune responses. *INOSR EXPERIMENTAL SCIENCES Учредители: International Digital Organization for Scientific Research*, *14*(2), 17–22.

de Thé, F. X. B., Baudier, C., Pereira, R. A., Lefebvre, C., & Moingeon, P.Patrimony Working Group. (2023). Transforming drug discovery with a high-throughput AI-powered platform: A 5-year experience with Patrimony. *Drug Discovery Today*, *28*(11), 103772.

Devaprasad, A., Radstake, T. R., & Pandit, A. (2021). Integration of immunome with disease-gene network reveals common cellular mechanisms between IMIDs and drug repurposing strategies. *Frontiers in Immunology*, *12*, 669400.

Dhillon, B. K., Smith, M., Baghela, A., Lee, A. H., & Hancock, R. E. (2020). Systems biology approaches to understanding the human immune system. *Frontiers in Immunology*, *11*, 1683.

Ding, K., Zhou, M., Metaxas, D. N., & Zhang, S. (2023). Pathology-and-genomics multimodal transformer for survival outcome prediction. In *International Conference on Medical Image Computing and Computer-Assisted Intervention* (pp. 622-631). Cham: Springer Nature Switzerland.

Doneva, N., Doytchinova, I., & Dimitrov, I. (2021). Predicting immunogenicity risk in biopharmaceuticals. *Symmetry*, *13*(3), 388.

Dounas, A., Cotet, T. S., & Yermanos, A. (2024). Learning immune receptor representations with protein language models. *arXiv preprint arXiv:2402.03823*.

Elemam, N. M., Talaat, I. M., Elmeligy, O. A. A., & Hundt, J. E. (2025). Cellular and molecular regulators in non-neoplastic immune-mediated diseases. *Frontiers in Immunology*, *16*, 1694308.

Enni, M. A., & Maraj, M. A. A. (2022). In silico drug repurposing for inflammatory diseases: A systematic review of molecular docking and virtual screening studies. *American Journal of Advanced Technology and Engineering Solutions*, *2*(04), 35–64.

Eslami, M., Fadaee Dowlat, B., Yaghmayee, S., Habibian, A., Keshavarzi, S., Oksenych, V., & Naderian, R. (2025). Next-generation vaccine platforms: Integrating synthetic biology, nanotechnology, and systems immunology for improved immunogenicity. *Vaccines*, *13*(6), 588.

Fatima, G., Siddiqui, Z., & Parvez, S. (2024). AI and precision medicine: paving the way for future treatment. https://doi.org/DOI: 10.20944/preprints202412.0036.v1

Fernandez, M. M., Motrich, R. D., Ostrowski, M., & De Marzi, M. (2024). Immune system disorders: From molecular mechanisms to clinical implications. *Frontiers in Immunology*, *15*, 1498830.

Folasole, A., Eshua, P. E., & Elesho, O. E. (2025). Modelling spatiotemporal immune dynamics in inflammatory diseases using integrative multi-modal analytics and high-dimensional longitudinal datasets. *World Journal of Biology Pharmacy and Health Sciences*, *23*(2), 196–218.

Gantla, M. R., Tsigelny, I. F., & Kouznetsova, V. L. (2023). Repurposing of drugs for combined treatment of COVID-19 cytokine storm using machine learning. *Medicine in Drug Discovery*, *17*, 100148.

Gao, J., Hu, J., Liu, L., Xue, Y., Zhu, K., Zhang, X., & Fang, X. (2024). Precise antigen-antibody structure predictions enhance antibody development with HelixFold-multimer. *arXiv preprint arXiv:2412.09826*.

Giriprasath, K. S., Pandiyarajan, P., Santhosh, C., Aneesh, K., & Vasanth, R. (2024). Revolutionizing drug development: navigating the convergence of artificial intelligence and pharmaceutical innovation. In *Analyzing Explainable AI in Healthcare and the Pharmaceutical Industry* (pp. 154–180). IGI Global Scientific Publishing.

Gopsill, J., Johns, G., & Hicks, B. (2021). Quantum combinatorial design. *Proceedings of the design society, 1*, 2511-2520.

Guedj, M., Swindle, J., Hamon, A., Hubert, S., Desvaux, E., Laplume, J., & Moingeon, P. (2022). Industrializing AI-powered drug discovery: Lessons learned from the patrimony computing platform. *Expert Opinion on Drug Discovery*, *17*(8), 815–824.

Gundappa, M., Arumugam, V. A., Hsieh, H. L., Balasubramanian, B., & Shanmugam, V. (2022). Expression of tissue factor and TF-mediated integrin regulation in HTR-8/SVneo trophoblast cells. *Journal of Reproductive Immunology*, *150*, 103473.

Guo, S., Guan, J., & Zhou, S. (2024). Diffusing on two levels and optimizing for multiple properties: A novel approach to generating molecules with desirable properties. *IEEE/ACM Transactions on Computational Biology and Bioinformatics*.

Guo, Z., Wang, Y., Liu, L., Sun, S., Feng, B., & Zhao, X. (2021). Siamese network-based few-shot learning for classification of human peripheral blood leukocyte. In *2021 IEEE 4th International Conference on Electronic Information and Communication Technology (ICEICT)* (pp. 818-822). IEEE.

Gupta, D., Sudhakar, R., Mujawar, S. S., Kadam, R., Patil, V., Kumar, A., & Gupta, K. (2026). The potential of generative AI in drug development. In *Applications of Artificial Intelligence in Pharmaceuticals* (pp. 125–156). IGI Global Scientific Publishing.

Gupta, P., Singh, A., & Mukherjee, D. (2025). Artificial intelligence based in silico clinical trials for vaccines. https://doi.org/DOI: 10.26434/chemrxiv-2025-3nh8w

Gupta, U., Pranav, A., Kohli, A., Ghosh, S., & Singh, D. (2024). The contribution of artificial intelligence to drug discovery: Current progress and prospects for the future. *Microbial data intelligence and computational techniques for sustainable computing, 47*, 1-23.

Haghighatlari, M., Marze, N., Seward, R., Ciarla, A., Hindin, R., Calderini, J., & Tourdot, S. (2025). HLAIIPred: Cross-attention mechanism for modelling the interaction of HLA class Ii molecules with peptides. *Communications Biology*, *8*(1), 1133.

Hassan, B. A. R., & Mohammed, A. H. (2024). Utilizing artificial intelligence in the development of medicinal drugs: Practical applications. *Journal of Innovations in Medical Research*, *3*(1), 22–25.

Henna, S. (2021). Modelling human innate immune response using graph neural networks. *IEEE Access : Practical Innovations, Open Solutions*, *9*, 167117–167127.

Hickey, S. L., McKim, A., Mancuso, C. A., & Krishnan, A. (2022). A network-based drug repurposing approach identifies new treatment opportunities for the systemic chronic inflammation underlying multiple complex diseases. *Frontiers in Pharmacology*, *13*, 995459.

Hoces, D., Miguens Blanco, J., & Hernández-López, R. A. (2023). A synthetic biology approach to engineering circuits in immune cells. *Immunological Reviews*, *320*(1), 120–137.

Hong, N., Jiang, D., Wang, Z., Sun, H., Luo, H., Bao, L., & Hou, T. (2024). TransfIGN: a structure-based deep learning method for modelling the interaction between HLA-A* 02: 01 and antigen peptides. *Journal of Chemical Information and Modeling*, *64*(13), 5016–5027.

Hou, J., Kouznetsova, V. L., & Tsigelny, I. F. (2022). Calming the storm: Identifying multi-cytokine inhibiting drugs with machine learning for COVID-19 induced cytokine storms. *Microbiology & Infectious Diseases (Wilmington, Del.)*, *6*(1), 1–7.

Hu, X. (2025). AI CAR Loop 1.0: A modular AI-driven platform for accelerated CAR-T therapy development, illustrated with CLDN18. 2-positive gastric cancer. https://doi.org/DOI: 10.21203/rs.3.rs-7350290/v1

Huang, K., Chandak, P., Wang, Q., Havaldar, S., Vaid, A., Leskovec, J., & Zitnik, M. (2024). A foundation model for clinician-centered drug repurposing. *Nature Medicine*, *30*(12), 3601–3613.

Huang, Q., He, Y., & Liu, K. (2025). Antibody immunogenicity prediction and optimization with ImmunoSeq. bioRxiv, 2025-08.

Iivanainen, S., Ekstrom, J., Virtanen, H., Kataja, V. V., & Koivunen, J. P. (2021). Electronic patient-reported outcomes and machine learning in predicting immune-related adverse events of immune checkpoint inhibitor therapies. *BMC Medical Informatics and Decision Making*, *21*(1), 205.

Imetkul, I., Kallow, Z. S., Edrees, A. E., Akram, S. A., Sabah, A., & Zhumagaliuly, A. (2025). Understanding the immunopathogenesis of autoimmune disorders: A comprehensive review. *Trends in Immunotherapy*, *9*(3), 47–60.

Islas-Avila, A. L., Martinez-Rebollar, A., Castrejon-Salgado, R., Avila-Jimenez, L., Estrada-Esquivel, H., & Sanchez-Gutierrez, A. F. (2025). Classification of generalized anxiety through life history strategies with random forest and explainable machine learning. In *Mexican International Conference on Artificial Intelligence* (pp. 115-128). Cham: Springer Nature Switzerland.

Ismail, S., & Barakat, K. (2025). Neoantigen mRNA cancer vaccines: how deep learning is advancing design and breaking barriers. https://doi.org/DOI: 10.5772/intechopen.1011567

Jarab, A. S., Abu Heshmeh, S. R., & Al Meslamani, A. Z. (2024). Bridging the gap: The future of biosimilars regulations. *Human Vaccines & Immunotherapeutics*, *20*(1), 2362450.

Ji, B., Wang, X., Wang, X., Xu, L., & Peng, S. (2024). scDCA: Deciphering the dominant cell communication assembly of downstream functional events from single-cell RNA-seq data. *Briefings in Bioinformatics*, *26*(1), bbae663.

Jokinen, E., Dumitrescu, A., Huuhtanen, J., Gligorijević, V., Mustjoki, S., Bonneau, R., & Lähdesmäki, H. (2023). TCRconv: Predicting recognition between T cell receptors and epitopes using contextualized motifs. *Bioinformatics (Oxford, England)*, *39*(1), btac788.

Kaur, S., & Sharma, H. (2025). Causal representation learning for predicting autoimmune disease progression from longitudinal multimodal clinical data. *13*, 150010-150027. *IEEE Access*.

Khater, T., Alkhatib, S. A., AlShehhi, A., Pitsalidis, C., Pappa, A. M., Ngo, S. T., & Truong, V. K. (2025). Generative artificial intelligence based models optimization towards molecule design enhancement. *Journal of Cheminformatics*, *17*(1), 116.

Kidd, B. A., & Dudley, J. T. (2015). Systems immunology. In *Translational Immunology: Mechanisms and Pharmacologic Approaches* (pp. 4-32). Academia Press.

Kim, H. Y., Kim, H. R., & Lee, S. H. (2014). Advances in systems biology approaches for autoimmune diseases. *Immune Network*, *14*(2), 73–80.

Kingham, R., Klasa, G., & Carver, K. H. (2010). Key regulatory guidelines for the development of biologics in the United States and Europe. *Pharmaceutical Sciences Encyclopedia: Drug Discovery, Development, and Manufacturing*, 1-36.

Komi, L. S., Mustapha, A. Y., Forkuo, A. Y., & Osamika, D. (2025). Reviewing pharmacovigilance strategies using real-world data for drug safety monitoring and management. *International Journal of Scientific Research in Computer Science. Engineering and Information Technology*, *11*(2), 3771–3779.

Koul, P., & Koul, I. B. (2025). Applications of artificial intelligence and robotics in pharmaceutical sciences: advancing drug discovery, personalized medicine, and pharmaceutical manufacturing. *Tropical Journal of Pharmaceutical and Life Sciences, 12*(2), 01-21.

Krishnan, K., Chugh, A., Rajaram, R., Sridharan, S., Setlur, A. S., Uttarkar, A., & Niranjan, V. (2025). Computational modelling and optimization of peptide-based CAR-T cell receptors targeting CD19 for enhanced efficacy and minimized toxicity. https://doi.org/DOI: 10.21203/rs.3.rs-6115435/v2

Kuang, Z., Thomson, J., Caldwell, M., Peissig, P., Stewart, R., & Page, D. (2016). Computational drug repositioning using continuous self-controlled case series. In *Proceedings of the 22nd ACM SIGKDD international conference on knowledge discovery and data mining* (pp. 491-500).

Kuchi Bhotla, H., Kaul, T., Balasubramanian, B., Easwaran, M., Arumugam, V. A., Pappusamy, M., Muthupandian, S., & Meyyazhagan, A. (2020). Platelets to surrogate lung inflammation in COVID-19 patients. *Medical Hypotheses*, *143*, 110098.

Kumar, M. A., & Sisir, A. T. (2025). Generative Ai: A new paradigm for antibody design and development. *Journal of Advances in Computational Sciences and Information Technology*, *13*(1), 37.

Kushwaha, V., Prabha, A., Sharma, V., Devi, A., Ramniwas, S., Sharma, A., & Kaur, D. (2024). Immunoinformatics: computational keys to immune system secrets. *Bioinformatics: Drug Discovery*, 123.

Laigle, L., Chadli, L., & Moingeon, P. (2023). Biomarker-driven development of new therapies for autoimmune diseases: Current status and future promises. *Expert Review of Clinical Immunology*, *19*(3), 305–314.

Laubenbacher, R., Niarakis, A., Helikar, T., An, G., Shapiro, B., Malik-Sheriff, R. S., & Glazier, J. A. (2022). Building digital twins of the human immune system: Toward a roadmap. *NPJ Digital Medicine*, *5*(1), 64.

Lax, T., Fallach, N., Stemmer, E., Shrem, G., & Salmon-Divon, M. (2025). Early risk prediction for biologic therapy in psoriasis using machine learning models based on routine health records. *Journal of Clinical Medicine*, *14*(18), 6421.

Lee, S. I., & Topol, E. J. (2024). The clinical potential of counterfactual AI models. *Lancet*, *403*(10428), 717.

Lee, T. H., Liu, P. S., Wang, S. J., Tsai, M. M., Shanmugam, V., & Hsieh, H. L. (2021). Bradykinin, as a reprogramming factor, induces transdifferentiation of brain astrocytes into neuron-like cells. *Biomedicines*, *9*(8), 923.

Lee, Y., Min, J., Kim, S., Park, W., Ko, J., & Jeon, N. L. (2025). Recapitulating the cancer-immunity cycle on a chip. *Advanced Healthcare Materials*, *14*(1), 2401927.

Lee, Y., Xu, Y., Gao, P., & Chen, J. (2024). Tenet: Triple-enhancement based graph neural network for cell-cell interaction network reconstruction from spatial transcriptomics. *Journal of Molecular Biology*, *436*(9), 168543.

Leung, H., Duan, C., Gou, W., Chen, J., Xin, Y., Zheng, Z., & Zhavoronkov, A. (2025). Advancing target discovery through disease-specific integration of multimodal target identification models and comprehensive target benchmarking system. bioRxiv, 2025-08.

Li, W., Wang, H., Zhao, J., Xia, J., & Sun, X. (2024a). scHyper: Reconstructing cell–cell communication through hypergraph neural networks. *Briefings in Bioinformatics*, *25*(5), bbae436.

Li, Y., Zhang, C., Zhang, X., & Zhang, Y. (2024b). TCRfinder: Improved TCR virtual screening for novel antigenic peptides with tailored language models. bioRxiv, 2024-06.

Lin, J., Zhu, S., Yin, M., Xue, H., Liu, L., Liu, X., & Zhu, J. (2024). Few-shot learning for the classification of intestinal tuberculosis and Crohn's disease on endoscopic images: A novel learn-to-learn framework. *Heliyon*, *10*(4).

Liu, W., Puri, A., Fu, D., Chen, L., Wang, C., Kellis, M., & Yang, J. (2024). Dissecting the tumor microenvironment in response to immune checkpoint inhibitors via single-cell and spatial transcriptomics. *Clinical & Experimental Metastasis*, *41*(4), 313–332.

Lu, T., Zhang, Z., Zhu, J., Wang, Y., Jiang, P., Xiao, X., & Wang, T. (2021). Deep learning-based prediction of the T cell receptor–antigen binding specificity. *Nature Machine Intelligence*, *3*(10), 864–875.

Ma, J., Wang, S., Zhao, C., Yan, X., Ren, Q., Dong, Z., & Liu, S. (2023). Computer-aided discovery of potent broad-spectrum vaccine adjuvants. *Angewandte Chemie International Edition*, *62*(18), e202301059.

Mahmoud, A., & Awad, W. A. (2025). AI-driven laboratory automation: transforming experimental phases of drug discovery. In *The Role of Artificial Intelligence in Advancing Applied Life Sciences* (pp. 361–378). IGI Global Scientific Publishing.

Mane, D. V., Deshmukh, A. N., Ambare, R. H., Solankar, A. A., & Madane, C. S. (2024). AI in autoimmune diseases: Transforming diagnosis and treatment. *Journal of Pharmaceutical and Biological Sciences*, *12*(2), 109–118.

Marinov, T. M., Abu-Shmais, A. A., Janke, A. K., & Georgiev, I. S. (2024). Design of antigen-specific antibody CDRH3 sequences using AI and germline-based templates. *bioRxiv*.

Martinelli, C., Repetto, M., & Curigliano, G. (2024). Artificial intelligence in small-molecule drug discovery. In *Artificial Intelligence for Medicine* (pp. 37–45). Academic Press.

Maxwell, G., & MacKay, C. (2008). Application of a systems biology approach to skin allergy risk assessment. *Alternatives to Laboratory Animals*, *36*(5), 521–556.

Medabalimi, V. (2024). Gradient oriented active learning for candidate drug design. bioRxiv, 2024-07.

Meyyazhagan, A., Balasubramanian, B., Easwaran, M., Alagamuthu, K. K., Shanmugam, S., Kuchi Bhotla, H., Pappusamy, M., Arumugam, V. A., Thangaraj, A., Kaul, T., Keshavarao, S., & Cacabelos, R. (2020). Biomarker study of the biological parameter and neurotransmitter levels in autistics. *Molecular and Cellular Biochemistry*, *474*(1-2), 277–284.

Meyyazhagan, A., Pushparaj, K., Balasubramanian, B., Kuchi Bhotla, H., Pappusamy, M., Arumugam, V. A., Easwaran, M., Pottail, L., Mani, P., Tsibizova, V., & Di Renzo, G. C. (2022). COVID-19 in pregnant women and children: Insights on clinical manifestations, complexities, and pathogenesis. *International Journal of Gynaecology and Obstetrics: the Official Organ of the International Federation of Gynaecology and Obstetrics*, *156*(2), 216–224.

Mohd, Y., Balasubramanian, B., Meyyazhagan, A., Kuchi Bhotla, H., Shanmugam, S.K., Ramesh Kumar, M.K., Pappusamy, M., Alagamuthu, K.K., Keshavarao, S., & Arumugam, V.A. (2021). Extricating the association between the prognostic factors of colorectal cancer. *J Gastrointest Cancer, 52*(3), 022-1028.

Mohd, Y., Kumar, P., Kuchi Bhotla, H., Meyyazhagan, A., Balasubramanian, B., Ramesh Kumar, M. K., Pappusamy, M., Alagamuthu, K. K., Orlacchio, A., Keshavarao, S., Sampathkumar, P., & Arumugam, V. A. (2021). Transmission jeopardy of adenomatosis polyposis coli and methylenetetrahydrofolate reductase in colorectal cancer. *Journal of the Renin-Angiotensin-Aldosterone System : JRAAS*, *2021*, 2021.

Moise, L., Marcello, A., Tassone, R., Cousens, L., Martin, W., & De Groot, A. S. (2013). Building better biotherapeutics and vaccines by design: EpiVax, Inc., an immunology company. *Rhode Island Medical Journal*, *1*(96), 19–21.

Monga, A., Jain, K., Popli, H., Telgote, P., Kaur, G., Rizwani, F., & Tuli, H. S. (2025). Organs-on-chips: Revolutionizing biomedical research. *Biophysica*, *5*(3), 38.

Morsink, M. A., Willemen, N. G., Leijten, J., Bansal, R., & Shin, S. R. (2020). Immune organs and immune cells on a chip: An overview of biomedical applications. *Micromachines*, *11*(9), 849.

Mortadha, M. M. (2024). GRNIX: A graph neural network framework for explainable gene regulatory network inference in autoimmune diseases using XAI. bioRxiv, 2024-11.

Moulange, R., Langenkamp, M., Alexanian, T., Curtis, S., & Livingston, M. (2023). Towards responsible governance of biological design tools. *arXiv preprint arXiv:2311.15936*.

Musnier, A., Dumet, C., Mitra, S., Verdier, A., Keskes, R., Chassine, A., & Poupon, A. (2024). Applying artificial intelligence to accelerate and de-risk antibody discovery. *Frontiers in Drug Discovery*, *4*, 1339697.

Nair, S. (2025). Explainable AI in Gxp validation: Balancing automation, traceability, and regulatory trust in the pharmaceutical industry. *Clinical Medicine and Health Research Journal*, *5*(05), 1430–1442.

Narang, V., Decraene, J., Wong, S. Y., Aiswarya, B. S., Wasem, A. R., Leong, S. R., & Gouaillard, A. (2012). Systems immunology: A survey of modelling formalisms, applications and simulation tools. *Immunologic Research*, *53*(1), 251–265.

Niarakis, A., Laubenbacher, R., An, G., Ilan, Y., Fisher, J., Flobak, Å., & Glazier, J. A. (2024). Immune digital twins for complex human pathologies: Applications, limitations, and challenges. *NPJ Systems Biology and Applications*, *10*(1), 141.

Nieto, P., Elosua-Bayes, M., Trincado, J. L., Marchese, D., Massoni-Badosa, R., Salvany, M., & Heyn, H. (2021). A single-cell tumor immune atlas for precision oncology. *Genome Research*, *31*(10), 1913–1926.

Nikolakis, D., Garantziotis, P., Sentis, G., Fanouriakis, A., Bertsias, G., Frangou, E., & Boumpas, D. T. (2023). Restoration of aberrant gene expression of monocytes in systemic lupus erythematosus via a combined transcriptome-reversal and network-based drug repurposing strategy. *BMC Genomics*, *24*(1), 207.

Noriega, H. A., & Wang, X. S. (2025). AI-driven innovation in antibody-drug conjugate design. *Frontiers in Drug Discovery*, *5*, 1628789.

Oktem, E. K., & Yazar, M. (2022). Drug repositioning identifies six drug candidates for systemic autoimmune diseases by integrative analyses of transcriptomes from scleroderma, systemic lupus erythematosus, and Sjogren's syndrome. *OMICS: A Journal of Integrative Biology*, *26*(12), 683–693.

Olawade, D. B., Clement David-Olawade, A., Adereni, T., Egbon, E., Teke, J., & Boussios, S. (2025). Integrating AI into cancer immunotherapy—A narrative review of current applications and future directions. *Diseases (Basel, Switzerland)*, *13*(1), 24.

Olawade, D. B., Teke, J., Fapohunda, O., Weerasinghe, K., Usman, S. O., Ige, A. O., & David-Olawade, A. C. (2024). Leveraging artificial intelligence in vaccine development: A narrative review. *Journal of Microbiological Methods*, *224*, 106998.

Omolayo, O., Aduloju, T. D., Okare, B. P., & Taiwo, A. E. (2022). Digital twin frameworks for simulating multiscale patient physiology in precision oncology: A review of real-time data assimilation, predictive tumor modelling, and clinical decision interfaces. *International Journal of Multidisciplinary Futuristic Development*, *3*(1), 1–8.

Orlando, G., Molon, B., Viola, A., Alaibac, M., Angioni, R., & Piaserico, S. (2022). Psoriasis and cardiovascular diseases: An immune-mediated cross talk? *Frontiers in Immunology*, *13*, 868277.

Ozdemir, Z., & Keles, H. Y., & ozgur Tanriover, O. (2025). Meta-transfer derm-diagnosis: Exploring few-shot learning and transfer learning for skin disease classification in long-tail distribution. *IEEE Journal of Biomedical and Health Informatics*. Advance online publication. DOI: 10.1109/JBHI.2025.3615479

Pandey, D. R., Dash, S. S., & Mishra, A. (2024). Advances of AI-driven drug design and discovery in pharmaceuticals-review. *Integrative Biomedical Research*, *8*(1), 1–10.

Papagiannopoulos, O. D., Papaloukas, C., & Fotiadis, D. I. (2023). Deep learning for biomarkers discovery in auto-inflammatory disorders. In *2023 IEEE EMBS Special Topic Conference on Data Science and Engineering in Healthcare, Medicine and Biology* (pp. 87-88). IEEE.

Papanastasiou, G., Scutari, M., Tachdjian, R., Hernandez-Trujillo, V., Raasch, J., Billmeyer, K., & Ivanov, V. (2024). Causal modelling in large-scale data to improve identification of adults at risk for combined and common variable immunodeficiencies. medRxiv, 2024-08.

Pappachan, P., Moslehpour, M., Bansal, R., & Rahaman, M. (2024). Transparency and accountability. In *Challenges in large language model development and AI ethics* (pp. 178–211). IGI Global Scientific Publishing.

Paranitharan, N., Kataria, S., Arumugam, V. A., Hsieh, H., Muthukrishnan, S., & Velayuthaprabhu, S. (2025). Integrin α1 upregulation by tf:fviia complex promotes cervical cancer migration through par2-dependent mek1/2 activation. *Biochemical and Biophysical Research Communications*, *742*, 151151.

Park, N., & Lee, J. H. (2025). A systematic multi-LLM AI framework for immunotherapy biomarker discovery and target identification. bioRxiv, 2025-06.

Patil, D. (2024). Explainable Artificial Intelligence (XAI): enhancing transparency and trust in machine learning models. *Available at SSRN* 5057400. http://dx.doi.org/ DOI: 10.2139/ssrn.5057400

Patil, S. P., Fattakhova, E., Hofer, J., Oravic, M., Bender, A., Brearey, J., & Smith, Z. (2022). Machine-learning guided discovery of bioactive inhibitors of PD1-PDL1 interaction. *Pharmaceuticals, 15*(5), 613.

Peng, J., Jury, E. C., Dönnes, P., & Ciurtin, C. (2021). Machine learning techniques for personalised medicine approaches in immune-mediated chronic inflammatory diseases: Applications and challenges. *Frontiers in Pharmacology*, *12*, 720694.

Peng, L., Wang, L., Chen, L., & Shen, Z. (2025). Machine learning-driven prediction models for brodalumab therapeutic effect and response speed in plaque psoriasis. *Psoriasis: Targets and Therapy*, 429-442.

Pennisi, M., Salanitri, F. P., Bellitto, G., Casella, B., Aldinucci, M., Palazzo, S., & Spampinato, C. (2024). FedER: Federated learning through experience replay and privacy-preserving data synthesis. *Computer Vision and Image Understanding*, *238*, 103882.

Peters, R., Rhrissorrakrai, K., Parthasarathy, P. B., Ratner, V., Gujarati, T. P., Tolunay, M., & Alban, T. J. (2025). Quantum convolutional HLA immunogenic peptide prediction (Q-CHIPP): next-generation neoantigen prediction with quantum neural networks. bioRxiv, 2025-07.

Petrovsky, N., & Brusic, V. (2002). Computational immunology: The coming of age. *Immunology and Cell Biology*, *80*(3), 248–254.

Pierini, E., Mazza, L., Petti, M., & Tieri, P. (2024). Exploring drug repurposing success stories through a network-based approach: insights from a case study. In *2024 IEEE International Conference on Bioinformatics and Biomedicine (BIBM)* (pp. 6959-6964). IEEE.

Puniya, B. L., Bessell, B., Zhao, Z., Loecker, J., Aghamiri, S. S., Mohanty, S., & Helikar, T. (2023). A computational pipeline for drug discovery in immunometabolism against autoimmune diseases. *The Journal of Immunology : Official Journal of the American Association of Immunologists*, *210*(Supplement_1), 85–15.

Pushparaj, K., Kuchi Bhotla, H., Arumugam, V. A., Pappusamy, M., Easwaran, M., Liu, W. C., Issara, U., Rengasamy, K. R. R., Meyyazhagan, A., & Balasubramanian, B. (2022). Mucormycosis (black fungus) ensuing COVID-19 and comorbidity meets - magnifying global pandemic grieve and catastrophe begins. *The Science of the Total Environment*, *805*, 150355.

Qu, Y., Siegler, E., Cheng, C., Liu, J., Cinay, G., Bagrodia, N., & Wang, P. (2019). Engineering CAR-expressing natural killer cells with cytokine signalling and synthetic switch for an off-the-shelf cell-based cancer immunotherapy. *MRS Communications*, *9*(2), 433–440.

Rajchenberg, D., Hess, R., Lins, M., Manor, A., Degany, O., & Shoenfeld, Y. (2025). Challenges, limitations, and ethical considerations of AI in immunology and healthcare. In *AI-Assisted Computational Approaches for Immunological Disorders* (pp. 393–426). IGI Global Scientific Publishing.

Raman, R., Pattnaik, D., Lathabai, H. H., Kumar, C., Govindan, K., & Nedungadi, P. (2024). Green and sustainable AI research: An integrated thematic and topic modelling analysis. *Journal of Big Data*, *11*(1), 1–28.

Ramya, S., Poornima, P., Jananisri, A., Geofferina, I. P., Bavyataa, V., Divya, M., Priyanga, P., Vadivukarasi, J., Sujitha, S., Elamathi, S., Anand, A. V., & Balamuralikrishnan, B. (2023). Role of hormones and the potential impact of multiple stresses on infertility. *Stresses*, *3*(2), 454–474.

Rappaport, N., Nogal, B., Perrott, K., Domina, V., Hood, L., & Price, N. D. (2026). Early detection of wellness-to-disease transitions in the AI era: Implications for pharmacology and toxicology. *Annual Review of Pharmacology and Toxicology*, •••, 66.

Robert, K., Kaium, O., & Alasa, L. (2025). Generative AI and pharmaceutical innovation: Accelerating drug discovery with deep learning and predictive analytics. *International Journal of Multidisciplinary Evolutionary Research*, *6*(2), 44–52.

Rossier, J. S., Baranek, S., Morier, P., Vollet, C., Vulliet, F., De Chastonay, Y., & Reymond, F. (2008). GRAVI: Robotized microfluidics for fast and automated immunoassays in low volume. *JALA: Journal of the Association for Laboratory Automation*, *13*(6), 322–329.

Roybal, K. T., & Lim, W. A. (2017). Synthetic immunology: Hacking immune cells to expand their therapeutic capabilities. *Annual Review of Immunology*, *35*(1), 229–253.

Sakhamuri, M. R., Henna, S., Creedon, L., & Meehan, K. (2023). graph modelling and graph-attention neural network for immune response prediction. In *2023 34th Irish Signals and Systems Conference (ISSC)* (pp. 1-6). IEEE.

Sanches, P. H. G., de Melo, N. C., Porcari, A. M., & de Carvalho, L. M. (2024). Integrating molecular perspectives: Strategies for comprehensive multi-omics integrative data analysis and machine learning applications in transcriptomics, proteomics, and metabolomics. *Biology (Basel)*, *13*(11), 848.

Sangeetha, T., Anand, A. V., & Begum, T. N. (2022). Assessment of inter-relationship between anemia and COPD in accordance with altitude. *The Open Respiratory Medicine Journal*, *16*, e187430642206270.

Sangeetha, T., Nargis Begum, T., Balamuralikrishnan, B., Arun, M., Rengasamy, K. R. R., Senthilkumar, N., Velayuthaprabhu, S., Saradhadevi, M., Sampathkumar, P., & Vijaya Anand, A. (2022). Influence of SERPINA1 gene polymorphisms on anemia and chronic obstructive pulmonary disease. *Journal of the Renin-Angiotensin-Aldosterone System : JRAAS*, *2022*, 2022.

Schöler, D., Kostev, K., Peters, M., Zamfir, C., Wolk, A., Roderburg, C., & Loosen, S. H. (2022). Machine learning can predict the probability of biologic therapy in patients with Inflammatory Bowel Disease. *Journal of Clinical Medicine*, *11*(15), 4586.

Sedeeq, F. S., & Arman, P. (2025). Human-centric AI governance: An adaptive public international law framework for ethical and inclusive AI regulation in public health. *The Journal of Law, Medicine & Ethics*, •••, 1–12.

Shafik, W. (2025). Ethical considerations in automated healthcare. In *Next-Generation Therapeutics Using Internet of Things and Machine Learning* (pp. 315–338). IGI Global Scientific Publishing.

Shah, D. K., Al Qaraghuli, F., & Zhang, W. (2020). PK/PD-driven starting and effective human dose determination for immuno-oncology drugs. In *Identification and Quantification of Drugs, Metabolites, Drug Metabolizing Enzymes, and Transporters* (pp. 657-667). Elsevier.

Shahid, S., Maity, D., & Chakrabarty, S. (2025). MTAN-ADMET: A multi-task adaptive neural network for efficient and accurate prediction of ADMET properties. *ChemRxiv*. http://dx.doi.org/DOI: 10.26434/chemrxiv-2025-zhrsk

Shahzadi, M., Rafique, H., Waheed, A., Naz, H., Waheed, A., Zokirova, F. R., & Khan, H. (2024). Artificial intelligence for chimeric antigen receptor-based therapies: A comprehensive review of current applications and future perspectives. *Therapeutic Advances in Vaccines and Immunotherapy*, *12*, 25151355241305856.

Shanehsazzadeh, A., Bachas, S., McPartlon, M., Kasun, G., Sutton, J. M., Steiger, A. K., & Meier, J. (2023). Unlocking de novo antibody design with generative artificial intelligence. BioRxiv, 2023-01.

Shanker, V. R., Bruun, T. U., Hie, B. L., & Kim, P. S. (2024). Unsupervised evolution of protein and antibody complexes with a structure-informed language model. *Science*, *385*(6704), 46–53.

Shanmugam, R., Thangavelu, S., Fathah, Z., Yatoo, M. I., Tiwari, R., Pandey, M. K., Dhama, J., Chandra, R., Malik, Y. S., Dhama, K., Sah, R., Chaicumpa, W., Shanmugam, V., & Arumugam, V. A. (2020). SARS-CoV-2 / COVID-19 pandemic – an update. *Journal of Experimental Biology and Agricultural Sciences, 8*(Special Issue 1), S219-S245.

Shi, J., Wei, X., Xun, Z., Ding, X., Liu, Y., Liu, L., & Ye, Y. (2024). The web-based portal SpatialTME integrates histological images with single-cell and spatial transcriptomics to explore the tumor microenvironment. *Cancer Research*, *84*(8), 1210–1220.

Shraim, R., Mooney, B., Conkrite, K. L., Hamilton, A. K., Morin, G. B., Sorensen, P. H., & Sacan, A. (2025). ImmunoTar—Integrative prioritization of cell surface targets for cancer immunotherapy. *Bioinformatics (Oxford, England)*, *41*(3), btaf060.

Sidhom, J. W., Oliveira, G., Ross-MacDonald, P., Wind-Rotolo, M., Wu, C. J., Pardoll, D. M., & Baras, A. S. (2022). Deep learning reveals predictive sequence concepts within immune repertoires to immunotherapy. *Science Advances*, *8*(37), eabq5089.

Singh, A. V., & Negi, A. (2019). Towards better drug repositioning using joint learning. In *2019 IEEE 16th India Council International Conference (INDICON)* (pp. 1-4). IEEE.

Singh, S., Shingatgeri, V., & Srivastava, P. (2024). Revolutionizing new drug discovery: Harnessing AI and machine learning to overcome traditional challenges and accelerate targeted therapies. *Artificial Intelligence in Health*, *2*(2), 29–40.

Snijder, B., Kandasamy, R. K., & Superti-Furga, G. (2014). Toward effective sharing of high-dimensional immunology data. *Nature Biotechnology*, *32*(8), 755–759.

Sobhani, N., Tardiel-Cyril, D. R., Chai, D., Generali, D., Li, J. R., Vazquez-Perez, J., & Li, Y. (2024). Artificial intelligence-powered discovery of small molecules inhibiting CTLA-4 in cancer. *BJC Reports*, *2*(1), 4.

Sobral, P. S., Luz, V. C., Almeida, J. M., Videira, P. A., & Pereira, F. (2023). Computational approaches drive developments in immune-oncology therapies for PD-1/PD-L1 immune checkpoint inhibitors. *International Journal of Molecular Sciences*, *24*(6), 5908.

Song, J., Kim, L., Shin, D., Kim, J., Um, T., Cho, A., & Chae, Y. K. (2025a). AI-based models integrating serum proteomics and clinical features to predict immune-related adverse events in NSCLC patients undergoing immunotherapy. *Cancer Research*, *85*(8, Supplement_1), 3667–3667.

Song, X., Liang, H., Nan, F., Chen, W., Li, J., He, L., & Zhang, D. (2025b). Autoimmune Diseases: Molecular Pathogenesis and Therapeutic Targets. *MedComm*, *6*(7), e70262.

Su, Y., Zeng, X., Zhang, L., Bian, Y., Wang, Y., & Ma, B. (2025). ABTrans: A transformer-based model for predicting interaction between anti-Aβ antibodies and peptides. *Interdisciplinary Sciences, Computational Life Sciences*, *17*(1), 140–152.

Subramanian, N., Torabi-Parizi, P., Gottschalk, R. A., Germain, R. N., & Dutta, B. (2015). Network representations of immune system complexity. *Wiley Interdisciplinary Reviews. Systems Biology and Medicine*, *7*(1), 13–38.

Sumit, M., & Dhara, V. G. (2025). Use of systems biology approaches toward target discovery, validation, and drug development. In *Biopharmaceutical Informatics* (pp. 281–305). CRC Press.

Sun, Z. Y., Yuan, J., Jaiswal, D., Ge, J., Liang, T., Wei, J., & Feng, Z. (2025). AntiB-MPNN: Structure-guided graph neural networks for precision antibody engineering. *Advancement of Science*, •••, 04278.

Swartz, M. A., Hirosue, S., & Hubbell, J. A. (2012). Engineering approaches to immunotherapy. *Science translational medicine, 4*(148), 148rv9-148rv9.

Tang, Y., Kim, J. Y., Carman, K. M., Bahmani, A., Chen, Q., Rosenberger, M. G., & Ferguson, A. L. (2023). Data-driven discovery of innate immunomodulators via machine learning-guided high throughput screening. *Chemical Science (Cambridge)*, *14*(44), 12747–12766.

Taroni, J. N., Grayson, P. C., Hu, Q., Eddy, S., Kretzler, M., Merkel, P. A., & Greene, C. S. (2018). MultiPLIER: a transfer learning framework reveals systemic features of rare autoimmune disease. *bioRxiv*.

Tavare, N., Singh, R., & Barage, S. H. (2025). AI-assisted vaccine design and development in immunological disorders. In *AI-Assisted Computational Approaches for Immunological Disorders* (pp. 181–204). IGI Global Scientific Publishing.

Thakkar, R., Upreti, D., Ishiguro, S., Tamura, M., & Comer, J. (2023). Computational design of a cyclic peptide that inhibits the CTLA4 immune checkpoint. *RSC Medicinal Chemistry*, *14*(4), 658–670.

Trares, K., Ackermann, J., & Koch, I. (2022). The canonical and non-canonical NF-κB pathways and their crosstalk: A comparative study based on Petri nets. *Bio Systems*, *211*, 104564.

Ujiie, H., Rosmarin, D., Schön, M. P., Ständer, S., Boch, K., Metz, M., & Ludwig, R. J. (2022). Unmet medical needs in chronic, non-communicable inflammatory skin diseases. *Frontiers in medicine*, *9*, 875492.

Upadhyay, J., Nandave, M., & Kumar, A. (2024). Role of artificial intelligence in pharmacovigilance. In *Pharmacovigilance Essentials: Advances, Challenges and Global Perspectives* (pp. 347–363). Springer Nature Singapore.

Vadde, R., & Gupta, M. K. (2025). Machine learning approaches for neuroblastoma risk prediction and stratification. *Critical Reviews™ in Oncogenesis, 30.*

Vázquez, N. G., Nada, H., Upadhyay, S., & Gabr, M. T. (2025). Phenotypic and targeted drug discovery in immune therapeutics: Challenges, opportunities, and future directions. *RSC Advances*, *15*(36), 29937–29951.

Velayuthaprabhu, S., & Archunan, G. (2005). Evaluation of anticardiolipin antibodies and antiphosphatidylserine antibodies in women with recurrent abortion. *Indian Journal of Medical Sciences*, *59*, 347–352.

Velayuthaprabhu, S., Archunan, G., & Balakrishnan, K. (2007). Placental thrombosis in experimental anticardiolipin antibodies-mediated intrauterine fetal death. *American Journal of Reproductive Immunology (New York, N.Y.)*, *57*, 270–276.

Velayuthaprabhu, S., Matsubayashi, H., & Archunan, G. (2016). Beta-2 GPI induced tissue factor and placental apoptosis for the pathophysiology of pregnancy loss in antiphospholipid syndrome. *International Journal of Research in Medical Sciences*, *4*(8), 3109–3113.

Velayuthaprabhu, S., Matsubayashi, H., Sugi, T., Nakamura, M., Ohnishi, Y., Ogura, T., & Archunan, G. (2013). Expression of apoptosis in placenta of experimental antiphospholipid syndrome (APS) mouse. *American Journal of Reproductive Immunology (New York, N.Y.)*, *69*(5), 486–494.

Velayuthaprabhu, S., Matsubayashi, H., Sugi, T., Nakamura, M., Ohnishi, Y., Ogura, T., Tomiyama, T., & Archunan, G. (2011). A unique preliminary study on fetal resorption and placental apoptosis in mice with passive immunization of anti-phosphatidylethanolamine antibodies and anti-Factor XII antibodies. *American Journal of Reproductive Immunology (New York, N.Y.)*, *66*, 373–384.

Vijayaragavan, V., Vijayakumar, M., Dharshini, P., Karunakaran, K., Kesavan, K., & Raj, R. D. S. (2025). AI and automation in organ-on-a-chip technology: advancing personalized medicine and disease modelling. In *2025 IEEE 6th International Conference in Robotics and Manufacturing Automation (ROMA)* (pp. 40-45). IEEE.

Vo, N. H. H., Phung, H. T. T., Chung, K. L., & Vu, T. Y. (2023). Design and evaluating the efficacy of novel antibodies enhancing binding on CTLA-4 and PD-1 immune checkpoints. *Journal of Advanced Engineering and Computation*, *7*(4), 224–236.

Wang, B., Tan, X., Guo, J., Xiao, T., Jiao, Y., Zhao, J., & Wang, Y. (2022a). Drug-induced immune thrombocytopenia toxicity prediction based on machine learning. *Pharmaceutics*, *14*(5), 943.

Wang, H., Hao, X., He, Y., & Fan, L. (2024a). AbImmPred: An immunogenicity prediction method for therapeutic antibodies using AntiBERTy-based sequence features. *PLoS One*, *19*(2), e0296737.

Wang, J. W., Dai, M. W., Liang, P., Hou, J., & Meng, M. (2025). Correlation does not equal causation: The imperative of causal inference in machine learning models for immunotherapy. *Frontiers in Immunology*, *16*, 1630781.

Wang, L., Zhou, Z., Yang, X., Shi, S., Zeng, X., & Cao, D. (2024b). The present state and challenges of active learning in drug discovery. *Drug Discovery Today*, *29*(6), 103985.

Wang, R., Wu, F., Gao, X., Wu, J., Zhao, P., & Yao, J. (2024c). Iggm: A generative model for functional antibody and nanobody design. bioRxiv, 2024-09.

Wang, T., Gao, X., Huai, Z., Gong, Z., Mao, T., Fan, X., & Huang, X. (2023). Revolutionizing antibody discovery industry with highly efficient and accurate AI-based epitope-specific antibody de novo design workflow. *Antibody Therapeutics*, *6*(Suppl 1), tbad014-024.

Wang, Z., Gao, C., Glass, L. M., & Sun, J. (2022b). Artificial intelligence for in silico clinical trials: A review. *arXiv preprint arXiv:2209.09023*.

Wasdin, P. T., Johnson, N. V., Janke, A. K., Held, S., Marinov, T. M., Jordaan, G., & Georgiev, I. S. (2025). Generation of antigen-specific paired chain antibody sequences using large language models. bioRxiv, 2024-12.

Weerasekara, S., Darras, N., Fernandez, N., Chen, M., Ainbinder, A., & Price, C. (2025). CellClique: Dissecting tumor microenvironments at the single cell level using generative AI and spatial transcriptomics. *Cancer Research*, *85*(8, Supplement_1), 2418–2418.

Xin, K., Wei, X., Shao, J., Chen, F., Liu, Q., & Liu, B. (2024). Establishment of a novel tumor neoantigen prediction tool for personalized vaccine design. *Human Vaccines & Immunotherapeutics*, *20*(1), 2300881.

Xu, B., Lu, Y., Li, C., Yue, L., Wang, X., Hao, N., & Chen, J. (2024). Smiles-mamba: Chemical mamba foundation models for drug admet prediction. *arXiv preprint arXiv:2408.05696*.

Yadav, K. L., Desai, N., Prajapati, A., Narkhede, S., & Luhar, S. (2025). From bench to bedside: AI-enabled drug repurposing for innovative therapies in complex diseases. *Asian Journal of Pharmaceutical Research*, *15*(1), 72–76.

Yang, D., Peng, X., & Peng, S. (2023). Transformer-based models for phla binding affinity prediction. In *2023 IEEE 14th International Conference on Software Engineering and Service Science (ICSESS)* (pp. 297-300). IEEE.

Ye, Y., Shen, Y., Wang, J., Li, D., Zhu, Y., Zhao, Z., & Wan, J. (2023). SIGANEO: Similarity network with GAN enhancement for immunogenic neoepitope prediction. *Computational and Structural Biotechnology Journal*, *21*, 5538–5543.

Yim, S., Hwang, W., Han, N., & Lee, D. (2022). Computational discovery of cancer immunotherapy targets by intercellular CRISPR screens. *Frontiers in Immunology*, *13*, 884561.

Yin, M., Zhou, H., Wu, J., Zhu, Y., Zhan, Y., Kong, Z., & Wu, J. (2025). S2alm: Sequence-structure pre-trained large language model for comprehensive antibody representation learning. *Research, 8*, 0721.

Yong, L., Fangmin, D., & Renbin, X. (2007). Path synthesis of rapid mechanisms by artificial immune networks. *Journal-Huazhong University of Science and Technology Nature Science Edition*, *35*(3), 70.

You, Z., Ma, J., Li, H., Hu, Y. F., & Huang, J. D. (2025). BConformeR: a conformer based on mutual sampling for unified prediction of continuous and discontinuous antibody binding sites. *arXiv preprint arXiv:2508.12029*.

Yousif, M. G., Fatima, G., Castro, H. J., Al-Amran, F. G., & Rawaf, S. (2023). Unraveling post-COVID-19 immune dysregulation using machine learning-based immunophenotyping. *arXiv preprint arXiv:2310.01428*.

Yuan, Q., Wei, X., Xiong, X., Li, M., & Zhang, Y. (2020). A hybrid neural collaborative filtering model for drug repositioning. In *2020 IEEE International Conference on Bioinformatics and Biomedicine (BIBM)* (pp. 515-518). IEEE.

Zhang, H., Zhu, T., Ren, M., He, Z., Tao, S., Li, M., & Bu, D. (2025a). Accurate immune protein structure prediction by large language model and transfer learning. https://doi.org/DOI: 10.21203/rs.3.rs-7153530/v1

Zhang, T., Lin, Y., & Gao, Q. (2023a). Bispecific antibodies targeting immunomodulatory checkpoints for cancer therapy. *Cancer Biology & Medicine*, *20*(3), 181–195.

Zhang, T., Zhang, X., Wu, Z., Ren, J., Zhao, Z., Zhang, H., & Wang, T. (2025b). VGAE-CCI: Variational graph autoencoder-based construction of 3D spatial cell–cell communication network. *Briefings in Bioinformatics*, *26*(1), bbae619.

Zhang, X., Rahnavard, A., & Crandall, K. A. (2025c). Machine learning enhances biomarker discovery: From multi-omics to functional genomics. *Medical Research Archives*, *13*(8).

Zhang, Y., Ari, S. L., Gupta, S., Zaemes, J., Shah, N. J., Alaoui, A., & Atkins, M. B. (2023b). 1317 Enhancing patient safety in melanoma treatment: Harnessing machine learning for predicting immune-related adverse events. *Journal for Immunotherapy of Cancer*, *11*(1, Supplement).

Zhao, L., He, Q., Song, H., Zhou, T., Luo, A., Wen, Z., & Lin, X. (2024). Protein A-like peptide design based on diffusion and ESM2 Models. *Molecules (Basel, Switzerland)*, *29*(20), 4965.

Zhao, Y., He, B., Xu, F., Li, C., Xu, Z., Su, X., & Yao, J. (2023). DeepAIR: A deep learning framework for effective integration of sequence and 3D structure to enable adaptive immune receptor analysis. *Science Advances*, *9*(32), eabo5128.

Zhou, M., Huang, Z., Ma, Z., Chen, J., Lin, S., Yang, X., & Zhong, J. (2025a). The next frontier in antibody-drug conjugates: Challenges and opportunities in cancer and autoimmune therapy. *Cancer Drug Resistance (Alhambra, Calif.)*, *8*, 34.

Zhou, X. J., Laouar, Y., & Tsoi, L. C. (2025b). Community series in towards precision medicine for immune-mediated disorders: Advances in using big data and artificial intelligence to understand heterogeneity in inflammatory responses, volume II. *Frontiers in Immunology*, *16*, 1553004.

Zhu, I., Piraner, D. I., & Roybal, K. T. (2023). Synthesizing a smarter CAR T cell: Advanced engineering of T-cell immunotherapies. *Cancer Immunology Research*, *11*(8), 1030–1043.

APPENDIX

Abbreviations

ADC - Antibody–Drug Conjugate
ADR - Adverse Drug Reactions
AI - Artificial Intelligence
AI-D3S - Drug Design and Discovery System
CAR - Chimeric Antigen Receptor
CDRs - Complementarity-Determining Regions
CIDs - Chronic Inflammatory Diseases
CRS - Cytokine Release Syndrome
CSCCS - Continuous Self-controlled Case Series
DACs - Disease-Associated Cells
DAGs - Disease-Associated Genes
DAS - Deep Antigen Sets
DIME - Disease-Gene Immune Cell Expression
DITP - Drug-Induced Immune Thrombocytopenia
DL - Deep Learning
DMTL - Design–Make–Test–Learn
GANs - Generative Adversarial Networks
GNNs - Graph Neural Networks
HER - Electronic Health Records
HTS - High-Throughput Screening
ICIs - Immune Checkpoint Inhibitors
IMIDs - Immune-Mediated Inflammatory Diseases
ISCTs - In-Silico Clinical Trials
LIME - Local Interpretable Model-Agnostic Explanations
LLMs - Large Language Models
MABEL - Minimal Anticipated Biological Effect Level
ML - Machine Learning
OoC - Organ-On-Chip
PAMP - Pathogen-Associated Molecular Pattern
PK/PD - Pharmacokinetic/Pharmacodynamic
PNVAC - Personalized Neoantigen Nano Vaccine
PRR - Pattern Recognition Receptor
Q-CHIPP - Quantum Convolutional Human Leukocyte Antigen Immunogenic Peptide Prediction
QML - Quantum Machine Learning

SHAP - Shapley Additive exPlanations
SQL - Structured Q-learning
TDM - Therapeutic Drug Monitoring
TID-Pro - Target Identification Pro
TMEs - Tumor Microenvironments
VAEs - Variational Autoencoders
XAI - Explainable AI

Chapter 5
AI-Driven Drug Development in Inflammatory Diseases

Balaji Esakkimuthu
Sudha Hospital, India

Manoj Mani
https://orcid.org/0009-0008-6601-0339
Bharathiar University, India

Prabakaran Dhashnamoorthy Subramanian
SRM Institute of Science and Technology, India

Balamuralikrishnan Balasubramanian
Sejong University, South Korea

Alwin Robert Asirvatham
Prince Sultan Military Medical City, Saudi Arabia

Antony Prabhu Jeyabal Philomenathan
Bharathiar University, India

Velayuthaprabhu Shanmugam
Bharathiar University, India

Vijaya Anand Arumugam
https://orcid.org/0000-0001-7485-1586
Bharathiar University, India

ABSTRACT

Artificial Intelligence in drug development for inflammatory diseases serves to enhance the overall efficiency, precision, and personalization of the process. AI integrates multi-omics, digital twins, and predictive modelling in order to identify therapeutic targets, accelerate molecular design, and optimize clinical translation of drugs. Machine learning and deep learning models help improve ADMET profiling, toxicity prediction, and the assessment of immunogenicity, while federated learning allows secure data collaboration across different institutions. Multi-modal AI with network pharmacology unravels complex disease mechanisms and supports systems-level drug modelling and optimization of multi-target therapy. Integration with automation,

DOI: 10.4018/979-8-3373-5258-9.ch005

closed-loop experimentation, and quantum computing is bound to accelerate both the processes of discovery and validation. Though ethical and regulatory challenges are at play, AI-driven frameworks will reshape translational medicine in driving equitable and explainable innovation in inflammation therapeutics.

1. INTRODUCTION

Inflammatory diseases are caused by a complex interplay of genetic, environmental, metabolic, and immune causes, imposing a major worldwide burden on health. Because of the diseases' complexity and their ever-changing pathways, traditional drug discovery in these inflammatory conditions has been time-consuming, expensive, and often characterized by low rates of clinical success. The apparent transformative solution for such needs is AI, through which computational power is added to accelerate early discovery, optimize molecular design, and enhance translational precision (Bindu *et al.,* 2025).

Machine learning (ML), deep learning (DL), and large language models (LLMs) currently enable high-accuracy prediction of drug-target interactions, modelling complex signaling networks, and de novo design of chemical structures with favorable pharmacological profiles. AlphaFold and AtomNet, among other tools, have transformed protein structure prediction and structure-based drug design by accurately modelling druggable conformations that accelerate target identification (Jarallah *et al.,* 2025). Graph neural networks (GNNs) and multimodal learning frameworks further enhance predictions of bioactivity, pathway involvement, and molecular behavior in diverse inflammatory settings (Patne *et al.,* 2024; Wang, 2025; Srinivas & Runkana, 2024).

AI has also advanced the field of precision medicine for inflammatory disorders by integrating multi-omics datasets of genomic, transcriptomic, proteomic, and metabolomic data with clinical and imaging information. Examples of such integrated models allow for molecular endotyping, stratification of patients, and prediction of therapeutic response, especially in complex diseases such as IBD and RA (Baldan-Martin *et al.,* 2025; Puentes-Osorio *et al.,* 2021). Moreover, AI-driven ADMET (Absorption, Distribution, Metabolism, Excretion, and Toxicity) prediction and toxicity assessment platforms enhance preclinical safety evaluation and thus immensely reduce the attrition rates during the inflammatory drug pipelines (Tian *et al.,* 2022; Swanson *et al.,* 2024).

The challenges yet remain despite such developments. Poor availability of high-quality annotated datasets, limited interpretability of complex AI models, data heterogeneity across platforms, and poor integration with experimental workflows continue to affect translational reliability (Goryanin *et al.,* 2025; Abed, 2025). Furthermore, there are ethical and regulatory barriers related to data privacy, model transparency, and algorithmic bias that raise a barrier to broad clinical adoption (Noor *et al.,* 2025). Most AI tools are validated in silico, and there remains the need for better coupling of computational predictions with biological or clinical validation.

This chapter reviews how AI is transforming drug development in inflammatory diseases in a focused, critically integrated manner. It describes the main AI technologies and rapidly emerging tools, along with their applications across the entire drug discovery pipeline, from target identification to clinical translation. The chapter further assesses current limitations, recent advances such as digital twins and federated learning (FL), and outlines future research directions needed to construct robust, explainable, clinically reliable AI-enabled frameworks for inflammation therapeutics.

2. MOLECULAR AND CELLULAR BASIS OF INFLAMMATION

The molecular mechanisms of chronic inflammation involve evolutionarily conserved systems, including NF-κB, JAK/STAT, the MAPK, and the NLRP3 inflammasome-signaling pathways to mutually regulate immune activation and the expression of inflammatory genes. Thus, NF-κB is a master transcription factor of pro-inflammatory cytokines, chemokines, and adhesion molecules, with its sustained activation contributing to chronic inflammation and tumorigenesis. JAK/STAT axis, in particular, the IL-6/JAK/STAT3 pathway, mediates cytokine-driven inflammatory responses in cancer, autoimmune diseases, and neurodegenerative disorders. Analogously, the MAPK, especially p38 MAPK, regulates stress response, apoptosis, and cell proliferation and impinges on the onset and persistence of various inflammatory pathologies (Kapoor *et al.,* 2025; Hou *et al.,* 2015; Yeung *et al.,* 2018). The NLRP3 inflammasome is a cytosolic multiprotein complex that controls the maturation of IL-1β and IL-18 and promotes low-grade chronic inflammation seen in obesity and IBD. Anti-inflammatory effects of natural compounds such as curcumin occur at least partly via modulation of these signaling cascades (Tian *et al.,* 2024).

At the cellular level, cytokine networks and crosstalk between immune cells regulate inflammatory processes. A number of chronic inflammatory disorders are underpinned by dysregulated cytokine secretion and altered interactions of immune cells. For instance, impaired interaction among NK cells, Tregs, and dendritic cells compromises hematopoiesis and enhances apoptosis in myelodysplastic syndrome (D'Silva *et al.,* 2019). Chronic immune activation promotes tissue damage, autoimmunity, and, in some instances, malignancy. Immune checkpoints, such as but not limited to PD-1 and CTLA-4, maintain tolerance and prevent excessive inflammation

(Mehta, 2025). Neuroendocrine stress pathways affect immune regulation via the gut-brain axis and enhance systemic inflammatory responses (Montgomery, 2024).

The dysregulation of NF-κB and JAK/STAT further contributes to systemic inflammation associated with metabolic imbalance and neuroimmune dysfunction. Recent insights into cellular contributors, including age-associated B cells and T follicular regulatory cells, have highlighted their role in chronic autoimmunity and defects in B-cell tolerance as new targets for therapeutic intervention (Long *et al.,* 2023). Advancement of multi-omics profiling continuously reveals predictive inflammatory biomarkers across diseases, including RA and IBD, strengthening system-biology approaches toward mechanistic understanding and the development of therapies (Baldan-Martin *et al.,* 2025; Puentes-Osorio *et al.,* 2021; Madrid-Paredes *et al.,* 2022; Chen *et al.,* 2025).

3. AI TECHNOLOGIES TRANSFORMING DRUG DISCOVERY

AI has now emerged as a strong driver for drug discovery transformation in inflammatory diseases by overcoming the traditional speed, cost, and efficiency bottlenecks of chemical queries. The architectures of DL, primarily Convolutional Neural Networks (CNNs) and Recurrent Neural Networks (RNNs), enable high-precision virtual screening and identification of targets by learning patterns in the spatial and sequential arrangement of chemical structures and biological sequences, respectively (Patne *et al.,* 2024). These models hasten rational drug design by accelerating hit discovery and determining structure-activity relationships important for anti-inflammatory therapeutics.

Another major advance now is the use of transformer-based architectures, which were developed originally for language modelling but are now put to use in "translating" molecular representations into novel chemical structures. Transformer-driven generative models may expand the chemical search space and allow de novo design of molecules with predefined biological properties. One example involves SN3-1, a potent NLRP3 inflammasome inhibitor generated through transformer-based DL in molecular generative modelling (Shi *et al.,* 2024). These models also enable scaffold hopping, chemical morphing, and optimization of ADMET properties; however, experimental validation has to be performed to work out metabolic complexity and off-target effects (Das, 2025).

GNNs introduce another stride toward the modelling of chemical and biological processes as interconnected graphs. GNNs capture molecular topology and protein-ligand interactions with high accuracy and further enable frameworks such as CSIP, which map chemical structures to imaging features for bioactivity prediction improvement. Multimodal models, such as MM-TCoCPIn, further integrate network topology, biomedical semantics, and 3D protein structure for state-of-the-art chemical-protein interaction predictions (Wang, 2025). Hybrid systems that are developed by integrating GNN with LLMs result in enhanced robustness and generalizability of these models for heterogeneous biomedical datasets (Srinivas & Runkana, 2024).

The state-of-the-art generative models, such as generative adversarial networks (GANs), variational autoencoders (VAEs), and reinforcement learning (RL)-based frameworks, can enable fully autonomous de novo drug design. Multi-objective optimization of molecules by RL balances potency, synthetic feasibility, and pharmacokinetics in frameworks such as Molecule Deep Q-Networks (MolDQN) and SHARP, which have already demonstrated synthesizable anti-inflammatory candidates validated both in vitro and in vivo (Zhou *et al.,* 2019; Kim *et al.,* 2025). It is, along with DL, transformers, and GNNs, that the generative models and RL coalesce into a potent ecosystem of computational tools, reshaping early discovery pipelines, reducing developmental attrition, and accelerating novel anti-inflammatory therapeutics identification. There is further integration of computational and experimental frameworks necessitated by biological complexity, data heterogeneity, and rigorous wet-lab validation.

4. AI IN TARGET IDENTIFICATION AND VALIDATION

AI-driven frameworks combining heterogeneous biological datasets, systems-level modelling, and knowledge-graph mining have revolutionized target identification and validation in inflammatory diseases. Modern computational methods identify the regulatory nodes whose perturbation is likely to yield therapeutic benefit by mapping complex inflammatory signalling pathways, including those driven by NF-κB, Hippo, and mTOR (Cucu, 2022). Some knowledge-graph platforms, including TARRAGON, deduce mechanistic links between diseases and candidate targets through the analysis of meta-paths deriving from curated molecular interactions (Beasley *et al.,* 2025).

Network pharmacology studies further support target prioritization by integrating protein–protein interaction networks, pathway enrichment, and disease-specific transcriptomic signatures. In IBD, network-based modelling has identified druggable targets across Crohn's disease (CD) and ulcerative colitis (UC) and pinpointed molecular checkpoints critical for the maintenance of host defense while keeping inflammation in check (Kitani *et al.,* 2020; O'Neill, 2006). There is also emerging evidence highlighting receptor clustering-for instance, the aggregation of IL-1 receptor complexes a therapeutic strategy for the modulation of inflammatory cascades (McCulloch *et al.,* 2006).

The ranking of targets improves significantly using ML-based prioritization frameworks that incorporate multi-omics datasets. Systems such as the F.O.R.W.A.R.D framework, which integrates transcriptomic and network connectivity data, have achieved 100% predictive accuracy when benchmarked against clinical trial outcomes in IBD (Figure 1) (Sinha *et al.,* 2025). In Multiple Sclerosis (MS), computational modelling that integrated structural dynamics with pathway-level enrichment identified TNFAIP3 as a high-confidence target (Yang *et al.,* 2021). Similarly, explainable ML methods have predicted patient-specific variation in drug response for IBD with an error margin as low as 4.98%, underlining their precision in mechanistic modelling (Okpete & Byeon, 2025).

The process of AI-driven immune target discovery is further accelerated by automated mining of voluminous biomedical literature. For instance, the tool Beegle applies gene-prioritization algorithms to extract genes implicated in diseases, whereas biomarkers and drug signatures of relevance to autoimmune and inflammatory disorders are inventoried in curated databases such as the autoimmune and inflammatory diseases biomarker database (ElShal *et al.,* 2016). Multi-omics data on the candidate targets are analyzed on ML-driven platforms such as Target Identification Pro to assess their translational value, while target predictions are ensured to be reliable and reproducible with benchmarking systems such as TargetBench 1.0 (Leung *et al.,* 2025).

A number of case studies underscore translational success with regard to AI-based target validation. Boolean gene-cluster network modelling identified gut-barrier-protective mechanisms in IBD, which were successfully validated in patient-derived organoids (Sahoo *et al.,* 2021). Boolean Network Explorer ranked PPARα and PPARγ as critical IBD regulators, and in vivo studies showed improvements in colitis and macrophage modulation (Katkar *et al.,* 2021). AI-guided drug repurposing has also been clinically validated: an RA drug predicted to show antiviral and anti-inflammatory effects was successfully repurposed for COVID-19 and validated by using organoid models and patient data (Schultz *et al.,* 2020).

Figure 1. F.O.R.W.A.R.D Framework for Predicting Drug Efficacy in Inflammatory Bowel Diseases

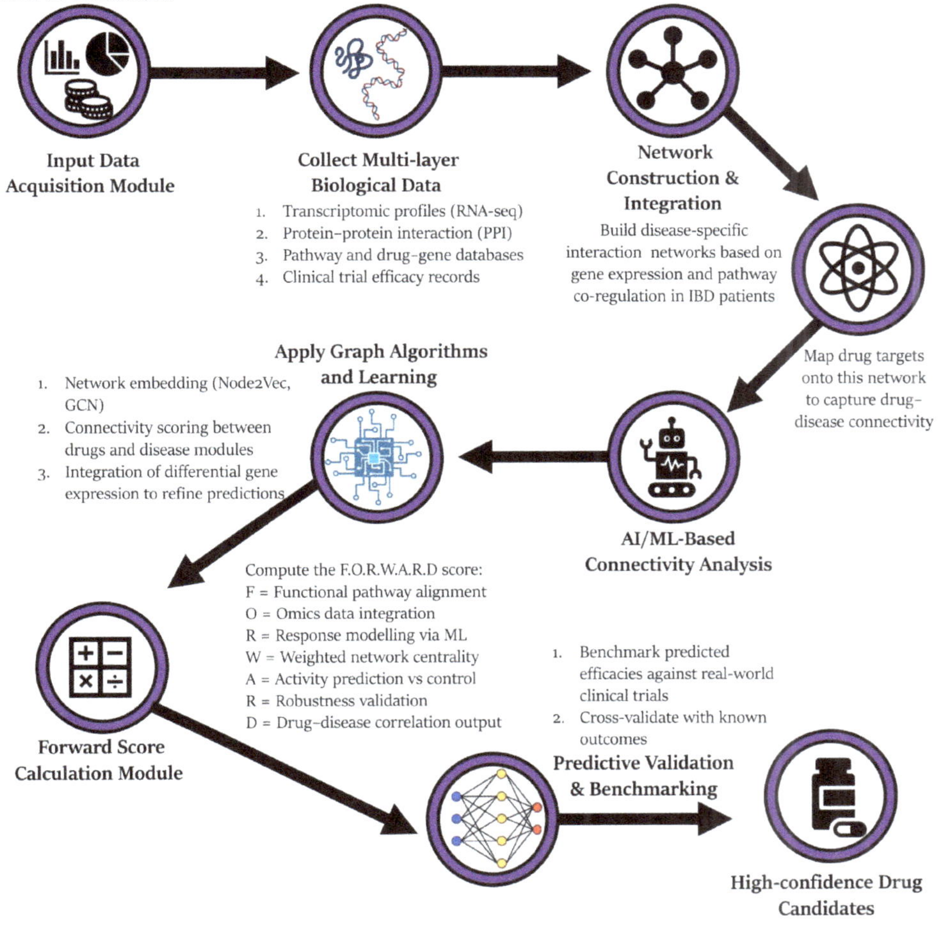

5. AI-DRIVEN DRUG DESIGN AND DISCOVERY

Generative AI models, including GANs, VAEs, and Transformers, are developing a paradigm for de novo anti-inflammatory drug design. These models efficiently navigate enormous chemical spaces in order to create new synthetically tractable molecular entities. The models learn high-dimensional patterns within wide chemical and biological datasets that allow compounds to be generated optimized for key biological targets implicated in inflammatory signaling. Working within latent chemical manifolds, the generative models allow for scaffold hopping and chemical morphing important for enhancing potency, selectivity, and structural diversity in anti-inflammatory agents. Integration with predictive analytics, including ADMET profiling and molecular docking, offers further refinement toward pharmacologically effective and safe design of drugs (Robert *et al.,* 2025; Das, 2025). Furthermore, RNNs of Long Short-Term Memory architecture enable the generation of valid SMILES strings of eventual drug candidates without the need for exhaustive virtual libraries (Gupta *et al.,* 2018). Such development has been further enhanced through RL together with GNNs, iteratively optimizing lead structures toward maximum bioactivity and drug-likeness (Das, 2025). Most impressively, these AI-driven approaches have allowed the synthesis of bioactive compounds with significant receptor-modulating properties, hence their applicability in anti-inflammatory drug discovery (Merk *et al.,* 2018).

RL coupled with hybrid symbolic-neural architectures, has given a big push to the lead optimization phase in anti-inflammatory compound development. Various RL-based frameworks have been proposed for balancing several objectives, such as binding affinity, synthetic feasibility, and pharmacokinetic properties, through reward-guided optimization. For example, one such RL model from Jiang et al. synthesizes new molecules against inflammation-related receptors, such as CXCR4, with commercially available chemical reaction templates and building blocks while ensuring synthesizability and drug-likeness through real-time docking and predictive evaluations (Jiang *et al.,* 2024). This is best epitomized by the framework of MolDQN, wherein domain-specific chemical knowledge is combined with RL for ensuring high chemical validity and optimal molecular performance (Zhou *et al.,* 2019). This optimization is further enhanced with the SHARP model, which uses a fragment-based hierarchical action space to overcome some of the major limitations of traditional RL in improving synthetic accessibility and allowing multi-objective optimization of binding affinity and drug-likeness (Kim *et al.,* 2025). Experimental validation through several in vitro and in vivo assays proved the efficacy of RL-generated compounds against inflammation-related processes (Jiang *et al.,* 2024). On another note, the integration of RL with systems pharmacology further empowers drug discovery with a personalized view and allows the development of inflammation therapies that can be tailored to patient genomic and molecular profiles (Tan *et al.,* 2022).

AI-assisted drug discovery has further been revolutionized by AlphaFold-based structural modelling, introducing atomic-level precision into the prediction of protein structure and, by extension, improving deep docking and virtual screening workflows. AlphaFold2 substantially increases predictive accuracy in structure-based drug design, particularly for those targets that do not have experimental crystal structures. This can be combined with ultra-large virtual screenings to allow the assessment of billions of compounds, which was so far impossible using the classical high-throughput screening methodologies (Gorgulla, 2024). AlphaFold2-RAVE extends this to capture metastable protein conformations very important in designing selective inhibitors. This framework models, with high accuracy, the interactions of the ligand in conformationally flexible targets, such as the DFG-out kinase states, via the combination of AlphaFold2 predictions with improved sampling molecular dynamics and induced fit docking (Gu *et al.*, 2024). Furthermore, AlphaFold2, coupled with molecular dynamics simulations and virtual screening, as highlighted in the identification of the inhibitors against SARS-CoV-2 main protease, underlines its potential for drug repositioning and fast lead identification (Zhao *et al.*, 2025).

AI applications in multi-target and polypharmacology modelling revolutionized the network-based strategies for inflammation control. The ML and DL frameworks introduce an opportunity for modelling protein-ligand interactions, and compound generation is possible with polypharmacological effects, which are necessary in targeting the interconnected networks of signalling in the inflammatory disease condition (Cichońska *et al.*, 2024). That also made a paradigm shift according to the principles of network pharmacology-from the "one-drug, one-target" model to a more effective "multi-target" therapeutic approach (Noor *et al.*, 2023). AI-assisted proteochemometric modelling and molecular docking can help in identifying synergistic co-targets while filtering out the anti-targets that are linked with the potential adverse effects (Cichońska *et al.*, 2024). Thus, network-based ranking algorithms analyze the topological properties of the disease networks in order to identify the synergistic combination of targets-as illustrated in Type 2 Diabetes Mellitus models (Vitali *et al.*, 2013). AI-driven in silico framework methods develop structure-based and ligand-based approaches, improving the predictions of polypharmacology for drug repositioning and multi-target drug discovery (Liu *et al.*, 2013). Network pharmacology on the inflammatory background encompasses the interaction between drugs and genes, expression profiles, and pathways to reveal the mechanisms of drugs, shed light on novel therapeutic uses, and assess the potential adverse drug reactions (ADRs)-this is facilitative of rational drug repurposing against inflammatory disorders (de Anda-Jáuregui *et al.*, 2018).

6. AI IN DRUG REPURPOSING FOR INFLAMMATORY DISEASES

The AI era has accelerated virtual screening in drug design, expanded the exploration of chemical space, and allowed for the rational optimization of anti-inflammatory therapeutics. Different DL frameworks now integrate structural biology information with cheminformatics and multi-omics datasets for the generation, evaluation, and refinement of molecules with better potency, selectivity, and superior pharmacokinetic characteristics (Patne *et al.,* 2024).

A major breakthrough includes the adoption of generative AI models, including GANs, VAEs, and RL systems for the independent design of new chemical entities. Examples of such RL-based platforms include MolDQN and ReLeaSE, while SHARP applies multi-objective RL to optimize the chemical structure in generating highly potent molecules with improved drug-likeness and synthetic feasibility (Zhou *et al.,* 2019; Kim *et al.,* 2025). In inflammatory disease, such architectures have enabled the creation of structurally diverse small molecules that were validated for anti-inflammatory activity both in vitro and in vivo (Jiang *et al.,* 2024).

Transformer-based molecular generators treat the chemical structures as a sort of "biological language" and further advance de novo drug design. This allows scaffold hopping, ADMET property optimization, and the design of molecules targeting complex inflammatory proteins. Of particular note, transformer-driven design produced SN3-1, a potent inhibitor of the NLRP3 inflammasome-exemplifying how foundation models will identify new anti-inflammatory scaffolds (Shi *et al.,* 2024)

GNNs have contributed much to structure-based drug design by accurately modelling molecular topology and protein-ligand interactions. GNN-enabled platforms, such as CSIP, integrate chemical structures with imaging features to predict bioactivity, while hybrid systems enable the optimization of properties and lead-likeness scoring through interpretable embeddings (Wang, 2025; Srinivas & Runkana, 2024).

Meanwhile, AI-driven virtual screening platforms accelerate hit identification by reducing the time and cost involved in wet-lab screens. Deep CNN-based scoring functions outperform classical docking by capturing fine-scale chemical-biophysical interactions important for inflammatory targets, such as NF-κB modulators, cytokine inhibitors, and metabolic regulators.

Generative and predictive AI models have now been integrated into automated closed-loop design workflows, bringing together:

1. Molecule generation
2. Property prediction, Potency, ADMET
3. Planning of synthesis
4. In vitro validation

Indeed, iterative design-test-learn systems of this kind have yielded optimized compounds that exhibit superior pharmacokinetics and reduced off-target interactions-all at the heart of challenges facing chronic inflammatory disorders. While AI-generated molecules are highly promising, further integration with medicinal chemistry expertise, robust experimental validation, and translation modelling is critical to further these candidates into clinical pipelines.

7. PREDICTIVE ADMET, TOXICOLOGY, AND SAFETY PROFILING

ML and DL models have become an important tool for predicting the ADMET profile and immunotoxicity properties of novel anti-inflammatory compounds, consequently contributing to the significant reduction of attrition rates during drug development (**Figure 2**). Extreme Gradient Boosting (XGBoost) was among the top performers in 18 out of 22 tasks on the Therapeutics Data Commons ADMET benchmark and is available via the web-based ADMETboost platform for the accurate optimization of ADMET properties. Similarly, admetSAR allows for rapid evaluation of pharmacokinetic and toxicological parameters by integrating a total of currently 51 different models on ADMET, thus providing early risk stratification within drug development. ADMET-AI represents another front-runner modelling platform that achieved the top average rank on the Therapeutics Data Commons Benchmark leaderboard and exhibits a 45% reduction in prediction time while supporting ultra-large chemical library screening in a high-throughput manner.

These microphysiological systems, replicating organ-level pharmacokinetics and toxicodynamics, present good clinical translatability, thus increasing the accuracy of toxicological prediction manifold and raising the overall translation reliability quotient (Cong *et al.,* 2020). Furthermore, AI- Organ-on-Chip (OOC) convergence allows for the interpretation of real-time biosensors, integration of multi-parameter data, and further modelling of organ-specific toxicity (Barua, 2024). AI-driven models, as seen with TransTox from GANs, execute cross-organ transcriptomic translation-that is, liver to kidney and vice versa-with toxicology prediction for multiple organs using their power (Li *et al.,* 2024). Integration of robotic automation with OOC enhances efficiency by allowing high-throughput fabrication and the reduction of human error in performing toxicology assays (Vijayaragavan *et al.,* 2025).

AI frameworks also demonstrate significant utility in the prediction of Cytokine Release Syndrome (CRS) and immune toxicity associated with biologics and cell-based therapies. A Mayo Clinic gradient-boosting ML model predicted CRS up to 72 hours in advance with a high degree of accuracy, with an AUC of 0.90; similarly, an XGBoost-based model presented a micro-average AUC of 0.94 for grading CRS severity (Pettinati *et al.,* 2022). Biomarkers such as IFN-γ and IL-6 remain strong predictors of severe CRS, offering quantitative metrics for early intervention (Teachey *et al.,* 2016).

Several regulatory issues dictate the need for standardized and transparent validation schemes. A four-phase external validation system was thus proposed to make the use of AI in toxicology reproducible and clinically reliable (Lopez-Perez *et al.,* 2024). European Crohn's and Colitis Organisation (ECCO) also emphasizes strong validation pipelines with a regulatory fit for the AI-based toxicological arms from the perspective of inflammatory diseases (Noor *et al.,* 2025).

Figure 2. AI-Based ADMET Prediction Pipeline for Inflammatory Disease Drug Development

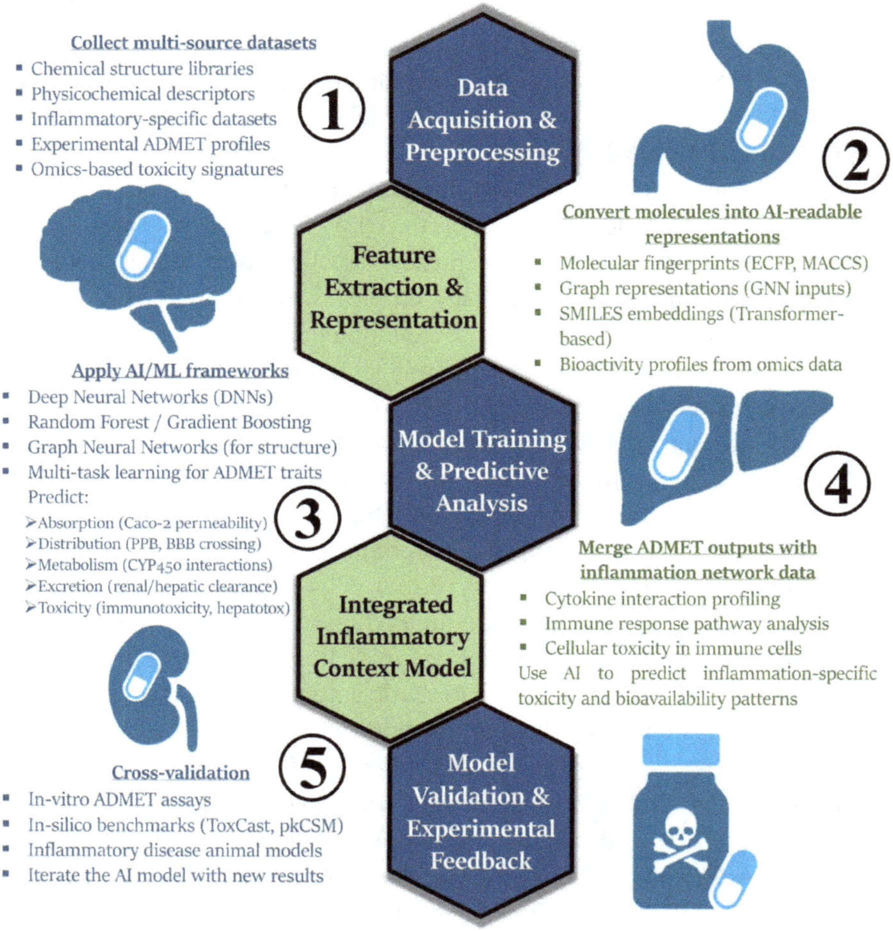

8. MULTI-OMICS AND SINGLE-CELL INTEGRATION IN INFLAMMATION

AI makes a difference in the ability of genomics, transcriptomics, proteomics, metabolomics, and metagenomics to integrate and decipher the heterogeneity of inflammatory diseases. In IBD, multi-omic AI models that incorporate genomic, transcriptomic, and proteomic features successfully differentiate between CD and UC by determining subtype-specific inflammatory signatures and molecular biomarkers (**Figure 3**). The integrative platforms overcome some of the main limitations of classical biomarker discovery in terms of reproducibility and scalability by offering the possibility to interpret disease-relevant features across different layers (Zhang *et al.,* 2025). AI-driven approaches also reveal shared and disease-specific immune signatures across autoimmune diseases and cancer, showing the power of ML/DL in extracting high-dimensional biological patterns in complex diseases such as IBD (Chinedu-Nzereogu *et al.,* 2025).

AI-based multi-omics analysis also provides host–microbiome research and therapeutic response prediction in IBD to support precision medicine strategies (Iacucci & Santacroce, 2024). Apart from bulk omics, single-cell and spatial multi-omics achieve finer resolution of immune heterogeneity. AI-enabled Single-Cell RNA Sequencing (scRNA-seq), ATAC-seq, and spatial transcriptomics chart immune-stromal interactions within inflamed tissues. Folasole et al. developed an integrated single-cell–spatial framework to characterize spatiotemporal immune responses in RA, IBD, and systemic lupus erythematosus (SLE), identifying early molecular perturbations and mechanistic therapeutic targets (Folasole *et al.,* 2025). In IBD, scRNA-seq highlighted macrophage–fibroblast communication as one of the key drivers of pathology (Garrido-Trigo *et al.,* 2023). Similarly, in psoriasis, spatial multi-omics identified pathogenic fibroblast–immune cell niches. Zhan et al. extended this latter approach by adopting Stereo-XCR-seq that coupled spatial transcriptomics with TCR/BCR sequencing, highlighting lymphocyte clonal architecture in IBD (Zhan *et al.,* 2025).

AI-driven temporal and causal modelling brings a new view into a dynamic temporal perspective on inflammation. Neural Stochastic Differential Equation models, reproducing factual and counterfactual disease trajectories, improve personalized prediction in chronic inflammatory diseases (Durso-Finley *et al.,* 2024). Temporal Transformer-based Causal Learning predicts disease course in autoimmune diseases while minimizing confounding variables (Kaur & Sharma, 2025). Similarly, nodes of immune signalling have been pinpointed as potential intervention points by means of mathematical models (Ugolkov *et al.,* 2024).

AI-driven multi-omics-to-drug target mapping links dysregulated pathways with druggable nodes. For example, network modelling identified TNFAIP3 as a therapeutic target in MS and was validated using pharmacophore-based virtual screening methods (Yang *et al.,* 2021). Boolean-network integration methods like mBONITA find genes that are consistently perturbed across multi-omic layers (Palshikar *et al.,* 2023). Explainable ML models integrate genomic, transcriptomic, and demographic features to yield a forecast of drug responses and stratify IBD patients into molecular endotypes (Gardiner *et al.,* 2022). Other tools, such as OmicsNet, further support multilayer network analysis for linking genes to functional phenotypes (Akhmedov *et al.,* 2017).

Figure 3. AI-Driven Multi-Omics Integration for IBD Subtype Differentiation

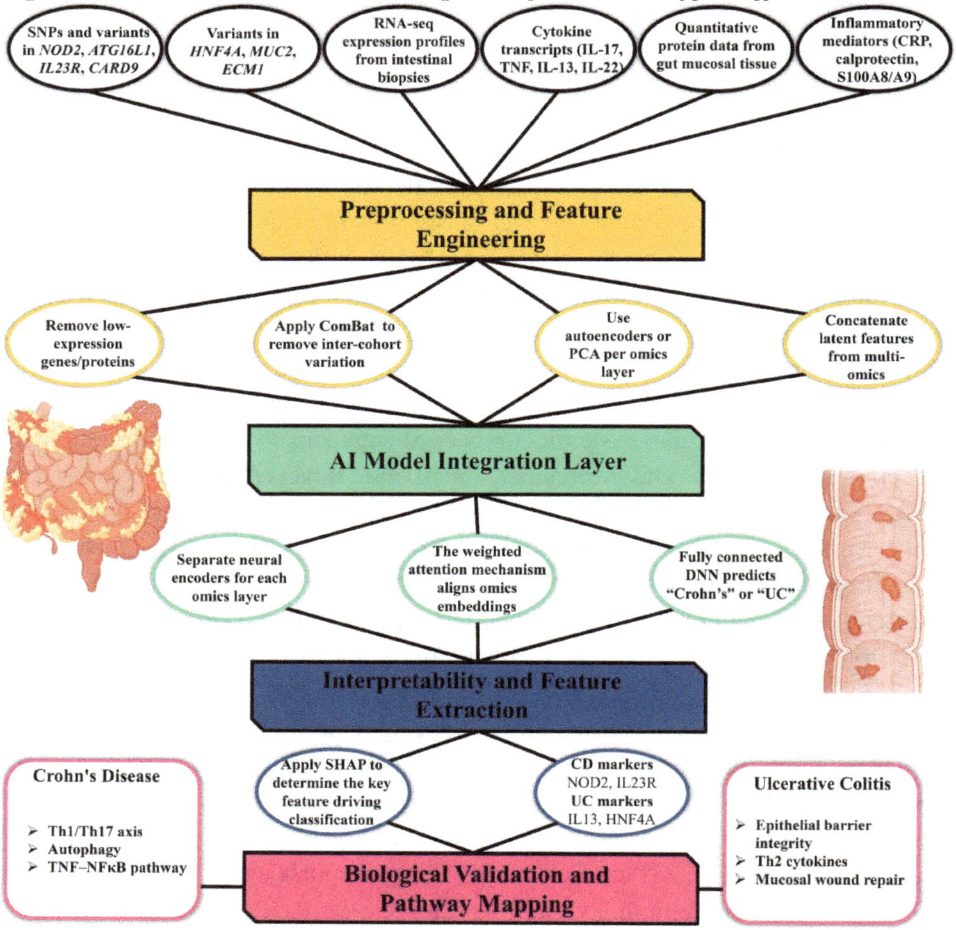

9. DIGITAL TWINS AND IN-SILICO MODELS

Of all the AI-driven innovations for modelling inflammatory diseases, one of the most transformational has been digital twins. Computational surrogates represent patient-specific immunological, molecular, and physiological states, enabling personalized simulations of disease progression and therapeutic interventions. Integrating genomics, transcriptomics, and clinical phenotypes, the digital twins capture complex immune variability across thousands of interacting genes, cell types, and tissue compartments (Benson, 2023). AI- and ML-enhanced frameworks further increase their capabilities in modelling heterogeneity, recognizing novel targets, and predicting patient-specific responses to anti-inflammatory agents (Moingeon *et al.,* 2024). Digital twin-guided advances in inflammation modelling outline how dynamic immune responses can be predicted with high fidelity for precision therapeutics (Sekaran *et al.,* 2025).

Mechanistic simulations of tissue-level biology under drug exposure complement digital twins through in-silico organs and virtual patient models. Such models embed individualized physiological and pharmacokinetic/pharmacodynamic (PK/PD) parameters, enabling virtual trials that enhance predictions about drug efficacy and safety (Alimguzhin *et al.,* 2020). Computational drug repurposing through molecular docking and virtual screening revealed modulators of key inflammatory mediators, including TNF-α and IL-6; in-silico validation increased their reliability before preclinical testing (Enni & Maraj, 2022). Also, integration with systems biology frameworks provides mechanistic insights into immune signalling, tissue injury, and therapeutic responses.

Large-scale virtual patient cohorts extend this paradigm by modelling population-level variability across molecular, clinical, and environmental factors. Such systems-patientomics approaches will help in predicting disease trajectories and optimization of therapeutic strategies with enhanced safety and at lower cost (Dimitrov, 2014). For instance, in cardiovascular inflammatory disorders, in-silico modelling allowed for therapeutic intervention assessment and the clarification of disease mechanisms (Angoulvant *et al.,* 2023)

Parallel developments are occurring in the ethical and regulatory spheres. Organizations such as ECCO emphasize the requirement for standardized validation and ethical governance of the AI-based modelling tools employed in IBD (Noor *et al.,* 2025). Organoid-based Non-Animal Testing Models (NAMs) provide a complementary technology but encounter serious challenges in terms of validation and regulatory acceptance (Fausch *et al.,* 2025). The global uptake of NAMs, including the in-silico, in-vitro, in-chemico, and ex-vivo approaches consistently hindered by a lack of clear unified standards of validation, which dictates the need to call for global harmonization frameworks along with open data sharing (Ouedraogo *et al.,* 2025; Athira *et al.,* 2022). These legislative undertakings, such as those in Australia, represent an attempt to bring national policy into line with international standards in relation to non-animal-based computational testing (Anderson & Smith, 2024).

Personalized digital twins are now redefining the prediction of treatment response in immune-mediated inflammatory diseases. These models integrate genomic, environmental, and lifestyle factors to simulate patient-specific disease dynamics with high accuracy, thus enabling adaptive and individualized therapeutic regimens. Their relevance is particularly evident in heterogeneous conditions like IBD, where patient-tailored predictions enable precision therapy and minimize side effects. Nevertheless, there are still formidable shortcomings regarding comprehensive modelling of genome-wide interactions and systemic effects that pose a major barrier to complete clinical translation.

10. AI FOR BIOLOGICS AND NEXT-GENERATION MODALITIES

The design of biologics and next-generation modalities for inflammatory diseases has depended increasingly on AI, which seamlessly models the protein structure, binding interfaces, developability, and immunogenicity with high accuracy. Today, DL architecture predicts antibody conformations, refines CDR loops, and assesses manufacturability to enable the rapid identification of high-affinity, low-liability candidates suitable for chronic inflammatory conditions. Transformer-based sequence models and AI-generated antibody libraries improved preclinical success rates by accelerating hit discovery and targeting optimization. These capabilities underpin the development of IL-23 and IL-17 inhibitors; guselkumab, risankizumab, and secukinumab showed >70% PASI-90 responses in psoriasis and demonstrated mucosal healing in CD (Rouyan *et al.,* 2025). Similar computational frameworks have also improved the therapeutic development of peptides. Ensemble models, CNNs, and gated recurrent units-based architectures furthered anti-inflammatory peptide activity predictions and offered insights into the structural determinants of bioactivity, guiding the development of peptide inhibitors against inflammasome components, including NLRP3 and caspase-1 (Guan *et al.,* 2023).

AI-driven immuno-engineering has also transformed protein optimization pipelines through the integration of mutational scanning, biophysical modelling, and language model predictions for improved binding specificity, stability, and safety. Computational affinity maturation has yielded antibodies with multi-fold enhancements in target binding, including reported improvements of 6.01-fold in IgG-binding performance and up to 160-fold affinity increases for SARS-CoV-2 spike-targeting antibodies through genetic algorithms and simulated annealing (Li *et al.,* 2025; Ashraf *et al.,* 2024). Immunogenicity prediction tools assessing sequence homology, MHC-binding motifs, and predicted epitope landscapes further help guide safe biologic design with translation to early mitigation of anti-drug antibody formation (Doneva *et al.,* 2021). Translation to the clinic has been direct, with optimized IL-2 muteins designed to preferentially expand regulatory T cells demonstrating improved safety and durable immunomodulation in early trials for UC and SLE. AI-guided engineering of IL-10 agonists and IL-1 receptor decoys has strengthened mucosal targeting and reduced cytokine-mediated toxicity in preclinical and early clinical studies, supporting their translation into therapies for chronic IBD.

The impact of AI extends beyond proteins into the RNA therapeutic space. Various ML frameworks are involved in the refinement of antisense oligonucleotide, siRNA, miRNA, and mRNA constructs by predicting stability, minimizing off-target effects, and modelling immunogenicity signatures critical for safe deployment in inflammatory conditions. These have underpinned clinically validated RNA therapeutics, givosiran, and accelerated ongoing programs targeting JAK/STAT and NF-κB mediators in autoimmune diseases (Vora *et al.,* 2023). AI-driven physicochemical modelling further enhances formulation through optimizing solubility, degradation kinetics, and nanoparticle compatibility. Predictive design of nanocarriers, supported by DL-driven material discovery, has enabled tissue-specific delivery whereby personalized nanoparticle functionalization enhances uptake within inflamed synovium or gut mucosa and reduces systemic toxicity (Zhu *et al.,* 2025; Liu *et al.,* 2025a).

These include the incorporation of structural, omics, imaging, and dynamic simulation data in emerging multimodal AI frameworks that build mechanistically interpretable models, linking molecular design to biological function. This has been particularly transformative in multispecific antibody engineering, where AI models characterize linker-mediated effects on quaternary structure, binding kinetics, and allosteric interactions that enable efficient optimization of multispecific antibodies for complex inflammatory networks (Occhipinti *et al.,* 2024; Singh *et al.,* 2025). Generative AI models such as GANs and VAEs accelerate scaffold design, hit identification, and affinity maturation, while high-throughput experimental coupling has substantially extended the druggable proteome (Liu *et al.,* 2025b). Clinically, this has guided the design of nanobody therapeutics such as ozoralizumab, an engineered anti-TNF nanobody with improved synovial penetration and reduced immunogenicity that demonstrates strong disease activity reduction in rheumatoid arthritis (RA) and is promising for IBD.

AI-enabled modelling has also entered cell-based therapy pipelines for inflammatory disease. Predictive antigen-selection tools and cytokine-release forecasting models support the development of low-toxicity CAR-T and CAR-macrophage platforms. These innovations have all contributed to the successful application of CD19 CAR-T therapy in refractory SLE, where several patients achieved drug-free remission, and now underpin early-stage exploration of engineered macrophages for chronic perianal fistulas and fibrotic complications of IBD (Son *et al.,* 2024). Across biologics, RNA therapeutics, and engineered cell therapies, therefore, AI has become central to accelerating design, improving clinical readiness, and enhancing mechanistic precision in the next generation of anti-inflammatory therapeutics.

11. CLINICAL TRANSLATION: AI IN PRECLINICAL AND CLINICAL DEVELOPMENT

AI-driven computational modelling is changing the face of preclinical drug development by enabling mechanistic simulation of the behavior of drugs in complex biological systems, thereby enhancing early prediction of efficacy, pharmacodynamics, and toxicity. Integrative ML models leverage molecular, structural, and multi-omics data to simulate PK/PD behavior and accelerate lead prioritization for biologics and pathway-specific agents (Dong *et al.,* 2022). This is especially the case in indications where poor translational relevance from animal models limits progress. These predictive frameworks further refine ADME estimates to provide dose-exposure predictions that will inform the rational optimization of therapeutic indices. Integration of patient-specific parameters further enables ML-supported PK/PD modelling to achieve superior levels of translational accuracy and allows for better forecasting of inter-individual variability (Pawar *et al.,* 2021). DL-based toxicity predictors complement this preclinical evaluation by predicting organ-specific toxicity from structural and physicochemical features, thus limiting the need for large-scale animal tests and risk of late-stage attrition (Malani *et al.,* 2023).

AI further empowers clinical monitoring through wearable biosensing platforms and digital biomarkers capable of continuous capture of physiological indicators of inflammation. Real-time wearable sensor streams, like VitalPatch, monitor heart rate, respiration rate, and skin temperature, thus allowing timely detection of flares in inflammation and dynamic treatment response assessment (Avey *et al.,* 2024). ML algorithms running on these data provide personalized digital twins that can help distinguish between inflammation-specific patterns and background physiological noise with enhanced diagnostic specificity (Mariam *et al.,* 2024). The modelling of AI biomarkers integrates the understanding of circulating inflammatory proteins together with physiological signatures for a holistic view of the inflammatory burden and facilitates data-driven therapeutic adjustments. Uniform data acquisition and interpretation protocols provided by standardized data frameworks, such as DACIA, improve the reproducibility of the development of digital biomarkers (Daniore *et al.,* 2024).

AI is part of adaptive trial design, synthetic control arm generation, and patient stratification during clinical development. The particular value of AI in inflammatory diseases lies in the fact that there is substantial inter-patient heterogeneity. AI-powered trial management platforms optimize dose selection, dynamic randomization, and targeted recruitment while performing analyses of high-dimensional immunological data to predict inflammatory responses in trial progression. Syntax integrates real-world datasets in constructing synthetic control arms (Makutam *et al.,* 2024; Zhou *et al.,* 2025), a concept extended to the creation of patient-specific digital twins by generative AI systems at Unlearn.AI, which allows for as much as a 34% reduction in size for the control arm with no loss of regulatory compliance (Turner *et al.,* 2024). Network-based disease modelling further enables the characterization and mechanistic refinement of targets in an early phase of development, as seen in studies identifying mechanisms protecting against gut barrier disruption in IBD (Sahoo *et al.,* 2021).

AI is also changing endpoint optimization and precision in chronic inflammatory diseases such as IBD, where trial outcomes are confounded by heterogeneous disease trajectories and variable treatment responses. Integration of multi-modal genomic, metabolomic, imaging, and clinical parameters allows predictive algorithms to forecast treatment response and early identification of non-responders, guiding refinement of endpoints to limit trial failure rates (Qian *et al.,* 2024). AI-enhanced endoscopic and histologic image analysis offers more homogeneous and quantitative assessment of inflammatory activity, improving diagnostic precision and disease grading in IBD (Ahmad *et al.,* 2023). ML tools integrating EHR, imaging, and multi-omics data promote personalized treatment selection for biologics and small molecules while continuously monitoring disease progression (Zand *et al.,* 2022). The integration challenges, heterogeneity of the analytical workflows, and overall limited prospective validation remain important barriers toward clinical adoption. Ongoing advances in model interpretability and data standardization are rapidly moving AI toward its regulatory-grade use in trials of inflammatory diseases.

12. REAL-WORLD DATA, FEDERATED LEARNING, AND PRECISION THERAPEUTICS

FL has become the cornerstone for developing privacy-preserving AI in inflammatory and autoimmune diseases. It allows model training across multi-institutional sites without actual data transfer. Instead of aggregating centralized data, it exchanges encrypted model parameters and, thus, maintains compliance with HIPAA and GDPR while enabling construction of the most robust models generalizable across heterogeneous cohorts (Ali *et al.,* 2022). Empirical studies have demonstrated that FL could attain up to 99% of centralized model performance, which provides clinical validation for high-fidelity medical AI. For example, in MS, the use of federated MRI lesion segmentation across different clinical sites yielded a strong accuracy despite diverse scanner types and acquisition protocols, and patient demographics (Sheller *et al.,* 2020). Large-scale efforts like Clinnova further underscore the translational prospects of FL in orchestrating cross-border data collaborations to advance precision medicine in chronic inflammatory diseases (Talebi & Azimi, 2025). However, communication burdens, site-specific heterogeneity in data, and disparities in computational resources continue to be several active challenges to improve scalability and deployment efficiency (Alekseenko *et al.,* 2024)

Building on this foundation, the integration of Real-World Evidence (RWE) with FL is already reshaping patient stratification, therapeutic prediction, and clinical decision-making. FL-enabled platforms support secure and regulatory-compliant integration of multimodal EHR, genomic, and imaging datasets at scale. The GenoMed4All Consortium exemplifies this potential through the use of an open-source FL infrastructure leveraging DeepSurv and generative AI for the purposes of modelling rare hematological diseases with higher accuracy, while it enables multi-centric collaboration (Asti *et al.,* 2025). In turn, NVIDIA FLARE trains models over international healthcare institutions using privacy-preserving cryptographic protocols, with its successful deployment in COVID-19 outcome prediction that may be adapted to inflammatory and autoimmune diseases (Roth *et al.,* 2025). FedBioMed furthers these features by adding transparency and reproducibility features expected in clinical research harmonization (Cremonesi *et al.,* 2025). Finally, at the level of complementary RWE-driven platforms, including Immunolab and PRISM, which integrate longitudinal clinical analytics, the trajectories of patients are characterized; treatment transitions are defined, and subgroups of patients showing differential responses to immunomodulators are uncovered (Hamelin *et al.,* 2022; Jemielita & Mehrotra, 2019).

Interpretability-driven models in explainable machine learning (XML) go further in advancing precision immunology by relating multi-omic, demographic, and pharmacologic features to treatment outcomes in inflammatory diseases. These approaches build upon trust and transparency by allowing clinicians to achieve feature contributions and biological plausibility. XML techniques have focused on the determination of transcriptomic and genomic signatures for stratifying patients with IBD into mechanistically different endotypes predictive of therapeutic efficacy (Gardiner *et al.,* 2022). Other interpretability tools, such as CODE-XAI (Lu *et al.,* 2024), leverage more granular estimates of Conditional Average Treatment Effects in order to provide personalized treatment attributions that support both precision dosing and choice of therapy. However, the performance of XML fundamentally remains limited by the scope and quality of available data, thus begging for harmonized phenotyping protocols and unified data pipelines in clinical immunology (Auger & Scott, 2025).

AI-driven, multimodal analytics are increasingly being integrated into clinical management for autoimmune and inflammatory diseases with real-time decision support and disease stratification capabilities. In SLE, AI models integrating clinical and serological data outperform traditional ANA assays by enhancing diagnostic precision and reducing false-negative rates (Park, 2024). In RA and systemic sclerosis, ML tools that integrate clinical, imaging, and omic profiles improve the prediction of therapeutic response, early disease progression, and organ involvement. In IBD, AI systems able to analyze endoscopic imagery have shown the ability to detect mucosal injury with high sensitivity, providing quantitative activity scoring superior to manual assessment. Decision-support platforms integrating EHR data, immunologic markers, and genetic features are now being validated for use in routine clinical practice in order to optimize biologic and small-molecule therapy selection (Silverman *et al.,* 2025). In parallel, AI accelerates drug discovery and repurposing mechanistically through target identification and viable candidate prioritization for inflammatory and autoimmune diseases, which dramatically reduces development timelines and costs. However, ethical transparency, data governance, and patient trust remain essential pillars for large-scale translation. Collaborative governance frameworks are increasingly required to ensure safe, equitable, and ethically aligned deployment of these technologies in precision immunology (Mane *et al.,* 2024).

13. NETWORK PHARMACOLOGY AND SYSTEMS-LEVEL DRUG MODELLING

AI-driven network pharmacology has transformed the way in which multi-target drug discovery for inflammatory diseases is pursued, through the use of computational methods for complex biological interaction mapping and the prediction of synergistic therapeutic effects. ML and DL models integrate bioactive compound libraries, protein-ligand interaction simulations, and pathway-level biological networks to identify multi-target compounds capable of modulating coordinated inflammatory cascades (Noor *et al.,* 2023). Systems pharmacology extends these approaches to multiscale modelling of drug action, wherein better personalization of therapy is achieved by predicting how molecular and physiological interactions change across patient populations (Van Hasselt & Iyengar, 2019). The utility of this latter framework is illustrated well by the rational repurposing of established anti-inflammatory agents: biomolecular network modelling, which integrated transcriptomic signatures and pathway associations, identified naproxen and meloxicam as candidates with favorable network topology features and low off-target toxicity, validating their potential for repositioning in chronic inflammatory disorders (de Anda-Jáuregui *et al.,* 2018). Such computational predictions resonate well with experience at the clinic-naproxen consistently demonstrating symptom improvement in ankylosing spondylitis, and meloxicam offering better gastrointestinal tolerability in RA-thereby validating the translational relevance of network-driven predictions.

Causal graph-based modelling further refines mechanistic predictions, connecting perturbations in molecular pathways to phenotypic outcomes across omics layers. Similarly, platforms integrating KEGG, Connectivity Map, and gene-set enrichment data map associations among targets, compounds, and ADRs, and give insight into system-level drug effects. The same models have been used in IBD to support the identification of gut barrier–protective pathways and predict drug combinations capable of restoring epithelial integrity; these findings are reflected clinically in the improved mucosal healing associated with combination therapy using anti-TNF agents and thiopurines in moderate-to-severe CD. Another advanced GNN framework-PDGrapher-embeds cellular states into causal networks to predict combinatorial perturbations of therapeutic potential (Gonzalez-Garcia *et al.,* 2015). Predictive power from these models is further enhanced by two-layer causal frameworks that integrate transcriptomic perturbation data and quantify the resultant molecular and phenotypic outcomes (Alfonso-González *et al.,* 2025). Consistently, mechanistic insights have translated to the clinically observed superior remission rates achieved by combination targeting of cytokine and adhesion molecule pathways in refractory UC, reinforcing the validity of system-level prediction.

RL reinforces the approach of systems pharmacology in optimising the combinations of drugs that maintain immune homeostasis while maximizing efficacy. Iterating simulations of pharmacodynamic interactions, RL models identify personalized multi-drug strategies for such complex immune-mediated diseases as RA, IBD, and lupus. Clinically, parallels in practice will be the combinations based on RL-like modelling strategies, such as methotrexate with TNF inhibitors in RA or ustekinumab following anti-TNF failure in CD. These reflect optimized therapeutic sequencing predicted by system-level modelling approaches. scRNA-seq further enriches these frameworks by profiling cell-state-specific responses to drug combinations, thus informing predictions of synergy in a clinically meaningful context (Jiang *et al.,* 2022). Network-based approaches, including NetPTP, apply gene-expression perturbation data to treatment personalization. The translation into clinical practice terms of decision-making regarding which therapy to use (Han *et al.,* 2021). Transcriptomic-guided therapy selection has enhanced the prediction of biologic response in a wide array of autoimmune and immune-mediated diseases, including RA and UC.

AI-driven network modelling represents a convergent framework through which systems immunology, multi-omics signatures, and computational pharmacology converge to expedite the development of immune-modulatory drugs. These models have identified shared molecular dysfunction across conditions such as lupus and RA that inform biomarker discovery and precision targeting (Alfonso-González *et al.,* 2025). In silico simulation of virtual patient populations strengthens translational relevance by predicting drug efficacy in heterogeneous cohorts in support of applications in disorders including trastuzumab-resistant HER2^{+} breast cancer and myocarditis (Hamano *et al.,* 2025). These predictions echo clinical observations when targeting interconnected inflammatory pathways, such as IL-1 and IL-6 blockade in cytokine storm syndromes, showing superior clinical response. In rheumatology, ML-based stratification tools integrating genetic, phenotypic, and serologic features support precision biologic selection based on clinical outcomes in which gene-expression-guided treatment assignment improved remission rates (Zhou *et al.*, 2025). Yet despite progress, substantial challenges pertain to data harmonization, mechanistic validation, and interpretability. The development of standardized integration pipelines and transparent decision-support systems will be imperative for the translation of AI-driven systems pharmacology frameworks into clinically actionable precision therapeutic strategies.

14. INTEGRATION OF AI WITH AUTOMATION AND CLOSED-LOOP EXPERIMENTATION

AI-driven automation and closed-loop experimentation will be key in the redefinition of how therapeutics will be discovered and optimized in translational development for inflammatory diseases. Advanced ML and DL models will probe enormous chemical spaces to forecast reaction outcomes, optimize synthesis routes, and identify high-value anti-inflammatory candidates at unprecedented speeds. Such automation-based platforms, capable of ingesting rich biological and chemical datasets, will be employed to identify disease-relevant targets, optimize physicochemical properties, and forecast pharmacokinetic and toxicological profiles, which are integral to safe and effective therapeutic design (Ghule *et al.*, 2024). Self-contained laboratories are the next acceleration along this pipeline through the implementation of ML-guided robotic synthesis within closed-loop systems that iteratively adjust reaction parameters in real time to minimize material waste and enhance precision in nanoparticle-based delivery (Jiang, 2025; Nematov & Raufov, 2025). In the clinical context, such advances are paralleled in IBD, where automated nanoparticle formulation systems have enhanced the reproducibility and scalability of orally delivered anti-TNF nanocarriers, leading to increased mucosal deposition and decreased systemic toxicity in early translational studies.

Active learning coupled with automation dramatically escalates the efficiency of anti-inflammatory scaffold discovery. ML models predict physicochemical, structural, and immune-modulatory properties of candidate molecules and guide navigation through extensive chemical landscapes (Tang *et al.*, 2023). Gaussian process regression and DL algorithms mapped quantitative structure-activity relationships that allowed the prioritization of scaffolds with favorable anti-inflammatory signatures, subsequently validated through high-throughput robotic screening (Kamuntavičius *et al.*, 2024). Continuous molecular refinement was achieved through closed-loop experimental cycles with iterative rounds of prediction, synthesis, testing, and model retraining; this expanded the accessible chemical space beyond capacities currently achievable through human-guided synthesis (Koscher *et al.,* 2023). Such approaches have echoes in translational immunology from efforts in combinatorial screening for IL-2 muteins and anti-IL-17 antibody variants, wherein automated evolution platforms identified candidates with improved drug-receptor affinity and decreased cytokine toxicity. There are, however, existing challenges: 'so far, so good' error quantification, scalability to multi-omic datasets, and the need for AI-automation workflows in active learning systems (Joshi & Kumar, 2021).

Digital laboratory twins extend these frameworks by generating high-fidelity virtual environments simulating biological systems and experimental processes. These digital twins will integrate genomic, proteomic, and clinical datasets and predict the course of disease, therapeutic response, and molecular behavior in inflammatory disorders (Vallée, 2025). Digital twins will support real-time immune monitoring, combined with automation, and will enable personalized treatment simulation through Bayesian inference and RL models with dynamic adjustment of interventions (Sen & Kılıç, 2025). Such work parallels emerging clinical applications in RA, where the development of simulations using digital twin models of synovial cytokine networks has been pursued to predict individualized response trajectories following TNF- or JAK-inhibitors. IoT-enabled laboratory integration further increases functionalities of such systems by enabling continuous data acquisition, feedback control, and automatic adjustment of experimental conditions (Eftimie *et al.,* 2023).

AI-driven feedback cycles represent a point of convergence for predictive analytics, automation, and closed-loop experimentation toward accelerating the development of therapeutics for inflammatory diseases. They rapidly screen molecular scaffolds, predict drug-target interactions, and prioritize compounds according to their pharmacological profile, with reduced dependency on animal testing (Serrano *et al.,* 2024; Ghule *et al.,* 2024). DL models strengthen virtual screening by enhancing the predictions of molecular interactions that will help in better optimization of the lead compounds and reduce attrition in late stages. Clinically, this capability corresponds to iterative refinement in small-molecule NLRP3 inhibitors, where closed-loop optimization frameworks achieved improved potency and metabolic stability that translated into improved preclinical efficacy in models of gouty arthritis and CAPS. Upon integration of model retraining with experimental feedback, closed-loop pipelines iteratively refine design hypotheses and reaction conditions, hence allowing adaptive high-precision medicine drug development (Joshi & Kumar, 2021).

15. ETHICAL, REGULATORY, AND TRANSLATIONAL CONSIDERATIONS

The integration of AI into research regarding inflammatory diseases and the development of treatments will therefore require strict ethical control, clear governance, and frameworks that ensure equity, accountability, and well-being for patients. Because diseases such as IBD, RA, and lupus result from multilevel factors, equitable data approaches in deploying AI consider bias and thus encourage the representation of groups and stand behind the reliability of clinical decision-making. Co-design and ethics stewardship will therefore be needed to instill trust in a variety of stakeholders so that AI-driven solutions are created in concert with realities in the clinic and with community values (Noor *et al.,* 2025). Bias mitigation strategies, including algorithmic audits, diverse dataset curation, and fairness-aware modelling, are important in reducing disparities, especially among those populations that, until recently, have been underrepresented in immunology research (Ratwani *et al.,* 2024). Inequity arising from structural and persistent data gaps informs the need for an interdisciplinary approach to innovation in striking a balance between speed and equity-driven outcomes in the care of inflammatory diseases (Muvva, 2021).

Regulatory frameworks for AI-driven drug discovery and clinical decision support increasingly focus on transparency, interpretability, and accountability as elements necessary for safe translational pathways. Application of adaptive standards, such as the meticulous transparency framework, evaluates an AI system based on performance capability, developer intent, and risk exposure, affording tiered regulatory oversight that evolves with technological advancement. Complementary frameworks, including IEEE P7001 and the CLeAR documentation model, advance the cause of standardized reporting of algorithmic behavior and model complexity (Lund *et al.,* 2025). Explainable AI (XAI) approaches, including gradient-based attribution and surrogate modelling, further facilitate interpretability and regulatory trust by exposing mechanistic features underlying model predictions (Lavecchia, 2025). However, a balance must be sought between transparency and protection of both intellectual property (IP) and data privacy, with adaptable governance systems needed to accommodate shifting AI architecture without compromising ethical safeguards (Qadri *et al.,* 2025).

Apart from the specific AI-generated drug discovery in inflammatory diseases, considerations of IP further contribute to the layers of complexity. Traditional IP frameworks fit into human inventorship and have problems accommodating emergent AI-driven molecular design and autonomous hypothesis generation. When AI unravels the molecular relationships that would be beyond the realm of conventional human inference, the establishment of novelty and nonobviousness becomes worse (Kumar, 2025). Data ownership further complicates questions of equitable licensing-

particularly when model development and dataset creation involve a diverse range of contributors, including clinical institutions and patient communities (Poddar & Rao, 2024). Dynamic IP policies will be required to keep pace with algorithmic evolution in AI-enabled discovery pipelines while continuing to uphold privacy, accountability, and fair benefit-sharing concerns. These are considered paramount in neglected inflammatory conditions, wherein limited data availability reduces generalizability and heightens the need for global standardization and collaborative governance (Nishan, 2025).

Needless to say, the responsible clinical translation of AI into the management of inflammatory diseases requires strict adherence to the principles of transparency, algorithmic equity, data protection, and human oversight. Global regulatory bodies, such as the EU AI Act, U.S. FDA, and WHO, among others so far, have presented frameworks that will ensure the validation and continuous performance monitoring and safeguards for high-risk medical AI systems, respecting patient autonomy and welfare (Panda & Ghosh, 2025). Interpretable choice pathways and fairness-aware model design accounting for demographic and clinical heterogeneity of the inflammatory disease populations would help build clinician and patient confidence in them (Ferroni & Parenti, 2024). Moreover, patient-centered, participatory design through interdisciplinary collaboration ensures the establishment of AI devices in line with real-world needs in clinical use and ethical considerations. There is no question about the fact that rapid evolution in AI technologies underpins and fragmented international regulations pose the imperative need for policies of iterative updates and harmonized governance frameworks. Global sustained cooperation might probably be necessary to ensure that this new wave of AI-driven innovation in inflammatory disease therapeutics is safely, equitably, and effectively implemented across diverse health systems (Jabarulla & Lee, 2021).

16. FUTURE PERSPECTIVES AND EMERGING FRONTIERS

Quantum Machine Learning (QML) is representative of a new frontier in the acceleration of molecular optimization, protein folding, and biomarker discovery in inflammatory diseases. By leveraging the computational advantages of quantum systems, QML allows the simulation of molecular energy states to a higher degree of accuracy while greatly reducing runtime compared to classical models. Algorithms such as the Variational Quantum Eigensolver allow high-resolution modelling of drug-target interactions and have been used in the rational optimization of compounds targeting inflammatory mediators (Gomase *et al.,* 2025). Quantum neural networks further accelerate early-stage discovery through the acceleration of compound screening and target identification workflows. Quantum-enhanced protein folding frameworks have reduced simulation times in modelling structural dynamics of inflammation-associated proteins. This, in turn, has enhanced the prediction of accuracy and unmasking of conformation states relevant to cytokine signalling (Akhi *et al.,* 2023). In parallel, QML's ability for analysis of high-dimensional biological datasets underpins rapid biomarker identification and creates new opportunities for precision treatment designs (Yenduri *et al.,* 2025). However, issues of qubit coherence, hardware scalability, and algorithmic stability represent ongoing scientific and engineering challenges and, therefore, create a need for an interdisciplinary collaboration for achieving quantum medicine in inflammatory therapeutics (Gomase *et al.,* 2025).

Large multimodal foundation models are similarly reshaping integrative drug discovery through the fusion of molecular structures, biological networks, and textual biomedical knowledge in unified representation systems. Systems like SPARK and InstructMol combine molecular graphs with natural language embeddings that enhance the mechanistic understanding of target identification and compound optimization across inflammatory pathways (Cao *et al.,* 2023). Large-scale datasets such as M33-20M have shown the value of multimodal learning in improved property prediction, virtual screening, and de novo molecule generation. LLM systems further mine biomedical literature and multi-omics datasets, enabling disease network mapping and novel therapeutic target identification of early utility for IBD, RA, and systemic inflammatory disorders (Liu *et al.,* 2025a). Such cross-attention and alignment mechanisms facilitate biologically grounded multimodal reasoning for the purpose of informing both preclinical exploration and real-world clinical decision-making. Nevertheless, there remain significant challenges regarding interpretability, avoidance of data leakage, and protection of patient privacy-all requiring appropriate and transparent governance and ethical oversight to ensure equitable technology adoption around the world (Choi *et al.,* 2025).

Integration of AI and CRISPR marks the other frontier of investigation of inflammatory mechanisms at a genomic and epigenomic level. AI-optimized gRNA design tools, of which CRISTA and DeepCRISPR are just some examples, predict off-target effects with very high precision while considering the genomic context to enhance editing specificity (Dixit *et al.,* 2024). Modelling DNA repair dynamics by AI-driven simulation predicts functional outcomes-allowing for stratified genome-editing strategies against immunogenetic disorders. Application of AI analytics to pooled CRISPR perturbation screens strengthens causal inference and exposes genetic drivers of inflammatory responses, usefully illustrated in the Perturbation Cell Atlas, modelling single-cell resolution of cellular states and pathway regulation (Rood *et al.,* 2024). So far, CRISPR-based epigenetic editing has held promise in reprogramming inflammatory loci such as IL1RN, thus modulating immune responses of therapeutic relevance across a number of inflammatory diseases (Valcárcel *et al.,* 2025).

The future of AI-driven inflammatory therapeutics rests very much on better coordination of collaboration among academia, industry, clinical institutions, and regulatory agencies. ML, DL, and generative AI integrated into experimentation and clinical trial pipelines at all levels of discovery-from target identification to the optimization of clinical trials-enable more powerful discovery. Cross-industry data sharing and frameworks of FL ensure secure utilization of multi-institutional datasets that are needed to make robust model development possible (Patel & Shah, 2022; Robert *et al.,* 2025). Generative models, including GANs and VAEs, accelerate ideation and optimization of molecules and allow tailored design of anti-inflammatory chemotypes with enhanced stability, potency, and safety. AI analytics is increasingly shaping clinical trial design through improved patient stratification, therapeutic response prediction, and attrition reduction, having a particular profound impact in diseases characterized by heterogeneous behavior of inflammation. Early regulatory engagement with transparent reporting means compliance, reproducibility, and public trust. While challenges like mitigation of bias, interpretability, global inequities in data infrastructure, and ethical accountability remain, standardized governance frameworks and continued interdisciplinary collaboration will be required for translation of AI-driven innovation into therapies that are safe, effective, and equitable for the management of inflammatory diseases (Liebman, 2022).

17. CONCLUSION

AI-driven innovation is redefining every stage of drug development for inflammatory diseases: from molecular design through clinical translation. It integrates predictive modelling, network pharmacology, and digital twins, enhancing the precision and personalization of therapeutic strategies. FL and real-world data frameworks enable privacy-preserving collaborations that expand access to a greater variety of datasets, increasing the robustness and generalizability of models. The integration of automation, active learning, and closed-loop experimentation has accelerated synthesis and preclinical validation, with advances in XAI and ethical governance enhancing transparency and patient trust. QML, CRISPR-integrated AI, and other emerging technologies have further expanded this frontier of precision therapeutics with new ways to enhance molecular simulation, genome editing, and biomarker discovery. Despite these remarkable advances, many challenges remain in data standardization, interpretability, and regulatory adaptation. Overcoming these limitations will require interdisciplinary collaboration and global regulatory alignment if AI is to fully transform inflammatory disease therapeutics into a truly predictive, ethical, and patient-centered paradigm.

ACKNOWLEDGEMENT

All the authors are thankful to their respective Universities and Institutions for their valuable supports.

REFERENCES

Abed, A. H. (2025). Artificial intelligence-driven pharmaceutical research: a comprehensive analysis of applications and challenges. *Journal of computers and digital business, 4*(1), 37-44.

Ahmad, H. A., East, J. E., Panaccione, R., Travis, S., Canavan, J. B., Usiskin, K., & Byrne, M. F. (2023). Artificial intelligence in inflammatory bowel disease: Implications for clinical practice and future directions. *Intestinal Research, 21*(3), 283–294.

Akhi, S. S., Hussain, A. H., Islam, S., Hasan, M. N., & Islam, M. M. (2023). Artificial intelligence–enhanced quantum computing for medical simulations: Accelerating drug discovery, protein folding, and personalized healthcare with performance optimization and predictive accuracy. *World Journal of Advanced Research and Review, 18*(01), 1328–1335.

Akhmedov, M., Arribas, A., Montemanni, R., Bertoni, F., & Kwee, I. (2017). Omicsnet: Integration of multi-omics data using path analysis in multilayer networks. *BioRxiv*, 238766.

Alekseenko, J., Stieltjes, B., Bach, M., Boerries, M., Opitz, O., Karargyris, A., & Padoy, N. (2024). Clinnova federated learning proof of concept: key takeaways from a cross-border collaboration. *arXiv preprint arXiv:2410.02443.*

Alfonso-González, L., Fernández, F. J., & Vega, M. C. (2025). Systems immunology: When systems biology meets immunology. *Frontiers in Immunology, 16*, 1630488.

Ali, M., Naeem, F., Tariq, M., & Kaddoum, G. (2022). Federated learning for privacy preservation in smart healthcare systems: A comprehensive survey. *IEEE Journal of Biomedical and Health Informatics, 27*(2), 778–789.

Alimguzhin, V., Mancini, T., Massini, A., Sinisi, S., & Tronci, E. (2020). In silico clinical trials through AI and statistical model checking. [). CEUR-WS.]. *CEUR Workshop Proceedings, 2509*, 17–22.

Anderson, N., & Smith, R. (2024). Rethinking the Three Rs: Growing momentum toward a new gold standard in Australian research. *Alternatives to Laboratory Animals, 52*(4), 224–231.

Angoulvant, D., Amarenco, P., Bastien, A., Bechet, E., Boccara, F., Boissel, J. P., & Steg, P. G. (2023). Design of a knowledge-based mechanistic model of atherosclerotic cardiovascular disease for in silico trials. *European Heart Journal, 44*(Supplement_2), ehad655–2944.

Ashraf, F. B., Zhang, Z., Paco, K., Mendivil, M. P., Lay, J. A., Ray, A., & Lonardi, S. (2024). A large language model guides the affinity maturation of variant antibodies generated by combinatorial optimization. *bioRxiv*, 2024.

Asti, G., Apellaniz, P. A., Carota, L., Casadei, F., Piscia, D., Delleani, M., & Álvarez Garcia, F. (2025). Development, implementation, and validation of an open-source federated learning platform to accelerate innovation and boost personalized medicine in rare and ultra-rare haematological diseases: an initiative by GenoMed4All Consortium. medRxiv, 2025-08.

Athira, R. K., Kripamol, R., Anju, M. S., Maya, B., Pai, R. R., Ajit, S., & Kasoju, N. (2022). Alternatives to animal testing: concepts, state of art, and regulations. *Biomedical product and materials evaluation*, 501-529.

Auger, S. D., & Scott, G. (2025). Machine learning detects hidden treatment response patterns only in the presence of comprehensive clinical phenotyping. *PLoS One*, *20*(10), e0334858.

Avey, S., Chatterjee, M., Manyakov, N. V., Cooper, P., Sabins, N., Mosca, K., & Pandis, I. (2024). Using a wearable patch to develop a digital monitoring biomarker of inflammation in response to LPS challenge. *Clinical and Translational Science*, *17*(2), e13734.

Baldan-Martin, M., Azkargorta, M., Aransay, A., Gil-Redondo, R., Moreno-Indias, I., & Iloro, I., & * Authors share co-senior authorship. (2025). OP04 multi-omics biomarkers for predicting therapeutic efficacy in inflammatory bowel disease: Advancing towards tailored treatments. *Journal of Crohn's and Colitis*, *19*(Supplement_1), i7–i8.

Barua, R. (2024). The emerging role of artificial intelligence in organ-on-a-chip (ooac) biomedical devices. In *Reshaping Healthcare with Cutting-Edge Biomedical Advancements* (pp. 369–381). IGI Global Scientific Publishing.

Beasley, J. M. T., Schatz, K., Ding, E., DeLuca, M., Zaid, N. A., Tucker, N. N., & Muratov, E. N. (2025). TARRAGON: Therapeutic target applicability ranking and retrieval-augmented generation over networks. bioRxiv, 2025-04.

Benson, M. (2023). Digital twins for predictive, preventive personalized, and participatory treatment of immune-mediated diseases. *Arteriosclerosis, Thrombosis, and Vascular Biology*, *43*(3), 410–416.

Bindu, C. H., Babu, R., Bhimana, S., Babu, M. K., Devadas, C., & Jalaiah, M. (2025). Revolutionizing pharmaceutical sciences: a comprehensive review of artificial intelligence's impact on drug discovery and development. *Genomics-Driven Drug Discovery Through Pharmacogenomics*, 217-246.

Cao, H., Liu, Z., Lu, X., Yao, Y., & Li, Y. (2023). Instructmol: Multi-modal integration for building a versatile and reliable molecular assistant in drug discovery. *arXiv preprint arXiv:2311.16208*.

Chen, L., Zhang, C., Niu, R., Xiong, S., He, J., Wang, Y., & Feng, R. (2025). Multi-omics biomarkers for predicting efficacy of biologic and small-molecule therapies in adults with inflammatory bowel disease: A systematic review. *United European Gastroenterology Journal*, *13*(4), 517–530.

Chinedu-Nzereogu, O. P., Olorunfemi, V. O., Osifeso, J. O., & John, T. (2025). Computational immunogenomics: Leveraging AI to uncover novel biomarkers for disease diagnosis and therapy. *International Journal of Life Science Research Archive*, *9*(1), 102–119.

Choi, H., Kang, E., Song, D., & Jung, G. (2025). Integrating Multimodal Data with Large Foundation Models in Healthcare. https://doi.org/DOI: 10.20944/preprints202508.0498.v1

Cichońska, A., Ravikumar, B., & Rahman, R. (2024). AI for targeted polypharmacology: The next frontier in drug discovery. *Current Opinion in Structural Biology*, *84*, 102771.

Cong, Y., Han, X., Wang, Y., Chen, Z., Lu, Y., Liu, T., & Zhang, X. (2020). Drug toxicity evaluation based on organ-on-a-chip technology: A review. *Micromachines*, *11*(4), 381.

Cremonesi, F., Vesin, M., Cansiz, S., Bouillard, Y., Balelli, I., Innocenti, L., & Lorenzi, M. (2025). Fed-biomed: Open, transparent and trusted federated learning for real-world healthcare applications. In *Federated Learning Systems: Towards Privacy-Preserving Distributed AI* (pp. 19–41). Springer Nature Switzerland.

Cucu, I. (2022). Signalling pathways in inflammation and cardiovascular diseases: An update of therapeutic strategies. *Immuno*, *2*(4), 630–650.

D'Silva, S., Rajadhyaksha, S. B., & Singh, M. (2019). *Immune dysregulation in MDS: the role of cytokines and immune cells. Recent Developments in Myelodysplastic Syndromes*. IntechOpen.

Daniore, P., Nittas, V., Haag, C., Bernard, J., Gonzenbach, R., & von Wyl, V. (2024). From wearable sensor data to digital biomarker development: Ten lessons learned and a framework proposal. *NPJ Digital Medicine*, *7*(1), 161.

Das, U. (2025). Transforming precision medicine through generative AI: Advanced architectures and tailored therapeutic design for patient-specific drug discovery. *ChemistrySelect*, *10*(36), e02448.

de Anda-Jáuregui, G., Guo, K., McGregor, B. A., & Hur, J. (2018). Exploration of the anti-inflammatory drug space through network pharmacology: Applications for drug repurposing. *Frontiers in Physiology*, *9*, 151.

Dimitrov, D. V. (2014). Systems patientomics: The virtual in-silico patient. *New Horizons in Translational Medicine*, *2*(1), 1–4.

Dixit, S., Kumar, A., Srinivasan, K., Vincent, P. D. R., & Ramu Krishnan, N. (2024). Advancing genome editing with artificial intelligence: Opportunities, challenges, and future directions. *Frontiers in Bioengineering and Biotechnology*, *11*, 1335901.

Doneva, N., Doytchinova, I., & Dimitrov, I. (2021). Predicting immunogenicity risk in biopharmaceuticals. *Symmetry*, *13*(3), 388.

Dong, S., Nessler, I., Kopp, A., Rubahamya, B., & Thurber, G. M. (2022). Predictive simulations in preclinical oncology to guide the translation of biologics. *Frontiers in Pharmacology*, *13*, 836925.

Durso-Finley, J., Barile, B., Falet, J. P., Arnold, D. L., Pawlowski, N., & Arbel, T. (2024). Probabilistic temporal prediction of continuous disease trajectories and treatment effects using neural SDEs. In *International Conference on Medical Image Computing and Computer-Assisted Intervention* (pp. 400-410). Cham: Springer Nature Switzerland.

Eftimie, R., Mavrodin, A., & Bordas, S. P. (2023). From digital control to digital twins in medicine: A brief review and future perspectives. *Advances in Applied Mechanics*, *56*, 323–368.

ElShal, S., Tranchevent, L. C., Sifrim, A., Ardeshirdavani, A., Davis, J., & Moreau, Y. (2016). Beegle: From literature mining to disease-gene discovery. *Nucleic Acids Research*, *44*(2), e18–e18.

Enni, M. A., & Maraj, M. A. A. (2022). In silico drug repurposing for inflammatory diseases: A systematic review of molecular docking and virtual screening studies. *American Journal of Advanced Technology and Engineering Solutions*, *2*(04), 35–64.

Fausch, I., Zeyer-Iyengar, D., Morales, R. M. C., Elger, B., Enzmann, V., & Früh, A. (2025). exploring alternatives to animal testing: scientific, legal and ethical challenges in developing novel alternative methods with a focus on organoids as potential NAMs. *LEOH-Journal of Animal Law, Ethics and One Health*, 81-99.

Ferroni, J. M., & Parenti, P. (2024). Ethical and regulatory challenges of Artificial Intelligence in medical research: reflections on intelligent regulation. *Binational Brazil-Argentina Journal: Dialogue between sciences, 14* (02), 103-119.

Folasole, A., Eshua, P. E., & Elesho, O. E. (2025). Modelling spatiotemporal immune dynamics in inflammatory diseases using integrative multi-modal analytics and high-dimensional longitudinal datasets. *World Journal of Biology Pharmacy and Health Sciences*, *23*(2), 196–218.

Gardiner, L. J., Carrieri, A. P., Bingham, K., Macluskie, G., Bunton, D., McNeil, M., & Pyzer-Knapp, E. O. (2022). Combining explainable machine learning, demographic and multi-omic data to inform precision medicine strategies for inflammatory bowel disease. *PLoS One*, *17*(2), e0263248.

Garrido-Trigo, A., Corraliza, A. M., Veny, M., Dotti, I., Melón-Ardanaz, E., Rill, A., & Salas, A. (2023). Macrophage and neutrophil heterogeneity at single-cell spatial resolution in human inflammatory bowel disease. *Nature Communications*, *14*(1), 4506.

Ghule, P. J., Kale, P. A., & Kale, S. P. (2024). Ai-enhanced drug discovery and pharmaceutical development. *Futuristic Trends in Pharmacy & Nursing. IIP: Chikkamagaluru, India*, *3*, 254–267.

Gomase, V. S., Ghatule, A. P., Sharma, R., & Dhamane, S. P. (2025). Quantum computing in drug discovery techniques, challenges, and emerging opportunities. *Current Drug Discovery Technologies.*

Gonzalez-Garcia, I., Irurzun-Arana, I., Ruiz-Cerda, L., Hu, C., Zhou, H., Vermeulen, A., & Gomez-Mantilla, J. D. (2015). Building an inflammatory bowel disease network, a systems pharmacology approach. In *6th American conference on Pharmacometrics (ACoP-6)* (Vol. 42, No. suppl. 1, pp. S83-S84).

Gorgulla, C. (2024). Structure-based ultra-large virtual screenings. *Computational Drug Discovery: Methods and Applications*, *2*, 441–470.

Goryanin, I., Goryanin, I., & Demin, O. (2025). Revolutionizing drug discovery: Integrating artificial intelligence with quantitative systems pharmacology. *Drug Discovery Today*, •••, 104448.

Gu, X., Aranganathan, A., & Tiwary, P. (2024). Empowering AlphaFold2 for protein conformation selective drug discovery with AlphaFold2-RAVE. *eLife*, *13*, RP99702.

Guan, J., Yao, L., Chung, C. R., Xie, P., Zhang, Y., Deng, J., & Lee, T. Y. (2023). Predicting anti-inflammatory peptides by ensemble machine learning and deep learning. *Journal of Chemical Information and Modeling*, *63*(24), 7886–7898.

Gupta, A., Müller, A. T., Huisman, B. J., Fuchs, J. A., Schneider, P., & Schneider, G. (2018). Generative recurrent networks for de novo drug design. *Molecular Informatics*, *37*(1-2), 1700111.

Hamano, H., Tanaka, Y., & Zamami, Y. (2025). An integrative drug discovery strategy using real-world data, in silico modelling, and network pharmacology. *Nihon yakurigaku zasshi. Folia pharmacologica Japonica, 160*(5), 352-359.

Hamelin, B., Rowe, P., Molony, C., Kruger, M., LoCasale, R., Khan, A. H., & Jacob, D. (2022). Immunolab: Combining targeted real-world data with advanced analytics to generate evidence at scale in immunology. *Frontiers in Allergy*, *3*, 951795.

Han, L., Sayyid, Z. N., & Altman, R. B. (2021). Modelling drug response using network-based personalized treatment prediction (NetPTP) with applications to inflammatory bowel disease. *PLoS Computational Biology*, *17*(2), e1008631.

Hou, X., Yang, F., Liu, W., Fu, Z., Chen, L., Li, Z., & Cao, G. (2015). Signalling pathways that facilitate chronic inflammation-induced carcinogenesis. *Journal of Cellular Signaling*, *1*, 9.

Iacucci, M., & Santacroce, G. (2024). Multi-OMICs orchestration enabled by artificial intelligence in inflammatory bowel disease: An exciting future. *United European Gastroenterology Journal*, *12*(10), 1350.

Jabarulla, M. Y., & Lee, H. N. (2021). A blockchain and artificial intelligence-based, patient-centric healthcare system for combating the COVID-19 pandemic: Opportunities and applications. [). Mdpi.]. *Health Care*, *9*(8), 1019.

Jarallah, S. J., Almughem, F. A., Alhumaid, N. K., Fayez, N. A., Alradwan, I., Alsulami, K. A., & Alshehri, A. A. (2025). Artificial intelligence revolution in drug discovery: A paradigm shift in pharmaceutical innovation. *International Journal of Pharmaceutics*, •••, 125789.

Jemielita, T. O., & Mehrotra, D. V. (2019). PRISM: patient response identifiers for stratified medicine. *arXiv preprint arXiv:1912.03337*.

Jiang, D. (2025). Optimizing drug synthesis driven by artificial intelligence. *Theoretical and Natural Science*, *131*, 80–87.

Jiang, J., Chen, S., Tsou, T., McGinnis, C. S., Khazaei, T., Zhu, Q., & Thomson, M. (2022). Therapeutic algebra of immunomodulatory drug responses at single-cell resolution. *arXiv preprint arXiv:2208.10661*.

Jiang, X., Lu, L., Li, J., Jiang, J., Zhang, J., Zhou, S., & Bai, R. (2024). Synthetically feasible De Novo molecular design of leads based on a reinforcement learning model: AI-assisted discovery of an Anti-IBD lead targeting CXCR4. *Journal of Medicinal Chemistry*, *67*(12), 10057–10075.

Joshi, R. P., & Kumar, N. (2021). Artificial intelligence for autonomous molecular design: A perspective. *Molecules (Basel, Switzerland)*, *26*(22), 6761.

Kamuntavičius, G., Prat, A., Paquet, T., Bastas, O., Aty, H. A., Sun, Q., & Norvaišas, P. (2024). Accelerated hit identification with target evaluation, deep learning and automated labs: Prospective validation in IRAK1. *Journal of Cheminformatics*, *16*(1), 127.

Kapoor, G., Prakash, S., Jaiswal, V., & Singh, A. K. (2025). Chronic inflammation and cancer: Key pathways and targeted therapies. *Cancer Investigation*, *43*(1), 1–23.

Katkar, G. D., Sayed, I., Anandachar, M. S., Castillo, V., Vidales, E., Toobian, D., & Ghosh, P. (2021). AI-guided use of balanced peroxisome proliferator-activated receptor a/g dual agonist finetunes macrophage responses in inflammatory bowel disease. *The Journal of Immunology : Official Journal of the American Association of Immunologists*, *206*(1, Supplement), 109–01.

Kaur, S., & Sharma, H. (2025). Causal representation learning for predicting autoimmune disease progression from longitudinal multimodal clinical data. *IEEE Access : Practical Innovations, Open Solutions*, *13*, 150010–150027.

Kim, J., Ryu, S., Park, H., & Seok, C. (2025). SHARP: generating synthesizable molecules via fragment-based hierarchical action-space reinforcement learning for pareto optimization. bioRxiv, 2025-07.

Kitani, T., Maddipatla, S. C., Madupuri, R., Baraniuk, J. N., Greco, C., Hartman, J., & Vasudevan, S. (2020). In search of newer targets for IBD: a systems and a network medicine approach. *arXiv preprint arXiv:2006.04181*.

Koscher, B. A., Canty, R. B., McDonald, M. A., Greenman, K. P., McGill, C. J., Bilodeau, C. L., & Jensen, K. F. (2023). Autonomous, multiproperty-driven molecular discovery: From predictions to measurements and back. *Science*, *382*(6677), eadi1407.

Kumar, R. (2025). AI-generated drug innovations and indian patent law: legal challenges and ethical responses. *Preprints*. https://doi.org/DOI: 10.20944/preprints202506.1166.v1

Lavecchia, A. (2025). Explainable artificial intelligence in drug discovery: Bridging predictive power and mechanistic insight. *Wiley Interdisciplinary Reviews. Computational Molecular Science*, *15*(5), e70049.

Leung, H., Duan, C., Gou, W., Chen, J., Xin, Y., Zheng, Z., & Zhavoronkov, A. (2025). Advancing target discovery through disease-specific integration of multimodal target identification models and comprehensive target benchmarking system. bioRxiv, 2025-08.

Li, T., Chen, X., & Tong, W. (2024). Bridging organ transcriptomics for advancing multiple organ toxicity assessment with a generative AI approach. *NPJ Digital Medicine*, *7*(1), 310.

Li, Y., Peng, H., Zhao, H., Han, X., Zhang, P., Ning, J., & Hao, F. (2025). A novel approach for antibody affinity maturation using AI-driven mutation prediction. *Cancer Research*, *85*(8, Supplement_1), 5679–5679.

Liebman, M. (2022). The role of artificial intelligence in drug discovery and development. *Chemistry International*, *44*(1), 16–19.

Liu, X., Zhang, J., Wang, X., Teng, M., Wang, G., & Zhou, X. (2025a). Application of artificial intelligence large language models in drug target discovery. *Frontiers in Pharmacology*, *16*, 1597351.

Liu, X., Zhu, F., & Ma, H, X., Shi, Z., Y Yang, S., Q Wei, Y., & Z Chen, Y. (2013). Predicting targeted polypharmacology for drug repositioning and multi-target drug discovery. *Current Medicinal Chemistry*, *20*(13), 1646–1661.

Liu, Y. T., Zhang, L. L., Jiang, Z. Y., Tian, X. S., Li, P. L., Wu, P. H., & Sun, C. (2025b). Applications of artificial intelligence in biotech drug discovery and product development. *MedComm*, *6*(8), e70317.

Long, A., Kleiner, A., & Looney, R. J. (2023). Immune dysregulation. *The Journal of Allergy and Clinical Immunology*, *151*(1), 70–80.

Lopez-Perez, L., Merino, B., Rujas, M., Maccaro, A., Guillén, S., Pecchia, L., & Fico, G. (2024). Regulatory frameworks and validation strategies for advancing artificial intelligence in healthcare. In *European Medical and Biological Engineering Conference* (pp. 260-265). Cham: Springer Nature Switzerland.

Lu, M., Covert, I., White, N. J., & Lee, S. I. (2024). CODE-XAI: construing and deciphering treatment effects via explainable ai using real-world data. medRxiv, 2024-09.

Lund, B., Orhan, Z., Mannuru, N. R., Bevara, R. V. K., Porter, B., Vinaih, M. K., & Bhaskara, P. (2025). Standards, frameworks, and legislation for artificial intelligence (AI) transparency. *AI and Ethics*, •••, 1–17.

Madrid-Paredes, A., Martín, J., & Márquez, A. (2022). -Omic approaches and treatment response in rheumatoid arthritis. *Pharmaceutics*, *14*(8), 1648.

Makutam, V., Achanti, S., & Doostan, M. (2024). Integration of artificial intelligence in adaptive trial designs: Enhancing efficiency and patientcentric outcomes. *International Journal of Advanced Research*, *12*(205215), 1021474.

Malani, M., Kasturi, A., Moinul, M., Gayen, S., Hota, C., & Nirmal, J. (2023). Role of artificial intelligence in the toxicity prediction of drugs. In *Biomedical Applications and Toxicity of Nanomaterials* (pp. 589–636). Springer Nature Singapore.

Mane, D. V., Deshmukh, A. N., Ambare, R. H., Solankar, A. A., & Madane, C. S. (2024). AI in autoimmune diseases: Transforming diagnosis and treatment. *Journal of Pharmaceutical and Biological Sciences*, *12*(2), 109–118.

Mariam, Z., Niazi, S. K., & Magoola, M. (2024). Unlocking the future of drug development: Generative AI, digital twins, and beyond. *BioMedInformatics*, *4*(2), 1441–1456.

McCulloch, C. A., Downey, G. P., & El-Gabalawy, H. (2006). Signalling platforms that modulate the inflammatory response: New targets for drug development. *Nature Reviews. Drug Discovery*, *5*(10), 864–876.

Mehta, P. (2025). System: A Delicate Balance. *Cell Death Regulation in Pathology*, 201.

Merk, D., Friedrich, L., Grisoni, F., & Schneider, G. (2018). De novo design of bioactive small molecules by artificial intelligence. *Molecular Informatics*, *37*(1-2), 1700153.

Moingeon, P., Garbay, C., Dahan, M., Fermont, I., Benmakhlouf, A., Gouyette, A., & Saint-Pierre, A. (2024). The revolution of AI in drug development. *Medecine Sciences. Ms*, *40*(4), 369–376.

Montgomery, R. M. (2024). Molecular mechanisms of chronic stress in immune dysregulation: From cytokine networks to clinical manifestations. *Wired Neurosci*, *1*, 24–53.

Muvva, S. (2021). Ethical AI and responsible data engineering: A framework for bias mitigation and privacy preservation in large-scale data pipelines. *International Journal of Scientific Research in Engineering and Management*, *5*(09).

Nematov, D., & Raufov, I. (2025). The bright future of materials science with ai: self-driving laboratories and closed-loop discovery. *Preprints*. https://doi.org/DOI: 10.20944/preprints202509.1369.v1

Nishan, M. N. H. (2025). AI-powered drug discovery for neglected diseases: Accelerating public health solutions in the developing world. *Journal of Global Health*, *15*, 03002.

Noor, F., Asif, M., Ashfaq, U. A., & Qasim, M., & Tahir ul Qamar, M. (2023). Machine learning for synergistic network pharmacology: A comprehensive overview. *Briefings in Bioinformatics*, *24*(3), bbad120.

Noor, N. M., Daperno, M., de Laffolie, J., Mookhoek, A., Sinonquel, P., Kopylov, U., & Baumgart, D. C. (2025). Results of the 9th scientific workshop of the european crohn's and colitis organisation (ECCO): artificial intelligence in IBD: regulatory and methodological considerations. *Journal of Crohn's and Colitis*, jjaf136.

O'Neill, L. A. (2006). Targeting signal transduction as a strategy to treat inflammatory diseases. *Nature Reviews. Drug Discovery*, *5*(7), 549–563.

Occhipinti, A., Verma, S., & Angione, C. (2024). Mechanism-aware and multimodal AI: Beyond model-agnostic interpretation. *Trends in Cell Biology*, *34*(2), 85–89.

Okpete, U. E., & Byeon, H. (2025). Explainable artificial intelligence for personalized management of inflammatory bowel disease: A minireview of recent advances. *World Journal of Gastroenterology*, *31*(35), 111033.

Ouedraogo, G., Alépée, N., Tan, B., & Roper, C. S. (2025). A call to action: Advancing new approach methodologies (NAMs) in regulatory toxicology through a unified framework for validation and acceptance. *Regulatory Toxicology and Pharmacology*, *162*, 105904.

Palshikar, M. G., Min, X., Crystal, A., Meng, J., Hilchey, S. P., Zand, M. S., & Thakar, J. (2023). Executable network models of integrated multiomics data. *Journal of Proteome Research*, *22*(5), 1546–1556.

Panda, P. K., & Ghosh, S. (2025). Ethical use of AI in infectious diagnostic decision and therapeutic stewardship. *IDCases*, •••, 02356.

Park, M. (2024). Improving the diagnosis of systemic lupus erythematosus with machine learning algorithms based on real-world data. *Mathematics*, *12*(18), 2849.

Patel, V., & Shah, M. (2022). Artificial intelligence and machine learning in drug discovery and development. *Intelligent Medicine*, *2*(3), 134–140.

Patne, A. Y., Dhulipala, S. M., Lawless, W., Prakash, S., Mohapatra, S. S., & Mohapatra, S. (2024). Drug discovery in the age of artificial intelligence: Transformative target-based approaches. *International Journal of Molecular Sciences*, *25*(22), 12233.

Pawar, V., Patil, A., Tamboli, F., Gaikwad, D., Mali, D., & Shinde, A. (2021). Harnessing the power of AI in pharmacokinetics and pharmacodynamics: A comprehensive review. *AAPS PharmSciTech*, *14*(2), 426–439.

Pettinati, M. J., Lajevardi-Khosh, A., Rajput, K. S., Majmudar, M., & Selvaraj, N. (2022). Towards remote continuous monitoring of cytokine release syndrome. In *2022 44th Annual International Conference of the IEEE Engineering in Medicine & Biology Society (EMBC)* (pp. 966-970). IEEE.

Poddar, A., & Rao, S. R. (2024). Evolving intellectual property landscape for AI-driven innovations in the biomedical sector: Opportunities in stable IP regime for shared success. *Frontiers in Artificial Intelligence*, *7*, 1372161.

Puentes-Osorio, Y., Amariles, P., Calleja, M. Á., Merino, V., Díaz-Coronado, J. C., & Taborda, D. (2021). Potential clinical biomarkers in rheumatoid arthritis with an omic approach. *Auto-Immunity Highlights*, *12*(1), 9.

Qadri, Y. A., Shaikh, S., Ahmad, K., Choi, I., Kim, S. W., & Vasilakos, A. V. (2025). Explainable artificial intelligence: A perspective on drug discovery. *Pharmaceutics*, *17*(9), 1119.

Qian, L., Lu, X., Haris, P., Zhu, J., Li, S., & Yang, Y. (2024). A Survey of Artificial Intelligence Methods for Clinical Trial Outcome Prediction. *ChemRxiv*. https://doi.org/DOI: 10.26434/chemrxiv-2024-08t4w

Ratwani, R. M., Sutton, K., & Galarraga, J. E. (2024). Addressing AI algorithmic bias in health care. *Journal of the American Medical Association*, *332*(13), 1051–1052.

Robert, K., Kaium, O., & Alasa, L. (2025). Generative AI and pharmaceutical innovation: Accelerating drug discovery with deep learning and predictive analytics. *International Journal of Multidisciplinary Evolutionary Research*, *6*(2), 44–52.

Rood, J. E., Hupalowska, A., & Regev, A. (2024). Toward a foundation model of causal cell and tissue biology with a perturbation cell and tissue atlas. *Cell*, *187*(17), 4520–4545.

Roth, H. R., Xu, Z., Chen, C., Xu, D., Dogra, P., Flores, M., & Feng, A. (2025). Overview of real-world applications of federated learning with NVIDIA FLARE. *Journal of Biopharmaceutical Statistics*, •••, 1–11.

Rouyan, A., Dudzic, P., Wilman, W., Satława, T., Wróbel, S., & Krawczyk, K. (2025). Applications of artificial intelligence and machine learning toward antibody discovery and development. In *Biopharmaceutical Informatics* (pp. 77–115). CRC Press.

Sahoo, D., Swanson, L., Sayed, I. M., Katkar, G. D., Ibeawuchi, S. R., Mittal, Y., & Ghosh, P. (2021). Artificial intelligence guided discovery of a barrier-protective therapy in inflammatory bowel disease. *Nature Communications*, *12*(1), 4246.

Schultz, M. B., Vera, D., & Sinclair, D. A. (2020). Can artificial intelligence identify effective COVID-19 therapies? *EMBO Molecular Medicine*, *12*(8), e12817.

Sekaran, S. D., Manikam, R., Thergerajan, G., Prasad, H., Alagar, M., & Tan, C. K. (2025). The role of personalized precision medicine in enhancing diagnostic accuracy and clinical outcomes. *Advances in Biomedical and Health Sciences*, *4*(2), 52–60.

Sen, S., & Kilic, K. D. (2025). Digital twins in medicine, AI-driven personalized healthcare, and predictive analytics. In *AI-Powered Digital Twins for Predictive Healthcare: Creating Virtual Replicas of Humans* (pp. 359-396). IGI Global Scientific Publishing.

Serrano, D. R., Luciano, F. C., Anaya, B. J., Ongoren, B., Kara, A., Molina, G., & Lalatsa, A. (2024). Artificial intelligence (AI) applications in drug discovery and drug delivery: Revolutionizing personalized medicine. *Pharmaceutics*, *16*(10), 1328.

Sheller, M. J., Edwards, B., Reina, G. A., Martin, J., Pati, S., Kotrotsou, A., & Bakas, S. (2020). Federated learning in medicine: Facilitating multi-institutional collaborations without sharing patient data. *Scientific Reports*, *10*(1), 12598.

Shi, C., Gao, T., Lyu, W., Qiang, B., Chen, Y., Chen, Q., & Liu, Z. (2024). Deep-Learning-Driven Discovery of SN3–1, a Potent NLRP3 Inhibitor with Therapeutic Potential for Inflammatory Diseases. *Journal of Medicinal Chemistry*, *67*(19), 17833–17854.

Silverman, A. L., Shung, D., Stidham, R. W., Kochhar, G. S., & Iacucci, M. (2025). How artificial intelligence will transform clinical care, research, and trials for inflammatory bowel disease. *Clinical Gastroenterology and Hepatology*, *23*(3), 428–439.

Singh, K., Gupta, A., Siddiqui, I., Sinha, A., Patwa, M. K., & Singh, U. (2025). Rational design of anti-inflammatory therapeutics. *Computational Methods for Rational Drug Design*, 389-402.

Sinha, S., McLaren, E., Mullick, M., Penrose, H. M., Tindle, C., Singh, S., & Ghosh, P. (2025). FORWARD: A data-driven framework for network-based target prioritization in drug discovery. bioRxiv, 2024-07.

Son, A., Park, J., Kim, W., Lee, W., Yoon, Y., Ji, J., & Kim, H. (2024). Integrating computational design and experimental approaches for next-generation biologics. *Biomolecules*, *14*(9), 1073.

Srinivas, S. S., & Runkana, V. (2024). Cross-modal learning for chemistry property prediction: large language models meet graph machine learning. *arXiv preprint arXiv:2408.14964*.

Swanson, K., Walther, P., Leitz, J., Mukherjee, S., Wu, J. C., Shivnaraine, R. V., & Zou, J. (2024). ADMET-AI: A machine learning ADMET platform for evaluation of large-scale chemical libraries. *Bioinformatics (Oxford, England)*, *40*(7), btae416.

Talebi, N., & Azimi, M. (2025). Federated learning for multi-institutional AI in healthcare via digital pathology. *Preprints*. https://doi.org/DOI: 10.20944/preprints202509.1352.v1

Tan, R. K., Liu, Y., & Xie, L. (2022). Reinforcement learning for personalized drug discovery and design for complex diseases: a systems pharmacology perspective. *arXiv preprint arXiv:2201.08894*.

Tang, Y., Kim, J. Y., Carman, K. M., Bahmani, A., Chen, Q., Rosenberger, M. G., & Ferguson, A. L. (2023). Data-driven discovery of innate immunomodulators via machine learning-guided high throughput screening. *Chemical Science (Cambridge)*, *14*(44), 12747–12766.

Teachey, D. T., Lacey, S. F., Shaw, P. A., Melenhorst, J. J., Maude, S. L., Frey, N., & Grupp, S. A. (2016). Identification of predictive biomarkers for cytokine release syndrome after chimeric antigen receptor T-cell therapy for acute lymphoblastic leukemia. *Cancer Discovery*, *6*(6), 664–679.

Tian, H., Ketkar, R., & Tao, P. (2022). Accurate admet prediction with xgboost. *arXiv preprint arXiv:2204.07532*.

Tian, W. W., Tang, B. H., Liu, L., Yu, D. M., & Hua, H. (2024). Research progress on curcumin improving chronic low-grade inflammation and related diseases. *Zhongguo Zhong yao za zhi= Zhongguo Zhongyao Zazhi=. Zhongguo Zhongyao Zazhi*, *49*(10), 2607–2618.

Turner, M., Millar, S., Kusiak, C., Fuller, F. D., Walsh, J., & Zhuang, R. (2024). Accelerating Crohn's Disease clinical trials using generative artificial intelligence. In *journal of crohns & colitis* (Vol. 18, pp. i1002-i1002). GREAT CLARENDON ST, OXFORD OX2 6DP, ENGLAND: OXFORD UNIV PRESS.

Ugolkov, Y., Nikitich, A., Leon, C., Helmlinger, G., Peskov, K., Sokolov, V., & Volkova, A. (2024). Mathematical modelling in autoimmune diseases: From theory to clinical application. *Frontiers in Immunology*, *15*, 1371620.

Valcárcel, G., Lazarenkov, A., López-Rubio, A. V., Berenguer, C., Calafell-Segura, J., Rodríguez-Ubreva, J., & Sardina, J. L. (2025). Modulating immune cell fate and inflammation through CRISPR-mediated DNA methylation editing. *Science Advances, 11*(29), eadt1644.

Vallée, A. (2025). Digital twins for personalized Medicine require epidemiological data and mathematical modelling. *Journal of Medical Internet Research*, *27*, e72411.

Van Hasselt, J. C., & Iyengar, R. (2019). Systems pharmacology: Defining the interactions of drug combinations. *Annual Review of Pharmacology and Toxicology*, *59*(1), 21–40.

Vijayaragavan, V., Vijayakumar, M., Dharshini, P., Karunakaran, K., Kesavan, K., & Raj, R. D. S. (2025). AI and automation in organ-on-a-chip technology: advancing personalized medicine and disease modelling. In *2025 IEEE 6th International Conference in Robotics and Manufacturing Automation (ROMA)* (pp. 40-45). IEEE.

Vitali, F., Mulas, F., Marini, P., & Bellazzi, R. (2013). Network-based target ranking for polypharmacological therapies. *Journal of Biomedical Informatics*, *46*(5), 876–881.

Vora, L. K., Gholap, A. D., Jetha, K., Thakur, R. R. S., Solanki, H. K., & Chavda, V. P. (2023). Artificial intelligence in pharmaceutical technology and drug delivery design. *Pharmaceutics*, *15*(7), 1916.

Wang, J. (2025). Multi-modal topology-aware graph neural network for robust chemical–protein interaction prediction. *International Journal of Molecular Sciences*, *26*(17), 8666.

Yang, J., Li, H., Wang, F., Xiao, F., Yan, W., & Hu, G. (2021). Network-based target prioritization and drug candidate identification for multiple sclerosis: From analyzing "Omics Data" to druggability simulations. *ACS Chemical Neuroscience*, *12*(5), 917–929.

Yenduri, L. K., Chaithra, M. H., Shahedhadeennisa, S., Annamalai, M., Rajesh, L., & Imran, S. M. (2025). Quantum computing and machine learning for transforming precision medicine and drug discovery. In *Modern SuperHyperSoft Computing Trends in Science and Technology* (pp. 339–366). IGI Global Scientific Publishing.

Yeung, Y. T., Aziz, F., Guerrero-Castilla, A., & Arguelles, S. (2018). Signalling pathways in inflammation and anti-inflammatory therapies. *Current Pharmaceutical Design*, *24*(14), 1449–1484.

Zand, A., Stokes, Z., Sharma, A., van Deen, W. K., & Hommes, D. (2022). Artificial intelligence for inflammatory bowel diseases (IBD); accurately predicting adverse outcomes using machine learning. *Digestive Diseases and Sciences*, *67*(10), 4874–4885.

Zhan, X., Liu, Y., Guo, Y., Zhou, W., Yan, Y., Zeng, H., & Feng, Y. (2025). Single cell resolved spatial immune repertoire unveils spatial heterogeneity of lymphoid aggregates in human immune disorders. bioRxiv, 2025-01.

Zhang, X., Rahnavard, A., & Crandall, K. A. (2025). Machine learning enhances biomarker discovery: From multi-omics to functional genomics. *Medical Research Archives*, *13*(8).

Zhao, H. X., Qi, W., Liu, K., Zhao, J., Hu, X., & Deng, W. Q. (2025). Accelerating drug discovery for Disease X via AlphaFold2 driven drug repositioning strategy. *Physical Chemistry Chemical Physics*.

Zhou, X. J., Laouar, Y., & Tsoi, L. C. (2025). Community series in towards precision medicine for immune-mediated disorders: Advances in using big data and artificial intelligence to understand heterogeneity in inflammatory responses, volume II. *Frontiers in Immunology*, *16*, 1553004.

Zhou, Z., Kearnes, S., Li, L., Zare, R. N., & Riley, P. (2019). Optimization of molecules via deep reinforcement learning. *Scientific Reports*, *9*(1), 10752.

Zhu, T., Liu, B., Chen, N., Liu, Y., Wang, Z., & Tian, X. (2025). Artificial intelligence-driven innovations in pharmaceutical development and drug delivery systems. *Current Topics in Medicinal Chemistry*.

APPENDIX

Abbreviations

AI - Artificial Intelligence
ML - Machine Learning
DL - Deep Learning
IBD - Inflammatory Bowel Disease
RA - Rheumatoid Arthritis
CNNs - Convolutional Neural Networks
RNNs - Recurrent Neural Networks
GNNs - Graph Neural Networks
LLMs - Large Language Models
XAI - Explainable AI
GANs - Generative Adversarial Networks
VAEs - Variational Autoencoders
RL - Reinforcement Learning
MolDQN - Molecule Deep Q-Networks
OOC - Organ-on-Chip
CRS - Cytokine Release Syndrome
ECCO - European Crohn's and Colitis Organisation
CD - Crohn's disease
UC - Ulcerative Colitis
scRNA-seq - Single-Cell RNA Sequencing
SLE - Systemic Lupus Erythematosus
MS - Multiple Sclerosis
PK/PD - Pharmacokinetic/Pharmacodynamic
NAMs - Non-Animal Testing Models
ADMET - Absorption, Distribution, Metabolism, Excretion, and Toxicity
FL - Federated Learning
RWE - Real-World Evidence
XML - Explainable Machine Learning
ADRs - Adverse Drug Reactions
MT - Meticulous Transparency
IP - Intellectual Property
QML - Quantum Machine Learning
XGBoost - Extreme Gradient Boosting

Chapter 6
Leveraging AI and ITRS in Drug Discovery for Inflammatory and Cardiovascular Diseases

N. L. Swathi
https://orcid.org/0000-0002-3695-0732
Manipal College of Nursing, Manipal Academy of Higher Education, India

Allenki Vineesh
https://orcid.org/0009-0005-3959-0276
Mallareddy Institute of Medical Sciences, India

Abhilash Dinesh Sadhankar
https://orcid.org/0009-0006-5520-0247
All India Institite of Medical Sciences, Rishikesh, India

Muhammad Muzzamil
https://orcid.org/0000-0001-9871-5837
Health Services Academy, Pakistan

Akhil Arun
https://orcid.org/0000-0003-1787-054X
Amrita School of Pharmacy, Amrita Vishwa Vidyapeetham, India

M. Karpakavalli
https://orcid.org/0000-0002-1907-2536
Karpagam College of Pharmacy, India

Dipanjan Maity
JSS College of Pharmacy, India

Ancelin Wilfy
https://orcid.org/0009-0002-4437-6782
JSS College of Pharmacy, India

J. Anto Musy Bosco
JSS College of Pharmacy, India

Gaurav Singh Pilkhwal
https://orcid.org/0009-0006-1000-6491
School of Pharmaceutical Sciences, SGRR University, Dehradun, India

DOI: 10.4018/979-8-3373-5258-9.ch006

ABSTRACT

Artificial Intelligence (AI) and Intelligent Translational Research Systems (ITRS) are reshaping drug discovery for inflammatory and cardiovascular diseases by enabling rapid, data-driven identification of novel therapeutic targets and optimization of drug development pipelines. These technologies integrate genomics, proteomics, and clinical data to accelerate translational insights and support personalized treatment strategies. AI models aid in virtual screening, biomarker identification, and adaptive clinical trial designs, reducing time and cost. ITRS further bridge pre-clinical and clinical domains, enhancing reproducibility and translational relevance. Despite their promise, challenges persist, including algorithmic bias, data privacy concerns, and the need for transparent validation processes. Ethical oversight is essential to ensure fairness and patient safety. Regulatory frameworks must adapt to the evolving digital landscape, emphasizing interoperability, accountability, and real-world applicability.

INTRODUCTION: EVOLVING PARADIGMS IN DRUG DISCOVERY

Burden of Inflammatory and Cardiovascular Diseases

The contemporary drug discovery paradigm addressing the dual burden of inflammation and cardiovascular disease (CVD) is shifting from single-target, organ-centric approaches to combination and mechanism-guided strategies. This includes repurposing anti-inflammatory and metabolic agents, such as probenecid and apremilast, and integrating cardio-renal-metabolic (CKM) therapies, including sodium-glucose cotransporter-2 inhibitors (SGLT2 inhibitors), glucagon-like peptide-1 receptor agonists (GLP-1RAs), and non-steroidal mineralocorticoid receptor antagonists (ns-MRAs), to exploit complementary mechanisms and mitigate safety signals (Alicic et al., 2025; Barbarroja et al., 2024; Onódi et al., 2023; Zollinger-Read & Filer, 2025).

This chapter outlines an integrative methodological framework that unites mechanistic, preclinical, and clinical evidence on inflammation-driven cardiovascular disease (CVD) to inform artificial intelligence (AI)-enabled and systems biology translational pipelines. A comprehensive literature search (PubMed, Scopus, Web of Science, Google Scholar; 2005-2025 + Historical articles) was performed with controlled vocabulary and free-text strings such as “cardiovascular inflammation,” “atherosclerosis inflammation,” and “microbial metabolism heart,” supplemented by citation tracing of high-impact reviews and trials. Studies were included if they detailed inflammatory pathways relevant to CVD, provided mechanistic insights into innate immune signaling, offered translational evidence from preclinical models, or reported clinical trials of anti-inflammatory interventions targeting cardiovascular endpoints. The exclusion criteria were non-inflammatory or non-cardiovascular reports, purely computational studies lacking drug discovery relevance, investigations without mechanistic or translational details, and anecdotal case-level data.

A parallel strategic axis involves targeting immunometabolic nodes, such as amino acid pathways and inflammasome/purinergic signalling, to modulate vascular and myocardial inflammation (Onódi et al., 2023; Shen & Zhang, 2025). Additionally, innovations in delivery modalities, such as plaque-directed nanotherapeutics, and advances in preclinical models are expected to increase translational yield and enhance mechanistic precision (Culver et al., 2025; Kanthi et al., 2020). The paradigm also emphasizes the coupling of advanced diagnostics, including oral and systemic biomarkers and multiplex platforms, with therapeutics to enable precise deployment and optimized patient stratification. Although current evidence is promising, it remains largely preclinical, narrative, or mechanistic in nature; therefore, high-quality randomized evidence testing multi-agent regimens on hard cardiovascular and renal endpoints is still lacking (Alicic et al., 2025; Kanthi et al., 2020; Onódi et al., 2023; Savira et al., 2020). The literature provided thus coalesces around a pragmatic, mechanistic, and translational shift defined by combination regimens, repurposing anti-inflammatory/metabolic agents, immunometabolic targeting, and new delivery/diagnostic innovations; however, the present body of work remains predominantly Level V evidence.

Contemporary cardiovascular drug discovery increasingly focuses on targeting the immune–inflammatory pathways that drive atherosclerosis, myocardial injury, and adverse remodeling. Therapeutically relevant nodes include innate immune sensors (TLRs, cGAS–STING), proinflammatory transcriptional hubs such as NF-κB and TBK1, the NLRP3 inflammasome, maladaptive macrophage polarization, and oxidant-defense circuits governed by Keap1–Nrf2 signaling. Clinical translation has demonstrated that suppressing vascular inflammation can modify cardiovascular outcomes; interleukin-1β blockade and low-dose colchicine provide event-reduction benefits across secondary prevention populations, establishing inflammation as a causal driver of atherosclerotic biology rather than a secondary marker (Lutgens et al., 2019; Nelson et al., 2023). These clinical signals also highlight therapeutic constraints, particularly the risk of infection with cytokine inhibition and drug-interaction liabilities with colchicine, underscoring the need for more selective pathway-directed intervention markers (Lutgens et al., 2019; Nelson et al., 2023).

Mechanistic evidence from multi-omic and transgenic studies further defines the inflammatory architecture of cardiovascular diseases. Macrophage-centered inflammatory circuits, including ILF3-driven NF-κB amplification and repression of the Keap1–Nrf2 antioxidant axis, accelerate vascular degeneration and aneurysm progression, whereas pharmacological restoration of Nrf2 signaling mitigates inflammatory injury (Z.-Y. Wang et al., 2024). Additional preclinical studies have demonstrated that immunometabolic modulation, such as semaglutide-mediated Sirt3-dependent restoration of RKIP with downstream inhibition of TBK1–NF-κB, attenuates diabetic cardiac inflammation, emphasizing the therapeutic promise of targeting upstream regulators rather than broad cytokine suppression (K. Lin et al., 2025). Upstream pattern recognition mechanisms are also applicable. Inhibition of TLR2/4–MYD88–TRAF–NF-κB and p38 MAPK signaling reduces myocardial inflammation and fibrosis in HFpEF and remodeling models (Dawuti et al., 2023; Fang et al., 2024), whereas cGAS–STING blockade suppresses NF-κB-driven microglial M1 polarization with organ-protective effects relevant to vascular inflammation (Shao et al., 2023).

Inflammasome biology is another translationally compelling research axis. NLRP3 activation orchestrates IL-1 family cytokine release and pyroptotic cell death. Rodent ischemic injury models have shown that NF-κB suppression and direct NLRP3 inhibition, including by compounds such as curcumin, reduce pyroptosis and improve structural outcomes (Ran et al., 2021). Given the clinical success of IL-1β targeting, the upstream interruption of inflammasome priming or direct NLRP3 inhibition constitutes a mechanistically justified next-generation anti-inflammatory strategy for cardiovascular disease.

MAPK and JAK-STAT signaling have emerged as recurrent modulators of plaque instability and fibrotic remodeling. Studies on small molecules and natural compounds have consistently demonstrated reduced macrophage M1 polarization and matrix metalloproteinase activity through the suppression of these stress-kinase pathways, supporting their relevance for drug discovery despite current preclinical limitations (Fang et al., 2024; Huang et al., 2024).

Similarly, Onódi et al. reviewed probenecid as a repurposed agent targeting pannexin-1/purinergic signalling, TRPV2 channels, and inflammasome pathways with potential cardiovascular benefits, yet emphasized gaps in human target validation and dose optimization, with efficacy unproven in broad randomized settings (Onódi et al., 2023). Barbarroja et al. highlighted the potential cardiometabolic benefits of apremilast in psoriatic diseases via PDE4-mediated anti-inflammatory and metabolic modulation, and Zollinger-Read and Filer summarized targeted immunomodulators in inflammatory disorders; however, direct evidence of CVD outcomes remains sparse (Barbarroja et al., 2024; Zollinger-Read & Filer, 2025). Shen and Zhang described immunometabolic pathways involving arginine, glutamine, branched-chain amino acids, and tryptophan metabolism as druggable axes influencing coronary inflammation and immune reprogramming; however, randomized data linking amino-acid-based interventions to major adverse cardiovascular events are unavailable (Shen & Zhang, 2025).

Kanthi et al. emphasized endothelial barrier heterogeneity, plaque biology, and immune-mediated uptake in advancing nanoparticle delivery and noted manufacturability and safety challenges that require refinement in mechanistic studies (Kanthi et al., 2020). Savira et al. reinforced the integrative systems perspective on cardiorenal interactions driven by neurohormonal, inflammatory, and metabolic pathways, and Foroughi et al. proposed periodontal inflammation as a modifiable systemic driver of cardiovascular risk, where multiplex diagnostics may support precision prevention, although prospective validation is limited (Foroughi et al., 2025; Savira et al., 2020). Culver et al. highlighted the translational lessons from GLP-1-based therapies, advocating for improved animal models and endpoints to increase predictive validity and avoid late-stage failures (Culver et al., 2025).

Limitations of Traditional Drug Development Approaches

Traditional drug development has historically followed a linear, target-centric paradigm in which a disease-associated molecular target is identified, small-molecule modulators are synthesized and screened, evaluated in cell-based and animal systems, and advanced through human clinical trials in phases. Although this model has generated many transformative therapeutics, it has several structural limitations. First, traditional discovery pipelines are time-intensive and resource-consuming, requiring sequential cycles of compound design, optimization, and protracted clinical evaluation, contributing to high attrition rates and delayed translation (Jia et al., 2024). The literature consistently highlights the labor-intensive nature of classical in vitro and in vivo validation and proposes computational augmentation to mitigate costs and accelerate development timelines (Azmal et al., 2025; Jia et al., 2024). Second, this approach is constrained by the limited "druggable" target space, as many pathobiologically critical proteins lack suitable binding sites for classical, small molecules.

The emergence of targeted protein degradation technologies, including PROTACs and related modalities, has expanded the therapeutic horizon but simultaneously underscores the inadequacy of traditional small-molecule strategies for historically "undruggable" targets (Valenza et al., 2025). Third, the translational fidelity from preclinical models to human diseases remains suboptimal. Mechanistic effects demonstrated in cell cultures or animal models frequently fail to recapitulate human clinical responses, reflecting insufficient physiological relevance and contributing to late-stage clinical failure (Kitchen et al., 2004; Parker & Pratt, 2020; Tu et al., 2023; Verma et al., 2010). Fourth, traditional systems often rely on indirect biochemical assays for target validation, leading to uncertainty regarding target engagement in complex biological environments. Although technologies such as CETSA, thermal proteome profiling, and bio-orthogonal click chemistry have begun to enable more direct and physiologically relevant target engagement assessments, their emergence highlights the limitations of classical methodologies (Parker & Pratt, 2020; Tu et al., 2023).

Fifth, screening and predictive techniques, including docking, scoring functions, and QSAR models, while foundational, still face recognized accuracy limitations when confronted with protein dynamics, solvation effects, and complex biochemical kinetics, emphasizing the need for rigorous experimental confirmation (Azmal et al., 2025; Kitchen et al., 2004; Verma et al., 2010).

Sixth, clinical progress is frequently hindered by biomarker variability and the limited reliability of surrogate endpoints, with the literature noting heterogeneity in circulating tumor DNA and measurable residual disease assays that constrain their immediate regulatory utility and reduce confidence in accelerated approval pathways (Kitchen et al., 2004; Valenza et al., 2025).

Seventh, traditional pipelines inadequately address the complexity of polypharmacy and host biological interactions, including metabolism, diet, and the microbiome, prompting the development of AI-driven models that can account for multidimensional pharmacological interactions beyond conventional capabilities (S. Chen et al., 2022). Eighth, the historical under-representation of diverse populations in trials and preclinical datasets restricts generalizability and delays equitable therapeutic applications, motivating the development of global and diverse real-world datasets to overcome population-specific evidence gaps (Galvin et al., 2024; Vollstedt et al., 2023). Ninth, the paradigm struggles to adequately generate dose and safety evidence in special populations, such as children, necessitating extrapolation from adult data through modeling approaches that remain imperfect and highlight systemic developmental constraints (Samant et al., 2015).

Collectively, these limitations mandate the strategic refinement of traditional discovery frameworks. Key opportunities include the systematic integration of emerging therapeutic modalities, such as degraders and LYTACs, and the routine application of direct target engagement assays to address mechanistic uncertainty (Parker & Pratt, 2020; Schneider et al., 2021; Tu et al., 2023; Valenza et al., 2025). Computational tools and AI-enabled models can accelerate early discovery but must be tightly coupled with physiologically relevant experimental validation to avoid false positive trajectories (Azmal et al., 2025; Kitchen et al., 2004; Verma et al., 2010). Standardization and external validation of biomarkers, assay platforms, and surrogate endpoints are necessary for reliable regulatory and clinical decision making. Furthermore, the early incorporation of system-scale modeling to anticipate polypharmacy and host interaction effects, diversification of clinical and preclinical cohorts, and judicious application of adaptive trial designs can strengthen translational fidelity and equity.

The Emergence of AI and Intelligent Translational Research Systems (ITRS)

The integration of Artificial Intelligence (AI) and Intelligent Translational Research Systems (ITRS) is transforming drug discovery in inflammatory and cardiovascular diseases, with the capacity to accelerate therapeutic development, strengthen precision medicine strategies, and improve patient outcomes. These technologies leverage large-scale biological, clinical, and molecular datasets to streamline translational workflows. However, its implementation requires careful navigation of clinical, ethical, and regulatory complexities to ensure transparent, equitable, and safe adoption.

From a clinical standpoint, AI enhances several phases of drug development. In target identification and validation, predictive modeling and machine-learning frameworks enable the rapid interrogation of complex biological datasets to uncover disease-associated pathways and forecast compound-target interactions, thus expediting early discovery processes (Barcelos & de Paula da Silva, 2024; Saeed & Alajlan, 2025; Saleem, 2025). Within clinical development pathways, AI facilitates trial optimization by supporting real-time data monitoring, algorithm-guided patient recruitment, and adaptive study designs, which collectively reduce trial duration, lower costs, and strengthen endpoint accuracy (Gadade et al., 2024; Saeed & Alajlan, 2025; Saleem, 2025). In precision medicine applications, AI integrates molecular and clinical signatures to tailor interventions, particularly for cardiovascular diseases, where it supports novel biomarker identification and informs individualized therapeutic strategies (A.-T. Chen et al., 2025; Krittanawong et al., 2017; Sabry et al., 2025). Furthermore, in cardiovascular applications, AI advances metabolic pathway analysis to elucidate the mechanisms of heart failure and coronary artery disease(A.-T. Chen et al., 2025; Sabry et al., diagnosis, and stratification of disease progression and treatment response (GALLONE et al., 2022; Krittanawong et al., 2017).

Ethical considerations are central to the deployment of AI in drug discovery. Algorithmic transparency and bias mitigation are essential, given the inherent risk of "black-box" decision-making systems; ensuring interpretability protects equity and clinical reliability (Barcelos & de Paula da Silva, 2024; Warokar & Lote, 2024). Safeguarding patient confidentiality is equally critical, as AI modules rely on extensive health and genomic datasets, necessitating stringent data protection controls and compliance with privacy laws, such as the GDPR and Health Insurance Portability and HIPAA (Alshehade et al., 2026; Mirakhori & Niazi, 2025; Warokar

& Lote, 2024). Therefore, ethical governance frameworks must enforce informed consent, equitable data use, and algorithmic fairness, supported by multidisciplinary collaboration among clinicians, technologists, bioethicists, and policymakers (Al Zo'ubi, 2025).

This regulatory perspective underscores the need for adaptive oversight. Traditional regulatory processes do not fully accommodate AI's dynamic learning capabilities and continuous validation requirements, creating gaps in their suitability for digital biomedical innovation (Pasas-Farmer & Jain, 2025). Therefore, regulatory bodies must define standardized validation criteria and quality benchmarks to ensure the reliability and clinical relevance of these models (Pasas-Farmer & Jain, 2025; Warokar & Lote, 2024). Risk-based regulatory approaches can balance innovation and safety by assessing the risks and benefits of AI systems and enforcing performance standards, whereas harmonized global frameworks support interoperable data standards, transparent algorithms, and unified compliance pathways (Alshehade et al., 2026; Mirakhori & Niazi, 2025; Pasas-Farmer & Jain, 2025).

AI and ITRS represent a paradigm shift in the development of therapeutics for inflammatory and cardiovascular disorders, offering substantial benefits in terms of discovery efficiency, mechanistic insights, and personalized care for patients. The realization of this potential depends on integrating ethical safeguards, advancing regulatory modernization, and fostering interdisciplinary collaboration to ensure the safe, equitable, and transparent deployment of AI.

The primary objective of this chapter is to examine the paradigm shift in drug discovery for inflammatory and cardiovascular diseases, transitioning from traditional linear, target-centric development pipelines toward integrated, AI-driven, and Intelligent Translational Research System (ITRS)-based models. This chapter aims to contextualize the burden of inflammatory and cardiovascular diseases, evaluate the constraints of conventional drug discovery systems, and articulate how emerging computational and multi-omic intelligence frameworks can enhance target validation, therapeutic precision, and translational efficiency. A key goal is to explore how AI-based platforms and ITRS architectures accelerate mechanistic understanding, biomarker discovery, drug repurposing, clinical trial optimization, and real-time decision support while maintaining clinical relevance and patient-centric outcomes.

This chapter encompasses the mechanistic, clinical, ethical, and regulatory dimensions of integrating AI and ITRS into cardiovascular and inflammation-focused drug development. It includes a systematic discussion of traditional limitations, the emergence of computational and intelligent translational models, multimodal data integration, real-world case examples, and future-ready applications in precision therapeutics. This chapter also addresses the challenges associated with data quality, interpretability, algorithmic fairness, interoperability, and regulatory adaptation required for digital-first translational ecosystems to be effective. Through this analysis, we delineate how AI and ITRS converge with next-generation multimodal biomarker strategies, adaptive trial frameworks, and mechanistic disease modeling to ultimately enable individualized, predictive, and preventive therapies for complex inflammatory and cardiovascular conditions.

Inflammatory Disorders: Mechanistic and Translational Challenges

Inflammatory disorders encompass a broad spectrum of diseases characterized by dysregulated immune responses that lead to tissue damage. Mechanistically, these disorders involve complex interactions between immune cells, cytokines, and signaling pathways that vary according to the disease context, making it difficult to identify universal targets. A critical translational challenge is the heterogeneity of patient responses and incomplete understanding of inflammation resolution processes. This complexity hampers the development of effective targeted therapies and necessitates integrated approaches using multi-omics and systems biology to uncover disease-specific mechanisms of action. Moreover, bridging preclinical findings with clinical efficacy remains a significant hurdle, emphasizing the need for advanced models, such as patient-derived organoids and digital twins, for personalized intervention strategies (L. Chen et al., 2017).

Cardiovascular Diseases: Mechanistic and Translational Challenges

Cardiovascular diseases (CVDs), the leading cause of morbidity and mortality worldwide, present intricate mechanistic challenges involving endothelial dysfunction, inflammation, metabolic disturbances, and genetic predisposition. Translational barriers include the long latency of disease progression, variations in phenotypes such as heart failure subtypes, and comorbidities that affect the treatment response. The integration of big data from genomic, proteomic, and metabolomic studies is still evolving and provides actionable insights into clinical practice. Digital twin models and AI-driven multi-omics analyses hold promise for improving risk stratification, early diagnosis, and personalized therapy for CVDs. However, successful translation requires overcoming challenges related to data standardization, model validation, and clinical implementation to effectively enhance patient outcomes (Frąk et al., 2022).

AI in Drug Discovery: From Data to Decision

The conventional drug discovery process is extensive and demanding, often requiring up to 15 years and expenditures exceeding $1 to $2 billion for each sanctioned drug (Hinkson et al., 2020). This is mostly attributable to increasing attrition rates and prolonged clinical trial durations (Barker, 2010). The failure rate is exceedingly high, with less than 10% of the medication candidates successfully reaching the market (Wouters et al., 2020). Considering these figures, there is an urgent need to discover methods for reducing and optimizing the overall drug development process. Most failures in clinical development are linked to safety concerns and insufficient efficacy, highlighting the need for enhancements in preclinical processes, such as target selection and drug discovery (Paul et al., 2010).

A growing number of our daily interactions rely on artificial intelligence (AI), which is one of the most discussed subjects. Applications and programs in the domains of diagnostics, text classification, and recommendation systems were common in our study. When people, especially the general public, refer to anything as artificial intelligence, it is usually machine learning (ML). ML is a data processing, prediction, and decision support tool that integrates methods and ideas from computer science and statistics (Jordan, 2019). The ability to analyze and understand massive amounts of data, which are inaccessible using conventional statistical approaches, has led to an exponential increase in the popularity of artificial intelligence (AI) in the health sector in recent years (Murmu & Győrffy, 2024). Despite the effectiveness of traditional methods in drug discovery and early clinical development, as seen by the approval and development of new agents, there is still a great possibility of refining these models with AI. Additionally, AI may introduce new methods that can revolutionize and accelerate these operations (Ocana et al., 2011).

The practical Implementation of Intelligent Translational Research Systems (ITRS) involves comprehensive infrastructure, workflow optimization, skilled personnel, and adherence to data standards. Infrastructure needs encompass high-performance computing resources, cloud platforms, and secure data storage systems capable of managing large-scale multiomics and clinical data. Integration with electronic health records (EHRs) and laboratory systems ensures a continuous real-time data flow, which is vital for translational research. Data security and compliance with privacy regulations such as GDPR and HIPAA are fundamental to protect sensitive health information and maintain trust (Mayrink et al., 2022).

In pharmaceutical and hospital contexts, the ITRS workflow begins with the acquisition of omics and clinical data, followed by AI-powered integration and analysis to generate hypotheses, identify biomarkers, and support clinical decision-making. The cycle is iterative, with clinical outcomes feeding back into system refinement. Essential personnel include translational scientists, bioinformaticians, clinicians, and data engineers, all of whom are trained in ITRS technologies and domain-specific standards. The use of FAIR data principles and HL7 messaging standards guarantees data interoperability, accessibility, and reproducibility across platforms and institutions (Ioachimescu & Shaker, 2025).

Clinical applications have demonstrated the impact of the ITRS. In oncology, multi-omics integrated with digital twin modeling enhance personalized therapy selection and toxicity prediction. In cardiology, patient-specific digital twins simulate disease progression and optimize interventions, such as stent placement or tailored pharmacotherapy, leading to improved clinical outcomes and cost-effectiveness. These examples signify the translational promise of the ITRS in accelerating bench-to-bedside research and precision medicine (Ooka, 2025).

Target Identification and Pathway Mapping Using AI

The discovery of potential new drugs can be aided by the efficient evaluation of massive datasets using algorithms based on systems biology and artificial intelligence (AI). Drug development success rates increase and project risks decrease when new targets are chosen based on a solid biological justification for their disease-related mechanisms and the known signaling pathways that these targets affect. The primary application of AI in drug research is the identification of drug targets (Vijayan et al., 2022). Artificial Intelligence can examine extensive datasets of genetic information, protein structures, and signaling pathways to identify prospective therapeutic targets. Through the analysis of these data, AI systems recognize targets implicated in disease progression that can be altered by drugs (Schork, 2019). This knowledge can facilitate the development of novel medicines for diseases with limited therapeutic alternatives (Dubey, 2020).

AI can assist with treatment planning and identifying the most effective treatments will work best for certain patients (R. Wang et al., 2022). Using a patient's genetic composition and medical history, this process entails teaching algorithms to anticipate how several medications may interact with one another. The use of AI in personalized medicine has the potential to enhance treatment outcomes while decreasing the likelihood of side effects (Johnson et al., 2022). More tailored treatments for a wide range of illnesses may soon be within reach, thanks to an AI-powered revolution in the drug development process that can identify pharmacological targets and pathways. The use of AI and ML in drug development can help identify therapeutic targets faster, predict the efficacy of medications, identify biomarkers for illness diagnosis, and monitor and enhance treatment outcomes by making treatment options more personalized for each patient. It can facilitate the creation of more efficacious medicines for many diseases and disorders, achieving this more rapidly and at a reduced cost compared with conventional research methodologies.

Virtual Screening and Molecular Optimization

The goal of drug discovery is to create new substances with desirable chemical characteristics that can be used to treat specific diseases. An essential part of the development of new drugs is improving the physical and chemical characteristics of molecules through a process called molecular optimization. Artificial intelligence (AI) methodologies have recently shown impressive effectiveness in this area as a novel strategy to address the intricacies of drug design, including molecular optimization, and to drastically reduce the costs and time required for drug discovery. New developments in molecular optimization for AI-powered drug discovery include data sources, molecular traits, optimization methods, and assessment standards for molecular improvements. Optimization techniques can be categorized into three groups: those based on molecular mapping, those based on molecular distribution matching, and those based on guided search. There are various perspectives on the potential future research directions offered by current molecular optimization problems, including interpretability, multidimensional optimization, and model generalization (Xia et al., 2024).

Conventional computer approaches to molecular optimization break down molecules into their component parts and optimize them by adding, removing, or replacing molecules in accordance with quantitative structure–activity relationships (QSAR). Given the abundance of molecular fragments, their combination gives rise to a vast chemical space; nevertheless, extracting the desired molecules from this space is difficult. Molecular optimization was shown to be inefficient; thus, researchers have created molecular optimization methods based on artificial intelligence (AI) that use swarm intelligence, reinforcement learning, and generative adversarial networks (Muhammad et al., 2018). In drug discovery, key molecular, pharmacokinetic, medicinal chemistry, physicochemical, and pharmacological properties are often optimized through Absorption, Distribution, Metabolism, Excretion, and Toxicity (ADMET) (Hefti, 2008). Recent advances in deep learning algorithms, specialized hardware (e.g., GPUs and TPUs), and big data have rapidly accelerated the application of AI in this domain.

Predictive Modeling for Pharmacodynamics and Toxicity

Interventional pharmacology is one of the most potent tools that contemporary medicine can utilize to combat diseases. Conversely, these drugs may produce significant side effects, necessitating vigilant monitoring of their use. Pharmacovigilance is a scientific subject dedicated to the monitoring, detection, and prevention of adverse drug reactions (ADRs) (Zhavoronkov et al., 2020). The integration of machine learning and artificial intelligence has led to pivotal advancements in the detection of early adverse medication responses and toxicity. These computer methods provide swift, comprehensive, and accurate forecasts of potential adverse drug responses and toxicity prior to drug production, preclinical evaluation, and clinical trials. This paradigm shift aims to develop more efficient and safer pharmaceuticals, thereby reducing the probability of drug withdrawal. This study examined the essential functions of machine learning and artificial intelligence in the rapid identification of adverse medication responses and toxicity, encompassing methodologies from data mining to deep learning. It enumerates the critical databases, modeling methodologies, and software applicable for modeling and forecasting various toxicities and drug reactions (Panda & Mohapatra, 2024). Recent applications of machine learning and artificial intelligence in toxicology include physiologically based pharmacokinetic (PBPK) modeling, quantitative structure–activity relationship (QSAR) modeling for toxicity prediction, adverse outcome pathway analysis, high-throughput screening, toxicogenomics, big data, and toxicological databases. By harnessing these approaches, it is now possible to efficiently generate PBPK models for hundreds of chemicals, underscoring their transformative potential for advancing predictive toxicology and accelerating drug discovery (Z. Lin & Chou, 2022).

AI-Enabled Biomarker Discovery

Biomarkers are essential for advancing clinical research and facilitating the development of tailored therapies. The amalgamation of Artificial Intelligence, Machine Learning, and Digital Biomarkers has the potential to transform clinical research by delivering enhanced disease detection and therapy methodologies. Artificial Intelligence and Machine Learning algorithms can discern patterns in extensive datasets, uncover new biomarkers, and enhance the precision of existing biomarkers. Digital biomarkers, with the extensive integration of digital health technology, provide objective and measurable data for health care evaluations. The breakthroughs in bioinformatics and numerous "omics" methodologies suggest a promising future for clinical research, with the potential for more focused therapies for diverse illnesses.(Raikar et al., 2023).

Figure 1. Applications of Artificial Intelligence in Drug Discovery.

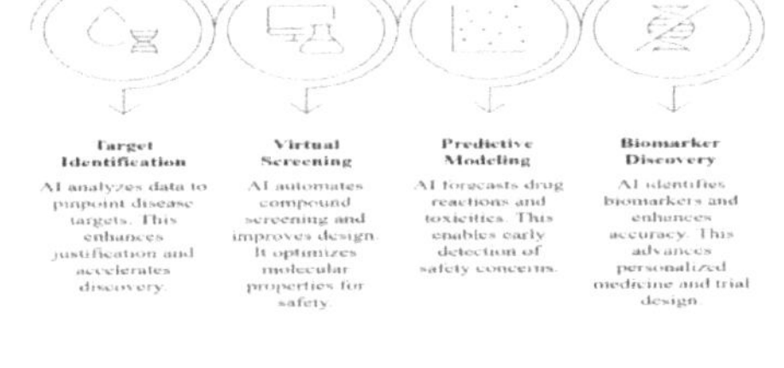

The figure explains how artificial intelligence (AI) is included in several phases of the drug discovery process. AI facilitates target identification and pathway mapping by analyzing extensive biological data, supports virtual screening and molecular optimization via sophisticated algorithms for compound design and ADMET profiling, enhances predictive modeling for pharmacodynamics and toxicity, enables early identification of adverse effects, and propels AI-driven biomarker discovery. This advances personalized medicine through innovative biomarker identification and the integration of digital health. These applications collectively underscore AI's transformational capacity of AI to expedite drug discovery, lower costs, and enhance therapeutic precision.

The integration of artificial intelligence and drug discovery signifies a significant advancement that overcomes the constraints of traditional methods. AI has the potential to significantly expedite timeframes, diminish attrition, and provide safer and more accurate medicines through sophisticated applications in target selection, virtual screening, predictive toxicity modeling, and biomarker development. Despite the ongoing challenges related to data quality, interpretability, and clinical integration, the advancement of AI-driven innovation indicates a transformation of the drug development paradigm, facilitating a future in which life-saving treatments can be identified and administered with an unparalleled speed and precision.

INTELLIGENT TRANSLATIONAL RESEARCH SYSTEMS (ITRS): INTEGRATING OMICS AND CLINICAL INTELLIGENCE

Definition and Architecture of ITRS

An Intelligent Translational Research System (ITRS) is a structured, technology-enabled continuum that transforms biological discoveries into clinically actionable interventions. In simple terms, an ITRS is a coordinated pipeline that integrates experimental platforms, standardized multimodal data capture, computational intelligence, and harmonized clinical validation to ensure that discoveries are efficiently translated into patient care. Such systems integrate tissue- and organ-scale experimental models, high-resolution analytical assays, electronic health record (EHR)-linked clinical data, and artificial intelligence-driven analytic frameworks to support rapid, reproducible, and context-aware translation into practice.

A core defining principle of ITRSs is multimodal data capture and integration, linking clinical outcomes, imaging, radiomic signatures, molecular omics profiles, and spatial cellular contexts into a harmonized dataset. This cross-scale integration enables context-aware biological interpretation, exemplified by spatial profiling that preserves tissue structure and cell–cell interactions, thereby strengthening mechanistic validity and translational hypothesis generation (Gong et al., 2024; Liu et al., 2025). Diagnostic individual patient data (IPD) meta-analysis frameworks further demonstrate that pooled harmonized datasets sharpen diagnostic performance boundaries and decision thresholds (Adamo et al., 2025).

The ITRS architecture requires physiologically relevant, scalable experimental platforms capable of modeling human pathophysiology with fidelity, such as organoids, engineered hydrogels, and organoid-based disease states that recapitulate structure–function relationships and support drug testing (Frattini et al., 2025; Mun et al., 2019; Zhu et al., 2025). These platforms provide mechanistic insights that can be linked to clinically relevant therapeutic interventions.

The analytical layer of the ITRS incorporates advanced computational pipelines, including machine learning, multimodal data fusion, model validation frameworks, and interpretable radiomics pipelines. Evidence from systematic reviews demonstrates that performance varies; however, methods such as gradient boosting and structured feature engineering perform effectively when externally validated and are accompanied by robust interpretability and monitoring frameworks (Parsaei et al., 2024). Similarly, ultrasound radiomics studies have shown that quantitative imaging features improve the detection of metastatic disease when they are embedded in high-quality methodological frameworks (Guerrisi et al., 2024).

Successful ITRSs relies on standardized diagnostic and outcome definitions to ensure comparability and reproducibility. Harmonized algorithms, consensus diagnostic thresholds, and rigorously defined clinical endpoints enable pooled evidence evaluation and consistent translation to clinical trial testing, as demonstrated by meta-analytic studies of imaging classification frameworks (Adamo et al., 2025). In contrast, fragmented clinical outcome definitions hinder synthesis and impede translation (Saboya-Galindo et al., 2025).

A defining architectural feature involves closed-loop learning, in which real-world outcomes and trial data are fed back into model retraining, meta-analytic updates, and experimental hypothesis refinement. High-quality pooled outcome analyses and meta-analyses illustrate how iterative evidence synthesis continually recalibrates diagnostic thresholds and informs trial designs (Adamo et al., 2025; Pala et al., 2024).

The operational backbone of an ITRS includes governance, interoperability, and reproducibility standards, ensuring harmonized data structures, secure data-sharing mechanisms, algorithmic transparency, and ethical compliance in workflows. Heterogeneity in imaging protocols, assay definitions, and trial outcomes across studies demonstrates the need for standardization and cross-institutional reproducibility infrastructure (Guerrisi et al., 2024; Saboya-Galindo et al., 2025). Ethical oversight and algorithmic transparency are required for responsible deployments.

Finally, ITRSs are fundamentally multidisciplinary ecosystems that unite clinical experts, experimental biologists, computational scientists, informaticians, biostatisticians, and regulatory specialists. Translational reviews consistently highlight that durable clinical translation requires the coupling of biologically grounded modeling with trial-aligned outcome design and pragmatic clinical deployment strategies (Kaur et al., 2023; Pala et al., 2024).

Structurally, ITRSs comprise the following layered components:

- **Data layer:** standardized clinical data, imaging archives, radiomic data, and molecular datasets with preserved provenance (Adamo et al., 2025; Gong et al., 2024; M. Liu et al., 2025).
- **Experimental layer:** Scalable organoids and organ-on-chip systems with high-throughput perturbation and multiomic readouts (Frattini et al., 2025; Mun et al., 2019; Zhu et al., 2025).
- **Analytics layer:** validated machine learning and radiomics pipelines with cross-site calibration (Guerrisi et al., 2024; M. Liu et al., 2025; Parsaei et al., 2024).
- **Evidence synthesis layer:** Continuous meta-analysis and pooled analytical pipelines (Adamo et al., 2025; Pala et al., 2024).
- **Clinical translation layer:** standardized diagnostic criteria, harmonized endpoints, adaptive trials, and real-world registries (Pala et al., 2024; Saboya-Galindo et al., 2025).
- **Governance layer:** Data privacy frameworks, interoperability standards, explainable AI modules, and clinical decision support pathways.
- **Feedback loop:** Prospective real-world learning and experimental reiteration mechanisms.

Integration of Genomics, Proteomics, and Clinical Data

Integrating genomics, proteomics, and clinical data within an Intelligent Translational Research System (ITRS) framework is both technically feasible and clinically promising, with the potential to substantively enhance preoperative diagnostic and prognostic performance. When such systems are engineered with rigorous data harmonization, explainable artificial intelligence (AI) models, and prospective validation pipelines, they demonstrate measurable improvements in clinical decision making. The multicenter PRAC-PTC study [1] serves as a key empirical proof-of-concept, reporting a high discriminative capability with an AUC of 0.925 in the discovery cohort and 0.787 and 0.799 in the retrospective and prospective external validation cohorts, respectively, across 558 patients. Complementary methodological analyses and domain reviews [2–4] outline the computational strategies necessary for

ITRS implementation, including multiview learning, network-based fusion, graph models, and FAIR-compliant data infrastructures, alongside essential translational safeguards related to explainable outputs, data provenance, and the definition of clinically meaningful end points.

From an evidence-driven perspective, a clinically functional ITRS must integrate multi-omics data streams with immune phenotypes and structured clinical variables within a transparent modular computational architecture. The PRAC-PTC model (Li et al., 2024) exemplifies this approach by combining clinical parameters, blood immune indices, BRAFV600E mutation status, and high-throughput proteomics to develop a 17-variable classifier for PTC. Performance gains were observed when clinicians used PRAC-PTC support, with accuracy increasing to 84.4 percent (95 percent CI: 82.9–84.4) in retrospective evaluation and 83.5 percent (95 percent CI: 82.2–84.2) in prospective testing. Key strengths include multicenter enrollment, blinded external validation, and validation across different sample types, mapping directly onto foundational ITRS requirements such as cross-site interoperability and heterogeneous data integration.

However, the observed AUC attenuation between the discovery and external cohorts indicates model optimism and real-world heterogeneity in clinical practice, assay conditions, and disease prevalence. Although the sample size (n=558) and feature count (17 variables) were methodologically reasonable, the power remained limited for rare disease subtypes and high-resolution calibration assessments. Moreover, the lack of reported decision-curve analysis, calibration plots, and net benefit estimates restricts claims regarding clinical utility and highlights the need for prospective impact studies before routine clinical deployment. Additionally, conflict of interest disclosures necessitate independent replication prior to embedding such systems into a regulated ITRS clinical infrastructure.

Assay and data-quality considerations represent another critical dimension. While proteomic assessment across FFPE and fine-needle aspiration (FNA) samples demonstrates feasibility, the absence of systematic reproducibility metrics (including inter-run variance and batch effect quantification) indicates the need for standardized quality control pipelines within ITRS architectures. Reliance on a single genomic marker (BRAFV600E) in this demonstration model, while practical, underscores the need for expanded genomic signatures and robust missing data handling strategies to improve generalizability.

Methodological reviews have reinforced that successful ITRSs must incorporate multi-omics integration pipelines with modality-specific pre-processing, feature-selection strategies, dimensionality-reduction techniques, and nested validation frameworks (Sathyanarayanan et al., 2023). Precision medicine-oriented integration requires deep phenotyping, linkage to standardized clinical ontologies, and access to validated biological knowledge bases (Ahmed, 2022). Furthermore, explainability and mechanistic interpretability are essential, as highlighted by critiques of opaque AI models; interpretable models linked to biological knowledge graphs and causal inference are central to ensuring clinical trust and facilitating hypothesis generation (Jurisica, 2024).

Pragmatically, an operational ITRS requires

(i) Standardized sample processing and assay quality-control pipelines
(ii) A modular computational integration stack supporting multiview fusion methods, graph learning, and rigorous cross-validation
(iii) Explainable clinical decision interfaces providing calibrated risk estimates and biologically interpretable outputs.
(iv) prospective validation including decision-analytic assessment and real-world implementation studies; and
(v) Governance frameworks that address transparency, independent replication, conflict-of-interest management, and regulatory pathway planning.

The strength of evidence supporting genomics–proteomics–clinical integration within ITRSs is mixed: PRAC-PTC provides empirical validation, whereas the remaining sources provide high-quality methodological and conceptual guidance. Collectively, the literature affirms the feasibility but indicates the necessity for larger multisite prospective trials, domain-standardized preprocessing pipelines, and transparent evaluation metrics before widespread clinical deployment. Ultimately, integrated omics–clinical systems aligned with structured governance, reproducible analytics, and clinician-centered interfaces can yield meaningful diagnostic and prognostic improvements; however, sustainable implementation requires meticulous methodological discipline and robust independent validation.

Enhancing Translational Relevance and Reproducibility

An Intelligent Translational Research System (ITRS) can strengthen translational relevance, rigor, and reproducibility by enforcing standardized methodological practices and embedding prospective validation pipelines across the discovery-to-clinic continuum. Specifically, such a system enables (i) standardized reporting and metadata capture spanning model selection, data provenance, preprocessing procedures, and performance metrics derived from established reporting frameworks (Kolbinger et al., 2024; Théry et al., 2018); (ii) incorporation of domain-specific minimal information checklists, such as MISEV for extracellular vesicle research (Théry et al., 2018), minimal-information elements for murine myocardial infarction models (Lindsey et al., 2021), and dosimetry/treatment-planning system (TPS) requirements for ultrahigh-dose-rate radiotherapy (FLASH) (Giannini et al., 2024);

(iii) systematic automation of external validation, out-of-distribution (OOD) testing, and hold-out design, addressing the artificial single-image evaluation paradigm observed in skin-lesion AI studies (Haggenmüller et al., 2021) and the scarcity of external validation in pregnancy-AI applications (Davidson & Boland, 2020); (iv) alignment with multi-scale molecular reference resources, including high-quality genomic assemblies and genome-wide association study (GWAS) loci, to minimize biological irreproducibility and annotation drift (Rhie et al., 2021; Vitanza et al., 2023; Wuttke et al., 2019); and (v) establishment of prospective, harmonized first-in-human translational registries that standardize reporting of potency, biodistribution, and adverse-event signals, similar to early CAR-T therapy development workflows, while addressing their limitations (Vitanza et al., 2023).

Evidence synthesis has demonstrated persistent and actionable translational gaps in this area. First, inconsistent reporting and incomplete external validation in AI systems remain major barriers (Davidson & Boland, 2020; Haggenmüller et al., 2021; Kolbinger et al., 2024), highlighting the need for the automated enforcement of reporting criteria and validation procedures within the ITRS. Second, the heterogeneity of preclinical models undermines their predictive fidelity. Zebrafish and murine cardiovascular and behavioral studies have shown protocol variability and insufficient sex-stratified analyses, emphasizing the need for standardized experimental metadata and reproducible stress/ischemia induction paradigms (Lindsey et al., 2021; Sarapultsev et al., 2025). Third, FLASH radiotherapy research illustrates technological constraints related to beam delivery, industrial LINAC modification, and incomplete dosimetric reporting, which impede mechanistic inference and clinical extrapolation; thus, the ITRS must enforce comprehensive dosimetric and TPS metadata capture (Giannini et al., 2024). Fourth, the scalable integration of high-confidence population-scale resources is essential. Near-complete reference genomes reduce annotation ambiguity (Rhie et al., 2021), kidney and breast cancer genetic consortia provide robust effect-size estimates for target prioritization (Haggenmüller et al., 2021; Wuttke et al., 2019), and the The MEGAVCID meta-analysis supports dementia-gene associations across nearly one million samples (Mega Vascular Cognitive Impairment and Dementia (MEGAVCID) consortium, 2024). Spatial transcriptomics further underscores the necessity of subcellular-to-tissue-level contextualization for accurate target mapping (Benjamin et al., 2024). Finally, first-in-human translation requires harmonized biospecimen sampling and potency-tracking. Early intracranial B7-H3 CAR-T cell studies have demonstrated feasibility but underscored sample size limitations and the need for standardized biomarker frameworks linking preclinical potency to clinical pharmacodynamics (Vitanza et al., 2023). The variability in FMT efficacy highlights the importance of quantifying donor/recipient microbiome compatibility, engraftment kinetics, and procedural consistency (Porcari et al., 2023).

Collectively, these data justify an ITRS architecture that (i) enforces machine-readable minimal reporting schemas synthesizing cross-study requirements (Kolbinger et al., 2024; Lindsey et al., 2021; Théry et al., 2018); (ii) operationalizes external and OOD validation requirements to correct artificial test set artifacts (Davidson & Boland, 2020; Haggenmüller et al., 2021); (iii) mandates complete technical provenance for device- and beam-based interventions (Giannini et al., 2024); (iv) links high-quality genomic, spatial, and molecular annotation resources to maintain biological accuracy; and (v) establishes prospective translational registries capturing bridging biomarkers, preclinical potency metrics, and harmonized clinical endpoints.

Applications and Case Examples in Inflammation and Cardiovascular Medicine

Cardiovascular diseases remain the leading cause of global morbidity and mortality posing the significant economic and social burden one healthcare systems worldwide.(Arnold et al., 2021)(*Cardiovascular Diseases (CVDs)*, n.d.) Over the years, there have been significant advances in pharmacotherapy and clinical care to improve treatment approaches; however, the "one size fits all" approach is often utilized, which fails to account for various factors and their interplay in disease management. This limitation necessitates the introduction of precision medicine to treat and deliver targeted individual interventions.

The combination of Artificial Intelligence (AI) and Integrated Translational Research Systems (ITRS) (Klee et al., 2021)shows a promising future in the management of such complex diseases. By integrating diverse datasets from genetic to imaging data and real world clinical records AI Driven tools can potentially aid in identifying disease patterns, predict disease trajectories and optimise strategies to treat the diseases appropriately.(Canuel et al., 2015)This approach can bring a significant breakthrough In the way in which the patients are treated given the disease heterogeneity and variable progression of disease.

This chapter explores how AI and ITRS can be utilized together as powerful tools to improve inflammation and cardiovascular medicine. Together, these applications highlight the potential of AI not only to expedite scientific discovery but also to bring healthcare closer to the vision of precision medicine, which is delivering the right therapy to the right patient at the right time.

Personalised Treatment Strategies via AI and ITRS

While conventional therapies have improved outcomes, they often undermine the importance of various factors that could potentially impact therapeutic efficacy, including variability in genetics, coexisting conditions, and lifestyle factors. (Su et al., 2024) Precision and personalized medicine uses various data acquired through multiple sources to design therapy that is more patient-specific and individualized (Gray et al., 2019). Heterogeneity in patients with cardiovascular disease is very evident as ischemic and non-ischemic heart failure arise from different yet distinct mechanisms requiring different modalities of treatment, although genetic variation influences individual susceptibility to atherosclerosis. (Soremekun et al., 2023)In various inflammatory disorders the variability is predominantly observed with respect to the underlying dominant cytokine pathway for example whether the information is driven by IL-6 or TNF-alpha explaining the variability in response to the same biologic therapy.(Kany et al., 2019; Xiang et al., 2023)

Role of AI

AI Enables the fusion of genomics, proteomics, metabolomics, imaging, and EHR data to provide a deeper understanding of the cardiovascular risk underlying disease mechanisms and treatment, particularly in the context of inflammation and complex disease phenotypes.

Data Fusion Strategies: AI uses early, intermediate and late fusion approaches to blend omics, imaging and health record data.(Mohsen et al., 2022) The early fusion combines raw features from all data; intermediate fusion derives data from individual modality before integration and late fusion combines outputs from each model . In this way Data from various sources are integrated to create specific models.(Athieniti & Spyrou, 2023)

Feature extraction: Deep learning models are utilised to derive and assimilate relevant features and decrease the complexity of high dimensional omics and imaging data allowing for better and effective integration with the electronic health records in a feasible manner.(M. Lin et al., 2025; Mohsen et al., 2022, 2023)

Multimodal Medical Fusion Networks: These medical fusion networks process the information and learn from a wide range of clinical data allowing for identification of molecular patterns and pathways, disease subtypes and thereby predict patient specific risk profiles.(Kiessling & Kuppe, 2024)

Role of ITRS

ITRS are designed to unify and amalgamate diverse biomedical datasets, including genetic, imaging, and EHR data, into usable patient-specific models for precision medicine implementation.

Mechanism for ITRS Integration

Data Standardization: ITRS platforms standardize data from various sources and clinical records into a uniform and well-equipped interoperable format. This integration and unification plays a vital role in linking molecular inflammation with image findings and clinical outcomes in cardiovascular disease.(Alfaddagh et al., 2020)

Multilayer Data Coupling: ITRS incorporates hierarchical model to connect metadata to connect biological samples, imaging studies and EHR derived clinical events for each patients enabling the mapping of inflammatory pathways to structural and functional cardiac changes observed in imaging and clinical phenotypes. (Zhazykbayeva et al., 2020)

AI-Driven Extraction and Modelling: Upon successful integration, AI and machine learning algorithm are used for extraction of features across various modalities.(Zhazykbayeva et al., 2020) These features are then utilised to build predictive models for disease risk progression and therapeutic response.(Guan et al., 2025)

Figure 2. Personalised treatment strategies via AI and ITRS

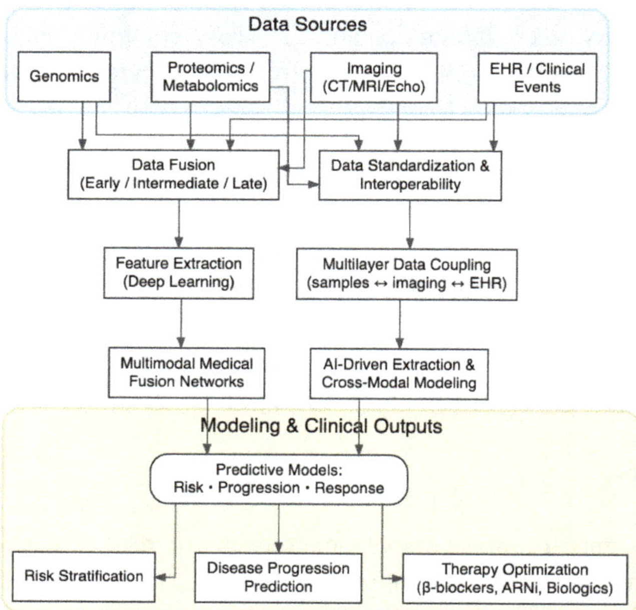

AI- Driven Adaptive Clinical Trials in CVD and Inflammatory Disorders

Randomized controlled trials (RCT) remain the gold standard for evaluating new therapies. Adaptive clinical trials guided by artificial intelligence offer a paradigm shift by enabling real-time modification in trial designs. AI algorithm can integrate the existing data to optimise patient recruitment by identifying subgroups most likely to respond.(Bothwell et al., 2018).The table below is a summary of the studies highlighting the integration of AI in the treatment of CVD and inflammatory disorders.

Table 1. Trial exhibiting Successful implementation of AI in CVD and inflammatory disorder

Trial/Study Name	Disease Area	AI Application	Outcome/Success	Reference
MIT-BIH Arrhythmia AI Study	Cardiac Arrhythmias	Deep learning ECG interpretation	Improved diagnostic accuracy compared to cardiologists	(Midani et al., 2023)(Zhang et al., 2021)
AI4HF Pilot Trial	Heart Failure	AI-based digital twin models	Personalized prediction of decompensation, reduced hospitalization rates	(Man et al., 2024)
RA-BioPredict	Rheumatoid Arthritis	AI-driven biomarker discovery	Identified gene expression predictors for biologic DMARD response	(Tomer et al., 2025)
UK Biobank AI Analysis	Atherosclerosis & CVD risk	Machine learning risk prediction	Enhanced early detection of CVD events over traditional risk scores	("Actionable Absolute Risk Prediction of Atherosclerotic Cardiovascular Disease Based on the UK Biobank," 2025; Omarov et al., 2024)

Case Studies of Drug Discovery Success Stories and Pipeline Acceleration

Artificial intelligence (AI) has already demonstrated success in accelerating drug discovery pipelines for cardiovascular and inflammatory diseases. By integrating high-throughput screening, molecular modeling, and real-world patient data, AI platforms have shortened discovery timelines from years to months and improved target validation accuracy. Below are the selected case studies.

Table 2. AI-Accelerated Cardiovascular & Cardiometabolic Drug-Discovery Case Studies

Case Study	Disease Area	AI Contribution	Timeline Impact	Outcome	References
BenevolentAI – Baricitinib	Rheumatoid arthritis / COVID-19	AI knowledge graph for drug repurposing	Identified in weeks	FDA EUA approval	(Smith et al., 2021)
Insilico Medicine – Anti-fibrotic drug	Fibrosis (CVD relevance)	Generative AI for novel molecules	<18 months to Phase I	First AI-discovered molecule in trials	(Medicine, 2025)
Exscientia – EXS21546	Oncology / Inflammation	AI-designed molecule optimization	27 months from target → trials	Ongoing Phase I	(*Exscientia - Exscientia Reports Topline Data From EXS-21546 Phase 1a Study Demonstrating Targeted A2A Receptor Signaling Inhibition in Healthy Volunteers*, n.d.)
AI-driven PCSK9 / lipid targets	Atherosclerosis / CVD	Genetics + docking + AI pipelines	Accelerated preclinical validation	Multiple RNA-based candidates in development	(Yepez et al., 2025)

Early Diagnostics and Disease Progression

Early diagnosis and timely prediction of disease progression are central to improving the outcomes of both cardiovascular and inflammatory disorders. Conventional approaches rely on clinical symptoms and biochemical markers, which often manifest at later stages of the disease, limiting the window for early intervention. Artificial Intelligence (AI) combined with Integrated Translational Research Systems (ITRS) enables the integration of multi-source data, including genomics, proteomics, metabolomics, imaging, and electronic health records (EHR), to identify early disease signatures and predict trajectories well before overt clinical manifestation.

Role of AI in Early Disease Diagnosis

AI-driven models leverage the recognition of battle, and deep learning is utilized to detect minute variations in imaging or molecular data that may otherwise remain unnoticed in conventional analysis.

Predictive Imaging Analytics: Deep convolutional neural networks (CNNs) Can easily identify early stages of atherosclerosis, myocardial patterns or inflammation head vascular level by using various imaging modalities like cardiac MRI, CT and echocardiography.(L. Wang et al., 2025; Yu & Chen, 2025)

Omic-based Biomarker Discovery: Machine learning algorithms screen high-dimensional data to detect new biomarkers with the potential to predict inflammatory or cardiovascular disease onset. Data compiled using various clinical records as well as biological samples serves as the primary source of information and on significant analysis reveals better predictors of both therapeutic and disease outcomes.(E et al., 2025)(C. Liu et al., 2025)

EHR-based Risk Stratification: By delving deeper into patient records and clinical data AI models can help in predicting individuals at elevated risk of stroke, myocardial infarcts or rheumatoid arthritis flare ups which indeed would enable in quicker therapy and faster resolution or remission of symptoms.(Momtazmanesh et al., 2022)(Al-Maini et al., 2023)

Role of ITRS in Disease Progression Prediction

ITRS serves as a comprehensive framework to unify patient-level multi-omics and clinical data into dynamic disease models.

Dynamic disease model: by combining the patient risk profile using genetic predisposition data with environmental and clinical data, ITRS can generate potential predictive maps of how disease progresses in different patients of groups and hence treatment can be more specific based on the patients demographics and the sub group he or she belongs to.(Hassan et al., 2022; Jain et al., 2022)

Digital twin for disease simulation: Integration with AI allows for creation of digital twins of patients and also aids in simulating disease evolution under various clinical scenarios to optimise long term treatment planning and therapeutic regimen design.(Chaparro-Cárdenas et al., 2025; Sadée et al., 2025)

Inflammatory pathway marking: Creating a link between the various inflammatory signalling pathways with imaging markers of organ dysfunction can enable clinicians to anticipate disease flares or cardiac remodelling before the damage is severe and irreversible. (Pfortmueller et al., 2017)

Clinical Impact

This integration of AI and ITRS early diagnosis will not only reduce delays but also shift healthcare towards a predictive and preventive treatment strategy, marking a significant breakthrough transition from reactive to proactive treatment plans. By leveraging multimodal data, these systems will encourage clinicians to intervene at the early stages where pathological changes are still reversible, thereby reducing the chances of morbidity and long-term healthcare costs. For example, early identification of subclinical myocardial infarct or inflammation in patients with autoimmune disorders through utilizing advanced image analysis and cytokine profiling will aid in guiding prophylactic therapy regimen design before the onset of cardiac dysfunction.

Similarly, predictive modelling can be utilized in forecasting disease progression, for example, in a patient in the prehypertensive stage to overt cardiovascular diseases, allowing clinicians to implement tailored lifestyle changes to optimize pharmacological therapy and close monitoring for higher-risk individuals.

Combining this predictive and preventive approach fosters healthcare models that emphasis on continuous monitoring personalised intervention and long term Disease Control ultimately bringing clinical practice closer to the vision of precision medicine

While challenges persist, including data interoperability, algorithm transparency, ethical use of patient data, and clinical validation, the trajectory of current research underscores immense promise. AI and ITRS together hold the potential to redefine inflammation and cardiovascular medicine, bringing healthcare closer to its ultimate vision: delivering the right therapy, to the right patient, at the right time.

CHALLENGES, LIMITATIONS, AND ETHICAL CONSIDERATIONS

Data Quality, Integration, and Standardization Issues

Integrated Translational Research Systems (ITRS) currently face three deeply interlinked barriers: (Porter et al., 2025) heterogeneous data capture and insufficient metadata/standardization, which compromise interoperability and analytic validity; (Landais et al., 2025) variable data quality, provenance, and completeness that erode clinician confidence and restrict the clinical utility of real-world evidence (RWE); and (Tomlinson et al., 2008) unresolved ethical and governance tensions, including consent models, re-identification risk, and commercial conflicts, which inhibit data sharing and broad deployment. Existing operational exemplars, such as RaDiCo and MiMiR, demonstrate technically feasible frameworks that incorporate unique identifiers, active curation, FAIR alignment, secure middleware, and cloud deployment. However, they simultaneously revealed ongoing challenges related to scalability, integration with contemporary genomics, and governance rigor. Physician acceptance remains conditional on demonstrable methodological standards and targeted training (Landais et al., 2025; Porter et al., 2025; Tomlinson et al., 2008).

Evidence from these studies exposes persistent translational bottlenecks. Regarding data quality and provenance, the national clinician survey (n = 128) illustrates a striking disconnect between awareness and use: although 94 percent (n = 120) of respondents reported familiarity with RWE, only 14 percent (n = 18) reported frequent use and just 3 percent (n = 4) used RWE daily, with only 49 percent (n = 63) expressing confidence in interpreting RWE outputs (Porter et al., 2025). Lower reliance scores for treatment-selection scenarios (mean 3.0 ±1.7) compared to dosing and outcome prediction (3.7 ±2.0, and 3.8 ±2.0, respectively) reflect persistent clinician preference for randomized controlled trial evidence when therapeutic stakes are highest. These quantitative signals demonstrate that data quality, analytic rigor, and interpretability remain gating factors for ITRS-enabled RWE adoption.

RaDiCo provides a structured model emphasizing continuous data quality monitoring, unique rare-disease identifiers, and FAIR compliance, with a robust accrual of 8,063 patients across 180 specialized sites (Landais et al., 2025). However, RaDiCo's claims are procedural rather than empirically validated: the platform description does not report phenotype sensitivity, missingness rates, or longitudinal completeness metrics, limiting the ability to assess real analytic reliability (Landais et al., 2025). Similarly, MiMiR highlights the benefits of active curation, standardized annotation, and middleware security, achieving MIAME compliance across >150 studies and ~3,000 hybridizations. However, MiMiR's architecture predates high-throughput sequencing, multi-omics, and complex clinical EHR data structures, and therefore necessitates modernization to meet ITRS requirements (Tomlinson et al., 2008).

Interoperability and standardization remain partial. RaDiCo adopts unique identifiers and aligns with European Reference Networks but lacks explicit documentation of mapping to global standards such as OMOP CDM, FHIR, CDISC, or HPO, limiting the evaluation of semantic portability (Landais et al., 2025). MiMiR's controlled vocabularies and Data Mapping Tool represent early ontology efforts, yet they do not provide the versioned provenance and automated ETL pipelines are needed for contemporary federated analytics (Tomlinson et al., 2008). Importantly, survey respondents prioritized improved analytic standards and guideline integration, reinforcing the requirement for common data models, standardized covariate frameworks, causal-inference pipelines, and benchmarking systems to reconcile RWE with RCT findings (Porter et al., 2025).

Ethical and governance constraints are significant. Although RaDiCo reports GDPR-compliant workflows, consent waivers for some cohorts without the disclosure of opt-in/out rates or dynamic consent approaches introduce transparency and trust limitations (Landais et al., 2025). Clinicians' concerns regarding commercial influence are reinforced by conflicts of interest disclosures in the survey study (Porter et al., 2025). MiMiR's secure middleware provides an early reference for controlled access, yet does not meet modern expectations for granular auditability, dynamic role-based controls, and HIPAA-equivalent protections (Tomlinson et al., 2008). Demographic representativeness remains under-reported on both platforms, limiting the generalizability of population-wide translational decision support.

Operational scalability and clinician readiness also impose certain constraints. The design of MiMiR is not optimized for streaming, containerized pipelines, or multi-omic and imaging workloads (Tomlinson et al., 2008), whereas RaDiCo lacks published throughput benchmarks and federated query latency data required for large-scale clinical integration (Landais et al., 2025). Survey evidence further demonstrates that late-career clinicians exhibit lower confidence in interpreting RWE, highlighting the importance of structured training, user-centric decision support tools, and transparent uncertainty communication to ensure equitable uptake (Porter et al., 2025).

Ethical Oversight, Patient Consent, and Privacy

The increasing integration of artificial intelligence and Intelligent Translational Research Systems in cardiovascular and inflammatory drug discovery necessitates rigorous ethical oversight, patient-centered consent structures, and privacy safeguards to maintain trust and regulatory integrity. Unlike traditional biomedical research models that rely on predefined datasets and static protocols, ITRS frameworks operate through continuous data accrual, multimodal integration, and iterative learning, raising complex ethical considerations related to autonomy, transparency, and data custodianship. In this context, patient consent is evolving from a one-time transactional agreement to a dynamic and adaptive model that enables longitudinal data use, secondary research, and federated learning while retaining participant autonomy. Evidence from longitudinal precision-medicine initiatives demonstrates that dynamic consent frameworks enhance participant understanding, increase willingness to share multi-omic and clinical data, and strengthen patient trust in research systems, particularly in chronic disease cohorts (Goncharov et al., 2022).

A central ethical imperative in ITRS deployment concerns privacy protection, as multi-source biological and clinical datasets, including imaging, genomics, and behavioral health records, inherently increase the risk of re-identification even after de-identification measures. This challenge is magnified when integrating hospital-linked Electronic Health Records, spatial omics, imaging biobanks, wearable-derived biomarkers, and social-determinants-of-health datasets. Techniques such as secure multiparty computation, homomorphic encryption, and differential privacy have demonstrated meaningful protection against re-identification risks while preserving analytic fidelity in biomedical research settings. Moreover, federated-learning paradigms deployed in multi-institutional cardiovascular imaging and EHR pipelines illustrate the feasibility of privacy-preserving AI architectures without centralizing patient data (Muller et al., 2023).

Ethical oversight mechanisms must also address risks associated with algorithmic bias, opaque decision logic, and inequitable model performance across demographic subgroups, which could perpetuate structural disparities in cardiovascular and inflammatory disease outcomes. Regulatory and ethical bodies emphasize transparency, explainability, and governance as prerequisites for AI-assisted clinical research and decision-support applications. In cardiovascular imaging, for example, studies have underscored that AI models trained on demographically homogenous datasets may degrade in accuracy across ethnic or sex subgroups, reinforcing the need for representative data and fair monitoring within ITRS pipelines. Additionally, genomic-based cardiovascular risk estimators, such as polygenic risk scores, demonstrate variable predictive accuracy across ancestry groups, demanding equitable model design and validation (Dankar et al., 2019).

Collectively, ethical oversight in ITRS adoption demands transparent consent mechanisms, robust privacy engineering, equitable model performance, and an accountable governance structure. Sustained trust will depend not only on compliance with legal mandates but also on proactive ethical stewardship and ongoing patient engagement.

Regulatory Challenges and the Need for Digital-First Frameworks

The rapid expansion of AI-enabled drug discovery and ITRS-driven translational ecosystems challenges traditional regulatory paradigms that are optimized for linear development cycles, static algorithms, and predefined data environments. Continuous learning algorithms, multimodal data fusion, adaptive trial designs, and real-time evidence generation require regulatory frameworks that are capable of iterative oversight, algorithmic version control, and performance monitoring throughout the product lifecycle. Regulatory authorities, including the U.S. The Food and Drug Administration, European Medicines Agency, and UK MHRA have acknowledged the limitations of legacy review processes and have initiated guidance for AI-enabled systems, emphasizing transparency, traceability, audit logs, and model-change control plans (Health, 2025). Digital-first regulatory pathways must reconcile innovation and safety by integrating real-world evidence pipelines, federated data structures, and adaptive clinical trial protocols. For instance, adaptive Bayesian trials and platform-trial frameworks such as RECOVERY and I-SPY have demonstrated accelerated therapeutic validation in high-burden disease settings and serve as regulatory models for dynamic evaluation pathways. In cardiovascular and inflammatory-drug development, the acceptance of real-world evidence for post-marketing surveillance and label expansion signals a regulatory willingness to incorporate continuous learning systems. However, systematic reviews emphasize variability in real-world data quality and analytical standards, requiring harmonized evidence-generation workflows and standardized data-fitness criteria.

Regulators increasingly require demonstration of algorithm robustness, fairness, and reproducibility, particularly when systems influence diagnostic interpretation or therapeutic selection. Studies have documented performance drift and accuracy degradation in clinical models over time, underscoring the necessity of lifecycle surveillance, dataset shift monitoring, and recalibration protocols within regulatory frameworks. Furthermore, algorithm auditability is essential; explainable-AI principles are being mandated to ensure that clinicians and regulators can interrogate model logic and evaluate safety risks (Singh et al., 2025).

Digital-first frameworks also require alignment with global interoperability standards, including HL7 FHIR, OMOP Common Data Model, and EMA Big Data Steering Group recommendations, enabling cross-site harmonization and regulatory reproducibility. Emerging global initiatives, such as the FDA's Real-World Evidence Program and EMA/HTA joint data guidance, signal a progressive shift toward digital-native regulatory science. Nonetheless, barriers persist, including legacy system fragmentation, limited regulatory expertise in machine learning validation, and a lack of unified international governance for AI-assisted drug development (Editor, 2025).

Ultimately, the establishment of digital-first regulatory environments must balance innovation with rigorous evidence standards, ensuring that AI-enabled therapies and decision support systems are safe, effective, transparent, and equitably deployed. Sustained collaboration between regulators, industry, clinicians, informatics experts, and patient groups is necessary to formalize regulatory science for learning health systems and ITRS-enabled precision therapeutics.

CONCLUSION

Across contemporary biomedical innovation, the central challenge is not discovery, but translation. This chapter demonstrates that ITRS represent a structurally and scientifically differentiated response to longstanding translational inefficiencies by replacing siloed, sequential research pathways with harmonized, iterative, and intelligence-enabled pipelines. The synthesis of multi-omics platforms, spatial and single-cell analytics, validated AI systems, clinician-in-the-loop interfaces, and standardized metadata creates higher-resolution mechanistic insights and improves predictive fidelity for clinical success. However, the feasibility demonstrated in multi-center pilot studies and systematic methodological reviews exists alongside systemic constraints: inconsistent reporting, limited out-of-distribution testing, fragmented ethical frameworks, variable clinician trust, and immature regulatory pathways.

Overcoming these gaps requires embedding enforceable data standards, a dynamic consent infrastructure, prospective external validation, governance transparency, and digital-first regulatory models capable of evaluating learning systems. When fully implemented, ITRS can materially reduce late-stage therapeutic failure, improve mechanistic certainty, elevate the evidentiary value of real-world data, and support equitable precision medicine. In doing so, they offer a path toward next-generation cardiovascular and inflammatory disease therapeutics founded not only on discovery excellence but also on reproducibility, integrity, and clinical impact.

REFERENCES

Actionable absolute risk prediction of atherosclerotic cardiovascular disease based on the UK Biobank. (2025, July 2). *UK Biobank.* https://www.ukbiobank.ac.uk/publications/actionable-absolute-risk-prediction-of-atherosclerotic-cardiovascular-disease-based-on-the-uk-biobank/

Adamo, R. G., van der Pol, C. B., Alabousi, M., Lam, E., Salameh, J.-P., Abedrabbo, N., Lerner, E., Naringrekar, H., Bashir, M. R., Costa, A. F., Osman, H., Ansari, D., Levis, B., Polikoff, A., Furlan, A., Tang, A., Kierans, A. S., Singal, A. G., Arvind, A., & McInnes, M. D. F. (2025). Diagnostic Performance of CT/MRI LI-RADS Version 2018 Major Feature Combinations: Individual Participant Data Meta-Analysis. *Radiology*, *315*(3), e243450. DOI: 10.1148/radiol.243450

Ahmed, Z. (2022). Precision medicine with multi-omics strategies, deep phenotyping, and predictive analysis. *Progress in Molecular Biology and Translational Science*, *190*(1), 101–125. DOI: 10.1016/bs.pmbts.2022.02.002

Al-Maini, M., Maindarkar, M., Kitas, G. D., Khanna, N. N., Misra, D. P., Johri, A. M., Mantella, L., Agarwal, V., Sharma, A., Singh, I. M., Tsoulfas, G., Laird, J. R., Faa, G., Teji, J., Turk, M., Viskovic, K., Ruzsa, Z., Mavrogeni, S., Rathore, V., & Suri, J. S. (2023). Artificial intelligence-based preventive, personalized and precision medicine for cardiovascular disease/stroke risk assessment in rheumatoid arthritis patients: A narrative review. *Rheumatology International*, *43*(11), 1965–1982. DOI: 10.1007/s00296-023-05415-1

Al Zo'ubi, M. (2025). Review of 2024 publications on the applications of artificial intelligence in rheumatology. *Clinical Rheumatology, 44*(4), 1427–1438. *Scopus.* Advance online publication. DOI: 10.1007/s10067-025-07382-3

Alfaddagh, A., Martin, S. S., Leucker, T. M., Michos, E. D., Blaha, M. J., Lowenstein, C. J., Jones, S. R., & Toth, P. P. (2020). Inflammation and cardiovascular disease: From mechanisms to therapeutics. *American Journal of Preventive Cardiology*, *4*, 100130. DOI: 10.1016/j.ajpc.2020.100130

Alicic, R. Z., Neumiller, J. J., & Tuttle, K. R. (2025). Combination therapy: An upcoming paradigm to improve kidney and cardiovascular outcomes in chronic kidney disease. *Nephrology, Dialysis, Transplantation*, *40*(Supplement_1), i3–i17. DOI: 10.1093/ndt/gfae212

Alshehade, S. A., Al Zarzour, R. H., Bitar, A. N., Alshehadeh, A. R., Tamilwanan, S., & Safni, S. (2026). Ethical Considerations in the Application of Artificial Intelligence in the Pharmaceutical Industry. In Alshehadeh A.R., El-Qirem I.A., & Ghaleb Awad Elrefae G.A. (Eds.), *Lect. Notes Networks Syst.: Vol. 1503 LNNS* (pp. 326–335). Springer Science and Business Media Deutschland GmbH; Scopus. https://doi.org/DOI: 10.1007/978-3-031-96631-6_32

Arnold, N., Lechner, K., Waldeyer, C., Shapiro, M. D., & Koenig, W. (2021). Inflammation and Cardiovascular Disease: The Future. *European Cardiology Review*, *16*, e20. DOI: 10.15420/ecr.2020.50

Athieniti, E., & Spyrou, G. M. (2023). A guide to multi-omics data collection and integration for translational medicine. *Computational and Structural Biotechnology Journal*, *21*, 134–149. DOI: 10.1016/j.csbj.2022.11.050

Azmal, M., Paul, J. K., Shohan, M. N. H., Haque, A. N. M. S. N. B., Mrinmoy, M., Talukder, O. F., & Ghosh, A. (2025). Evaluating computational and experimental approaches in early-stage Alzheimer's drug discovery: A systematic review. *Journal of Computer-Aided Molecular Design*, *39*(1), 27. DOI: 10.1007/s10822-025-00610-7

Barbarroja, N., López-Medina, C., Escudero-Contreras, A., & Arias-de la Rosa, I. (2024). Clinical and molecular insights into cardiovascular disease in psoriatic patients and the potential protective role of apremilast. *Frontiers in Immunology*, *15*, 1459185. DOI: 10.3389/fimmu.2024.1459185

Barcelos, M. P., & de Paula da Silva, C. H. T. (2024). The Role of Artificial Intelligence in the Discovery of New Drugs. In *Eng. Mater.: Vol. Part F3949* (pp. 353–370). Springer Science and Business Media Deutschland GmbH; Scopus. https://doi.org/DOI: 10.1007/978-3-031-75984-0_14

Barker, R. (2010). A flexible blueprint for the future of drug development. *Lancet*, *375*(9712), 357–359. DOI: 10.1016/S0140-6736(10)60141-9

Benjamin, K., Bhandari, A., Kepple, J. D., Qi, R., Shang, Z., Xing, Y., An, Y., Zhang, N., Hou, Y., Crockford, T. L., McCallion, O., Issa, F., Hester, J., Tillmann, U., Harrington, H. A., & Bull, K. R. (2024). Multiscale topology classifies cells in subcellular spatial transcriptomics. *Nature*, *630*(8018), 943–949. DOI: 10.1038/s41586-024-07563-1

Bothwell, L. E., Avorn, J., Khan, N. F., & Kesselheim, A. S. (2018). Adaptive design clinical trials: A review of the literature and ClinicalTrials.gov. *BMJ Open*, *8*(2), e018320. DOI: 10.1136/bmjopen-2017-018320

Canuel, V., Rance, B., Avillach, P., Degoulet, P., & Burgun, A. (2015). Translational research platforms integrating clinical and omics data: A review of publicly available solutions. *Briefings in Bioinformatics, 16*(2), 280–290. DOI: 10.1093/bib/bbu006

Cardiovascular diseases (CVDs). (n.d.). Retrieved August 27, 2025, from https://www.who.int/news-room/fact-sheets/detail/cardiovascular-diseases-(cvds)

Chaparro-Cárdenas, S. L., Ramirez-Bautista, J.-A., Terven, J., Córdova-Esparza, D.-M., Romero-Gonzalez, J.-A., Ramírez-Pedraza, A., & Chavez-Urbiola, E. A. (2025). A Technological Review of Digital Twins and Artificial Intelligence for Personalized and Predictive Healthcare. *Health Care, 13*(14), 1763. DOI: 10.3390/healthcare13141763

Chen, A.-T., Zhang, Y., & Zhang, J. (2025). Artificial intelligence in cardiac metabolism: The next frontier in cardiovascular health. *Metabolism and Target Organ Damage, 5*(1). *Scopus.* Advance online publication. DOI: 10.20517/mtod.2024.82

Chen, L., Deng, H., Cui, H., Fang, J., Zuo, Z., Deng, J., Li, Y., Wang, X., & Zhao, L. (2017). Inflammatory responses and inflammation-associated diseases in organs. *Oncotarget, 9*(6), 7204–7218. DOI: 10.18632/oncotarget.23208

Chen, S., Li, T., Yang, L., Zhai, F., Jiang, X., Xiang, R., & Ling, G. (2022). Artificial intelligence-driven prediction of multiple drug interactions. *Briefings in Bioinformatics, 23*(6), bbac427. Advance online publication. DOI: 10.1093/bib/bbac427

Culver, A., Stayrook, K., Comerota, M., Oblak, A., & Burris, T. (2025). Animal models for development of anti-obesity drugs in the age of GLP-1 agents. *Expert Opinion on Drug Discovery, 20*(7), 913–925. DOI: 10.1080/17460441.2025.2507766

Dankar, F. K., Gergely, M., & Dankar, S. K. (2019). Informed Consent in Biomedical Research. *Computational and Structural Biotechnology Journal, 17*, 463–474. DOI: 10.1016/j.csbj.2019.03.010

Davidson, L., & Boland, M. R. (2020). Enabling pregnant women and their physicians to make informed medication decisions using artificial intelligence. *Journal of Pharmacokinetics and Pharmacodynamics, 47*(4), 305–318. DOI: 10.1007/s10928-020-09685-1

Dawuti, A., Sun, S., Wang, R., Gong, D., Liu, R., Kong, D., Yuan, T., Zhou, J., Lu, Y., Wang, S., Du, G., & Fang, L. (2023). Salvianolic acid A alleviates heart failure with preserved ejection fraction via regulating TLR/Myd88/TRAF/NF-κB and p38MAPK/CREB signaling pathways. *Biomedicine & Pharmacotherapy = Biomedecine & Pharmacotherapie, 168*, 115837. https://doi.org/DOI: 10.1016/j.biopha.2023.115837

Dubey, A. (2020). Showcasing the Impact of Machine Learning in Healthcare. *Bioinformatics & Proteomics Open Access Journal*, *4*(1). Advance online publication. DOI: 10.23880/bpoj-16000131

Exscientia—Exscientia Reports Topline Data From EXS-21546 Phase 1a Study Demonstrating Targeted A2A Receptor Signaling Inhibition in Healthy Volunteers. (n.d.). Retrieved August 27, 2025, from https://investors.exscientia.ai/press-releases/press-release-details/2022/Exscientia-Reports-Topline-Data-From-EXS-21546-Phase-1a-Study-Demonstrating-Targeted-A2A-Receptor-Signaling-Inhibition-in-Healthy-Volunteers/default.aspx

Fang, R., Zhou, R., Ju, D., Li, M., Wang, H., Pan, L., Wang, X., Han, M., & Yu, Y. (2024). Zhen-wu-tang protects against myocardial fibrosis by inhibiting M1 macrophage polarization via the TLR4/NF-κB pathway. *Phytomedicine*, *130*, 155719. DOI: 10.1016/j.phymed.2024.155719

Foroughi, M., Torabinejad, M., Angelov, N., Ojcius, D. M., Parang, K., Ravnan, M., & Lam, J. (2025). Bridging oral and systemic health: Exploring pathogenesis, biomarkers, and diagnostic innovations in periodontal disease. *Infection*. Advance online publication. DOI: 10.1007/s15010-025-02568-y

Frąk, W., Wojtasińska, A., Lisińska, W., Młynarska, E., Franczyk, B., & Rysz, J. (2022). Pathophysiology of Cardiovascular Diseases: New Insights into Molecular Mechanisms of Atherosclerosis, Arterial Hypertension, and Coronary Artery Disease. *Biomedicines*, *10*(8), 1938. DOI: 10.3390/biomedicines10081938

Frattini, E., Faustini, G., Lopez, G., Carsana, E. V., Tosi, M., Trezzi, I., Magni, M., Soldà, G., Straniero, L., Facchi, D., Samarani, M., Martá-Ariza, M., De Luca, C. M. G., Vezzoli, E., Pittaro, A., Stepanyan, A., Silipigni, R., Rosety, I., Schwamborn, J. C., & Di Fonzo, A. (2025). Lewy pathology formation in patient-derived GBA1 Parkinson's disease midbrain organoids. *Brain*, *148*(4), 1242–1257. DOI: 10.1093/brain/awae365

Gadade, D. D., Kulkarni, D. A., Raj, R., Patil, S. G., & Modi, A. (2024). Pushing Boundaries: The Landscape of AI-Driven Drug Discovery and Development with Insights Into Regulatory Aspects. In *Artificial Intelligence and Machine Learning in Drug Design and Development* (pp. 533–561). wiley; Scopus. https://doi.org/ DOI: 10.1002/9781394234196.ch17

Gallone, G., Bruno, F., D'Ascenzo, F., & Ferrari, G. M. D. (2022). What will we ask to artificial intelligence for cardiovascular medicine in the next decade? *Minerva Cardiology and Angiology*, *70*(1), 92–101.

Galvin, J. E., Cummings, J. L., Benea, M. L., de Moor, C., Allegri, R. F., Atri, A., Chertkow, H., Paquet, C., Porter, V. R., Ritchie, C. W., Sikkes, S. A. M., Smith, M. R., Grassi, C. M., & Rubino, I. (2024). Generating real-world evidence in Alzheimer's disease: Considerations for establishing a core dataset. *Alzheimer's & Dementia, 20*(6), 4331–4341. DOI: 10.1002/alz.13785

Giannini, N., Gadducci, G., Fuentes, T., Gonnelli, A., Di Martino, F., Puccini, P., Naso, M., Pasqualetti, F., Capaccioli, S., & Paiar, F. (2024). Electron FLASH radiotherapy in vivo studies. A systematic review. *Frontiers in Oncology, 14*, 1373453. DOI: 10.3389/fonc.2024.1373453

Goncharov, L., Suominen, H., & Cook, M. (2022). Dynamic consent and personalised medicine. *The Medical Journal of Australia, 216*(11), 547–549. DOI: 10.5694/mja2.51555

Gong, D., Arbesfeld-Qiu, J. M., Perrault, E., Bae, J. W., & Hwang, W. L. (2024). Spatial oncology: Translating contextual biology to the clinic. *Cancer Cell, 42*(10), 1653–1675. DOI: 10.1016/j.ccell.2024.09.001

Gray, I. D., Kross, A. R., Renfrew, M. E., & Wood, P. (2019). Precision Medicine in Lifestyle Medicine: The Way of the Future? *American Journal of Lifestyle Medicine, 14*(2), 169–186. DOI: 10.1177/1559827619834527

Guan, X., Li, H., Zhang, L., & Zhi, H. (2025). Mechanisms of mitochondrial damage-associated molecular patterns associated with inflammatory response in cardiovascular diseases. *Inflammation Research, 74*(1), 18. DOI: 10.1007/s00011-025-01993-x

Guerrisi, A., Miseo, L., Falcone, I., Messina, C., Ungania, S., Elia, F., Desiderio, F., Valenti, F., Cantisani, V., Soriani, A., & Caterino, M. (2024). Quantitative ultrasound radiomics analysis to evaluate lymph nodes in patients with cancer: A systematic review. *Ultraschall in Der Medizin (Stuttgart, Germany: 1980), 45*(6), 586–596. https://doi.org/DOI: 10.1055/a-2275-8342

Haggenmüller, S., Maron, R. C., Hekler, A., Utikal, J. S., Barata, C., Barnhill, R. L., Beltraminelli, H., Berking, C., Betz-Stablein, B., Blum, A., Braun, S. A., Carr, R., Combalia, M., Fernandez-Figueras, M.-T., Ferrara, G., Fraitag, S., French, L. E., Gellrich, F. F., Ghoreschi, K., … Brinker, T. J. (2021). Skin cancer classification via convolutional neural networks: Systematic review of studies involving human experts. *European Journal of Cancer (Oxford, England: 1990), 156*, 202–216. https://doi.org/DOI: 10.1016/j.ejca.2021.06.049

Hassan, M., Awan, F. M., Naz, A., deAndrés-Galiana, E. J., Alvarez, O., Cernea, A., Fernández-Brillet, L., Fernández-Martínez, J. L., & Kloczkowski, A. (2022). Innovations in Genomics and Big Data Analytics for Personalized Medicine and Health Care: A Review. *International Journal of Molecular Sciences, 23*(9), 4645. DOI: 10.3390/ijms23094645

Health, C. for D. and R. (2025). Artificial Intelligence in Software as a Medical Device. *FDA*. https://www.fda.gov/medical-devices/software-medical-device-samd/artificial-intelligence-software-medical-device

Hefti, F. F. (2008). Requirements for a lead compound to become a clinical candidate. *BMC Neuroscience, 9*(S3), S7. DOI: 10.1186/1471-2202-9-S3-S7

Hinkson, I. V., Madej, B., & Stahlberg, E. A. (2020). Accelerating Therapeutics for Opportunities in Medicine: A Paradigm Shift in Drug Discovery. *Frontiers in Pharmacology, 11*, 770. DOI: 10.3389/fphar.2020.00770

Huang, R., Sun, Y., Liu, R., Zhu, B., Zhang, H., & Wu, H. (2024). ZeXieYin formula alleviates atherosclerosis by inhibiting the MAPK/NF-κB signaling pathway in APOE-/- mice to attenuate vascular inflammation and increase plaque stability. *Journal of Ethnopharmacology, 327*, 117969. DOI: 10.1016/j.jep.2024.117969

Ioachimescu, O. C., & Shaker, R. (2025). Translational science and related disciplines. *Journal of Investigative Medicine, 73*(1), 3–26. DOI: 10.1177/10815589241283515

Jain, N., Nagaich, U., Pandey, M., Chellappan, D. K., & Dua, K. (2022). Predictive genomic tools in disease stratification and targeted prevention: A recent update in personalized therapy advancements. *The EPMA Journal, 13*(4), 561–580. DOI: 10.1007/s13167-022-00304-2

Jia, Z.-C., Yang, X., Wu, Y.-K., Li, M., Das, D., Chen, M.-X., & Wu, J. (2024). The Art of Finding the Right Drug Target: Emerging Methods and Strategies. *Pharmacological Reviews, 76*(5), 896–914. DOI: 10.1124/pharmrev.123.001028

Johnson, M., Albizri, A., & Simsek, S. (2022). Artificial intelligence in healthcare operations to enhance treatment outcomes: A framework to predict lung cancer prognosis. *Annals of Operations Research, 308*(1–2), 275–305. DOI: 10.1007/s10479-020-03872-6

Jordan, M. I. (2019). Artificial Intelligence—The Revolution Hasn't Happened Yet. *Harvard Data Science Review*. Advance online publication. DOI: 10.1162/99608f92.f06c6e61

Jurisica, I. (2024). Explainable biology for improved therapies in precision medicine: AI is not enough. *Best Practice & Research. Clinical Rheumatology*, *38*(4), 102006. DOI: 10.1016/j.berh.2024.102006

Kanthi, Y., de la Zerda, A., & Smith, B. R. (2020). Nanotherapeutic Shots through the Heart of Plaque. *ACS Nano*, *14*(2), 1236–1242. DOI: 10.1021/acsnano.0c00245

Kany, S., Vollrath, J. T., & Relja, B. (2019). Cytokines in Inflammatory Disease. *International Journal of Molecular Sciences*, *20*(23), 6008. DOI: 10.3390/ijms20236008

Kaur, R., Bhardwaj, A., & Gupta, S. (2023). Cancer treatment therapies: Traditional to modern approaches to combat cancers. *Molecular Biology Reports*, *50*(11), 9663–9676. DOI: 10.1007/s11033-023-08809-3

Kiessling, P., & Kuppe, C. (2024). Spatial multi-omics: Novel tools to study the complexity of cardiovascular diseases. *Genome Medicine*, *16*(1), 14. DOI: 10.1186/s13073-024-01282-y

Kitchen, D. B., Decornez, H., Furr, J. R., & Bajorath, J. (2004). Docking and scoring in virtual screening for drug discovery: Methods and applications. *Nature Reviews. Drug Discovery*, *3*(11), 935–949. DOI: 10.1038/nrd1549

Klee, E. W., Cousin, M. A., Pinto, E., Vairo, F., Morales-Rosado, J. A., Macke, E. L., Jenkinson, W. G., Ferrer, A., Schultz-Rogers, L. E., Olson, R. J., Oliver, G. R., Sigafoos, A. N., Schwab, T. L., Zimmermann, M. T., Urrutia, R. A., Kaiwar, C., Gupta, A., Blackburn, P. R., Boczek, N. J., & Lazaridis, K. N. (2021). Impact of integrated translational research on clinical exome sequencing. *Genetics in Medicine: Official Journal of the American College of Medical Genetics*, *23*(3), 498–507. DOI: 10.1038/s41436-020-01005-9

Kolbinger, F. R., Veldhuizen, G. P., Zhu, J., Truhn, D., & Kather, J. N. (2024). Reporting guidelines in medical artificial intelligence: A systematic review and meta-analysis. *Communications Medicine*, *4*(1), 71. DOI: 10.1038/s43856-024-00492-0

Krittanawong, C., Zhang, H., Wang, Z., Aydar, M., & Kitai, T. (2017). Artificial Intelligence in Precision Cardiovascular Medicine. *Journal of the American College of Cardiology*, *69*(21), 2657–2664. DOI: 10.1016/j.jacc.2017.03.571

Landais, P., Gueguen, S., Clement, A., & Amselem, S., & RaDiCo Program. (2025). The RaDiCo information system for rare disease cohorts. *Orphanet Journal of Rare Diseases*, *20*(1), 166. DOI: 10.1186/s13023-025-03629-z

Li, Y., Wu, F., Ge, W., Zhang, Y., Hu, Y., Zhao, L., Gou, W., Shi, J., Ni, Y., Li, L., Fu, W., Lin, X., Yu, Y., Han, Z., Chen, C., Xu, R., Zhang, S., Zhou, L., Pan, G., & Luo, D. (2024). Risk stratification of papillary thyroid cancers using multidimensional machine learning. *International Journal of Surgery (London, England)*, *110*(1), 372–384. DOI: 10.1097/JS9.0000000000000814

Lin, K., Wang, A., Zhai, C., Zhao, Y., Hu, H., Huang, D., Zhai, Q., Yan, Y., & Ge, J. (2025). Semaglutide protects against diabetes-associated cardiac inflammation via Sirt3-dependent RKIP pathway. *British Journal of Pharmacology*, *182*(7), 1561–1581. DOI: 10.1111/bph.17327

Lin, M., Guo, J., Gu, Z., Tang, W., Tao, H., You, S., Jia, D., Sun, Y., & Jia, P. (2025). Machine learning and multi-omics integration: Advancing cardiovascular translational research and clinical practice. *Journal of Translational Medicine*, *23*(1), 388. DOI: 10.1186/s12967-025-06425-2

Lin, Z., & Chou, W.-C. (2022). Machine Learning and Artificial Intelligence in Toxicological Sciences. *Toxicological Sciences*, *189*(1), 7–19. DOI: 10.1093/toxsci/kfac075

Lindsey, M. L., Brunt, K. R., Kirk, J. A., Kleinbongard, P., Calvert, J. W., de Castro Brás, L. E., DeLeon-Pennell, K. Y., Del Re, D. P., Frangogiannis, N. G., Frantz, S., Gumina, R. J., Halade, G. V., Jones, S. P., Ritchie, R. H., Spinale, F. G., Thorp, E. B., Ripplinger, C. M., & Kassiri, Z. (2021). Guidelines for in vivo mouse models of myocardial infarction. *American Journal of Physiology. Heart and Circulatory Physiology*, *321*(6), H1056–H1073. DOI: 10.1152/ajpheart.00459.2021

Liu, C., Wang, Y., Zhou, L., Cai, F., Tang, X., Wang, L., & Zhang, X. (2025). Exploration of potential biomarkers and immune cell infiltration characteristics for peripheral atherosclerosis in sjögren's syndrome based on comprehensive bioinformatics analysis and machine learning. *Frontiers in Genetics*, *16*, 1546315. DOI: 10.3389/fgene.2025.1546315

Liu, M., Yue, Y., Chen, X., Xian, K., Dong, C., Shi, M., Xiong, H., Tian, K., Li, Y., Zhang, Q. C., & He, A. (2025). Genome-coverage single-cell histone modifications for embryo lineage tracing. *Nature*, *640*(8059), 828–839. DOI: 10.1038/s41586-025-08656-1

Lutgens, E., Atzler, D., Döring, Y., Duchene, J., Steffens, S., & Weber, C. (2019). Immunotherapy for cardiovascular disease. *European Heart Journal*, *40*(48), 3937–3946. DOI: 10.1093/eurheartj/ehz283

Man, J. P., Koole, M. A. C., Meregalli, P. G., Handoko, M. L., Stienen, S., de Lange, F. J., Winter, M. M., Schijven, M. P., Kok, W. E. M., Kuipers, D. I., van der Harst, P., Asselbergs, F. W., Zwinderman, A. H., Dijkgraaf, M. G. W., Chamuleau, S. A. J., & Schuuring, M. J. (2024). Digital consults in heart failure care: A randomized controlled trial. *Nature Medicine*, *30*(10), 2907–2913. DOI: 10.1038/s41591-024-03238-6

Mayrink, N. N. V., Alcoforado, L., Chioro, A., Fernandes, F., Lima, T. S., Camargo, E. B., & Valentim, R. A. M. (2022). Translational research in health technologies: A scoping review. *Frontiers in Digital Health*, *4*, 957367. DOI: 10.3389/fdgth.2022.957367

Medicine, I. (2025, March 7). *Insilico Medicine's AI-driven drug Rentosertib receives official generic name*. News-Medical. https://www.news-medical.net/news/20250307/Insilico-Medicines-AI-driven-drug-Rentosertib-receives-official-generic-name.aspx

Mega Vascular Cognitive Impairment and Dementia (MEGAVCID) consortium. (2024). A genome-wide association meta-analysis of all-cause and vascular dementia. *Alzheimer's & Dementia*, *20*(9), 5973–5995. DOI: 10.1002/alz.14115

Midani, W., Ouarda, W., & Ayed, M. B. (2023). DeepArr: An investigative tool for arrhythmia detection using a contextual deep neural network from electrocardiograms (ECG) signals. *Biomedical Signal Processing and Control*, *85*, 104954. DOI: 10.1016/j.bspc.2023.104954

Mirakhori, F., & Niazi, S. K. (2025). Harnessing the AI/ML in Drug and Biological Products Discovery and Development: The Regulatory Perspective. *Pharmaceuticals, 18*(1). *Scopus*. Advance online publication. DOI: 10.3390/ph18010047

Mohsen, F., Al-Saadi, B., Abdi, N., Khan, S., & Shah, Z. (2023). Artificial Intelligence-Based Methods for Precision Cardiovascular Medicine. *Journal of Personalized Medicine*, *13*(8), 1268. DOI: 10.3390/jpm13081268

Mohsen, F., Ali, H., El Hajj, N., & Shah, Z. (2022). Artificial intelligence-based methods for fusion of electronic health records and imaging data. *Scientific Reports*, *12*(1), 17981. DOI: 10.1038/s41598-022-22514-4

Momtazmanesh, S., Nowroozi, A., & Rezaei, N. (2022). Artificial Intelligence in Rheumatoid Arthritis: Current Status and Future Perspectives: A State-of-the-Art Review. *Rheumatology and Therapy*, *9*(5), 1249–1304. DOI: 10.1007/s40744-022-00475-4

Muhammad, U., Uzairu, A., & Ebuka Arthur, D. (2018). Review on: Quantitative structure activity relationship (QSAR) modeling. *Journal of Analytical & Pharmaceutical Research*, *7*(2). Advance online publication. DOI: 10.15406/japlr.2018.07.00232

Muller, S. H., van Thiel, G. J., Mostert, M., & van Delden, J. J. (2023). Dynamic consent, communication and return of results in large-scale health data reuse: Survey of public preferences. *Digital Health*, *9*, 20552076231190997. DOI: 10.1177/20552076231190997

Mun, S. J., Ryu, J.-S., Lee, M.-O., Son, Y. S., Oh, S. J., Cho, H.-S., Son, M.-Y., Kim, D.-S., Kim, S. J., Yoo, H. J., Lee, H.-J., Kim, J., Jung, C.-R., Chung, K.-S., & Son, M. J. (2019). Generation of expandable human pluripotent stem cell-derived hepatocyte-like liver organoids. *Journal of Hepatology*, *71*(5), 970–985. DOI: 10.1016/j.jhep.2019.06.030

Murmu, A., & Győrffy, B. (2024). Artificial intelligence methods available for cancer research. *Frontiers of Medicine*, *18*(5), 778–797. DOI: 10.1007/s11684-024-1085-3

Nelson, K., Fuster, V., & Ridker, P. M. (2023). Low-Dose Colchicine for Secondary Prevention of Coronary Artery Disease: JACC Review Topic of the Week. *Journal of the American College of Cardiology*, *82*(7), 648–660. DOI: 10.1016/j.jacc.2023.05.055

Ocana, A., Pandiella, A., Siu, L. L., & Tannock, I. F. (2011). Preclinical development of molecular-targeted agents for cancer. *Nature Reviews. Clinical Oncology*, *8*(4), 200–209. DOI: 10.1038/nrclinonc.2010.194

Omarov, M., Zhang, L., Jorshery, S. D., Malik, R., Das, B., Bellomo, T. R., Mansmann, U., Menten, M. J., Natarajan, P., Dichgans, M., Raghu, V. K., Anderson, C. D., & Georgakis, M. K. (2024). Deep Learning-Based Detection of Carotid Plaques Informs Cardiovascular Risk Prediction and Reveals Genetic Drivers of Atherosclerosis. *medRxiv*, 2024.10.17.24315675. https://doi.org/DOI: 10.1101/2024.10.17.24315675

Onódi, Z., Koch, S., Rubinstein, J., Ferdinandy, P., & Varga, Z. V. (2023). Drug repurposing for cardiovascular diseases: New targets and indications for probenecid. *British Journal of Pharmacology*, *180*(6), 685–700. DOI: 10.1111/bph.16001

Ooka, T. (2025). The Era of Preemptive Medicine: Developing Medical Digital Twins through Omics, IoT, and AI Integration. *JMA Journal*, *8*(1), 1–10. DOI: 10.31662/jmaj.2024-0213

Pala, L., Pagan, E., Sala, I., Oriecuia, C., Oliari, M., De Pas, T., Specchia, C., Cocorocchio, E., Zattarin, E., Rossi, G., Catania, C., Ceresoli, G. L., Laszlo, D., Canzian, J., Valenzi, E., Viale, G., Gelber, R. D., Mantovani, A., Bagnardi, V., & Conforti, F. (2024). Outcomes of patients with advanced solid tumors who discontinued immune-checkpoint inhibitors: A systematic review and meta-analysis. *EClinicalMedicine*, *73*, 102681. DOI: 10.1016/j.eclinm.2024.102681

Panda, P., & Mohapatra, R. (2024). Revolutionizing Patient Safety: Machine Learning and AI for the Early Detection of Adverse Drug Reactions and Drug-Induced Toxicity. *Current Artificial Intelligence*, *02*, e29503752308394. DOI: 10.2174/01295037523083942410131 65241

Parker, C. G., & Pratt, M. R. (2020). Click Chemistry in Proteomic Investigations. *Cell*, *180*(4), 605–632. DOI: 10.1016/j.cell.2020.01.025

Parsaei, M., Arvin, A., Taebi, M., Seyedmirzaei, H., Cattarinussi, G., Sambataro, F., Pigoni, A., Brambilla, P., & Delvecchio, G. (2024). Machine Learning for prediction of violent behaviors in schizophrenia spectrum disorders: A systematic review. *Frontiers in Psychiatry*, *15*, 1384828. DOI: 10.3389/fpsyt.2024.1384828

Pasas-Farmer, S., & Jain, R. (2025). From discovery to delivery: Governance of AI in the pharmaceutical industry. *Green Analytical Chemistry, 13. Scopus.* Advance online publication. DOI: 10.1016/j.greeac.2025.100268

Paul, S. M., Mytelka, D. S., Dunwiddie, C. T., Persinger, C. C., Munos, B. H., Lindborg, S. R., & Schacht, A. L. (2010). How to improve R&D productivity: The pharmaceutical industry's grand challenge. *Nature Reviews. Drug Discovery*, *9*(3), 203–214. DOI: 10.1038/nrd3078

Pfortmueller, C. A., Meisel, C., Fux, M., & Schefold, J. C. (2017). Assessment of immune organ dysfunction in critical illness: Utility of innate immune response markers. *Intensive Care Medicine Experimental*, *5*(1), 49. DOI: 10.1186/s40635-017-0163-0

Porcari, S., Benech, N., Valles-Colomer, M., Segata, N., Gasbarrini, A., Cammarota, G., Sokol, H., & Ianiro, G. (2023). Key determinants of success in fecal microbiota transplantation: From microbiome to clinic. *Cell Host & Microbe*, *31*(5), 712–733. DOI: 10.1016/j.chom.2023.03.020

Porter, T. M., Andersen, K. M., Paez, W., Corr, P., & Figueiredo, S. (2025). Acceptance and Utilization of Real-World Evidence among Cancer Care Physicians in the USA: A National Survey. *Pharmaceutical Medicine*, *39*(6), 453–463. DOI: 10.1007/s40290-025-00586-7

Raikar, G. V. S., Raikar, A. S., & Somnache, S. N. (2023). Advancements in artificial intelligence and machine learning in revolutionising biomarker discovery. *Brazilian Journal of Pharmaceutical Sciences*, *59*, e23146.

Ran, Y., Su, W., Gao, F., Ding, Z., Yang, S., Ye, L., Chen, X., Tian, G., Xi, J., & Liu, Z. (2021). Curcumin Ameliorates White Matter Injury after Ischemic Stroke by Inhibiting Microglia/Macrophage Pyroptosis through NF-κB Suppression and NLRP3 Inflammasome Inhibition. *Oxidative Medicine and Cellular Longevity*, *1552127*. Advance online publication. DOI: 10.1155/2021/1552127

Rhie, A., McCarthy, S. A., Fedrigo, O., Damas, J., Formenti, G., Koren, S., Uliano-Silva, M., Chow, W., Fungtammasan, A., Kim, J., Lee, C., Ko, B. J., Chaisson, M., Gedman, G. L., Cantin, L. J., Thibaud-Nissen, F., Haggerty, L., Bista, I., Smith, M., & Jarvis, E. D. (2021). Towards complete and error-free genome assemblies of all vertebrate species. *Nature*, *592*(7856), 737–746. DOI: 10.1038/s41586-021-03451-0

Saboya-Galindo, P., Cifuentes-González, C., Rojas-Carabali, W., Mejía-Salgado, G., Le Tong, Y., Putera, I., Song, X. Y. R., Walter, C. F. Y., Shengjuan, Z., Chan, R., La Distia Nora, R., Biswas, J., Gangaputra, S., Pulido, J. S., Kempen, J. H., Nguyen, Q. D., de-la-Torre, A., Gupta, V., Rosenbaum, J. T., … REVISE-IUSG study group. (2025). Clinical trials and quasi-experimental studies in the treatment of noninfectious retinal vasculitis: A systematic review from the International Uveitis Study Group (IUSG) Retinal Vasculitis Study (ReViSe) - Report 4. *Survey of Ophthalmology*, S0039-6257(25)00173-0. https://doi.org/DOI: 10.1016/j.survophthal.2025.09.013

Sabry, Z., Arora, H. S., Chandrasekaran, S., & Wang, Z. (2025). AI-driven drug discovery and repurposing using multi-omics for myocardial infarction and heart failure. *Exploration of Medicine, 6. Scopus.* Advance online publication. DOI: 10.37349/emed.2025.1001340

Sadée, C., Testa, S., Barba, T., Hartmann, K., Schuessler, M., Thieme, A., Church, G. M., Okoye, I., Hernandez-Boussard, T., Hood, L., Shmulevich, I., Kuhl, E., & Gevaert, O. (2025). Medical digital twins: Enabling precision medicine and medical artificial intelligence. *The Lancet. Digital Health*, *7*(7), 100864. DOI: 10.1016/j.landig.2025.02.004

Saeed, A., & Alajlan, S. A. (2025). The Dawn of AI in Pharmaceutical Research: AI Transforming Pharma-Ethics, Trials, and Beyond. In *Transforming Pharmaceutical Research With Artificial Intelligence* (pp. 1–26). IGI Global; Scopus. https://doi.org/DOI: 10.4018/979-8-3693-6270-9.ch001

Saleem, R. (2025). Revolutionizing Pharmaceutical Engineering: A Deep Dive Into AI- Driven Drug Discovery and Development. In *Transforming Pharmaceutical Research With Artificial Intelligence* (pp. 113–139). IGI Global; Scopus. https://doi.org/DOI: 10.4018/979-8-3693-6270-9.ch004

Samant, T. S., Mangal, N., Lukacova, V., & Schmidt, S. (2015). Quantitative clinical pharmacology for size and age scaling in pediatric drug development: A systematic review. *Journal of Clinical Pharmacology*, *55*(11), 1207–1217. DOI: 10.1002/jcph.555

Sarapultsev, A., Gusev, E., Hu, D., & Komelkova, M. (2025). Experimental PTSD Models in Zebrafish: A Systematic Review of Behavioral, Neurochemical, and Molecular Outcomes. *Biology (Basel)*, *14*(5), 456. DOI: 10.3390/biology14050456

Sathyanarayanan, A., Mueller, T. T., Ali Moni, M., & Schueler, K., ECNP TWG Network members, Baune, B. T., Lio, P., Mehta, D., Baune, B. T., Dierssen, M., Ebert, B., Fabbri, C., Fusar-Poli, P., Gennarelli, M., Harmer, C., Howes, O. D., Janzing, J. G. E., Lio, P., Maron, E., … Xicota, L. (2023). Multi-omics data integration methods and their applications in psychiatric disorders. *European Neuropsychopharmacology: The Journal of the European College of Neuropsychopharmacology*, *69*, 26–46. DOI: 10.1016/j.euroneuro.2023.01.001

Savira, F., Magaye, R., Liew, D., Reid, C., Kelly, D. J., Kompa, A. R., Sangaralingham, S. J., Burnett, J. C., Kaye, D., & Wang, B. H. (2020). Cardiorenal syndrome: Multi-organ dysfunction involving the heart, kidney and vasculature. *British Journal of Pharmacology*, *177*(13), 2906–2922. DOI: 10.1111/bph.15065

Schneider, M., Radoux, C. J., Hercules, A., Ochoa, D., Dunham, I., Zalmas, L.-P., Hessler, G., Ruf, S., Shanmugasundaram, V., Hann, M. M., Thomas, P. J., Queisser, M. A., Benowitz, A. B., Brown, K., & Leach, A. R. (2021). The PROTACtable genome. *Nature Reviews. Drug Discovery*, *20*(10), 789–797. DOI: 10.1038/s41573-021-00245-x

Schork, N. J. (2019). Artificial Intelligence and Personalized Medicine. In Von Hoff, D. D., & Han, H. (Eds.), *Precision Medicine in Cancer Therapy* (Vol. 178, pp. 265–283). Springer International Publishing., DOI: 10.1007/978-3-030-16391-4_11

Shao, J., Meng, Y., Yuan, K., Wu, Q., Zhu, S., Li, Y., Wu, P., Zheng, J., & Shi, H. (2023). RU.521 mitigates subarachnoid hemorrhage-induced brain injury via regulating microglial polarization and neuroinflammation mediated by the cGAS/STING/NF-κB pathway. *Cell Communication and Signaling : CCS*, *21*(1), 264. DOI: 10.1186/s12964-023-01274-2

Shen, R., & Zhang, Y. (2025). Relationship between amino acid metabolism and inflammation in coronary heart disease [Review]. *International Journal of Molecular Medicine*, *56*(2), 120. DOI: 10.3892/ijmm.2025.5561

Singh, R., Zhou, K., & Auclair, J. R. (2025). Reimagining drug regulation in the age of AI: A framework for the AI-enabled Ecosystem for Therapeutics. *Frontiers in Medicine*, *12*. Advance online publication. DOI: 10.3389/fmed.2025.1679611

Smith, D. P., Oechsle, O., Rawling, M. J., Savory, E., Lacoste, A. M. B., & Richardson, P. J. (2021). Expert-Augmented Computational Drug Repurposing Identified Baricitinib as a Treatment for COVID-19. *Frontiers in Pharmacology*, *12*, 709856. DOI: 10.3389/fphar.2021.709856

Soremekun, O., Dib, M.-J., Rajasundaram, S., Fatumo, S., & Gill, D. (2023). Genetic heterogeneity in cardiovascular disease across ancestries: Insights for mechanisms and therapeutic intervention. *Cambridge Prisms. Precision Medicine*, *1*, e8. DOI: 10.1017/pcm.2022.13

Su, J., Yang, L., Sun, Z., & Zhan, X. (2024). Personalized Drug Therapy: Innovative Concept Guided With Proteoformics. *Molecular & Cellular Proteomics*, *23*(3), 100737. DOI: 10.1016/j.mcpro.2024.100737

Théry, C., Witwer, K. W., Aikawa, E., Alcaraz, M. J., Anderson, J. D., Andriantsitohaina, R., Antoniou, A., Arab, T., Archer, F., Atkin-Smith, G. K., Ayre, D. C., Bach, J.-M., Bachurski, D., Baharvand, H., Balaj, L., Baldacchino, S., Bauer, N. N., Baxter, A. A., Bebawy, M., & Zuba-Surma, E. K. (2018). Minimal information for studies of extracellular vesicles 2018 (MISEV2018): A position statement of the International Society for Extracellular Vesicles and update of the MISEV2014 guidelines. *Journal of Extracellular Vesicles*, *7*(1), 1535750. DOI: 10.1080/20013078.2018.1535750

Tomer, R., Jain, S., Gahlot, P. S., Bajiya, N., & Raghava, G. P. S. (2025). In Silico Tool for Predicting and Scanning Rheumatoid Arthritis-Inducing Peptides in an Antigen (p. 2025.03.19.644081). *bioRxiv*. https://doi.org/DOI: 10.1101/2025.03.19.644081

Tomlinson, C., Thimma, M., Alexandrakis, S., Castillo, T., Dennis, J. L., Brooks, A., Bradley, T., Turnbull, C., Blaveri, E., Barton, G., Chiba, N., Maratou, K., Soutter, P., Aitman, T., & Game, L. (2008). MiMiR—an integrated platform for microarray data sharing, mining and analysis. *BMC Bioinformatics*, *9*, 379. DOI: 10.1186/1471-2105-9-379

Tu, Y., Tan, L., Tao, H., Li, Y., & Liu, H. (2023). CETSA and thermal proteome profiling strategies for target identification and drug discovery of natural products. *Phytomedicine*, *116*, 154862. DOI: 10.1016/j.phymed.2023.154862

Valenza, C., Saldanha, E. F., Gong, Y., De Placido, P., Gritsch, D., Ortiz, H., Trapani, D., Conforti, F., Cremolini, C., Peters, S., Mateo, J., Subbiah, V., Parsons, H. A., Partridge, A. H., & Curigliano, G. (2025). Circulating tumor DNA clearance as a predictive biomarker of pathologic complete response in patients with solid tumors treated with neoadjuvant immune checkpoint inhibitors: A systematic review and meta-analysis. *Annals of Oncology : Official Journal of the European Society for Medical Oncology*, *36*(7), 726–736. DOI: 10.1016/j.annonc.2025.03.019

Verma, J., Khedkar, V. M., & Coutinho, E. C. (2010). 3D-QSAR in drug design—A review. *Current Topics in Medicinal Chemistry*, *10*(1), 95–115. DOI: 10.2174/156802610790232260

Vijayan, R. S. K., Kihlberg, J., Cross, J. B., & Poongavanam, V. (2022). Enhancing preclinical drug discovery with artificial intelligence. *Drug Discovery Today*, *27*(4), 967–984. DOI: 10.1016/j.drudis.2021.11.023

Vitanza, N. A., Wilson, A. L., Huang, W., Seidel, K., Brown, C., Gustafson, J. A., Yokoyama, J. K., Johnson, A. J., Baxter, B. A., Koning, R. W., Reid, A. N., Meechan, M., Biery, M. C., Myers, C., Rawlings-Rhea, S. D., Albert, C. M., Browd, S. R., Hauptman, J. S., Lee, A., & Park, J. R. (2023). Intraventricular B7-H3 CAR T Cells for Diffuse Intrinsic Pontine Glioma: Preliminary First-in-Human Bioactivity and Safety. *Cancer Discovery*, *13*(1), 114–131. DOI: 10.1158/2159-8290.CD-22-0750

Vollstedt, E.-J., Madoev, H., Aasly, A., Ahmad-Annuar, A., Al-Mubarak, B., Alcalay, R. N., Alvarez, V., Amorin, I., Annesi, G., Arkadir, D., Bardien, S., Barker, R. A., Barkhuizen, M., Basak, A. N., Bonifati, V., Boon, A., Brighina, L., Brockmann, K., Carmine Belin, A., & Klein, C. (2023). Establishing an online resource to facilitate global collaboration and inclusion of underrepresented populations: Experience from the MJFF Global Genetic Parkinson's Disease Project. *PLoS One*, *18*(10), e0292180. DOI: 10.1371/journal.pone.0292180

Wang, L., Wang, L., Wu, P., & Ding, L. (2025). Cardiovascular Magnetic Resonance imaging analysis using neural networks. *Journal of Radiation Research and Applied Sciences*, *18*(4), 101874. DOI: 10.1016/j.jrras.2025.101874

Wang, R., Jiao, Z., Yang, L., Choi, J. W., Xiong, Z., Halsey, K., Tran, T. M. L., Pan, I., Collins, S. A., Feng, X., Wu, J., Chang, K., Shi, L.-B., Yang, S., Yu, Q.-Z., Liu, J., Fu, F.-X., Jiang, X.-L., Wang, D.-C., & Bai, H. X. (2022). Artificial intelligence for prediction of COVID-19 progression using CT imaging and clinical data. *European Radiology*, *32*(1), 205–212. DOI: 10.1007/s00330-021-08049-8

Wang, Z.-Y., Cheng, J., Wang, Y., Yuan, H.-T., Bi, S.-J., Wang, S.-X., Hou, Y.-M., Zhang, X., Xu, B.-H., Wang, Z.-Y., Zhang, Y., Jiang, W.-J., Chen, Y.-G., & Zhang, M.-X. (2024). Macrophage ILF3 promotes abdominal aortic aneurysm by inducing inflammatory imbalance in male mice. *Nature Communications*, *15*(1), 7249. DOI: 10.1038/s41467-024-51030-4

Warokar, P., & Lote, S. (2024). Ethical and Regulatory Consideration in AI-Assisted Drug Development. *DMIHER Int. Conf. Artif. Intell. Healthc., Educ. Ind., IDICAIEI*. 2024 2nd DMIHER International Conference on Artificial Intelligence in Healthcare, Education and Industry, IDICAIEI 2024. Scopus. https://doi.org/DOI: 10.1109/IDICAIEI61867.2024.10842700

Wouters, O. J., McKee, M., & Luyten, J. (2020). Estimated Research and Development Investment Needed to Bring a New Medicine to Market, 2009-2018. *Journal of the American Medical Association*, *323*(9), 844. DOI: 10.1001/jama.2020.1166

Wuttke, M., Li, Y., Li, M., Sieber, K. B., Feitosa, M. F., Gorski, M., Tin, A., Wang, L., Chu, A. Y., Hoppmann, A., Kirsten, H., Giri, A., Chai, J.-F., Sveinbjornsson, G., Tayo, B. O., Nutile, T., Fuchsberger, C., Marten, J., Cocca, M., & Pattaro, C. (2019). A catalog of genetic loci associated with kidney function from analyses of a million individuals. *Nature Genetics*, *51*(6), 957–972. DOI: 10.1038/s41588-019-0407-x

Xia, Y., Wang, Y., Wang, Z., & Zhang, W. (2024). A comprehensive review of molecular optimization in artificial intelligence-based drug discovery. *Quantitative Biology*, *12*(1), 15–29. DOI: 10.1002/qub2.30

Xiang, Y., Zhang, M., Jiang, D., Su, Q., & Shi, J. (2023). The role of inflammation in autoimmune disease: A therapeutic target. *Frontiers in Immunology*, *14*, 1267091. DOI: 10.3389/fimmu.2023.1267091

Yepez, D. B., Porta, D. S., Aguas, L. M., & Jattin, F. M. (2025). Optimizing treatment to control LDL cholesterol using machine learning. *Computers in Biology and Medicine*, *195*, 110599. DOI: 10.1016/j.compbiomed.2025.110599

Yu, T., & Chen, K. (2025). Enhancing cardiac disease detection via a fusion of machine learning and medical imaging. *Scientific Reports*, *15*, 26269. DOI: 10.1038/s41598-025-12030-6

Zhang, D., Yang, S., Yuan, X., & Zhang, P. (2021). Interpretable deep learning for automatic diagnosis of 12-lead electrocardiogram. *iScience*, *24*(4), 102373. DOI: 10.1016/j.isci.2021.102373

Zhavoronkov, A., Vanhaelen, Q., & Oprea, T. I. (2020). Will Artificial Intelligence for Drug Discovery Impact Clinical Pharmacology? *Clinical Pharmacology and Therapeutics*, *107*(4), 780–785. DOI: 10.1002/cpt.1795

Zhazykbayeva, S., Pabel, S., Mügge, A., Sossalla, S., & Hamdani, N. (2020). The molecular mechanisms associated with the physiological responses to inflammation and oxidative stress in cardiovascular diseases. *Biophysical Reviews*, *12*(4), 947–968. DOI: 10.1007/s12551-020-00742-0

Zhu, M., Zhang, H., Zhou, Q., Sheng, S., Gao, Q., Geng, Z., Chen, X., Lai, Y., Jing, Y., Xu, K., Bai, L., Wang, G., Wang, J., Jiang, Y., & Su, J. (2025). Dynamic GelMA/DNA Dual-Network Hydrogels Promote Woven Bone Organoid Formation and Enhance Bone Regeneration. *Advanced Materials (Deerfield Beach, Fla.)*, *37*(24), e2501254. DOI: 10.1002/adma.202501254

Zollinger-Read, C., & Filer, A. (2025). Therapeutics update in immune-mediated rheumatic diseases: Rheumatoid arthritis, idiopathic inflammatory myositis and ANCA-associated vasculitis. *Clinical Medicine (London, England)*, *25*(5), 100507. DOI: 10.1016/j.clinme.2025.100507

Chapter 7
Integrating AI Models for Predicting Drug Efficacy and Toxicity:
Toward Safer and Faster Pharmaceutical Development

Muhammad Usman Tariq
https://orcid.org/0000-0002-7605-3040
Abu Dhabi University, UAE & University College Cork, Ireland

ABSTRACT

The incorporation of artificial intelligence (AI) in drug research holds the potential for making transformative predictions of drug efficacy and toxicity with unprecedented speed and accuracy. Traditional pipelines for the discovery and development of medicinal products are time-consuming, expensive, and susceptible to breakdowns, especially at the clinical stage of research, which often result in adverse effects or inadequate therapeutic benefits. AI models, particularly those utilizing deep learning, machine learning, and systems biology, are employed to simulate complex biological interactions, predict pharmacokinetics and pharmacodynamics, and assess molecular security profiles early in the development cycle. By analyzing large datasets from genomics, proteomics, electronic health records, and preclinical assays, these models facilitate better-informed decision-making, including drug development, precision medicine, and adaptive clinical research design.

DOI: 10.4018/979-8-3373-5258-9.ch007

INTRODUCTION

Traditional drug discovery and security assessments are notoriously known for their time-consuming and expensive, often extending over a decade and requiring billions of dollars to develop a single treatment. Despite these investments, the failure rates remain high. However, there are not a significant number of candidates due to inefficiency and unexpected toxicity during clinical trials. A significant bottleneck exists in the linear and sealed nature of traditional pipelines (Singh et al., 2024). It is often based on preclinical models, such as in vitro assays and animal studies, which may not fully capture the complexity of human biology. This interruption between early detection models and actual patient responses can lead to slow adoption rates and represent immeasurable financial and human costs to the healthcare system. Furthermore, current strategies for assessing toxicity have limited scalability and prediction and are often significantly more responsive than they are proactive. They rely heavily on retrospective analysis and empirical rule-based systems, which are insufficient for capturing the subtle and large dynamics of biological systems and chemical interactions. The inability to predict reliable drug responses (ADRs) to predict organ-specific toxicity or dose-effect curves contributes to early developmental risk and regression. In contrast to traditional methods, AI enables data control, hypothesis-generating approaches, identification of hidden patterns, drawing predictive conclusions, and dynamic learning from new data (Malheiro et al., 2025). The integration of these technologies into medicinal product discovery and security assessment creates unprecedented opportunities for speed, accuracy, and adaptability. AI models, particularly those rooted in machine learning, deep learning, learning enrichment, and generative algorithms, can now handle large heterogeneous datasets that extend post-marketing molecular structures, OMICS profiles, clinical records, and monitoring reports. This ability allows researchers to simulate complex biological interactions, predict toxic outcomes, and predict efficacy profiles before connections reach the laboratory. For example, deep learning algorithms show great promise in classifying toxicological endpoints with high accuracy.

In contrast, augmented learning frames can optimize complex synthesis strategies based on effectiveness and security. This advancement is not only a technological improvement but also a paradigm shift towards a predictive, repetitive, and integrated drug development cycle (Singh et al., 2024). Effectiveness, the ability of connections to determine the desired biological responses and toxicity, is a key aspect of pharmaceutical development. Even the most promising treatment candidates can be estimated. The AI control approach aims to compensate for this equation more accurately than the traditional approach. It utilizes computational models to predict how connections between different biological contexts and patient populations function. AI models support early stage target identification, ligand-binding prediction, and pharmacodynamic simulation. All of these factors help in choosing better candidates and optimizing them in silico. In the case of toxicity, AI enables early warnings against organ-specific toxicity, predicting hepatotoxicity, cardiotoxicity, genotoxicity, and immunotoxicity, as well as the integration of actual evidence and security signal flags that are not recorded in clinical research. The AI model must incorporate feedback from each phase of the pipeline and become increasingly refined and contextually relevant over time (Suriyaamporn et al., 2024). First, AI models must inform how they can predict drug efficacy and toxicity at different stages of the drug pipeline by bringing together compounds and guiding optimizations for market-specific preclinical evaluation and monitoring. Second, the technical, biological, and data-oriented foundations of these models, including the required data, functional engineering strategies, model architectures, and validation frames, are explored. Special attention is paid to the role of real-world clinical inputs in enhancing multi-omic integration, the utilization of high-throughput screening data, and generalization of models. Third, this chapter aims to explore new tools, such as explainable AI (XAI), Digital Twins, and federated learning, as enablers of transparency, cooperation, and privacy in model development and delivery. These devices are crucial for overcoming the regulatory, ethical, and clinical adoption barriers that have previously hindered the use of AI.

Consortia and initiatives such as Melloddy, Open Goals, and the Accelerating Medicines Partnership (AMP) demonstrate how distributed expertise and data exchange accelerate the development and validation of forecast AI models. These joint frameworks not only enhance the robustness of individual models but also democratize access to tools and knowledge, enabling small organizations and academic institutions to contribute to the development of AI-controlled drugs. Issues such as data heterogeneity, annotation distortions, lack of standardization in model benchmarks, and the opaque nature of many black-box algorithms raise concerns about reproducibility, accountability, and regulatory acceptance. Ethical and legal considerations, such as data protection, algorithm bias, and explanations, are also considered, particularly in the context of patient safety and frequent decision making. These concerns highlight the importance of developing governance frameworks and technically robust models. This ensures the integration of responsibility and AI in the pharmaceutical work process. This chapter comprehensively investigates how AI shifts can be effectively enabled to predict drug efficacy and toxic changes (Malheiro et al., 2025). The development of AI applications in pharmaceutical research and development focuses on the underlying technologies and data strategies that enhance predictive models while considering the practical and regulatory implications of deploying these models at scale. By highlighting opportunities and obstacles, this chapter aims to provide researchers, developers, clinicians, and political decision-makers with a clear and nuanced understanding of how the future of AI-controlled drug safety and efficacy assessments can be navigated.

OVERVIEW OF AI IN PHARMACEUTICAL R&D

Artificial Intelligence (AI) has revolutionized drug research and development (R&D) and transformed traditional workflows into more efficient, data-driven, and predictive systems. The increased volume and complexity of biomedical data, along with advances in computing power and algorithm innovation, position AI as a central tool for the discovery, development, and translation of medicinal products. Numerous AI techniques are available, including machine learning, reinforcement learning, growth enhancement, generative model development, viable drug target identification, molecular design optimization, pharmacokinetic and toxicity prediction, and clinical research result simulation. This shift is not only a technological development but also a fundamental rethinking of how scientific knowledge is extracted and applied in pharmaceutical science. Machine learning (ML) refers to an algorithm that learns from data and makes predictions or decisions based on them (Suriyaamporn et al., 2024). It includes monitored learning, where the model is trained with marked data (such as connectivity or toxicity effectiveness), and unattended learning, which finds essential patterns without predefined results in the algorithm (helps clustering of patient subgroups or gene expression profiles). These have been applied to tasks such as bioactivity prediction, unwanted event classification, and estimation of molecular properties.

Deep learning models, such as convolutional neural networks (CNNs) and recurrent neural networks (RNNs), are primarily adept at processing high-dimensional and unstructured data, including molecular diagrams, protein structures, and clinical records with time-series data. These models demonstrate cutting-edge performance in areas such as image-based phenotypic screening, protein-ligand binding prediction, and generation of synthetic molecular libraries. For example, CNNs can be used to identify visual biomarkers from histological images, while graph neural networks (GNNs) have proven to be effective for understanding complex topological relationships within molecules. In the drug context, RL is used to optimize the dynamic adjustment of drug synthesis pathways, design combination therapies, and develop drug plans based on simulated patient responses. The adaptability of the RL model creates a vast decision-making space, making it suitable for contexts in which the outcome of selection occurs over time. Optimizing pharmaceutical schemes or navigating through complex chemical reaction trees. These models can be used to design entirely new connections that meet predefined properties, such as solubility, effectiveness, and security. Figure 1 provides overview of AI-Driven drug development ecosystem.

Figure 1. The AI-Driven Drug Development Ecosystem

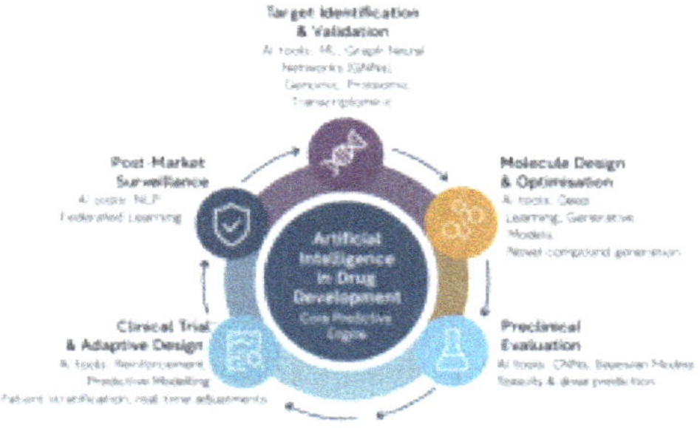

In contrast to traditional databases based on known chemical scaffolds, generative models can examine untapped areas of chemical space and allow for the design of "de -de-novo." Some generative models integrate property predictors into the generation process. It controls the creation of molecules with the desired bioactivity profile or connection, ensuring low predictive toxicity (Suriyaamporn et al., 2024). These AI systems surpass the limits of creativity in medical chemistry, shortening the path between ideas and viable drug candidates. In the past, pharmacology was analyzed by rule-based modeling and quantitative structure-activity relationships (QSAR), which attempted to correlate chemical features with biological effects using linear or polynomial regression. These methods are fundamental and are often limited by their inability to capture small datasets and nonlinear interactions. The advent of high-throughput screening (HTS), systems biology, and large-scale OMICS technology has created large, multidimensional datasets that require more complex analytical methods. Predictive modeling in the discovery and development of medicinal products is often based on data from three major domains: chemical, biological (OMIC), and clinical domains. Chemical data include structural information (e.g., SMILES, InChI, and 3D conformations), physicochemical properties (e.g., solubility, logP, and molecular weight), and bioactivity profiles resulting from the assay. These data are transferred to molecular properties, virtual screening pipelines, and chemical models. These data records provide insights into disease mechanisms, biomarker discovery, and target identification. For example, transcriptome data from RNA-seq can be used to create models that predict how drugs alter gene expression patterns. The integration of multi-omic data, sometimes referred to as system pharmacology, enables the creation of an overall model that captures the interactions among genetic mutations, cellular pathways, and therapeutic interventions. AI models trained with these data records can predict patient outcomes and identify candidates for the reuse and personalization of treatment recommendations (Suriyaamporn et al., 2024). Tools for natural language processing (NLP) extract structured information from unstructured clinical notes, thereby extending the available data. Linking molecular and OMICS data with clinical outcomes enables accurate and personalized predictions concerning drug and security modeling. Data records from different sources often vary in scale, format, and quality, requiring careful preprocessing and normalization. Functional engineering, including the creation of effective descriptors and embedding, plays a crucial role in developing models that can be learned efficiently. Data curation is increasingly automated using AI, with models recognizing anomalies, identifying missing values, and detecting fraud.

Finally, migration to a collaborative cloud-based platform accelerates the integration of AI in Pharma. Initiatives such as the Open Targets Platform, Cancer Genome Atlas (TCGA), and British Biobank provide large, curated data records. Similarly, consortiums such as Melloddy (Orchestration of Machine Learning Books for Drug Discovery) and the Joint AI Infrastructure, supported by the Federal Learning Framework, allows companies to train models together on distributed data without compromising privacy (Mottaghi-Dastjerdi & Soltany-Rezaee-Rad, 2024). This coalition approach is fundamental in healthcare systems, where databases, confidentiality, and regulatory restrictions limit data exchange. The maturation of various AI technologies, including machine learning for structured data analysis, deep learning for unstructured high-dimensional data, reinforcement learning for dynamic decision-making, and generative models for chemical innovation, has enabled the pharmaceutical industry to achieve greater speed, accuracy, and personalization in drug discovery and development. The success of AI implementation depends not only on model architecture but also on access to high-quality, integrated datasets and interdisciplinary collaboration between computer scientists, pharmacologists, and clinical researchers.

AI MODELS FOR PREDICTING DRUG EFFICACY

The AI model was developed as a powerful tool to predict the efficacy of pharmaceuticals, providing unprecedented accuracy and scalability in identifying viable treatment candidates for various diseases. Traditional drug discovery processes are based on methods that are time-consuming and expensive and often result in low success rates in clinical studies owing to inaccurate predictions of drug efficacy. Key dimensions in which AI contributes to predicting drug efficacy include target identification and validation, predictive modeling of biological activity and pharmacodynamics, in silico screening, and case-specific modeling, such as in oncology and antiviral drug development, which can impact the downstream success of treatment development (Suriyaamporn et al., 2024). AI plays a key role in accelerating this process by analyzing vast biological data records, such as genomics, proteomics, transcriptomics, and epigenomics, to provide new insights and confirm existing findings. Traditional bioinformatics pipelines often struggle with data complexity and noise issues. However, AI models, such as unattended clustering, graph-based learning, and representative learning, can guide higher-dimensional biological data into interpretable patterns of distillation. For example, network-based models, such as graph convolutional networks (GCNS), can identify the most influential nodes (genes or proteins) in disease-related pathways.

AI also helps in target validation through the integration of functional genomics screens (e.g., CRISPR- or RNAi-mediated knockdowns), which provide a reference for the causal relationship between the target and disease phenotypes. Deep learning models can be effectively prioritized for treatment by managing genetic disorders or correlating with proteomic responses. Biomobilization prediction models aim to estimate the strength of the interactions between a particular biological target and its connections. These predictions are typically based on data records, such as binding affinity (KD, AI, IC50), activation/inhibition profiles, and dose-effect relationships. The molecular representations used in these models range from traditional descriptors (such as molecular fingerprints and topology indices) to more complex coding-based graphs that preserve the 3D structural and physicochemical context of connections. Folding networks (CNNS) and GNNs are particularly effective in recording the spatial relationships between atoms and functional groups, which are crucial for understanding bioactivity.

In addition to assessing biological activity, AI models are increasingly used to simulate the pharmacodynamics of drugs and their effects on the body. This includes modeling receptor dynamics, downstream signaling effects, and dose-dependent efficacy (Mottaghi-Dastjerdi & Soltany-Rezaee-Rad, 2024). Reinforcement learning and recurrent neural networks (RNNs) have been used to simulate a set of drug responses in preclinical models or organoids derived from patients. These models are helpful not only for maximizing the effect of the drug but also for determining the duration and likelihood of tachycardia (loss of efficacy over time). Integration with pharmacokinetics (PK) is modeled on drug absorption, distribution, metabolism, and excretion (ADME). In combination with actual data from electronic health records (EHRs) or clinical research repositories, AI responder supply can identify and predict unnecessary events in patient structures and refine the strategies. Engagement. Structure-based virtual screening (SBV) and ligand-based virtual screening (LBV) have traditionally relied on molecular-docking algorithms and pharmacological models. These methods provide useful approximations but often do not capture the dynamic and multi-salient nature of molecular interactions. AI-enhanced in Silico screening overcomes these limitations by learning from empirical data and improving attachment prediction. Deep learning models such as DeepDock, AtomNet, and Gnina utilize 3D structural information to predict binding modes and evaluate binding free energy with greater accuracy than traditional docking scores.

Furthermore, attention-based models and transformers, inspired by the progression of natural language processing (e.g., the use of transformers in protein fitting), have been adapted to interpret the interactions between atomic-level details and protein leagues. Genetic models, such as the variation code (VAE) and generative adversarial networks (GANs), can suggest new connections that maximize the predicted effectiveness while simultaneously minimizing non-target interactions and toxicity (Mandlik et al., 2024). These models not only accelerate lead optimization but also support scaffolds that discover new chemical types that retain the biological functions. The combination of molecular dynamics simulations with AI predictions enables researchers to accurately assess sensitive solvent effects. In oncology, the complexity of tumor biology, characterized by heterogeneity, genetic instability, and the world factor of Microm, is a significant challenge in predicting efficacy of drugs.

AI models help navigate this complexity by integrating drug susceptibility screening and multi-omic tumor data (such as somatic mutations, gene expression, and methylation profiles) from patient-derived cancer cell lines and xenograft implants. For example, deep learning models trained on data from the Cancer Cell Line Encyclopedia (CCLE) and Genomics of Drug Sensitivity in Cancer (GDSC) projects can predict the likelihood of tumors responding to specific chemotherapy or targeted therapies. Transfer learning techniques enable these models to generalize from cell lines in patient tumors, thereby improving their clinical relevance. AI is also used to identify synergistic drug combinations, particularly to overcome resistance. By analyzing the paths affected by resistance mutations, reinforcement learning models can simulate a combination program that restores or improves efficacy (Tyagi et al., 2025). AI models have been used to model existing drugs, new connections, and viral wort protein interactions. For example, COVID-19 pandemic AI platforms such as Benevolentai and Nuclear examined rapid approval libraries of approved drugs to identify candidates with potential efficacy against SARS-Cov-2. Deep learning models trained on viral protease structures have predicted inhibitors that were later validated in vitro or underwent clinical testing.

Furthermore, AI models that integrate host gene expression profiles have helped identify the goals and connections that regulate host responses. These applications demonstrate how AI reduces the time between pathogen and therapeutic development while maintaining scientific rigor. By combining target identification, bioactivity modeling, in silico screening, and real-world case applications, AI enables faster, more accurate, and cheaper treatment development (Mottaghi-Dastjerdi & Soltany-Rezaee-Rad, 2024). The ability to integrate various biological data types, learn complex nonlinear patterns, and simulate biological systems enables AI to predict treatment outcomes at granular levels that were previously unattainable. As data availability continues to increase and model architectures arise, AI becomes even more critical in the design of more effective, personalized, and safe treatments throughout the treatment area. The synergistic effect of arithmetic modeling and experimental verification creates a robust ecosystem in which AI is not only a support tool but also the core engine of innovation in modern drug development.

AI MODELS FOR PREDICTING DRUG TOXICITY

Toxicity can manifest in various ways, including organ-specific damage (such as to the liver, heart, and kidneys), genotoxicity (causing DNA damage), immunotoxicity (effects on immune responses), and early, undetermined, and potentially fatal systemic effects. Historically, animal experiments and in vitro testing have been pivotal for toxicity prediction; however, these methods are resource-intensive, time-consuming, and sometimes challenging to translate into human biology. AI integration, particularly deep learning, has begun to redefine this landscape by modeling results with complex biological interactions, mining patterns from high-dimensional datasets, and predicting toxicity at high speeds with rapid scalability. Biological systems. The classification of subtype toxicity allows researchers to develop target models and predict specific outcomes (Mottaghi-Dastjerdi & Soltany-Rezaee-Rad, 2024). Organ-specific toxicity is one of the most frequently examined areas in computer toxicology. Hepatotoxicity (liver injury) and cardiotoxicity (cardiac-related toxicity) are significant, as they often play a role in late-stage drug use. Genotoxicity includes DNA mutations, chromosomal damage, and other genetic changes that can lead to cancer development. Immunotoxicity includes the unintended activation or suppression of immunotherapy and biologically related immune responses. Additionally, there are concerns such as nephrotoxicity (renal injury), neurotoxicity (brain and nervous system), and reproductive toxicity, all of which need to be predicted with certainty. The development of individual models tailored to each category ensures that researchers can concentrate on the dataset of the corresponding biomarkers, focusing on histopathological findings and chemical properties.

For example, CNNs are used for toxicity assessments, such as RNNs, which are suitable for temporal toxicity data and pursue the development of toxicity over time during chronic drug exposure. GNN is currently well-oriented to represent chemical structures. As atoms are chemical bonds with nodes, molecules can be encoded as diagrams so that models can be learned directly from the molecular topology. Accurate prediction of drug concentrations at which toxic effects occur (e.g., IC50 and LD50) can save time and reduce risks in the development pipeline. Regression-based deep learning models, including deep and Bayesian neural networks, are increasingly being applied to model dose-effect curves across multiple cell lines and assay systems. This enables deterministic predictions and quantification of uncertainties, where confidence intervals can influence decision-making. In combination with pharmacokinetic and pharmacodynamic data, these models contribute to a more comprehensive risk review and support the design of safer therapeutic schemes (Mettleq et al., 2024). Multiamics refers to the combined analysis of data on genomics, transcriptomics, proteomics, metabolomics, and epigenomics to capture a comprehensive image of the biological responses. A single biomolecular layer rarely determines the toxicological reactions. Rather, they have cascade effects at several levels. For example, toxic insults start with genomics (genomics), leading to abnormal RNA transcription (transcriptome), dysfunctional proteins (proteomics), and metabolic pathways (metabolism). These different data flows can be integrated, allowing AI models to build a wide range of mechanical representations of toxicity development using architectures such as automated encoders and multimodal transformers.

Deep learning models trained on multi-omic data from cell lines, animal studies, or human clinical samples can identify early organic markers for side effects, pinpoint affected pathways, and even generate mechanistic hypotheses regarding the behavioral effects, thereby constructing a deeper understanding. HTS assays often generate a wealth of data on how thousands of compounds interact with different biological targets under several concentration conditions (Mottaghi-Dastjerdi & Soltany-Rezaee-Rad, 2024). AI models can be trained with these data to recognize toxic signatures associated with a particular chemical scaffold or organic activity. For example, transcriptome signatures from LINCS databases (a library of integrated network-based cellular signatures) or cytotoxic data from the ToxCast and Tox21 initiatives can be used to train classifiers to identify sensitive and specific toxic connections. Therefore, it is essential to integrate HTS and deep learning to enable the real-time triggering of drug candidates. It utilizes molecules that are characterized as high-risk at the start of the pipeline or chemically modified molecules. Liver damage involves several mechanisms, including mitochondrial dysfunction, oxidative stress, inhibition of bile acid transporters, and immune-mediated responses. In combination with data connection structure data and clinically undesirable event reports, a deep learning model trained on liver-specific transcriptome responses has demonstrated promising results for predicting liver damage. For example, GNN-based models can recognize structural motifs associated with known hepatotoxins, whereas recurrence models trained on longitudinal biomarker data from in vivo studies can identify early warning signs of liver stress. Corresponding to Silico predictions with Vitro signatures (such as Alto Astenenzyme Mirror), researchers can provide three possible connections that cause liver violations and characterize them for further verification or redesigning.

Cardiotoxicity, particularly medication-induced QT dilation and arrhythmias, is another critical area in which AI can have significant effects. The electrophysiological stability of the heart is sensitive to subtle chemical interference, and compounds that extend the QT interval can cause fatal arrhythmias such as torsade de pointes (Suri et al., 2024). A deep learning model was developed that combined cardiomyocytes, ion channel assays, ECG waveform data, and data from human-induced chemical descriptors. CNNs and transformer models were used to analyze waveform features with early signs of toxicity, and GNN and ensemble models were trained on the structural characteristics associated with known cardiotoxic drugs. When these models are trained on integrated datasets, such as the Comprehensive in-vitro-pro-profit Massai (CIPA), they can achieve clinically related levels of sensitivity and specificity, providing alternatives with high throughput for traditional patch clamps and animal research.

Deep learning provides predictive power, but it is essential to understand why models need connections as toxic to accept them in a regulated manner. Methods such as SHAP, integrated gradients, and attention visualization enable researchers to identify the properties of molecular substructures, OMICS markers, or imaging regions that are most commonly associated with prediction. This interpretability will facilitate regulatory submissions, guide medical chemists in redesigning toxic scaffolds, and help clinicians understand the potential risks associated with the re-use of existing drugs. Open science initiatives such as Tox21, Openox, and ETOX provide publicly available data records, model benchmarks, and APIs for toxicity modeling. Integration with the principles of FAIR data (easy to find, accessible, interoperable, and reusable) ensures reproducibility and accelerates innovation. Pharmaceutical companies, regulators, and academic institutions must collaborate to standardize assessment protocols, validate model predictions against real-world results, and develop AI tools early in the life cycle (Mutha et al., 2024). By modeling complex biological processes based on toxicity responses, these tools accelerate the identification of uncertain connections, provide information on connection optimization, and reduce the dependency on tables. With continued advancements in model architecture, data availability, interpretability, and joint infrastructure, AI will play a central role in ensuring drug safety, improving patient outcomes, and improving efficiency and ethical rigor in drug development.

MODEL TRAINING, VALIDATION, AND INTERPRETATION

Model training, validation, and interpretation form the backbone of AI integration into the biomedical domain, particularly in tasks such as predicting drug efficacy and toxicity. The reliability, integrity, and ethical implications of AI models are deeply related to how data are curated, how functions are built, how models are trained and evaluated, and, above all, how results are interpreted and communicated. At each of these levels, there is considerable complexity, especially in biomedical applications, where decision-making can directly impact patient health and safety outcomes. The challenge is not only to build high-performance models but also to generalize them transparently across different population groups, thereby making them usable by domain experts without requiring deep technical knowledge. Biomedical data records are often fragmented, heterogeneous, and loud from a variety of sources, such as electronic health records (honor), clinical research, genomic databases, chemical connection libraries, and imaging studies. These data records need to be harmonized, cleaned, and commented on to ensure consistency and relevance. Essential parts of curation include the standardization of terms using vocabularies such as Snom CT, bitch, or MEDDRA, treatment of missing or inconsistent entries, and assurance of ethical and legal data regarding the origin.

Furthermore, biomedical data records are often imbalanced. For example, there may be far more non-toxic compounds than toxic predictions and far more non-toxic compounds than toxic predictions (Yingngam et al., 2024). To prevent past learning outcomes, it is essential to address this imbalance using techniques such as oversampling, undersampling, and class weight loss functions. Characteristics range from molecular fingerprints, gene expression profiles, and protein interaction networks to clinical variables, including laboratory results, demographic factors, and comorbidity values. Practical and functional engineering requires domain literacy to select biologically meaningful variables and reduce the dimensions of extensive data records without losing essential information. For example, pharmacogenomics studies can use principal component analysis (PCA) or automated encoders to distill meaningful patterns from thousands of gene-expression values. Time modeling is crucial for analyzing longitudinal patient data.

Characteristic extractions must preserve the time-dependent nature of treatment responses or side effects and often require repetitive neural networks or attention-based architectures to model these sequences with accuracy. This includes selecting the appropriate algorithm for molecular representation, ranging from methods with classic machine learning, such as random forests and gradient-based vector machines, to support deep learning architectures, including convolutional neural networks (CNNs), recurrent neural networks (RNNs), and graph neural networks (GNNs). The training process must be managed carefully to prevent overfitting, considering the relatively small size of many biomedical data records, particularly compared to data records in other areas, such as natural language and computer vision. Normalization techniques, breaking down layers of neuronal networks, and strategies for data augmentation (such as those used in chemical modeling) can help to mitigate excessive adaptation. In this context, cross-validation is often employed in k-fold or layered k-fold configurations. In biomedical chronology, such as clinical longitudinal measurements, time-oriented cross-validation respects the necessary time orders to avoid data leakage. External validation using completely independent data records from various institutions, countries, or patient populations is the gold standard for demonstrating generalizability. This is essential in biomedicine, where variations in demographics, clinical practice, and genetic background can significantly impact outcomes (Marques et al., 2024). Benchmarks for established models or traditional statistical methods also provide context for assessing the value-addedness of complex AI approaches. Metrics such as the area under the receiver operating characteristic curve (AUROC), precision-recall curve, F1 score, and Matthews correlation coefficient are often used. However, these results need to be interpreted with caution, especially in disproportionate scenarios where high aurochs can be misleading. Biomedical decisions often involve high stakes; therefore, it is essential to understand the limitations of model trust. Methods such as Monte Carlo faults, bootstrap ensembles, and Bayesian neural networks allow for estimates of predictive uncertainty that can affect decision thresholds and facilitate rapid human reviews. These techniques prevent the model from acting as a "black box" that always returns a deterministic result, but rather as a system to watch out for when predictions are made in diagnostic or therapeutic environments, where they are fundamental. Explainable AI (XAI) plays a central role in this context. Clinics, supervisors, and patients require a specific understanding of how and why AI models reach certain conclusions, particularly when these decisions impact health-related decisions. To this end, many XAI technologies have been developed from local descriptions, such as lime (locally interpretable models-logical explanations) and shapes (Shapley Additive explanations), as well as global descriptions, such as distinctive weight rankings and decision trees extracted from complex models. These methods help identify the best traits that contribute to a particular prediction (Zhang et al., 2025). They can indicate whether the model is based on clinically meaningful signals or on false correlations.

Figure 2. Framework for AI Model Development, Validation, and Governance

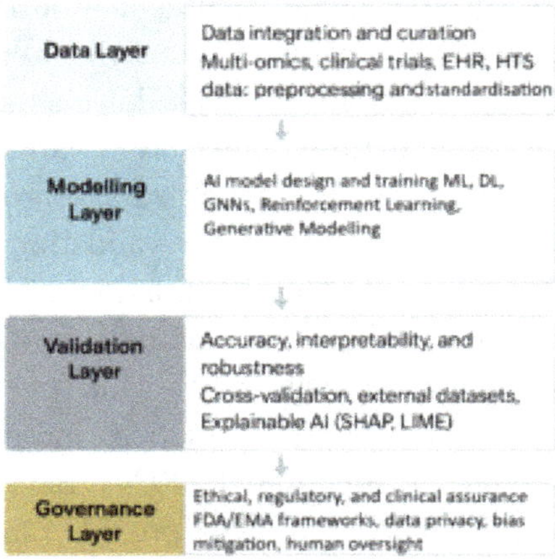

Chemical modeling can use XAI to highlight the molecular substrates that are most relevant to the predicted toxicity or efficacy. For image-based predictions (such as histopathology or radiation), heat and output cards can indicate the areas of the image that influenced the decision. In a clinical setting, tools such as SHAP can explain how variables, including blood pressure, creatinine, and genetic markers, influence treatment recommendations (Son et al., 2024). These interpretations not only build trust but also support hypothesis generation, regulatory verification and post-testing. However, it is essential to note that the interpretability technique itself is undoubtedly. Costs depend on assumptions and approximations and should be validated to align with the domain knowledge. These include rules-based systems, generalized additive models (GAMs), and sparse linear models, which may not achieve the same raw performance as deep learning systems but can provide clear inferences. In a specific regulatory context, such as B, transparency is preferred over complexity in those affecting security assessments and patient risks. A hybrid approach that combines powerful and interpretable models is gaining traction, allowing for in-depth reviews of deep model outputs based on simpler, human-readable models. Interpretations aimed at regulatory authorities must be more rigorous and testable, providing clinicians with quick insights into treatment decisions. The design of human-AI interfaces must consider these differences and ensure that the description is not only technically correct but also implementable and reliable. Interpretation also plays a role in the unstable cooperation in drug development. Pharmacologists, toxicologists, data scientists, and regulatory issues experts must align the model version to require joint vocabulary and precise documentation. Unexplainable models pose risks of algorithm distortion, lack of accountability, and increased reliance on errors. In areas with strict data protection regulations, such as the European Union, in accordance with the General Data Protection Regulation (GDPR), individuals may have the right to know whether they are exposed to algorithmic decisions. This regulatory trend underscores the importance of developing transparent and understandable AI systems not only for engineers but also for everyone involved in biomedical ecosystems. Care must be taken to ensure data quality, robust assessment frames, and transparent communication of knowledge. As AI advances in drug development and clinical decision-making, these fundamentals determine the reliability, acceptance, and actual impact of AI systems (Panda & Mohapatra, 2024). Compensating for predictive performance, with the interpretability and scalability of innovation, requires oversight and accountability, making it more than just a technical task. This is a socio-technical imperative for the future of AI in healthcare and drug discovery.

REGULATORY AND CLINICAL IMPLICATIONS

As AI tools evolve from research support to critical decision-making components, particularly in preclinical and early clinical development, regulatory frameworks must be adapted to maintain trust and protect patients' safety. Additionally, the role of AIS in Adaptive Clinical Study Designs offers new opportunities for dynamic data control research, while also providing clear guidelines for use, validation, and protection. Both the FDA and EMA have published early framework conditions and discussion papers recognizing the increasing use of AI/ML in drug development. For example, "Artificial Intelligence/Machine Learning Based Action Plans as Medical Devices" describes a risk-based approach that promotes transparency, robustness, and continuous surveillance. The plan focuses primarily on AI-based devices but presents a broader tone of expectations for pharmaceutical applications. Similarly, until 2025, the EMA recognized the growing importance of AI in regulatory science strategies, emphasizing the need for dialogue and collaboration among stakeholders from member states (Visan & Negut, 2024). These positions reveal that AI is welcomed as a transformative tool. However, it must be implemented in an interpretable, testable, and scientifically robust way. First, the data used to train and validate these systems must be of high quality, integrity, and relevance. Supervisors require certainty that the conclusions of AI analysis are grounded in solid evidence. In particular, these conclusions influence GO/NO-GO decisions in early stage testing or drug security assessments. Second, we need to explain the AI model to some extent. This requires regulators to understand how decisions are made in the industry. While this does not imply complete transparency of all neuronal network weights or decision paths, developers can provide a wise summary of the impact of input data and existing levels of trust. Third, AI model validation should follow rigorous statistical methods, ideally including external validation of independent datasets and sensitivity analysis to examine how model predictions change under various assumptions or conditions. For example, FDAs often require robust indications of reproducibility and generalization, especially when tools are intended to support central decisions in the drug development pipeline.

In preclinical and early clinical decision-making, AI tools can accelerate candidate screening, predict potential toxicity, and prioritize connections with preferred pharmacokinetic and pharmacodynamic profiles. These skills significantly reduce the time and cost of early development while simultaneously increasing the likelihood that successful candidates will make progress. AI also helps identify biomarkers that can predict responses to drugs or side effects, thereby improving strategies for patient stratification. However, the use of AI for these purposes requires thoughtful integration into traditional toxicology, pharmacology, and test design approaches (Mottaghi-Dastjerdi & Soltany-Rezaee-Rad, 2024). The supervisor expects sponsors to demonstrate that AI-derived knowledge is supported by biological validity, which replaces human expertise in the field. For example, suppose that sponsors use AI models to predict liver toxicity in new connections. In this case, the FDA will require both documentation of the model's power and supporting data from in vitro or in vivo studies that validate the predictions. Sponsors must utilize AI tools to generate hypotheses and ensure that these tools are used to select the endpoints or define the inclusion criteria. Traceability is essential when the data pipeline contains complex or iterative model updates. In preclinical submissions, such as new drug applications (NDAs), supervisors can request detailed documentation on how AI-supported analyses are conducted, which data records are used, and how conclusions are informed by the design of the first human research. It is insufficient to determine whether the AI model predicts low toxicity or high efficacy levels. Instead, regulatory experts require reasons, methodologies, confidence intervals, and boundaries associated with these predictions. Suppose that AI is used in test simulations to determine the appropriate dosage or population parameters. In such cases, this should be explicitly explained in the manuscript. The coordination of research that adjusts aspects of the research design according to interim data results in increased efficiency, ethical flexibility, and the possibility of accelerated scheduling.

AI improves adaptive research by providing real-time analytics, predictive modeling, and intelligent decision-making support. For example, AI algorithms can be used to monitor patient responses, adapt randomization probability, terminate ineffective treatments, or recommend changes to dosage schemes. These features are based on dynamic data analysis and predictive modeling, both of which must be specified and rigorously verified to meet the regulatory standards (Bhattacharjee et al., 2025). The FDA has provided guidelines for adaptive design clinical research, emphasizing the importance of starters, control of Type I errors, and data integrity. The same principles apply when AI is used to implement such adjustments. Test sponsors should clearly outline how AI algorithms are trained, validated, and monitored, as well as how their costs affect adaptive decisions. In particular, supervisors are looking for evidence that AI does not introduce distortion, damage glare, or damage the outcome of play. The EMA also recognizes the commitment to adaptive design and cooperation through platforms such as the International Council for Harmonization (ICH), which aims to create a unified global standard for its implementation. AI can analyze data at the patient level to optimize dose-effect curves, reduce dropout rates, and increase the likelihood of research success by early identification of responders. In the context of rare diseases, AI-enabled adaptive studies can contribute to the design of N-Von-1 studies or baskets that integrate several subtypes into a coherent frame. However, supervisors require robust control mechanisms to ensure that such personalizations do not compromise scientific accuracy or lead to cherry-picked results. Adaptation protocols using AI should be designed to require statistical validity when employing simulation-based control weapons and utilizing the appropriate hierarchical variables.

In many cases, AI systems learn and improve when new data records are used to train machine learning models for license plates. However, this dynamic nature makes regulatory oversight difficult (Mirakhori & Niazi, 2025). Unless there is a clear change control process and a continuous validation mechanism, regulators should take note before adaptive AIS shifting behavior becomes the center of action. The FDA proposed the concept of specific change control planning for AI-based devices, enabling similar strategies to be applied to devices used in drug development and other medical applications. This includes defining the aspects of the model. The model can be changed under specific circumstances, and these changes can be documented and reevaluated (Dhudum et al., 2024). Sponsors must coordinate the need for model development with the stability and predictability of regulatory trust. When AI is used to recruit or monitor experiments, it becomes part of the decision chain that affects patient risk factors. For example, suppose an AI system determines that a patient is an ideal candidate based on a predicted response, but the prediction is incorrect. In this case, questions of responsibility and ethical liability arise. Supervisory authorities require clear documentation of how patients are selected, which data are used, and how human investigators verify or override decisions. AI tools require regular checks to ensure consistent performance, and the mechanism of human supervision within the loop must be an integral part of the test management. Similarly, the procedure for declaring consent must consider the use of AI, particularly when prediction or layering decisions can affect patient participation or treatment pathways (Tariq, 2025).

From a clinical perspective, AI is promising for post-marketing surveillance and pharmacovigilance. Real-world data collected after a drug is approved can be analyzed using artificial intelligence (AI) to detect rare adverse events, monitor long-term efficacy, and identify unreported uses (Bhatt et al., 2024). These applications align with the growing approach of regulators in managing the life cycle and security after authorization. However, these systems must be transparent, validated, and integrated into existing pharmacovigilance frameworks. Regulators will want to know how safety signs derived from AI are generated, what thresholds activate alerts, and how these alerts are communicated to sponsors, doctors, and patients. Systems that automate the detection of adverse events or prioritize the review of cases based on the AI score must be demonstrated, fair, and auditable.

Ultimately, the integration of AI in regulatory and clinical decision-making necessitates a new collaborative paradigm among developers, regulators, physicians, and patients (Mottaghi-Dastjerdi & Soltany-Rezaee-Rad, 2024). This collaboration should be based on shared principles of transparency, scientific rigor, patient-centeredness, and continuous learning. As AI becomes a fixed element in pharmaceutical innovation, regulatory frameworks must evolve to maintain the rhythm, balancing innovation with responsibility and flexibility with supervision. Mutual education is key: regulators must develop literacy in AI technologies, and developers must internalize the ethical and legal standards that govern medical care.

CHALLENGES AND LIMITATIONS

The integration of artificial intelligence (AI) into drug research and development, particularly in predicting drug efficacy and toxicity, promises to be transformative. However, this technological revolution does not pose any significant challenges or limitations. These topics encompass technical, ethical, legal, and operational aspects. Nuance and foresight must be considered to ensure that AI realizes its full potential safely, fairly, and reliably (Gupta et al., 2024). The most urgent issues include data heterogeneity and quality concerns, distortions within AI models, concerns about reproducibility, and ethical and legal complexities associated with integrating human security forecasts into automated systems. Drug development encompasses a range of data types, including chemical structures, genomic sequencing, clinical research records, electronic health records, OMICS data records, adverse event reports, and preclinical toxicological results. These data records are not only extensive but also very foreign, with different structures, forms, granularities, origins, and reliabilities. Data from high-throughput screening assays are sparse and extensive. However, clinical laboratory data may be extensive in detail but limited in terms of their scope and diversity. Providing electronic health files can provide the longest insight into the effectiveness of drugs. However, such data are notoriously inconsistent because of differences in medical terminology, coding standards, medical practices, and documentation habits. Integrating these different sources into a coherent, high-quality training set for AI models is exceptionally complex. While efforts to standardize, such as the use of ontologies and interoperable data formats, will help mitigate these challenges, the task remains daunting.

Furthermore, incomplete, inaccurate, or fraudulent data can not only be ineffective but also lead to the development of potentially harmful models when informing decisions with high stakes, such as patient treatment and drug approval. Missing data, outliers, and noise can significantly affect the performance and reliability of the model. Data processing and preprocessing, although often underestimated, are crucial components of the structure of reliable AI systems in the pharmaceutical industry. In this context, distortions can manifest in various ways, including biases in the selection of training data, confirmation of model interpretations, or systemic distortions affecting underrepresented population groups. Suppose the training data disproportionately represent a particular demographic group, such as white middle-aged males. In this case, the model's outcome may be difficult for people outside this group to understand. It has a significant impact on medicine, where differences in genetics, physiology, and environmental pollution can substantially affect drug response. Although gender and racial discrepancies in unwanted event profiles are well documented, these nuances are not always well documented in the training dataset (Tariq, 2025). Consequently, AI models for specific population groups may systematically underestimate risk or overestimate effectiveness, thereby increasing existing health disparities instead of improving them. Reproducibility is a central concern in AI control research. Many AI research studies, particularly those published in highly influential journals, are based on unique datasets or black-box algorithms that cannot be independently verified or reproduced. This undermines scientific transparency and hinders progress, as other researchers cannot verify the results or build upon previous research. Additionally, reproducibility is reduced if the model is not well documented or if the same model yields different results under slightly different conditions owing to the stochastic nature of the training process (Gupta et al., 2024). Addressing these issues requires strict benchmark practices, the use of publicly available data records and code where possible, and the development of reproducible pipelines for model training and evaluation.

One ethical dilemma lies in the opacity of many AI models. Although deep learning systems are robust, they can be challenging to interpret and understand. If such models predict that a drug will likely cause liver acidity, it may not be immediately clear which function or data points led to this conclusion. This lack of explanation can make it difficult for supervisory authorities, clinics, and researchers to trust or respond to the model's performance. This description is fundamental when AI predictions have direct consequences for human health or are used to inform regulations. Without a clear justification for the decision, accountability is blurred. Who is responsible if AI-based forecasts lead to developers, pharmaceutical companies, or regulators who have approved their use? The regulatory framework for AI in healthcare and medicine is still developing, and there is considerable uncertainty regarding how existing laws apply to AI control models. For example, the issue of liability remains clear if an unwanted drug response occurs after an AI-recommended treatment. Data safety regulations, such as the European GDPR and US HIPAA, impose strict requirements for the use, sharing, and storage of personal health data. These regulations aim to collect extensive data records necessary for training robust AI models, particularly in joint or cross-border environments.

Additionally, you can verify that you use AI for security forecasting, following the Product Liability Act. If AI models are integrated into the drug development pipeline and their predictions are used to determine GO/NO-GO decisions in clinical research, all subsequent results could lead to legal disputes (Mak et al., 2024). Equity requires that AI models do not exacerbate existing differences in access to healthcare system outcomes. This includes intentional efforts to validate the model across various subgroups, including different populations represented in the training data. Charities demand that AI systems have been shown to improve human well-being. This includes rigorous testing, transparent reporting, and careful monitoring of real-world impacts. Respect for people means a declaration of consent that becomes complicated when AI is used to generate predictions from aggregated data or when it is not easy to understand the impact of AI-derived knowledge on patients or providers (Gupta et al., 2024). However, AI models trained on a particular context or narrow data records work well in this environment but are missing if used in other environments. For example, models for predicting drug responses cannot be generalized to patients in Asia or Africa using data from hospitals in North America because of differences in genetic makeup, dietary habits, and healthcare systems.

Similarly, models trained with controlled clinical experimental data should struggle to measure more measurements that lack entries and actual data in non-standard formats. This limitation poses a significant challenge to AI delivery in global pharmaceutical applications, where the need for generalized models that work across diverse population groups and environments is crucial. Transfer learning and domain adjustment techniques provide partial solutions but require careful calibration and verification. If the model is tuned but not tailored to the training data and not generalized, excessive adaptation occurs. Conversely, a lower adaptation indicates that the model is too simple to grasp the underlying patterns. Both issues are common in drug datasets, which may be high-dimensional, but are limited by cost and ethical limitations (Gupta et al., 2024). To avoid these pitfalls, it is essential to carefully select the model architecture, normalization techniques, and validation strategies (Tariq, 2025).

Furthermore, the compromise between interpretability and overview often complicates the model selection. A simpler model is easy to explain but may lack the predictive power. In contrast, complex models are more accurate but also more challenging to trust (Mak et al., 2024). Integrating AI into a highly regulated, risk-averse drug development environment requires cultural change, infrastructure investment and interdisciplinary collaboration. Scientists, clinicians, and regulatory experts require training to understand, validate, and interact effectively with artificial intelligence (AI) systems. Companies must establish robust data governance frameworks, adequate cybersecurity protection, and regular maintenance protocols to ensure that the model remains reliable and accurately maintains its data. There is also the challenge of version control to ensure that models are developed responsibly when new data become available without affecting previous decisions or records. A clear test track for the use of AI models in development, updates, and decision-making is essential for compliance and trust (Shaki et al., 2024). The path to integrating meaningful, safe, and ethical AI into drug development is challenging and requires interdisciplinary solutions. Technical issues related to data quality, bias, and reproducibility must be addressed using strict standards and transparent practices. Ethical concerns regarding fairness, accountability, and patient rights necessitate intentional design decisions and robust governance structures to ensure transparency and accountability in AI systems. Legal uncertainty requires clear formal guidelines and proactive risk management. Only by focusing on these challenges can we harness our full potential to build a safer, faster, and fairer future for medicines.

FUTURE DIRECTIONS AND OPPORTUNITIES

The convergence of quantum computing, federated learning, Digital Twin Technologies, and Open AI collaborations will transform the future of pharmaceutical research and development. The complexity of drug discovery often struggles to keep pace as it continues to grow in response to the requirements of precision medicine, increasingly complex biological data, and the need for faster, safer, and more scalable solution models. The integration of new technologies not only provides improved speed and accuracy but also introduces new paradigms for research. Knowledge and innovation are realized throughout the pharmaceutical ecosystem. At its core, quantum computing enables the modeling of complex molecular and biochemical systems with granularity and scale that classical computers cannot achieve efficiently. Traditional methods for simulating protein folding, enzyme-substrate interactions, and drug-target affinity are rooted in nature, particularly in the quantum behavior of electrons and molecular orbitals (Sampathi & Bhatia, 2024). Understanding the precise energy and conformational dynamics of biomolecules, which are central to drug efficacy and selectivity, is crucial for comprehending their roles. Quantum computing remains at the level of results, and actual implementations face limitations, such as error rates and qubit stability. However, hybrid quantum-classical models are already being considered in collaboration with pharmaceutical companies and academic institutions for drug design. These hybrid approaches enable quantum processors to solve the most mathematically intensive parts of molecular simulations while simultaneously delegating simple tasks to classical systems (Ahmad, 2025). When quantum hardware matures and becomes more accessible, it can dramatically accelerate the optimization of leads from hits, lead to rational drug designs, and reduce the confidence of broad testing and error testing.

Simultaneously, there will be coalition learning and robust solutions to one of the most depressing challenges in drug data calculations and data calculations (Vignesh, 2024). The healthcare and biopharmaceutical sectors operate in strictly regulated environments, making it challenging to exchange sensitive patient data between institutions, regions, and businesses. Federated Learning addresses this issue by enabling collaborative model training through distributed data sources via direct data exchange. In the federated learning framework, individual companies, such as hospitals, research centers, and pharmaceutical companies, have AI models within their data premises, with only model parameters or updates being used by a central aggregator. This approach preserves data sovereignty and privacy while simultaneously benefiting from the collective learning of multiple records.

Regarding drug efficacy and toxicity prediction, federal learning can utilize findings from global clinical records, test data, and genomics, without compromising patient confidentiality. It also enables the development of more generalizable models that reflect biological and demographic diversity, reduce distortions, and increase robustness. When spring-based learning is combined with techniques such as privacy-preserving differential privacy and secure multiparty computation, it provides a framework for responsible AI innovation that aligns with ethical and legal standards in healthcare and pharmaceuticals. With the rise of digital twins and virtual patients, another layer of conversion has been introduced into the development of medicines. In this context, a digital twin refers to a virtual representation of an actual biological system, such as an organ, physiological process, or entire patient profile (Sampathi & Bhatia, 2024). The idea is to simulate how a particular drug behaves in an individualized biological context before it is physically administered. A comprehensive digital structure of virtual patients based on real or synthetic clinical data can be used to model population-level variability and simulate clinical research in various scenarios. This technology holds significant promise for reducing the reliance on animal experiments, enhancing the early identification of side effects, and optimizing research design for maximum efficiency. Pharmaceutical companies can simulate hundreds or thousands of virtual patients with different comorbidities, genetic profiles, and lifestyle factors (Amorim et al., 2024). They can test how candidates develop under different real-world conditions. It accelerates the process of understanding the effectiveness and safety of the treatment while simultaneously minimizing risks, costs, and ethical concerns. Digital twin technology has also been integrated into regulatory science, with virtual models that can provide additional evidence to support the drug approval process and offer hope for long-term results after approval. The potential for combining digital twins with real-time health monitoring through wearable and networked devices could further enhance treatment plans and support dynamic adaptive therapeutics. The complexity and cost of drug discovery, exacerbated by global health crises such as COVID-19, have led to a shift towards a collaborative, transparent, and open approach to AI model development. Initiatives such as the Open Targets Platform, Melloddy (the orchestration of machine learning ledgers for pharmaceutical drilling rigs), and the COVID Moonshot project demonstrate how the industrial, scientific, and non-profit sectors can collaborate to bundle data, models, and expertise to address common challenges (Tariq, 2025).

Open-source AI frameworks, such as those based on deep learning and TensorFlow, reduce the barriers to entry for researchers and small organizations, allowing for broader participation in pharmaceutical innovation. These platforms not only improve reproducibility and model validation but also promote interdisciplinary contributions from data scientists, bioinformaticians, chemists and clinicians. Additionally, the Open AI ecosystem promotes transparency. This is essential for ethical oversight, trust in regulations, and public acceptance. When AI models used in drug development are openly accessible and interpretable, stakeholders can better assess their reliability, biases, and limitations. Furthermore, this collaboration often leads to the establishment of general benchmarks, data records, and evaluation criteria that standardize the development process and drive improvements. Scenery. These must not be isolated trends, however. Instead, they are increasingly used in concerts and other events. For example, federated learning models trained using digital twins in multiple hospitals can be used to predict personalized drug responses while simultaneously maintaining data protection periods. Quantum reinforcement simulations can inform the generation of digital twins with biophysical realism (Gupta et al., 2024). Open AI platforms can provide the common infrastructure required to coordinate these components in a coherent and scalable workflow. This integration at the system level will not only promote technological advancements but also systemic resilience, mobility, and the comprehensive development and testing of new therapies.

Finally, the future of pharmaceutical development is shaped by the technology's rock ecosystem, which expands the ability to expand AI capabilities. Timetable challenges regarding drug efficacy, security, and development are not only arithmetic problems but also multifactorial issues that require a holistic solution. Quantum computing addresses the bottleneck of molecular complexity, whereas spring-based learning overcomes the limitations of data silos (Abbas et al., 2024). Digital twins simulate biological individuality, and open AI initiatives have democratized innovation. Together, we enable a new era in which safer, faster, and more patient-oriented treatments can be developed not only through better science but also through better systems that are transparent, ethical, and deeply collaborative.

CONCLUSION

The conclusion of this chapter on AI-controlled predictions of the effectiveness and toxicity of medicinal products is not only an endpoint but also a window into the future of faster, safer, and more cost-effective therapeutic innovations. In the past, weakly scheduled drug development pipelines, high costs, and frequent failures in the late stages have been attributed to unexpected toxicity or inefficiency due to various challenges. AI provides a mechanism to tackle these long-term inefficiencies by improving the ability to predict, model, and understand biological complexities in previously impossible ways, particularly through machine learning, deep learning, and neural networks. Traditional methods, which rely on high-throughput screening and manual analysis of chemical libraries, are time-consuming and costly. AI models, particularly generative models and graph neural networks, can now simulate millions of drug-like compounds in silico, reducing the binding affinity and assessing potential biological interactions as targets (Kapustina et al., 2024). This shift significantly reduces the number of compounds that require physical synthesis and biological testing, resulting from the transition from wet laboratories to virtual screening. Furthermore, AI helps identify new molecular structures with desirable pharmacological profiles that may be overlooked using traditional methods.

Toxicity is one of the most common causes of drug shortages in clinical trials. AI offers an increasingly sophisticated approach to toxicity prediction by integrating a wide range of data from in vitro toxicity studies, OMICS data, and descriptors, ranging from historically undesirable event reports of chemical structures. By training predictive models for these data sources, researchers can estimate the likelihood of hepatotoxicity, cardiotoxicity, nephrotoxicity, or other side effects before the candidate drug undergoes animal experiments. AI must enable the development of models that are aware of the underlying disease states beyond the goal and are contextually capable of identifying interactions outside the goal that support subtle toxicity assessments, surpassing traditional standards-based systems. By analyzing transcriptome and proteome profiles, researchers can predict whether a drug binds to its intended target and whether this interaction leads to a therapeutic effect (Gholap et al., 2024). AI also facilitates the modeling of disease pathways and networks, enabling scientists to simulate how biological systems disrupt drug therapies. The biological perspective of this system is crucial for understanding the multifactorial nature of many diseases, particularly cancer, neurodegenerative disorders, and autoimmune diseases (Tariq, 2025).

Test simulation platforms using AI can help optimize research designs and predict fashion results across registration and ABRAS rates, as well as low-test results. Adaptive clinical research designs that operate in real-time using data and AI algorithms enable continuous adjustments to improve protocols based on preliminary outcomes, efficiency, and ethical considerations. Additionally, the AI-controlled pharmacovigilance system monitors real data from electronic health files (HONOR), social media, and portable devices. It recognizes unnecessary events more quickly than traditional systems, thereby improving monitoring and enhancing long-term security. Data quality, standardization, and integration are key hurdles in the development of reliable AI models. Drug data are often fragmented and heterogeneous, making it challenging to build a powerful and generalized model. In addition, the "Black Box Nature of many AI models, particularly profound architectures, raises concerns regarding interpretability, transparency, and regulatory acceptance (Bhatia et al., 2024). For clinical and regulatory stakeholders to trust AI predictions, especially in matters as serious as patient safety, mechanisms for explaining and validating them must be established. Explainable AI (XAI) aims to create models that are accessible to human users without compromising governance. Ensure that you are responsible and accountable for the tool in a way that significantly improves patient outcomes.

Another important consideration is the integration of AI into existing pharmaceutical workflows and cultures. AI should not be viewed as an alternative to human scientists, but rather as a powerful augmentation device. The most successful applications of AI occur when interdisciplinary teams, including data scientists, clinicians, pharmacologists, and regulatory experts, collaborate to interpret the results, validate the findings, and translate the predictions into actionable insights. In principle, this human approach guarantees scientific rigor and helps bridge the gap between theoretical modeling and practical applications. Drug reuse can now be accelerated by AI algorithms that match existing drugs with slower random processes and soon new indications based on molecular and clinical signatures (Gupta et al., 2024). The rise of digital virtual representations of individual patients or biological systems could potentially enable truly personalized drug testing before the first tablet is administered to a patient. As the availability of the Federated Learning approach increases, agencies can cooperate in model training without sharing sensitive patient data, thereby opening up possibilities for significant and private AI innovation across borders.

In summary, the integration of AI to predict drug efficacy and toxicity represents a transformative leap towards a more agile, well-informed, and patient-oriented drug development process. By using significant data sources, modeling biological complexity, and enabling faster decision-making (Amorim et al., 2024). AI provides the tools required to tackle some of the most firmly fixed challenges in drug discovery. To fully leverage this opportunity, stakeholders must commit to overcoming technical, regulatory, and ethical challenges, while fostering a culture of interdisciplinary collaboration and transparency. The future of medicine will become increasingly dependent not only on molecules and mechanisms but also on intelligently designed algorithms and insights, as well as on the discovery of new treatments.

REFERENCES

Abbas, M. K. G., Rassam, A., Karamshahi, F., Abunora, R., & Abouseada, M. (2024). The role of AI in drug discovery. *ChemBioChem*, *25*(14), e202300816. PMID: 38735845

Ahmad, F. (2025). Optimizing Treatment: The Role of Pharmacology, Genomics, and AI in Improving Patient Outcomes. *Drug Development Research*, *86*(3), e70093. PMID: 40285487

Amorim, A. M., Piochi, L. F., Gaspar, A. T., Preto, A. J., Rosário-Ferreira, N., & Moreira, I. S. (2024). Advancing drug safety in drug development: Bridging computational predictions for enhanced toxicity prediction. *Chemical Research in Toxicology*, *37*(6), 827–849. PMID: 38758610

Bhatia, N., Khan, M. M. U., & Arora, S. (2024). The Role of Artificial Intelligence in Revolutionizing Pharmacological Research. *Current Pharmacology Reports*, *10*(6), 323–329.

Bhatt, P., Singh, S., Kumar, V., Nagarajan, K., Mishra, S. K., Dixit, P. K., & Kumar, S. (2024). Artificial intelligence in pharmaceutical industry: Revolutionizing drug development and delivery. *Current Artificial Intelligence*, *2*(1), E051223224198.

Bhattacharjee, A., Kumar, A., Ojha, P. K., & Kar, S. (2025). Artificial intelligence to predict inhibitors of drug-metabolizing enzymes and transporters for safer drug design. *Expert Opinion on Drug Discovery*, *20*(5), 621–641. PMID: 40241626

Dhudum, R., Ganeshpurkar, A., & Pawar, A. (2024). Revolutionizing drug discovery: A comprehensive review of AI applications. *Drugs and Drug Candidates*, *3*(1), 148–171.

Gholap, A. D., Uddin, M. J., Faiyazuddin, M., Omri, A., Gowri, S., & Khalid, M. (2024). Advances in artificial intelligence in drug delivery and development: A comprehensive review. *Computers in Biology and Medicine*, •••, 108702. PMID: 38878397

Gupta, U., Pranav, A., Kohli, A., Ghosh, S., & Singh, D. (2024). The contribution of artificial intelligence to drug discovery: Current progress and prospects for the future. *Microbial Data Intelligence and Computational Techniques for Sustainable Computing*, 1-23.

Kapustina, O., Burmakina, P., Gubina, N., Serov, N., & Vinogradov, V. (2024). User-friendly and industry-integrated AI for medicinal chemists and pharmaceuticals. *Artificial Intelligence Chemistry.*, •••, 100072.

Mak, K. K., Wong, Y. H., & Pichika, M. R. (2024). Artificial intelligence in drug discovery and development. *Drug discovery and evaluation: safety and pharmacokinetic assays*, 1461-1498.

Malheiro, V., Santos, B., Figueiras, A., & Mascarenhas-Melo, F. (2025). The Potential of Artificial Intelligence in Pharmaceutical Innovation: From Drug Discovery to Clinical Trials. *Pharmaceuticals*, *18*(6), 788. PMID: 40573185

Mandlik, M. R., Pathan, N. H., & Mahanor, P. B. (2024). INTEGRATING ARTIFICIAL INTELLIGENCE INTO DRUG DEVELOPMENT AND MANUFACTURING: ADVANCEMENTS AND CHALLENGES.

Marques, L., Costa, B., Pereira, M., Silva, A., Santos, J., Saldanha, L., & Vale, N. (2024). Advancing precision medicine: A review of innovative in silico approaches for drug development, clinical pharmacology and personalized healthcare. *Pharmaceutics*, *16*(3), 332. PMID: 38543226

Mettleq, A. S. A., Akkila, A. N., Alkahlout, M. A., ALmurshidi, S. H., Abu-Nasser, B. S., & Abu-Naser, S. S. (2024). Revolutionizing Drug Discovery: The Role of Artificial Intelligence in Accelerating Pharmaceutical Innovation.

Mirakhori, F., & Niazi, S. K. (2025). Harnessing the AI/ML in Drug and Biological Products Discovery and Development: The Regulatory Perspective. *Pharmaceuticals*, *18*(1), 47. PMID: 39861110

Mottaghi-Dastjerdi, N., & Soltany-Rezaee-Rad, M. (2024). Advancements and Applications of Artificial Intelligence in Pharmaceutical Sciences: A Comprehensive Review. *Iranian Journal of Pharmaceutical Research : IJPR*, *23*(1), e150510. PMID: 39895671

Mutha, R. E., Bagul, V. S., Tade, R. S., & Vinchurkar, K. (2024). An Overview of Artificial Intelligence (AI) In Drug Delivery and Development. *AI Innovations in Drug Delivery and Pharmaceutical Sciences; Advancing Therapy through. Technology*, •••, 1–27.

Panda, P., & Mohapatra, R. (2024). *Revolutionizing Patient Safety: Machine Learning and AI for the Early Detection of Adverse Drug Reactions and Drug-Induced Toxicity*. Current Artificial Intelligence.

Sampathi, S., & Bhatia, N. (2024). AI-Enabled Models in the Restoration of Drug Efficacy and Drug Design. In *Biosystems, Biomedical & Drug Delivery Systems: Characterization, Restoration and Optimization* (pp. 83–103). Springer Nature Singapore.

Shaki, F., Amirkhanloo, M., & Chahardori, M. (2024). The Future and Application of Artificial Intelligence in Toxicology. *Asia Pacific Journal of Medical Toxicology*, *13*(1).

Singh, B., Crasto, M., Ravi, K., & Singh, S. (2024). *Pharmaceutical advances: Integrating artificial intelligence in QSAR, combinatorial and green chemistry practices*. Intelligent Pharmacy.

Son, A., Park, J., Kim, W., Yoon, Y., Lee, S., Ji, J., & Kim, H. (2024). Recent Advances in Omics, Computational Models, and Advanced Screening Methods for Drug Safety and Efficacy. *Toxics*, *12*(11), 822. PMID: 39591001

Suri, G. S., Kaur, G., & Shinde, D. (2024). Beyond boundaries: Exploring the transformative power of AI in pharmaceuticals. *Discover Artificial Intelligence*, *4*(1), 82.

Suriyaamporn, P., Pamornpathomkul, B., Patrojanasophon, P., Ngawhirunpat, T., Rojanarata, T., & Opanasopit, P. (2024). The artificial intelligence-powered new era in pharmaceutical research and development: A review. *AAPS PharmSciTech*, *25*(6), 188. PMID: 39147952

Tariq, M. U. (2025). Decolonizing Education Systems Through Action Research and Action Learning. In Mapotse, T., Tetteh, E., & Matsekoleng, T. (Eds.), *Enabling Indigenous Knowledge Systems in Action Research and Action Learning* (pp. 107–128). IGI Global Scientific Publishing., DOI: 10.4018/979-8-3693-3542-0.ch006

Tariq, M. U. (2025). Decolonising Education Systems Through Action Research and Action Learning Methodologies. In Mapotse, T., Tetteh, E., & Matsekoleng, T. (Eds.), *Enabling Indigenous Knowledge Systems in Action Research and Action Learning* (pp. 87–106). IGI Global Scientific Publishing., DOI: 10.4018/979-8-3693-3542-0.ch005

Tariq, M. U. (2025). AI in the Classroom: Revolutionizing Instruction and Student Engagement. In M. Kessinger, G. Nelson, L. Lennex, & K. Nettleton (Eds.), *Enhancing Classroom Instruction and Student Skills With AI* (pp. 35-62). IGI Global Scientific Publishing. https://doi.org/DOI: 10.4018/979-8-3373-4576-5.ch002

Tariq, M. U. (2025). The Challenge of Artificial Intelligence in Environmental Sustainability: Opportunities, Risks, and Policy Implications. In Ahmadi, A., & Mna, A. (Eds.), *Nexus of Environmental Quality and Technology Innovation* (pp. 267–292). IGI Global Scientific Publishing., DOI: 10.4018/979-8-3373-1822-6.ch012

Tariq, M. U. (2025). Machine Learning Techniques for Personalized Rehabilitation: Enhancing Patient Outcomes Through Predictive Algorithms. In Korupalli, V., Ranasinghe, P., & Feldman, D. (Eds.), *Predictive Algorithms for Rehabilitation and Assistive Systems* (pp. 221–252). IGI Global Scientific Publishing., DOI: 10.4018/979-8-3373-0194-5.ch009

Tyagi, E., Kumari, P., Prakash, A., & Bhuyan, R. (2025). Revolutionizing Anti-Cancer Drug Discovery: The Role of Artificial Intelligence. *International Journal of Bioinformatics and Intelligent Computing*, *4*, 1–38.

Vignesh, M. (2024). Al in Predictive. *AI-Powered Advances in Pharmacology*, 61.

Visan, A. I., & Negut, I. (2024). Integrating artificial intelligence for drug discovery in the context of revolutionizing drug delivery. *Life (Chicago, Ill.)*, *14*(2), 233. PMID: 38398742

Yingngam, B., Navabhatra, A., & Sillapapibool, P. (2024). AI-Driven Decision-Making Applications in Pharmaceutical Sciences. In *Using Traditional Design Methods to Enhance AI-Driven Decision Making* (pp. 1–63). IGI Global Scientific Publishing.

Zhang, K., Yang, X., Wang, Y., Yu, Y., Huang, N., Li, G., & Yang, S. (2025). Artificial intelligence in drug development. *Nature Medicine*, ●●●, 1–15. PMID: 39833407

KEY TERMS AND DEFINITIONS

Drug Efficacy: A compound's ability to produce the desired effect.

Machine Learning Models: Algorithms learning patterns from pharmaceutical data.

Toxicity Prediction: Forecasting harmful biological drug responses computationally.

Chapter 8
Artificial Intelligence in Clinical Trials of Drugs

Bancha Yingngam
https://orcid.org/0000-0001-7215-9123
Faculty of Pharmaceutical Sciences, Ubon Ratchathani University, Thailand

ABSTRACT

Artificial intelligence (AI) is revolutionizing the clinical trial paradigm in the pharmaceutical industry at a rapid pace. Machine learning, natural language processing, and real-time analytics enhance every phase of clinical trials—from protocol design and recruitment to monitoring, analysis, and regulatory submission. AI algorithms have been shown to reduce trial length and increase the probability of success. They also enable more personalized and effective strategies for patient engagement. Therefore, this chapter discusses the theoretical frameworks from major international regulatory perspectives and introduces some of the new innovations using AI through all phases (I–IV) of the trials. In addition, the chapter emphasizes the promise and challenges that await AI in clinical development pipelines.

INTRODUCTION

Clinical trials remain the backbone of evidence-based drug development and are notoriously inefficient, cumbersome, and expensive. A typical clinical trial lasts 6–8 years, costing $1.5–2.6 billion. Patient recruitment and data analysis are usually the most expensive stages (Kant et al., 2025; Yingngam & Sethabouppha, 2024). Nearly 80% of trials fail to meet their enrollment targets in a timely manner, and many are ultimately terminated owing to design or operational flaws, which could have been avoided. In recent years, the number of trials and their overall complexity have increased dramatically owing to personalized therapies and new modalities.

DOI: 10.4018/979-8-3373-5258-9.ch008

For example, in 2023, over 400,000 trials were registered worldwide; more than 80% faced enrollment delays, costing $200 billion annually, with success rates under 12% (Olawade et al., 2026). Artificial intelligence (AI) now offers transformative solutions across the entire clinical trial life cycle. Advanced modeling and machine learning platforms use historical trial data to optimize design, simulate enrollment, and analyze results in real time. Previous studies have occasionally suggested dramatic performance "uplifts," such as claims of 65% faster patient recruitment and 40% lower costs (Olawade et al., 2026). However, subsequent analyses indicated that these effects are highly context dependent, with average gains typically closer to 25–35% improvements in recruitment speed in oncology and metabolic trials and 15–30% reductions in operational costs when risk-based monitoring is implemented (Bikou et al., 2024; Goldberg Jana et al., 2024). In addition, digital biomarkers derived from social and sensor data allow continuous assessment and monitoring in real time, with ±90% sensitivity for the early detection of adverse events (Olawade et al., 2026). These advances promise safer clinical trials across all phases (I–IV), reducing attrition rates without compromising scientific rigor (Akbarialiabad et al., 2025). AI technologies are integrated across the entire clinical–trial lifecycle—from adaptive trial design and predictive recruitment to continuous safety monitoring and outcome prediction—transforming trial efficiency and success rates (Figure 1). While AI contributes substantial efficiency gains, such estimates must be framed within specific assumptions—the trial phase, data maturity, and regulatory environment—and not generalized across all therapeutic areas. The evidence base remains evolving; comparative trials and meta-analyses show consistent but variable effects, highlighting the importance of transparent reporting and multisource validation.

Figure 1. Overview of AI applications across clinical trial phases

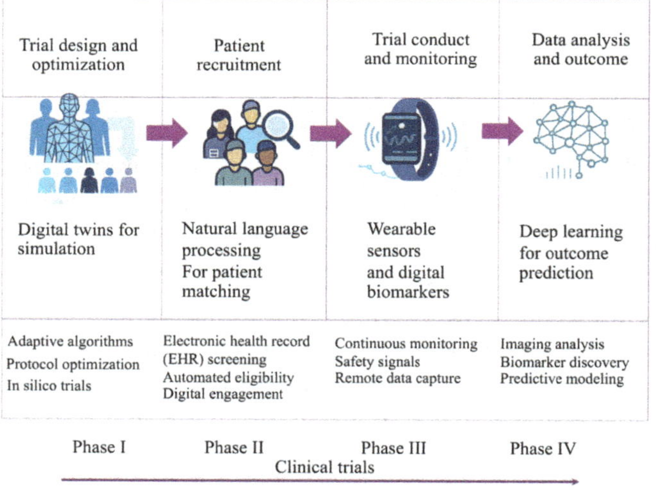

AI methods are actively applied from protocol planning in early-phase trials (Phases I–II) through patient recruitment, site selection, and operational execution in later phases (phases III–IV). In early clinical trials in which patients are recruited, ML-driven simulation and Bayesian modeling are utilized to optimize both dose–escalation decisions and calculations of sample size requirements, assisting in forms of adaptive designs. For example, in oncology trials, AI has been used to optimize inclusion criteria and biomarker endpoints, allowing smaller or more targeted cohorts with retained statistical power (Askin et al., 2023). Unsupervised learning and digital-twin technologies generate virtual patient cohorts for *in silico* testing of protocol variations, improving trial safety and efficiency. Digital twin technology espouses the definition of computational models of individual patients, which will allow the simulation of disease progression and the response to therapeutic modalities. This will provide improvements in safety assessment but will also allow for synthetic control arms in rare disease studies (Akbarialiabad et al., 2025). Indeed, one review of AI methods noted that AI was capable of systematic predications of clinical trial phase transitions (e.g., phase II trials complete to efficacy) and optimal design solutions for phases of clinical trials suited to speedier assessments or trials with reduced financial risk (Cho et al., 2025; Teodoro et al., 2025).

Patient identification and recruitment is yet another phase in which AI is rapidly making inroads into trial design. Advanced natural language processing (NLP) and ML algorithms are actively employed to analyze electronic health records (EHRs), clinical notes, laboratory data, and even social media data, with the aim of matching patients suitably to trials. Thus, natural language models can automatically optimize certain unstructured eligibility criteria against suitable patient profiles, thus improving prescreening of clinical EHRs. Large language models (LLMs), for example, have been shown to provide optimal solutions for the automation of patient–trial matching for the extraction of certain trial-oriented features from text, with the goal of decreasing the amount of human activity demanded for this exercise and the associated costs (Askin et al., 2023; Lin et al., 2025). Targeted AI-driven recruitment tools and networks have increased in diversity and reach through identifying suitably underrepresented subgroups. In a recent analysis, it was demonstrated that recruiting tools described as AI-driven provided a two-thirds improvement in overall recruitment efficiency (Olawade et al., 2026). Various studies have shown that certain predictive algorithms can identify likely drop outs or noncompliance with protocols ahead of time, so potential early interventions can be made or dynamic adjustments can be made to the inclusion criteria (Cho et al., 2025; Teodoro et al., 2025). These tools are now being integrated into the management of trial operations. For example, AI-driven referral networks can identify and contact potential participants via email or social media, but conversational agents can also provide prequalification of patients prior to visits to clinical sites.

Once the trial is running, AI-powered monitoring and real-time analytics will improve the safety and data quality of trials (phases II–IV). Sensor networks and mobile health technologies provide the opportunity for the collection of continuous data related to vital signs, degree of activity and patient-reported outcome data. ML systems analyze these identified "digital markers" in real time, with the potential elimination of either trial safety signals or protocol deviation points. For example, deep learning on computer-aided ECG or activity data can provide alerts for investigators to detect adverse trends much faster than scheduled attendance at clinics for visits. AI-driven anomaly detection tools highlight inconsistencies or missing data in data banks for a clinical trial, reducing the chances of human error in data entry. Notably, advanced risk-based monitoring frameworks leverage data to utilize AI methods to select site audits that focus appropriately on the most vulnerable cases. A review of qualitative methodologies revealed that AI-driven risk assessment tools (safety, efficacy and operational risk) are a burgeoning field, e.g., predictive models of the risk of adverse events or clinical dropout, vastly improving operational oversight across phases II–III of the trail (Teodoro et al., 2025). Predictive models (e.g., neural survival models) have been reported to optimize clinical trial duration forecasts and decision-making so that they expedite clinical trial testing and allow much better resource allocation (Cho et al., 2025).

Thus, the gross summary is that AI and related technologies are radically changing in all phases of clinical trials across phases I–IV. In the design of protocols, ML and simulation-driven tools allow adaptive and efficient study designs (Askin et al., 2023). In relation to recruitment, NLP and AI analytic features vastly improve the speed of recruitment into clinical trials and patient matching for inclusion in clinical trials (Lin et al., 2025; Olawade et al., 2026). In the actual conduct of a clinical trial, AI-driven real-time analytics are dominated by wearable physical devices for the capture of both safety assessments and the dynamic management of clinical trials (Akbarialiabad et al., 2025; Olawade et al., 2026). The enabling of systems for predictive modeling includes the discharge and transferability of divergent data (genomics, imaging and real-world evidence, etc.) for the prediction of different outcomes at scientific levels and the assistance of alert-providing decision-making (Cho et al., 2025). The maturation of the AI toolkit, which is popular in drug development, suggests that its application in clinical trials should lead to vastly increased efficiency, increased patient safety and shorter times to market for new therapies (Olawade et al., 2026).

This chapter aims to provide a practitioner-focused overview of AI and its incorporation into each of the various human-involved parts of trial design and delivery. A core review of the main theoretical paradigms in AI is provided, for example, under the headings of supervised learning models in relation to features of patient selection and recruitment, deep learning methods employed to greatly affect digital biomarker analysis, etc. How various AI toolkits interact with regulatory issues, ethical ones and the transition to decentralized and hybrid trials are also discussed. Two case studies are analyzed in a comprehensive fashion as demonstrative real-life examples of clinical trials enhanced through AI: Pfizer's REMOTE trial in overactive bladder and Verily's Baseline Health Study, a long-term major digital, phenotyping study. These findings provide suitable and wide-ranging examples regarding the operational, technical and regulatory dynamics when implementing such AI-enhanced trials. The chapter concludes with an analysis of areas of present shortcomings and future developments in context, for example, ranging from issues of algorithmic transparency to issues of data interoperability and the changing role that regulators will take in the approval process of AI-enabled protocols. In essence, at a time when the pharmaceutical industry is entering an exciting era of digital therapeutics and personalized medicine, understanding the practical applications of AI in clinical trials is not merely advantageous but vital. This chapter not only reviews each AI paradigm individually but also emphasizes their synergistic integration across the clinical trial continuum. For example, natural language processing (NLP) identifies eligible participants, federated learning (FL) preserves privacy during multisite analysis, and digital twin modeling enables adaptive simulation. Together, these methods form an integrated "AI trial ecosystem" in which data flow continuously between the design, recruitment, monitoring, and analysis phases.

THEORETICAL FRAMEWORKS FOR AI IN CLINICAL TRIALS

Clinical trials produce complex and multimodal data through various phases, from early safety assessments to postmarketing surveillance. AI methods are categorized into primary paradigms—supervised learning, unsupervised learning (including generative models), reinforcement learning, deep learning, federated learning, natural language processing (NLP) and digital twins (digital representations)—with each paradigm suited to specific tasks. Supervised learning models are trained on known trial data (such as outcomes or eligibility) to perform classification or regression analyses (Miller et al., 2023). In practice, for example, if one wishes to predict patient responses and trial success, logistic regression or ensemble classifiers could be employed. For example, supervised random forest algorithms have been used to predict the likelihood of drug approval in phases II and III (Lin et al., 2025) and show how patient features and early phase results can be used in the construction of models to predict future outcomes. Such models can assist in protocol design by simulating the endpoint probability, evaluating which criteria to include and which subpopulations to stratify according to risk.

Unsupervised learning techniques work on unlabeled data to find hidden structural features, such as clustering patients according to profiles of their biomarkers or assays for anomalous behavior. Techniques such as k-means clustering or principal component analysis can assist in identifying clusters of trial participants with similar characteristics, perhaps indicating subpopulations for rigorous analysis. To create synthetic trial data or augment datasets that may be limited, generative models (a form of unsupervised learning), such as variational autoencoders or GANs, are able to create synthetic trial data. Such models "work to produce novel data products", converting structured inputs or noise to realistic samples (Miller et al., 2023). The generative networks are used in the area of clinical trials, and simulations of patient trajectories or the creation of high-resolution images from low-resolution data images have been explored, allowing *in silico* experimentation without any risk to patients. By extracting hidden structures (latent mappings) (for example, disease subtypes or hidden phenotypes), unsupervised or AI may assist with exploratory evaluations of trial data in later studies and even suggest changes to eligibility rules to increase cohort diversity.

Reinforcement learning (RL) uses strategies to explore problems of sequential decision making, achieving a policy that maximizes the cumulative reward. The RL strategy has an "agent" (for example, a trial decision algorithm) exploring actions (for example, assigning doses or boosting the level of recruitment) and obtaining feedback (reward) as feedback (generally reward) on the basis of performance in the trial (Miller et al., 2023). For example, an RL agent may modify the dose escalation rules in a phase I dose evaluation trial or pair patients adaptively with certain treatment arms in a phase III trial, aiming to enhance results on the basis of either efficacy or safety. Although the use of RL in clinical trials is in its infancy, early explorations revealed how this approach may be used to optimize adaptive trial designs and to personalize treatment regimens. RL models "respond to rewards by … adjusting parameters (of the model)" (Miller et al., 2023). This approach renders RL particularly suited for the monitoring of trial conduct with the ability for real-time adjustments, for example, dynamically altering the plan of treatment or modifying randomization ratios as new data come to hand. Deep learning involves multilayer architectures of neural networks that are capable of producing mappings that are complex and high dimensional.

Convolutional neural networks (CNNs), recurrent networks and transformers fall into this category of models. Such techniques are well developed for working with those large, unstructured data streams that arise in trials—imaging, genomics, time series from sensors or free format text. In imaging trials, CNNs have been shown to produce spectacular results, such as the ability of CNNs to analyze retinal angiography/radiography images to quantify treatment effects (Lin et al., 2025). Deep networks require millions of parameters and specialized hardware (GPUs) for effective training. However, these techniques learn how to tease apart nonobvious features. A neural network might analyze continuous biometric signals or electrocardiograms that might be obtained during the monitoring process or could learn about complex interrelations of an electronic health record (EHR). Deep learning is also utilized in the production of large language models (LLMs) for the area of NLP. Generally, the area of deep learning produces very powerful and end-to-end learning tools for trial data (classifying responders, automatic endpoint detection, image segmentation and so on), which simply cannot be matched by conventional techniques (Lin et al., 2025; Miller et al., 2023).

Federated learning is a privacy-preserving strategy for the collaborative analysis of (training of) models of multiple centers. In federated learning, each trial site (or data owner) trains a local model on its local patient dataset, and these local model updates (not data) are transmitted to a server (which coordinates the federated process) where a global model may be produced (Hu et al., 2024). This is particularly useful from a patient privacy and data sovereignty point of view in multisite phase III and larger studies. The strategy works by "jointly training a global model while preserving the privacy of their local data" (Hu et al., 2024), meaning that diverse, geographically distributed trial data can be used without the need to centralize sensitive data. In the area of clinical trials, this means that predictive models (either of recruitment or of outcomes) can be improved on from the quality of experience in the area of that many hospitals, without requiring patient-level data from any one institution. The use of federated learning techniques may thus be a suitable methodology for the data analytics of multicenter trials (for example, shared learning of common eligibility scoring frameworks or prediction models with enormous databases) while embodying the necessary regulatory framework issues.

Natural language processing (NLP) and its most recent avatar, which is represented by large language models (LLMs), is necessary for cutting through the analysis of unstructured data and text data within clinical trials. NLP algorithms extract meaningful information from sources such as literature, clinical notes or reports written in normal language. As an example of such analysis, NLP may look at EHRs (clinical notes) or trial registries, compare notes, match patients with trial opportunities and assist in recruitment. As has been observed in recent trials, NLP has been applied to "screening" of "unstructured" clinical text, which allows automated patient–trial matching, resulting in vastly accelerated enrollment (Miller et al., 2023). IBM's Watson is illustrative and is able to combine patient ascertainment with target eligibility criteria, leading to a greater than 80% increase in patient enrollment rates in oncology trials (Miller et al., 2023). LLMs can also, in a more general sense, be trained with a corpus of biological data to automatically extract PICO elements (which represent protocol definitions) or wording inclusion or exclusion rules during the course of protocol design (Lin et al., 2025). During the course of a clinical trial, NLP can produce real-time alerts (for example, identifying the elements of EHRs that use updated criteria for new studies). NLP can also process narrative safety reports (Miller et al., 2023). Language models therefore offer techniques to automatically read, write and generate clinical trial documentation (protocols, case report forms, regulatory information) during the inputs of a clinical trial process and allow for the rapid application of tasks such as cohort identification and data curation.

Digital twins are virtual copies of the patient, organ or trial and are the mechanism for permitting *in silico* experimentation. In a clinical trial context, a digital twin can work by using mechanistic models (physiological simulators, etc.) and patient data to predict how an individual or cohort would respond to or be affected by a proposed intervention. Trial designers can therefore experiment with protocol variations, testing the designs before human studies are performed, by developing "digital replicas of physical systems" that are computably tried in trial scenarios. Digital twins can model processes that involve drug actions at the molecular level to organ responses, thereby increasing the understanding of a disease and the discovery of novel biomarkers. In practical terms, a digital twin approach may simulate thousands of virtual patients undergoing experimental protocols to provide a picture of the expected results of the action on such groups or individuals or to identify safety profiles (Bordukova et al., 2024; März et al., 2025). This technique has the potential to lower phases of trials (both cost and risk) by consolidating resource focus to those designs most likely to produce a favorable result. The careful use of digital twins could mean that trial burdens could be lowered in virtual trials of early phases, increasing the ease of stratifying patients and even allowing *in silico* arms to trials to reinforce human–man control arms (März et al., 2025). Newer techniques involve generative AI as a form of AI to create digital twins of specific patients along the way of trials. The merging of mechanistic forms of experimentation with data-driven methods has the capacity to create improved effects when addressing dosing techniques and the likelihood of comprehensively individualized treatment regimens at the later phases of trials.

The applications of AI frameworks in clinical trials can be conceptualized into several major paradigms, each with unique analytical and operational advantages throughout the trial life cycle. These include supervised, unsupervised, reinforcement and deep learning paradigms as well as federated learning, natural language processing and digital twin technologies. These paradigms are summarized in Table 1, which presents their basic principles of learning, foremost applications in clinical research, and representative examples from the literature. These paradigms also enable data-driven design of clinical trials, optimal recruitment processes, continuous monitoring, and outcome prediction but retain patient privacy and regulatory compliance. Thus, traditional trials have been transformed from a linear process into a continuum of adaptive intelligent paradigms for trial management, enabling real-time decision making for optimal patient management.

Table 1. Summary of artificial intelligence paradigms applied in clinical trials

AI paradigm	Core principle/learning type	Typical applications in clinical trials	Key advantages	References
Supervised learning	Model learns from labeled datasets to predict known outcomes (classification/ regression)	Predicting trial success rates, patient response modeling, endpoint prediction, safety signal classification	Improves accuracy of trial outcome prediction; enhances protocol design through simulation of endpoints	Lin et al. (2025); Miller et al. (2023)
Unsupervised learning	Discovers hidden patterns or clusters in unlabeled data	Identifying patient subgroups, discovering hidden phenotypes, outlier detection, exploratory data analysis	Enables discovery of new biomarkers or subpopulations; augments diversity and precision in cohort selection	Ali et al. (2025); Miller et al. (2023)
Reinforcement learning (RL)	Algorithm optimizes sequential decision-making by maximizing cumulative reward	Adaptive trial design, dose-escalation optimization, dynamic treatment allocation	Supports real-time adjustments and adaptive randomization, improving ethical and statistical efficiency	Miller et al. (2023); Park and Nycklemoe (2025)
Deep learning (DL)	Multilayer neural networks extract complex, nonlinear features from high-dimensional data	Imaging analysis, signal processing from wearables, endpoint detection, multimodal data fusion	Automates image and sensor analysis with high accuracy; identifies digital biomarkers	Houssein et al. (2025); Lin et al. (2025)
Federated learning (FL)	Distributed model training without sharing raw data; local updates aggregated into a global model	Multicenter trials, privacy-preserving data integration, real-world data analytics	Enhances collaboration across sites while maintaining patient privacy and data sovereignty	Hu et al. (2024); Madathil et al. (2025)

continued on following page

Table 1. Continued

AI paradigm	Core principle/learning type	Typical applications in clinical trials	Key advantages	References
Natural language processing (NLP)/large language models (LLMs)	Algorithms extract meaning from unstructured text data (e.g., EHRs, protocols, literature)	Eligibility screening, protocol generation, patient-trial matching, automated documentation	Reduces manual screening workload; accelerates recruitment and protocol review	Lin et al. (2025); Su et al. (2023)
Digital twins	Virtual representations of patients or trials simulating biological and clinical processes	*In silico* trials, synthetic control arms, dose optimization, safety assessment	Enables simulation of trial outcomes, reduces sample size, improves safety and ethics	Akbarialiabad et al. (2025); Bordukova et al. (2024); März et al. (2025)

AI IN TRIAL DESIGN AND OPTIMIZATION

Study Planning

Innovative AI methods are essential for designing resource-efficient clinical trials. For example, ML methods can analyze historical clinical trial data and EHRs, suggesting optimal sample sizes, endpoints, and populations (Askin et al., 2023; Kant et al., 2025). AI-enhanced feasibility tools that estimate enrollment rates and site performance assist sponsors in determining if a purported protocol is feasible. *In silico* simulations are key innovations: Digital twin frameworks provide cohorts of virtual patients who simulate real patients. Generative models synthesize "complementary-patient" twins of realistic clinical features, facilitating whole intervention and placebo arms *in silico* (Akbarialiabad et al., 2025; Kleeberger, 2025). AI-driven methods such as digital twin simulation and adaptive randomization frameworks are increasingly being used to improve trial precision and efficiency across phases I–III. As shown in Figure 2, AI makes it possible to generate patient-specific models from real-world data and assign these models to either control or interventional arms, simulating outcomes (Akbarialiabad et al., 2025). Such *in silico* trials give investigators the ability to test dosing-sensitive projected efficacy and safety signals without exposing real patients to risk, frequently reducing both the required sample size and trial duration.

Figure 2. AI-driven trial–design frameworks. (Left) Digital twin simulation: Virtual patients are generated from patient data and used to simulate both the placebo (control) and intervention arms. (Right) Adaptive randomization: Machine learning models continuously update treatment-assignment probabilities on the basis of interim outcome predictions

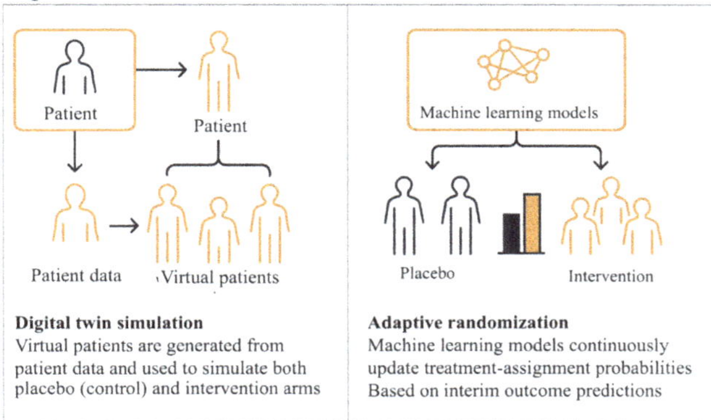

Artificial intelligence tools are now integrated into every step of a clinical trial, from the design of the protocol to postmarketing surveillance. Table 2 shows the application of these technologies throughout Phases I to IV. Digital twins and reinforcement learning modify design and dosage through adaptive design. In the phase of large-scale testing for efficacy, federated learning and NLP improve the efficiency of recruitment and the quality of the data. After marketing, deep learning and analytics on real-world data allow for rapid detection of safety signals. Thus, these technologies overall change clinical trials from static, linear processes to dynamic, data-driven systems that allow for real-time decision-making processes and oversight of individual participants.

Adaptive methods involve further trials via adaptive algorithms. In adaptive randomization, AI-based models predict which treatment is thought to be more effective, and future assignments are biased accordingly. For example, an ML method for adaptive design (MARGO) has been created that dynamically updates patient-allocation weights to bias them toward treatments with a higher predicted chance of success, all while controlling type I error rates rigorously (Park & Nycklemoe, 2025). Additionally, it has recently been noted that response-adaptive methods supervised by ML may optimize treatment effect estimation in real time (Teodoro et al., 2025). Overall, AI-saturated adaptive designs, which learn from cumulative data dictatorial for trials, ultimately improve patient-provided benefits if they are part of the trials, complementing the complimentary simulations to maximize the optimization efficiency.

Table 2. AI-enabled innovations across clinical trial phases (I–IV)

Clinical trial phase	Primary objectives	AI technologies/ tools applied	Key innovations and impacts	References
Phase I – trial design and feasibility	Assess safety, tolerability, pharmacokinetics, and determine initial dosing	• Machine learning (ML) simulation models • Bayesian adaptive design • Digital twin *in silico* simulations • Reinforcement learning for dose-escalation	• Optimizes dose-escalation and sample-size requirement • Predicts safety events before occurrence • Reduces participant exposure through virtual cohorts	Akbarialiabad et al. (2025); Askin et al. (2023)
Phase II – proof-of-concept and dose optimization	Evaluate preliminary efficacy and refine dose–response relationships	• Supervised learning (regression, decision trees) • Deep neural networks for biomarker discovery • Predictive analytics platforms	• Identifies responders/ nonresponders early • Improves adaptive endpoint selection • Shortens cycle time by early futility detection	Arango-Argoty et al. (2025); Cho et al. (2025)
Phase III – efficacy confirmation and large-scale validation	Confirm therapeutic efficacy and monitor adverse events across diverse populations	• Natural language processing for eligibility screening • Federated learning for multisite data integration • AI-driven adaptive randomization • Risk-based monitoring dashboards	• Accelerates patient recruitment by ≈ 65% • Enhances diversity and inclusion • Improves data integrity and early anomaly detection	Madathil et al. (2025); Olawade et al. (2026); Park and Nycklemoe (2025)
Phase IV – postmarketing surveillance and real-world evidence	Monitor long-term safety, effectiveness, and rare adverse events	• Deep learning for signal detection • Natural language models for pharmacovigilance • Federated analytics across registries • Digital biomarkers from wearable sensors	• Detects safety signals 30–50% faster than traditional methods • Generates real-world evidence continuously • Supports regulatory decisions with transparent, explainable AI	Ferreira and Carneiro (2025); Pedroso and Khera (2025); Teodoro et al. (2025)

Protocol Review

Natural language processing (NLP) involves changing the writing and reviewing of trial protocols, especially eligibility criteria. A 2023 review stated that NLP and computable query generation are at the cutting edge of trial eligibility research (Su et al., 2023). Modern NLP pipelines can read unstructured inclusion/exclusion texts and map them to standard clinical concepts. For example, automated systems such as CriteriaMapper normalize free text criteria into structured attributes, which can then be matched to patient records. One study showed concordance, with $\kappa \approx 0.82$ for manual curation, and the F1 patient-matching score was 0.94 (Lee et al., 2024). The AI accurately identified more than half of the unique criteria (e.g., Stage III lung cancer, laboratory ranges), and this method identified eligible patients with a high degree of accuracy.

Simultaneously, large language models and rule-based systems that generate EHR queries from protocol text are under development. These tools, which are based on Criteria2Query, can use GPT4 to turn complex phrases of criteria into executable SQL or OMOP-CDM queries. These systems allow clinical researchers to interactively review and edit the mapped logic. By converting free text criteria into computable forms, AI allows rapid patient–trial matching and flags inconsistencies or prohibitive criteria. In practice, NLP-enhanced review will allow for the discovery of latent biases or gaps in the protocol and ensure that the trial meets its targeted population effectively.

In conclusion, AI-enhanced analysis of protocol documents makes the review and site selection processes more efficient. By validating eligibility logic against real-world data, sponsors can iteratively optimize criteria for recruitment. Tools to convert narrative criteria into formal queries not only speed but also gather metrics on the feasibility of patient screening for trials. These developments make the review of the protocol more data driven and therefore decrease the likelihood of delays and improve the chances of successful recruitment (Su et al., 2023).

AI IN PATIENT RECRUITMENT

Patient enrollment in clinical trials is often slow and prone to error, delaying nearly 80% of studies by an average of 6–8 months. Approximately one-third of all trial sites do not enroll any subjects without some special measures. AI-completed tools are beginning to relieve this bottleneck by automating and improving various steps in the recruitment process. For example, NLP and machine-learning models can scour large EHR databases to identify potentially eligible participants with a level of speed and precision previously inconceivable (Olawade et al., 2026; Yingngam, 2025). A recent review revealed that AI-activated recruitment tools increased enrollment by approximately 65%, whereas predictive analytics produced an 85% improvement in predictiveness, leading to a reduction in trial completion time of as much as 50% (Olawade et al., 2026). In practical terms, structured and unstructured clinical data (such as diagnostic codes, laboratory results, and clinical notes) are analyzed by algorithms to speed up the matching of patients with trials, allowing clinical personnel to devote themselves to outreach rather than review. Predictive matching models also classify patients with respect to enrollment in and completion of trials, allowing sponsors to focus their outreach on the most likely candidates (Olawade et al., 2026).

By incorporating AI-augmented workflows, modern patient recruitment pipelines frequently conform to a three-phase scheme, namely, (A) EHR/NLP screening, where advanced NLP engines run automated evaluations to assess EHR data for inclusion/exclusion criteria to provide information on trial eligibility (Olawade et al., 2026). Most systems employ structured approaches (diagnostic codes, limits to lab values) to perform noninflammatory selection, whereas NLP systems address the reading of clinical notes for various subtle clues. One survey of EHR-enabled support systems revealed that more than 50% of them relied on querying structured data to match patients with trials (Vaterkowski et al., 2025). By placing the trial protocol into the EHR, these tools may work continuously in the background, functioning autonomously and informing investigators when matching patients to light. (B) Digital engagement: where identified patients receive tailored digital outreach. Chatbots, apps, and web portals can provide personalized information about a trial and facilitate the consent process. Conversational AI interfaces answer patient questions and respond to their literacy and cultural reading assessments in real time (Olawade et al., 2026).). This outreach is advantageous because it is 24/7 accessible and facilitates the education and consent process without burning out clinical personnel. Ultimately, (C) automated retention and the enlisted assistants are reminded to stay committed via personalized touchpoints. Intelligent reminders, health tips and updates via text and email are individualized according to patient preference. Studies show that retention is greatly improved through tailored outreach; one platform in use "helps to identify the patients best suited for recurrent trials" and informs them in a way that boosts adherence (Olawade et al., 2026).

As outlined in Figure 4, an AI-enabled patient recruitment pipeline integrates these characteristics fluidly. At (A) EHR/NLP screening, ML exploits algorithmic approaches to information in electronic form to identify members of the required cohort with accuracy. At (B) digital engagement, interactive supporting technologies (chatbots, apps, purpose-designed messaging) provide candidates with information about ongoing trials and help them with enrollment as needed. At (C) automated retention, the same or related technologies continue to be made available for support systems — e.g., reminders, supporting information) to patients, aiding their commitment during ongoing trials. This entire pipeline accelerates patient enrollment for trials while meeting the additional requirement of patients being enrolled long enough in the trials to provide significant results (Olawade et al., 2026). An integrated, AI-powered pipeline from EHR screening to personalized engagement and adaptive retention forms the core of modern recruitment strategies (Figure 3).

Figure 3. Schematic of an AI-driven clinical trial recruitment pipeline

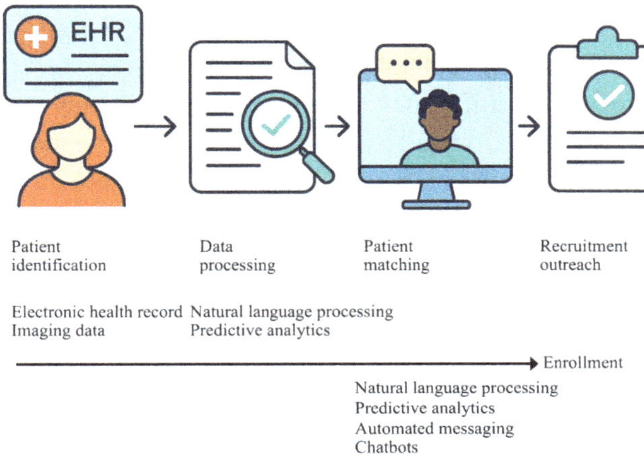

Most significantly, AI brings diversity and inclusion. By analyzing demographic fields and social determinants in real-world data, algorithms can identify underrepresented groups and tag any potential barriers to participation (Olawade et al., 2026). For example, NLP-enabled tools can also note information that indicates transportation difficulties or limited language skills in patient notes, thereby informing trialists of features of outreach necessary for those populations (e.g., offering language help and transport) needed. AI algorithms that are "fairness aware" contain demographic and diverse features for patient matching as a specific feature (Shams et al., 2025). Thus, AI helps address the biases in traditional recruitment, which results in cohorts that are homogenous (Olawade et al., 2026; Shams et al., 2025). Evidence is that adding electronic features (digital means of support) and targeting (AI-enabled) improves the recruitment of racial/ethnic minorities and women, allowing trials to be more reflective of real-world populations. Diversity principles can be embedded in all stages of patient outreach problems and EHR screening through communication; hence, AI-enabled recruitment can be made to be inclusive without losing efficiency. The fusion of electronic health records analytics with predictive matching and individualized digital outreach is changing the recruitment of patients for participation in clinical trials. Clearly, machine learning models reduce the list rapidly of eligible candidates, NLP-assisted chatbots inform and consent to the patients thus selected, and continue messaging keeps the attention of the patients thus selected. Thus,

AI-enabled processes lead to greater enrollment rates, reduced costs and greater participant diversity (Olawade et al., 2026).

AI IN TRIAL CONDUCT AND MONITORING

AI systems can interpret continuously collected streams of digital data to monitor the conduct of clinical trials in real time. Recent studies have shown that AI-enabled monitoring systems can identify safety signals up to 30–50% faster than traditional review cycles can and reduce overall trial timelines by the same margin (Olawade et al., 2026). For example, digital markers of health and disease can be derived from wearable devices (pulse rates, accelerometry, ECG, etc.) via deep learning models (Olawade et al., 2026). Similar techniques can be applied to imaging and laboratory data whereby quantitative markers of patient status are obtained automatically. This pipeline is illustrated in Figure 4. Thus, data from wearables, smartphones, imaging and laboratory sensors are fed into AI/ML algorithms, which derive predictive biomarkers and provide alerts to monitors. This enables 24-hour monitoring for adverse medical events and clinical changes, far surpassing traditional site visits (Olawade et al., 2026). In practice, AI applied to streams of digital biomarkers has shown remarkably high sensitivity (e.g., ≈90 % in the detection of early untoward events) through learning to ascertain patterns in continuous data (Olawade et al., 2026).

Figure 4. AI-driven monitoring tool pipeline

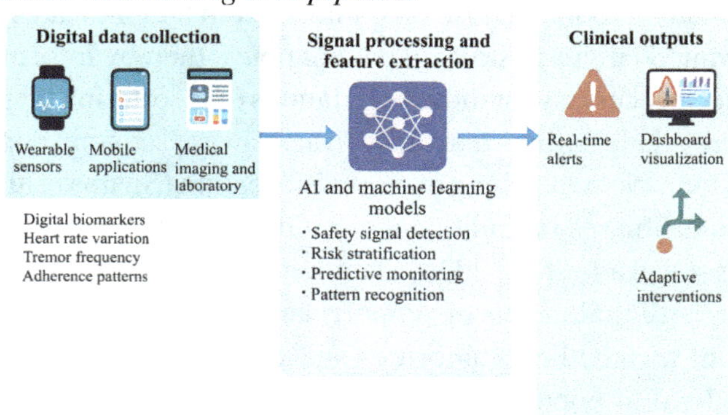

Continuous Digital Biomarkers

Modern trials are increasingly using intelligent sensors for data collection: wearable sensors collect physiologic measurements (ECG, actigraphy, pulse oximetry), smartphone-based apps record both behavior and speech, and even ingestible sensors ("digital pills") can measure when ingestion occurs (Liu et al., 2022; Reis et al., 2025). AI algorithms can fuse these input signals into actionable digital biomarkers (e.g., tremor frequency, gait metrics, and cardiac variability). These biomarkers can be continuously calculated and input into monitoring dashboards for trials. In Parkinson's disease studies, AI-based gait analysis using wearable sensors has achieved over 90% sensitivity and specificity, enabling earlier symptom detection (Twala, 2025). Thus, any concerning trend (e.g., arrhythmia episodes, symptom spikes) can be flagged immediately (Pedroso & Khera, 2025). The result is almost real-time safety surveillance without the need for manual review of logs or for scheduled visits.

Risk-Based Monitoring

AI enables a risk-based approach to monitoring trials since it can detect anomalies/deviations early. Machine learning techniques are capable of reviewing multisite trial data (CRFs, laboratory data, ePROs, etc.) to identify outliers, protocol deviations and data integrity problems (Teodoro et al., 2025). As an illustration, unsupervised models may identify a site with patterns of data that diverge from the norm of the study. In practice, AI-enhanced central monitoring has shown the ability to identify problems in 24–48 hours rather than weeks (Teodoro et al., 2025). These systems also predict which sites or patients are at the highest risk of noncompliance (by looking at past performance as well as real-time metrics) and allow monitors to intervene before (Cho et al., 2025). Early AI pilot studies have shown that timelines of trials can be 30–50% faster and greatly improve the quality of the data by targeting monitoring efforts to high-risk areas (Olawade et al., 2026; Teodoro et al., 2025).

Decentralized Trial Support

In decentralized trials or virtual trials, AI-enhanced apps and devices remotely validate behavior patterns in subjects. The smartphone apps utilize machine vision and/or sensor fusion to verify pill swallowing and other behavioral changes (subjects can, for example, record videos of themselves swallowing pills, and ML on the devices verifies it). Ingestible sensors tested in human trials have verified heart and respiration signals with ~92.7% accuracy, confirming adherence and physiological metrics in decentralized trials (Reis et al., 2025). Other AI apps utilize speech or movement analytics of phone calls or wearable data to verify missed doses or symptoms. These ML verifications minimize the need for or reliance on self-report or manual reconciliation methods, thus improving adherence tracking. In one study, AI-assisted digital interventions (video/voice prompts and monitoring) improved adherence by as much as ~30% (Reis et al., 2025).

Privacy-Preserving Integration

Combining heterogeneous sources of data—such as imaging, wearable, EHR, and registry datasets—often raises concerns about patient privacy and data security. Federated learning, a key AI paradigm, addresses this challenge by training machine learning models across distributed data silos without moving any raw patient data (Hu et al., 2024). In a typical FL framework, each trial site or hospital builds and trains a local model via its own dataset. Instead of sharing the underlying data, sites send only encrypted model parameters (weights) to a central aggregation server. The server then computes a weighted average of these parameters to produce a unified global model, which is subsequently redistributed back to all participating sites for further training. This iterative process continues until convergence, allowing the model to improve collaboratively while fully preserving patient privacy (Madathil et al., 2025). (see Figure 5 for an overview of the federated model aggregation process.)

In this way, AI models learn across metrics that might be real-world and remote data without violating patient confidentiality. Federated AI methods have been developed from consortiums spawned for rare diseases and multicenter trials, producing richer models of patient response without the transport or transfer of sensitive data (Madathil et al., 2025). Such usage of privacy-secure AI techniques facilitates such integration of onsite and real-world data flows into the conduct of decentralized trials, propagating security and monitoring capacity outside or beyond the walls of clinics (e.g., by means of smartphone health applications) and still conforming to guidelines set down in the GDPR/HIPAA regulations (Hu et al., 2024; Madathil et al., 2025).

Therefore, AI improves efforts at trial monitoring by transforming raw sensor and clinical data metrics into real-time predictive insights. These techniques produce improved monitoring methods, including continuous surveillance capacity, rapidity in the determination of anomalies, automated scoring of site performance, and patient verification methods that are usable in traditional or decentralized trials. The introduction of approaches such as federated learning and on-device AI serves to provide convincing argumentation that these advances inevitably contribute to fulfilling patients' sense of privacy even while enhancing or merging (even) remote data and real-world evidence into monitoring methods (Hu et al., 2024; Madathil et al., 2025).

Figure 5. Federated learning framework for privacy-preserving model aggregation across clinical trial sites

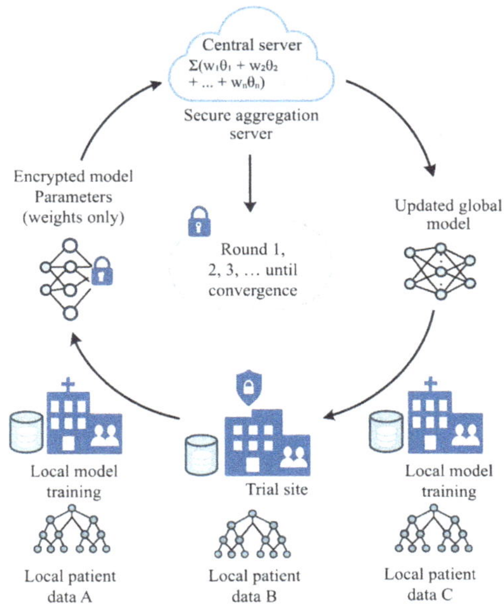

AI IN DATA ANALYSIS AND OUTCOME PREDICTION

Following a trial's conclusion, AI-enabled analytics can extract rich clinical and biomarker data to yield insights. For example, deep learning models can integrate multimodal datasets (such as imaging, genomics, and laboratory data) to reveal hidden patient subtypes and predictive signatures. One review reported that AI can recognize "subpopulations of patients who respond to particular treatments" and can find biological signatures involved in disease progression and drug response (Ali et al., 2025). Meta-learning algorithms (such as "meta-learners") are also used to estimate individualized treatment effects and assess heterogeneity in randomized trial data, thus answering the question of "what works for whom" by determining covariate-defined subpopulations with differing outcomes (Salditt et al., 2024).

Imaging and Biomarkers

CNNs facilitate the analysis of diagnostic images (MRIs, CT scans, and pathological slides) to derive new imaging biomarkers (tumor volume, lesion texture, etc.) that are related to trial endpoints. Importantly, explainability tools (Grad-CAM, SHAP, LIME, etc.) allow for the identification of the image features driving a prediction, which facilitates clinicians' interpretation of abnormalities detected by artificial intelligence (Houssein et al., 2025; Mohammad et al., 2025). Simply put, AI will no longer just segment or score lesions. Rather, it will be able to backtrack predictions to pixels or regions, which provides insight into imaging-based endpoints and risks.

For example, Figure 6 depicts a chest radiograph processed by a CNN that predicts the likelihood of treatment efficacy for pulmonary tuberculosis (TB). The colored overlay is a Grad-CAM heatmap: warm colors (red/orange) mark the regions that most influenced the model's prediction; cooler colors (green/blue) contributed less. In this example, salient regions include cavitations and dense consolidations in the right upper lobe—typical TB phenotypes associated with high bacillary burden. The model integrates these patterns into a probabilistic score indicating whether the current regimen is likely to succeed (e.g., sputum culture conversion by week 8).

Figure 6. Explainable convolutional neural network (CNN) for chest X-ray-based tuberculosis drug-response prediction. (A) Preprocessed PA chest radiograph with a lung-field mask (not shown). (B) CNN prediction head output probability of week-8 culture conversion under the current regimen. (C) Grad-CAM heatmap overlays highlight model-salient regions (red/orange) corresponding to cavitations and dense consolidations in the right upper lobe. (D) Derived biomarkers—cavity volume, lesion burden index, and upper-lobe weighting—are summarized alongside the predicted probability and its calibrated confidence interval. This visualization enables clinicians to relate model outputs to observable pathology and to track imaging-based endpoints on serial scans.

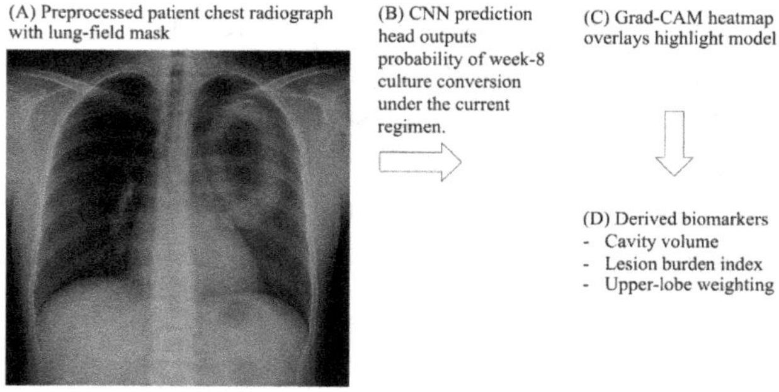

Subgroup Discovery

Unsupervised machine learning (ML) and clustering approaches applied to data collected after trial termination revealed hidden subgroups of patients (responders vs nonresponders) that were not prespecified. These approaches evaluate the genomics, proteomics and clinical covariates available during the trial to identify candidate predictive biomarker(s). For example, neural networks have been shown to identify interpretable predictive biomarkers from early-phase data that allow for better prediction of survival in phase III trials retrospectively. One such network led to a 15% increase in the predicted survival hazard in a phase III oncology trial when patients were stratified on the basis of early-phase data (Arango-Argoty et al., 2025). Similarly, flexible data-driven models can be used to explore many different combinations of covariates for the purpose of identifying effect modifiers for trial interventions, complementing traditional subgroup analysis while ensuring that any important subgroup is not neglected (Ali et al., 2025; Salditt et al., 2024).

Federated Meta-analyses

Federated learning (FL) frameworks allow for analyses across many centers or trials without pooling the subjects at the individual patient level. A 2021 multi-institution study demonstrated that FL improved model accuracy across diverse datasets without transferring patient data (Twala, 2025). In FL, each center (hospital or trial) trains its own local model on its own data and sends only model updates (not data) to a collective server. This distributed ML preserves privacy while enabling modeling of global knowledge that traverses all datasets (Madathil et al., 2025). For pharmaceuticals, FL can replicate a patient-level meta-analysis, as the investigators can collectively produce powerful models across trials (even in different countries) while protecting data governance. Essentially, FL allows for insights (new biomarkers or new risk factors) that are collective across studies while preserving the integrity of individual data (Madathil et al., 2025).

Predictive Endpoints

AI-based predictive analytics can be used to predict clinical endpoints or long-term outcomes from interim data. Machine learning time series or survival (if early-off treatment biomarkers or surrogate end points are used) can predict final efficacy end points. Recent work has emphasized that "AI models for predicting trial outcomes" can reduce failures and hasten decision-making (Qian et al., 2025; Yingngam et al., 2024). One study contained a neural network modeling framework that identified an early-interim predictive biomarker (based on routine data) that, if used to stratify patients, would have provided a 15% relative increase in the predicted survival hazard (Arango-Argoty et al., 2025). In practice, this approach allows sponsors to adjust the trial design (adaptive endpoints or enrollment) on the fly or to plan subsequent studies on the basis of AI projections.

Explainable AI (XAI) is critical to all of these applications. Efficacy techniques that are model-agnostic (such as Shapley additive exPlanations (SHAPs) and LIME) can decompose a prediction to identify how each feature contributes (Miller et al., 2023; Mohammad et al., 2025). For example, SHAP has been employed with wearable sensors and clinical data to clarify the key variables that explain a risk score (Mohammad et al., 2025). It is now recommended that "white-box" models or post hoc XAI be adopted: a recent review recommends that more stress be placed on 'white box' implementations, with models having interpretable outputs using… XAI" so outputs can be trusted (Ferreira & Carneiro, 2025). Additionally, regulatory authorities are now stressing transparency. The FDA and EMA are developing guidelines to delineate clear documentation for AI model validation and model interpretability for decision support tools. This means in practice that AI-driven predictions (new biomarkers or predictors) should be put forth with an explanation—showing what the causatives (e.g., lab results or image markers) are—so that the predictors or findings can be seen as applied to be probably respectable for regulators and clinicians.

The integration of AI transforms the way in which clinical trials are designed, conducted, and analyzed. Table 3 presents the contrasts between traditional and AI-based workflows from six key areas of trial activity: design, recruitment, monitoring, data for management, outcome analysis, and interaction with regulators. Conventional trials utilize static protocols and episodic supervision, whereas AI involves adaptive, automated and real-time intelligence at each point. These enhancements serve to shorten the time and cost of the trials while simultaneously improving the quality, diversity and transparency of the data. Overall, AI-based workflows heighten the speed of the transition of drug candidates into their postdiscovery phase and thus mark a change in the paradigm of clinical development into something that is both quicker and more efficacious, evidential and patient oriented.

Table 3. Comparison of traditional vs. AI-driven clinical trial workflows

Workflow dimension	Traditional clinical trials	AI-driven clinical trials	Measured or reported impact	References
Study design	Static protocol; fixed inclusion/exclusion criteria determined manually	Adaptive, data-driven design using ML simulation, Bayesian modeling, and digital twins	20–40% reduction in trial duration through adaptive simulation	Akbarialiabad et al. (2025); Askin et al. (2023)
Patient recruitment	Manual screening of limited site databases; slow enrollment	NLP and predictive analytics automatically match EHRs and demographics to trial criteria	~65% faster recruitment; improved participant diversity	Olawade et al. (2026); Su et al. (2023)
Monitoring & data capture	Periodic site visits; manual CRF entry; lagging adverse-event detection	Continuous real-time data from wearables and IoT sensors analyzed by deep-learning algorithms	30–50% faster safety-signal detection; improved data integrity	Pedroso and Khera (2025); Teodoro et al. (2025)
Data management	Centralized databases; manual cleaning and reconciliation; privacy risks	Federated learning integrates decentralized datasets without sharing raw data	Preserves patient confidentiality; enables global model accuracy gains of 10–20%	Hu et al. (2024); Madathil et al. (2025)
Outcome analysis	Conventional biostatistics; limited handling of complex or multimodal data	Deep and meta-learning integrate imaging, omics, and clinical data for predictive modeling	15% gain in predictive accuracy for survival and efficacy endpoints	Arango-Argoty et al. (2025); Qian et al. (2025)
Regulatory interaction	Manual documentation and delayed reporting	Automated report generation and explainable AI (XAI) ensure transparency for regulators	Faster review cycles; enhanced traceability and reproducibility	Ferreira and Carneiro (2025); Houssein et al. (2025)

In the past ten years, an increasing amount of research data has shown the real-world applicability of artificial intelligence in managing clinical investigations. Various trial types, from early digital biomarker feasibility studies to fully decentralized AI-assisted randomized controlled trials, have demonstrated noticeable improvements in recruitment efficiency, data quality, compliance and patient outcome. Table 4 shows selected clinical trials and pilot studies using AI techniques involving various therapeutic areas. These include arrhythmia detection via wearable sensor technology, digital twin-guided metabolic therapy, AI-assisted recruitment and monitoring and decentralized virtual trial methodology. The collective impact of these findings shows that AI-enabled systems yield operational improvements consistently, e.g., a reduction in enrollment periods of 30--50%, predictive accuracy over 90%, and retention of patients beyond 90%, while retaining or improving clinical validity.

These experimental data provide empirical evidence of the practical applicability and regulatory acceptability of AI-enabled innovations in modern clinical development.

Table 4. Selected clinical trials/studies using AI with experimental values

Trial/program (sponsor)	Year	Therapeutic area	Trial design and sample size	Artificial intelligence method used	Key experimental findings	Reference
Apple heart study (Stanford University and Apple Inc.)	2019	Cardiology – detection of atrial fibrillation	Prospective, single-arm, approximately 419,297 participants using smartwatches	Machine-learning algorithm analyzing pulse irregularity from wearable photoplethysmography	Positive predictive value for detecting atrial fibrillation was 0.84 (95% confidence interval 0.76–0.92); alert rate 0.52 percent of participants	Perez et al. (2019)
Fitbit irregular heart rhythm study	2022	Cardiology – detection of atrial fibrillation	Prospective digital-device cohort	Machine-learning–based rhythm classification on wearable sensor data	Participants who received irregular rhythm notifications showed a high probability of atrial fibrillation confirmation on electrocardiogram	Lubitz et al. (2022)
Verily study watch atrial fibrillation validation	2023	Cardiology – ambulatory rhythm monitoring	Multicenter ambulatory study, 117 participants (91,857 intervals analyzed)	Deep-learning model combining photoplethysmography and electrocardiography	Detection sensitivity 96.1%, specificity 98.1%, correlation for atrial fibrillation burden $R^2 = 0.986$	Poh et al. (2023)
Smartwatch early-warning COVID-19 trial	2020	Infectious disease – COVID-19 prediction	Observational, multidevice	Machine-learning algorithm on continuous physiological data	Physiological change detected in 81% of infected individuals before symptom onset	Mishra et al. (2020)
mSToPS continuous electrocardiogram trial	2024–25	Cardiology – atrial fibrillation detection	Randomized comparative study	Artificial-intelligence analysis of continuous patch electrocardiogram	Continuous electrocardiogram monitoring detected atrial fibrillation approximately ten times more often than standard home blood-pressure screening	Park and Bae (2025)
RECTIFIER artificial-intelligence prescreening trial	2024–25	Clinical trial operations – participant recruitment	Randomized implementation trial, 4,476 records screened	Natural-language processing and machine-learning applied to electronic health records	Artificial-intelligence prescreening produced 20.4% eligibility versus 12.7% with manual screening; time-to-eligibility improved by a factor of 1.78 ($p < 0.001$)	Unlu et al. (2025)
Digital twin diabetes real-world cohort	2024	Endocrinology – type 2 diabetes	Observational, 1,853 participants	Whole-body digital-twin platform integrating clinical and lifestyle data	89% achieved glycated hemoglobin below 7% at one year with sustained metabolic improvement	Shamanna et al. (2024)

continued on following page

Table 4. Continued

Trial/program (sponsor)	Year	Therapeutic area	Trial design and sample size	Artificial intelligence method used	Key experimental findings	Reference
Decentralized cardiovascular monitoring trial	2025	Cardiology – cardiovascular risk screening	Prospective multicenter	Artificial-intelligence algorithms applied to consumer device data for cardiovascular prediction	Enabled scalable population screening; improved detection of early cardiovascular risk patterns by 30–50% versus standard screening	Pedroso and Khera (2025)
HIV antiretroviral therapy adherence study	2022	Infectious disease – HIV treatment	Randomized controlled trial	Ingestible sensor system with artificial-intelligence-verified dose ingestion	Medication adherence significantly improved compared with standard self-report; sustained viral suppression correlated with digital-adherence data	Liu et al. (2022)

EMERGING TRENDS AND INNOVATIONS

AI-enabled technologies have extended throughout the pharmaceutical pipeline, from early drug discovery through the execution of clinical trials to clinical practice. For example, digital twin and synthetic control models utilizing AI to simulate patient trajectories can replace or augment the control arms in trials (Akbarialiabad et al., 2025). *In silico* cohorts created by deep models allow researchers to explore dosing and endpoints while performing traditional numbers of subjects and patient exposure (Akbarialiabad et al., 2025). Generative models (GANs, VAEs, LLMs) can also synthesize realistic patient data and images, providing large datasets for trials that are statistically indistinguishable from real-world records (Bordukova et al., 2024; Ferreira & Carneiro, 2025). Moreover, AI-augmented remote monitoring (wearables, biosensors) feeds into the above simulations, allowing for decentralized trials that improve participant engagement and retention through home-based telehealth (Alsabah et al., 2025). Together, the technologies in Figure 7 show how AI-based analytics and modeling can work together to make trials more efficient, adaptive and patient-centered.

Figure 7. AI-based analytics and modeling for trial innovation

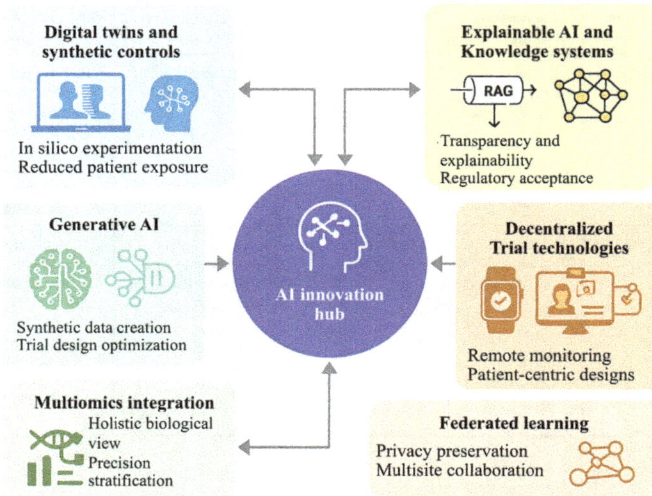

Digital Twins and Synthetic Controls

Both digital twins and synthetic control arms are novel AI-enabled innovations in clinical research, but they serve distinct purposes. A digital twin is a computationally engineered digital model of a human patient who is continuously fed with a math-digestible dataset of multimodal data that includes genomic, imaging and physiologic parameters to build the model continuously (Khumsikiew et al., 2025). This allows researchers to simulate separate patient disease and therapeutic progression scenarios to model patient-specific dosing functions, safety forecasts, and adaptive protocol improvements (Yingngam et al., 2025). A synthetic control arm is a virtual comparator arm built from aggregated real-world evidence data from historical or other methods, such as analysis of prior completed trials, or digital twins that can fill in or substitute for the placebo control arm in the trial design. While a digital twin models the progression of an individual patient, a synthetic control arm represents the aggregate trajectory of a comparable control population. Hence, digital twins function at the micro (single patient simulation, mechanistic modeling approach) level, whereas synthetic control arms are at the macro (population-controlled statistical testing) level (Chaiburi & Yingngam, 2025). In practical terms, digital twins can be used to construct synthesized synthetic control arm outcomes, but they are not interchangeable. The former is focused on dynamically generated patient-specific modeling, whereas the synthetic control arm models are focused on regulatory-level evidence generation through the alignment of either historic or digitized data with trial endpoints. Understanding this distinction is of paramount importance where transparency of trial design features is concerned with avoiding confusion and methodological conflations when reporting on AI-generated *in silico* evidentiary dataset evidence to regulators.

Patient-specific digital twins, computational avatars made from a person's genetics, physiology, and health data, are being developed as powerful trial innovations (Akbarialiabad et al., 2025). In essence, each real patient can be coupled with a labeled digital twin, the clinical course of which is predicted according to the standard of care; this digital course provides a synthetic control arm (Bordukova et al., 2024). By employing digital twins instead of or in conjunction with placebo groups, studies can lower necessary sample sizes, shorten timeframes and spare participants unnecessary risk (März et al., 2025). These authors noted that these twins not only increase efficiency but also elevate ethical standards (safety, justice, informed consent) by reducing the burden on patients (Akbarialiabad et al., 2025; März et al., 2025). Models driven by simulations can allow for ad hoc optimization of dosing and endpoint selection within adaptive designs.

Recent peer-reviewed studies have provided concrete demonstrations of digital-twin applications in real-world clinical research. For example, Voigt et al. (2021) discussed the development of digital–twin frameworks for multiple sclerosis (MS) research, highlighting how longitudinal magnetic resonance imaging and clinical data can be used to simulate patient-specific disease trajectories. Their work emphasized conceptual validation—showing that digital twin modeling could reproduce typical patterns of disease progression and treatment response observed in clinical trials, thereby illustrating the feasibility of constructing virtual comparators for neurological disorders. More recently, Katsoulakis et al. (2024) conducted a comprehensive scoping review of digital-twin technologies in health care and reported emerging use cases in oncology, including non-small cell lung cancer (NSCLC), where deep-learning-based survival models trained on large real-world datasets were employed to emulate clinical outcomes. These examples underscore that, when grounded in diverse and well-curated data, digital-twin systems can complement conventional trial designs by generating scientifically reliable and ethically advantageous synthetic control arms, particularly in data-rich and high-cost therapeutic areas.

The qualification of synthetic controls generally involves several layers of statistical validation: (1) covariate balance assessments using standardized mean differences; (2) calibration via bootstrap resampling or Bayesian posterior predictive checks; and (3) sensitivity analyses to test robustness against unmeasured confounding. Regulatory pilot programs, including the U.S. FDA's 2023 "Innovation in Clinical Trial Design" initiative and the EMA's Big Data Task Force reflection paper, now acknowledge digital twins as supportive rather than substitutive evidence for pivotal trials (EMA, 2023; U.S. FDA, 2023). From a regulatory perspective, digital twins are most acceptable when they augment, not replace, control arms—particularly in rare diseases, pediatric populations, or when randomization is ethically constrained. Complete replacement remains confined to exploratory or hypothesis-generating trials until methodological standards for transparency, bias control, and independent validation are universally established. These approaches, however, pose new regulatory issues related to the validity and bias in the models of twins. Regulators and IRBs need to assess the extent to which digital twins yield real outcomes and ensure transparency (e.g., via explainable algorithms), as these inferential syllogisms are based on digital twins that enter submissions (Ferreira & Carneiro, 2025).

Generative AI for Trial Design and Data Generation

Recent generative AI algorithms are changing how trials are designed and recruited for. Large models, along with generative adversarial networks (GANs), can suggest entirely new patient profiles, along with trial scenarios, for planning purposes. For example, generative frameworks have successfully produced synthetic health records, imaging outcomes, and tabular clinical trial datasets that are statistically indistinguishable from real data (Bordukova et al., 2024; Ferreira & Carneiro, 2025). Such synthetic data can serve as both historical controls and poorly represented subgroups so that trial power is increased without the need for more patients. Generative AI can also be used to simulate complete outcomes of trials for alternative permutations of the protocol, which allows for rapid optimization of eligibility criteria and endpoint selection. Such AI-driven simulations make *in silico* trial runs possible, whereby the sponsor can discern the most appropriate designs prior to costly real-world implementations. Notably, the level of quality control and validation checks are paramount, whereby the models must be calibrated to confirm that the generated patients represent the population needed, a challenge being addressed by current research and "good machine learning practice" guidelines that are emerging (Askin et al., 2023; Ferreira & Carneiro, 2025).

Explainable and Trustworthy AI (RAG Pipelines, Knowledge Graphs)

As AI takes on more critical trial tasks, explainability and trust become paramount. One promising paradigm is retrieval-augmented generation (RAG), which grounds AI outputs in curated scientific databases. In a RAG pipeline, a clinical query first retrieves relevant literature or database entries (using traditional search or vector similarity), and then an LLM generates answers on the basis of that evidence. This architecture can dramatically improve accuracy and traceability in medicine. For example, RAG can ensure that synthetic data generation or trial predictions are linked to known pharmacology or previous trial results. Crucially, researchers emphasize that RAG systems must include interfaces for auditing the evidence retrieval and reasoning process (Abo El-Enen et al., 2025). Abo El-Enen et al. (2025) outlined future work on visualizing the chain of retrieved facts and providing natural-language explanations that clinicians can validate. Similarly, knowledge graphs—structured networks of biomedical entities and relationships—can be used alongside a RAG to support transparency. By representing the provenance of a prediction (e.g., linking a model's hypothesis to specific pathways or prior studies), knowledge-graph embeddings help regulators and investigators inspect AI reasoning. Overall, integrating the RAG and graph-based methods promises more trustworthy AI in trial design and decision-making, but it also adds engineering complexity and computational cost (e.g., building and maintaining large medical corpora).

Decentralized Trials with Telehealth and Remote Sensors

Modern advances in AI are in line with the decentralized clinical trial (DCT) movement. By taking advantage of IoT devices, applications and telehealth services, researchers can monitor patients on a continuous basis away from traditional sites. High-quality biosensors (wearables, ingestables, and at-home lab kits) can feed real-time data into AI systems that can report adherence issues or adverse events immediately (Alsabah et al., 2025). For example, smart health monitors can obtain readings of vital signs and activity levels, and these readings can allow algorithms to highlight early safety signals or protocol deviations. Telemedicine visits via secure videos and digital consent increase trial access and diversity (e.g., rural or mobility-limited patients may be able to participate). Most importantly, AI-based analytics support the unification of those disparate streams of data — from cloud-based surveys on smartphones to at-home device reading — into a whole patient profile. As Akbarialiabad et al. noted, combining digital twins with mobile health and wearables has been shown to lead to increased engagement and data quality in decentralized contexts (Akbarialiabad et al., 2025). This synergy has led to improved retention and more granular patient monitoring. However, it also asks for high-level data security: patient privacy must be protected by the growing mass of personal data (geolocation, biometrics) that are needed. Encryption, federated learning and strong governance are needed to help protect sensitive data. A unified systems approach—combining patient monitoring, AI-driven decision support, and decentralized infrastructure—is central to modern decentralized trials (Figure 8).

Figure 8. AI-enabled decentralized trial ecosystem

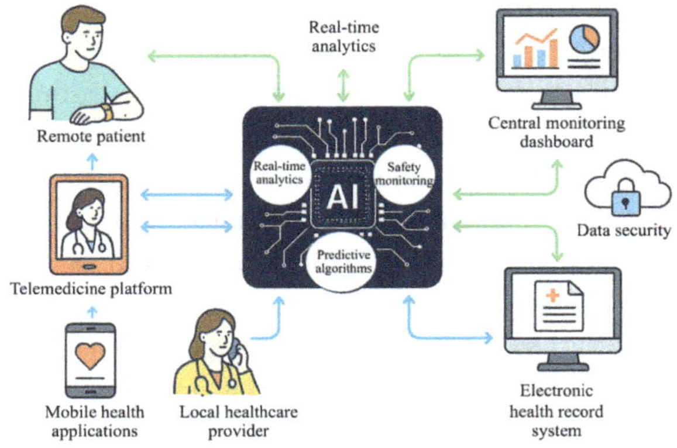

Multi-Omics Integration and AI

Another burgeoning trend is AI-enabled multiomics integration. More robust AI models can leverage the genomic, transcriptomic, proteomic, metabolomic, and other molecular layers to create a holistic view of the biology of each individual patient (Prashar et al., 2026). Deep phenotyping of patients provides the possibility for different levels of precision stratification in clinical trials, for example, choosing patients with a specific pathway signature or predicting differences in drug response derived from combined gene and protein data. Prashar et al. described how AI integration allows seamless merging of disparate data sources to elucidate complex disease relationships to direct therapy selection (Prashar et al., 2026). In practice, deep neural networks and graph algorithms are being developed to take advantage of learning from multiomics, EHR data and published literature simultaneously. The result will be the availability of better predictive biomarkers and adaptive trial arms. Unfortunately, the traditional problems associated with the complexity of multiomics are also great, as the data are both heterogeneous and high dimensional, and robust computational and sophisticated algorithms are needed to harmonize the findings of all the datasets. In particular, the high demand for aligning and analyzing genomic and clinical data at a large scale will require robust infrastructure and data types that are standardized (Hu et al., 2024; Madathil et al., 2025). As researchers note, the question of data integration and interoperability must be addressed to fully optimize AI-driven trials on technology platforms, and this can be accomplished only by significant investment in IT infrastructure development and data curation.

As clinical development evolves to encompass more data and more patient-centered workstreams, many assets arise as accelerants of speed, robustness, and inclusivity.

Table 5 summarizes these assets—digital twin technology, generative AI, RAG with knowledge graph-enabled knowledge bases, decentralized trial toolchains, federated analytics, unified multiomics, and XAI pipelines—where they add the most value, where they stand on the readiness continuum, and what their respective risks are. All of these aims include enabling auditable evidence synthesis, privacy-enabled collaboration across sites, continual real-world monitoring, and stratification while shortening study cycles, improving safety oversight, and increasing transparency in the regulatory process.

Table 5. Emerging AI technologies transforming clinical trials

Technology	What it is	High-Value Clinical Trial Use Cases	Readiness/ notes	Key Risks/ Limitations	References
Digital twins and synthetic controls	Virtual patient/ trial replicas built from mechanistic models + real data	In-silico arms; dose/endpoint optimization; safety forecasting; rare-disease controls	Rapidly piloted in planning and phase I–II; growing regulatory interest	Model validity, bias, transparency, and acceptance by regulators/IRBs	Akbarialiabad et al. (2025); Bordukova et al. (2024); März et al. (2025)
Generative AI and synthetic data	GAN/VAE/LLM methods that generate realistic patient records, images, and time series	Data augmentation; scenario simulation; bolstering underrepresented subgroups; privacy-preserving sharing	Accelerating; used in planning and methods development	Distribution shift, privacy leakage, and fidelity/ traceability of synthetic cohorts	Bordukova et al. (2024); Ferreira and Carneiro (2025)
Retrieval-augmented generation (RAG)	LLMs grounded with curated, citable sources at inference	Evidence-linked protocol drafting; rapid literature synthesis; auditable trial decisions	Emerging best-practice for trustworthy LLM use	Corpus quality, retrieval bias, and provenance auditing at scale	Abo El-Enen et al. (2025)
Biomedical knowledge graphs	Graphs linking entities (drugs, targets, phenotypes) for reasoning and discovery	Hypothesis generation; signal triage; subgroup discovery; explainable decision support	Growing adoption alongside RAG and XAI dashboards	Incompleteness, ontology drift, maintenance burden	Lin et al. (2025)
Decentralized trials with telehealth and remote sensors	IoT wearables, ePRO apps, telemedicine integrated with AI analytics	Continuous safety monitoring; adherence verification; inclusive recruitment/ retention	Deployed today in hybrid/virtual designs	Device variability, data quality, connectivity, and privacy governance	Alsabah et al. (2025); Chodankar et al. (2024); Daly et al. (2024)
Federated learning and privacy-preserving analytics	Collaborative model training without sharing raw patient data	Multisite harmonization; cross-registry signal detection; RWE integration	Increasingly practical for phase III/IV networks	Systems complexity; heterogeneity across sites; secure aggregation	Hu et al. (2024); Madathil et al. (2025)

continued on following page

Table 5. Continued

Technology	What it is	High-Value Clinical Trial Use Cases	Readiness/ notes	Key Risks/ Limitations	References
Multiomics integration (graph and multimodal deep learning)	Joint modeling of genomics, transcriptomics, proteomics, metabolomics with clinical data	Precision stratification; predictive biomarkers; adaptive arm selection	Active research; entering early-phase trials	High dimensionality, data harmonization, compute needs, standardization	Prashar et al. (2026)
Explainable/ trustworthy AI (XAI) pipelines	SHAP/LIME/ Grad-CAM and documentation for transparent decisions	Regulator-ready model explanations; clinician trust; audit trials	Strongly recommended by regulators and journals	Added engineering overhead; risk of superficial explanations	Houssein et al. (2025); Mohammad et al. (2025)

REGULATORY, PRIVACY, AND FEASIBILITY CONSIDERATIONS

These innovations carry important regulatory and privacy implications. To date, regulatory guidance on AI in trials is still evolving. The lack of clear standards is a major hurdle: for example, one survey revealed that drug developers are eager to use AI to reduce sample sizes and accelerate studies, but they lack formal FDA/EMA criteria for acceptable AI tools (Askin et al., 2023). Agencies have begun issuing draft frameworks (e.g., the FDA's 2023 discussion paper on AI/ML, EMA reflection papers) that emphasize transparency, validation, and risk management. In practice, sponsors must demonstrate that any AI-generated insight is reliable: this means thorough internal validation, explainability (as above), and often parallel testing against traditional analyses. Data privacy is another critical issue. Synthetic data and digital twins must be deidentified and checked to prevent reidentification of real patients. As Akbarialiabad et al. reported, maintaining privacy and informed consent is an ethical requirement when trials become data intensive (Akbarialiabad et al., 2025). Methods such as federated learning or differential privacy may help alleviate concerns when combining patient sensor or omics data. Finally, technical feasibility must be addressed: many of these AI systems require specialized computing (GPUs for deep learning, high-bandwidth links for the IoT, and secure cloud platforms). Organizations need to invest in infrastructure and workforce training. Prashar et al. noted that handling large multiomic datasets and real-time streams demands robust computational pipelines (Prashar et al., 2026). In sum, while AI-driven trials promise efficiency and insight, their success hinges on regulatory acceptance, data governance, and the readiness of technical ecosystems.

CHALLENGES AND CONSIDERATIONS

Data Quality and Bias

AI models require large representative datasets. If the training datasets do not have the right mix of populations, the predictions are not useful. For example, an AI designed to detect adverse events that is trained almost entirely on younger populations would not be useful in older populations. Therefore, datasets that represent diverse populations need to be used. Privacy and security: Clinical trial data constitute one of the most highly sensitive sets of information (genetic make-up of patients, records, etc.). Dedicated systems must be developed to maintain the integrity of AI applications. Encryption, federated learning, differential privacy and other mechanisms are being developed. For example, mechanisms such as federated learning and differential privacy can protect participant confidentiality while allowing distributed model training (Hu et al., 2024; Madathil et al., 2025).

Explainability and Reproducibility

The clinical and regulatory environments require transparency. Black-box models have greatly slowed the use of AI in many areas. However, new developments, such as SHAP, LIME and others, are being developed in which it becomes possible to understand the reasoning behind the model's conclusions. These tools are increasingly recommended by both journals and regulators for trustworthy AI in medicine (Ferreira & Carneiro, 2025; Houssein et al., 2025).

Regulatory Hurdles

Frameworks for the approval of general AI tools to be used in clinical trials are still being developed. Regulatory bodies (FDAs, EMAs) are developing guidance, but no general regulation has yet been developed. There will need to be collaboration among the various stakeholders to establish a validation protocol and guidelines for the use of AI systems (Askin et al., 2023; Teodoro et al., 2025).

Operational Integration

Many of the clinical trial infrastructure systems (EHRs, CTMSs, etc.) are not ready for AI interfacing. The upgrading of systems and training of personnel is not a trivial task. Integration studies have shown that AI-ready systems improve efficiency and reduce errors in multicenter operations (Olawade et al., 2026; Su et al., 2023).

Although artificial intelligence in clinical trials can resolve many issues, some challenges remain related to the quality of the data, algorithmic bias, privacy, regulations and ethics. Table 6 summarizes the principal challenges, indicating some of the possible methods reported in the literature for meeting these challenges. Meeting these challenges will require a multidisciplinary approach that incorporates technical solutions (for example, federated learning, explainable AI) as well as institutional readiness and oversight in ethical matters. Transparency, fairness and interoperability need to be instilled into each part of the lifecycle of AI so that digital transformation in the pharmaceutical ecosystem can be assured to support scientific integrity and public trust.

Table 6. Challenges and mitigation strategies in implementing ai in clinical trials

Challenge category	Description of the issue	Proposed mitigation strategies	Expected outcomes	References
Data quality and representativeness	Clinical trial datasets often lack diversity or completeness, leading to biased or unreliable AI models	• Standardize data formats and ontologies • Employ diverse, multicenter data sources • Use synthetic data or generative AI for underrepresented subgroups	Reduces bias; improves generalizability and external validity of AI predictions	Akbarialiabad et al. (2025); Ali et al. (2025)
Algorithmic bias and explainability	Black-box models hinder interpretability and regulatory trust	• Adopt explainable AI (XAI) frameworks such as SHAP, LIME, and Grad-CAM • Require transparent model documentation • Apply fairness-aware algorithms	Enhances interpretability and accountability; fosters clinician and regulator confidence	Ferreira and Carneiro (2025); Houssein et al. (2025)
Data privacy and security	Aggregating multisource data increases privacy risks and regulatory complexity	• Use federated learning and differential privacy mechanisms • Encrypt communication between sites • Employ blockchain for audit trails	Ensures compliance with GDPR/HIPAA; protects patient confidentiality while enabling collaboration	Hu et al. (2024); Madathil et al. (2025)

continued on following page

Table 6. Continued

Challenge category	Description of the issue	Proposed mitigation strategies	Expected outcomes	References
Regulatory acceptance and validation	Lack of standardized guidelines for AI model validation and auditability in clinical settings	• Engage early with regulatory bodies (FDA, EMA) • Use Good Machine Learning Practice (GMLP) frameworks • Conduct parallel validation using conventional analytics	Accelerates AI tool approval; ensures transparent and reproducible validation pipelines	Askin et al. (2023); Teodoro et al. (2025)
Operational integration	Existing EHR, CTMS, and ePRO systems lack interoperability with AI tools	• Develop interoperable APIs and standardized data exchange formats (FHIR, OMOP-CDM) • Provide workforce training for digital competencies	Streamlines implementation; enhances efficiency of AI-supported workflows across trial sites	Olawade et al. (2026); Su et al. (2023)
Ethical and social consideration	AI may unintentionally reinforce inequalities or erode patient autonomy	• Include diverse demographic representation • Ensure informed consent for AI use • Establish ethics review committees with AI expertise	Promotes fairness, trust, and social accountability in clinical AI deployment	März et al. (2025); Shams et al. (2025)

CONCLUSION AND FUTURE DIRECTIONS

Artificial intelligence is set to evolve clinical drug development into more rapid, intelligent and patient-centric processes by deploying AI algorithms at all steps. These steps include designing, recruiting, conducting and analyzing where sponsors benefit from decreasing costs, increasing success rates, and accelerating the delivery of drugs to patients. Theoretical (adaptive algorithms, digital twins, predictive analytics) models are being developed, and real-life evidence (Pfizer, Verily) demonstrates where achievement is occurring. However, continued success depends on solving the data quality, bias, ethics and regulatory issues that beset these areas. Collaborative attitudes among physicians, AI practitioners and regulators are necessary. In the future, it is envisaged that AI will be built into routine processes so that AI can monitor areas such as reactogenicity/safety data in real time (*in vivo*) and digital lifelines (*in silico*) in protocol simulations. Once the AI tools are validated and their workings expressed more transparently, they will also allow clinical trials to change their rigid protocol structures to nonlinear and evolving ones, which will in turn hasten medicines to the market on the basis of better, safer outcomes.

Even with notable advances, a number of research frontiers still have to be explored. These include the validation of digital-twin models against real-world clinical outcomes, the development of standardized proactive explainability metrics for regulatory audits, and benchmarking of federated-learning performance in heterogeneous data environments. Further work is necessary to integrate causal inference modeling, evaluate the fair distribution among demographic subgroups, and develop interoperable data streams that facilitate continuous model retraining. The closure of these research gaps will determine the extent and effectiveness of the potential changes predicted for future clinical development pipelines as a consequence of harnessing AI technologies.

REFERENCES

Abo El-Enen, M., Saad, S., & Nazmy, T. (2025). A survey on retrieval-augmentation generation (RAG) models for healthcare applications. *Neural Computing & Applications*, *37*, 28191–28267. DOI: 10.1007/s00521-025-11666-9

Akbarialiabad, H., Pasdar, A., Murrell, D. F., Mostafavi, M., Shakil, F., Safaee, E., . . . Grada, A. (2025). Enhancing randomized clinical trials with digital twins. *npj Systems Biology and Applications, 11*(1), 110. DOI: PMID: 41044102DOI: 10.1038/s41540-025-00592-0

Ali, N., Hanif, N., Khan, H. A., Waseem, M. A., Saeed, A., Zakir, S., & Saleem, A. (2025). Deep learning and artificial intelligence for drug discovery, application, challenge, and future perspectives. *Discover Applied Sciences*, *7*(6), 533. DOI: 10.1007/s42452-025-06991-6

Alsabah, M., Naser, M. A., Albahri, A. S., Albahri, O. S., Alamoodi, A. H., Abdulhussain, S. H., & Alzubaidi, L. (2025). A comprehensive review on key technologies toward smart healthcare systems based IoT: Technical aspects, challenges and future directions. *Artificial Intelligence Review*, *58*(11), 343. DOI: 10.1007/s10462-025-11342-3

Arango-Argoty, G., Bikiel, D. E., Sun, G. J., Kipkogei, E., Smith, K. M., Carrasco Pro, S., & Jacob, E. (2025). AI-driven predictive biomarker discovery with contrastive learning to improve clinical trial outcomes. *Cancer Cell*, *43*(5), 875–890. e878. DOI: 10.1016/j.ccell.2025.03.029

Askin, S., Burkhalter, D., Calado, G., & El Dakrouni, S. (2023). Artificial Intelligence applied to clinical trials: Opportunities and challenges. *Health and Technology*, *13*(2), 203–213. DOI: 10.1007/s12553-023-00738-2

Bikou, A. G., Deligianni, E., Dermiki-Gkana, F., Liappas, N., Teriús-Padrón, J. G., Beltrán Jaunsarás, M. E., & Kontogiorgis, C. (2024). Improving participant recruitment in clinical trials: Comparative analysis of innovative digital platforms. *Journal of Medical Internet Research*, *26*, e60504. DOI: 10.2196/60504

Bordukova, M., Makarov, N., Rodriguez-Esteban, R., Schmich, F., & Menden, M. P. (2024). Generative artificial intelligence empowers digital twins in drug discovery and clinical trials. *Expert Opinion on Drug Discovery*, *19*(1), 33–42. DOI: 10.1080/17460441.2023.2273839

Chaiburi, C., & Yingngam, B. (2025). Digital twin technology fundamentals. In Iyer, S., Nayyar, A., Paul, A., & Naved, M. (Eds.), *Digital Twins for Smart Cities and Villages* (pp. 1–35). Elsevier., DOI: 10.1016/B978-0-443-28884-5.00001-4

Cho, J., Xu, Q., Wong, C. H., & Lo, A. W. (2025). Predicting clinical trial duration via statistical and machine learning models. *Contemporary Clinical Trials Communications*, *45*, 101473. DOI: 10.1016/j.conctc.2025.101473

Chodankar, D., Raval, T. K., & Jeyaraj, J. (2024). The role of remote data capture, wearables, and digital biomarkers in decentralized clinical trials. *Perspectives in Clinical Research*, *15*(1), 38–41. DOI: 10.4103/picr.picr_219_22

Daly, B., Brawley, O. W., Gospodarowicz, M. K., Olopade, O. I., Fashoyin-Aje, L., Smart, V. W., & Li, B. T. (2024). Remote monitoring and data collection for decentralized clinical trials. *JAMA Network Open*, *7*(4), e246228–e246228. DOI: 10.1001/jamanetworkopen.2024.6228

EMA. (2023). *European Medicines Agency (EMA): Reflection paper on the use of artificial intelligence in the lifecycle of medicines*. Retrieved 1 November 2023 from https://www.ema.europa.eu/en/documents/scientific-guideline/reflection-paper-use-artificial-intelligence-ai-medicinal-product-lifecycle_en.pdf

Ferreira, F. J. N., & Carneiro, A. S. (2025). AI-driven drug discovery: A comprehensive review. *ACS Omega*, *10*(23), 23889–23903. DOI: 10.1021/acsomega.5c00549

Goldberg Jana, M., Amin Nivee, P., Zachariah Krista, A., & Bhatt Ami, B. (2024). The introduction of AI into decentralized clinical trials. *JACC Advances*, *3*(8), 101094. DOI: 10.1016/j.jacadv.2024.101094

Houssein, E. H., Gamal, A. M., Younis, E. M. G., & Mohamed, E. (2025). Explainable artificial intelligence for medical imaging systems using deep learning: A comprehensive review. *Cluster Computing*, *28*(7), 469. DOI: 10.1007/s10586-025-05281-5

Hu, K., Gong, S., Zhang, Q., Seng, C., Xia, M., & Jiang, S. (2024). An overview of implementing security and privacy in federated learning. *Artificial Intelligence Review*, *57*(8), 204. DOI: 10.1007/s10462-024-10846-8

Kant, S., Deepika, & Roy, S. (2025). Artificial intelligence in drug discovery and development: Transforming challenges into opportunities. *Discover Pharmaceutical Sciences*, *1*(1), 7. DOI: 10.1007/s44395-025-00007-3

Katsoulakis, E., Wang, Q., Wu, H., Shahriyari, L., Fletcher, R., Liu, J., & Deng, J. (2024). Digital twins for health: A scoping review. *npj. Digital Medicine*, *7*(1), 77. DOI: 10.1038/s41746-024-01073-0

Khumsikiew, J., Netthong, R., & Yingngam, B. (2025). Research advancements in quantum computing and digital twins. In Iyer, S., Nayyar, A., Paul, A., & Naved, M. (Eds.), *Digital Twins for Smart Cities and Villages* (pp. 103–125). Elsevier., DOI: 10.1016/B978-0-443-28884-5.00005-1

Kleeberger, J. A. (2025). Virtual patients in clinical trials for drug development: A narrative review. *Cureus*, *17*(6), e85380. DOI: 10.7759/cureus.85380

Lee, K., Mai, Y., Liu, Z., Raja, K., Jun, T., Ma, M., & Wang, X. (2024). Criteria-Mapper: Establishing the automatic identification of clinical trial cohorts from electronic health records by matching normalized eligibility criteria and patient clinical characteristics. *Scientific Reports*, *14*(1), 25387. DOI: 10.1038/s41598-024-77447-x

Lin, A., Wang, Z., Jiang, A., Chen, L., Qi, C., Zhu, L., & Luo, P. (2025). Large language models in clinical trials: Applications, technical advances, and future directions. *BMC Medicine*, *23*(1), 563. DOI: 10.1186/s12916-025-04348-9

Liu, H., Wang, Y., Huang, Y., Xiong, D., Shen, J., Siqueiros, L., & Daar, E. S. (2022). Ingestible sensor system for measuring, monitoring and enhancing adherence to antiretroviral therapy: An open-label, usual care-controlled, randomized trial. *EBioMedicine*, *86*, 104330. DOI: 10.1016/j.ebiom.2022.104330

Lubitz, S. A., Faranesh, A. Z., Selvaggi, C., Atlas, S. J., McManus, D. D., Singer, D. E., & Foulkes, A. S. (2022). Detection of atrial fibrillation in a large population using wearable devices: The fitbit heart study. *Circulation*, *146*(19), 1415–1424. DOI: 10.1161/circulationaha.122.060291

Madathil, N. T., Dankar, F. K., Gergely, M., Belkacem, A. N., & Alrabaee, S. (2025). Revolutionizing healthcare data analytics with federated learning: A comprehensive survey of applications, systems, and future directions. *Computational and Structural Biotechnology Journal*, *28*, 217–238. DOI: 10.1016/j.csbj.2025.06.009

März, J. W., Baumgartner, M., Blau, N., & Biller-Andorno, N. (2025). Digital twins for children with rare diseases: An exploration of the legal and ethical issues. *Ethics and Information Technology*, *27*(3), 44. DOI: 10.1007/s10676-025-09848-z

Miller, M. I., Shih, L. C., & Kolachalama, V. B. (2023). Machine learning in clinical trials: A primer with applications to neurology. *Neurotherapeutics; the Journal of the American Society for Experimental NeuroTherapeutics*, *20*(4), 1066–1080. DOI: 10.1007/s13311-023-01384-2

Mishra, T., Wang, M., Metwally, A. A., Bogu, G. K., Brooks, A. W., Bahmani, A., & Snyder, M. P. (2020). Presymptomatic detection of COVID-19 from smartwatch data. *Nature Biomedical Engineering*, *4*(12), 1208–1220. DOI: 10.1038/s41551-020-00640-6

Mohammad, A. A. S., Mohammad, S. I. S., Al Oraini, B., Vasudevan, A., Hindieh, A., Altarawneh, A., & Ali, I. (2025). Strategies for applying interpretable and explainable AI in real world IoT applications. *Discover Internet of Things*, *5*(1), 71. DOI: 10.1007/s43926-025-00155-z

Olawade, D. B., Fidelis, S. C., Marinze, S., Egbon, E., Osunmakinde, A., & Osborne, A. (2026). Artificial intelligence in clinical trials: A comprehensive review of opportunities, challenges, and future directions. *International Journal of Medical Informatics*, *206*, 106141. DOI: 10.1016/j.ijmedinf.2025.106141

Park, Y., & Nycklemoe, S. (2025). MARGO: Machine learning-assisted adaptive randomization for group sequential trials based on overlap weights. *Statistics in Medicine*, *44*(15-17), e70158. DOI: 10.1002/sim.70158

Park, Y. J., & Bae, M. H. (2025). Screening and diagnosis of atrial fibrillation usinwearable devices. *The Korean Journal of Internal Medicine*, *40*(1), 7–14. DOI: 10.3904/kjim.2023.521

Pedroso, A. F., & Khera, R. (2025). Leveraging AI-enhanced digital health with consumer devices for scalable cardiovascular screening, prediction, and monitoring. *npj Cardiovascular Health, 2*(1), 34. DOI: PMID: 40620667DOI: 10.1038/s44325-025-00071-9

Perez, M. V., Mahaffey, K. W., Hedlin, H., Rumsfeld, J. S., Garcia, A., Ferris, T., & Turakhia, M. P. (2019). Large-scale assessment of a smartwatch to identify atrial fibrillation. *The New England Journal of Medicine*, *381*(20), 1909–1917. DOI: 10.1056/NEJMoa1901183

Poh, M. Z., Battisti, A. J., Cheng, L. F., Lin, J., Patwardhan, A., Venkataraman, G. S., & Ghanbari, H. (2023). Validation of a deep learning algorithm for continuous, real-time detection of atrial fibrillation using a wrist-worn device in an ambulatory environment. *Journal of the American Heart Association*, *12*(19), e030543. DOI: 10.1161/jaha.123.030543

Prashar, A., Singh, M., Sharma, S., Kuna, S. S., Putha, S., Gudekota, S., . . . Joshi, R. (2026). AI-driven multi-omics analysis for personalized healthcare. In: Goar, V., Gajrani, J., Yousuf, M. A., R. s. Tavares, J. M. (eds) Proceedings of International Conference on Computational Complexity and Intelligent Algorithms. IC3IA 2025. Algorithms for Intelligent Systems. Springer, Singapore. DOI: DOI: 10.1007/978-981-96-7473-2_21

Qian, L., Lu, X., Haris, P., Zhu, J., Li, S., & Yang, Y. (2025). Enhancing clinical trial outcome prediction with artificial intelligence: A systematic review. *Drug Discovery Today*, *30*(4), 104332. DOI: 10.1016/j.drudis.2025.104332

Reis, Z. S. N., Pereira, G. M. V., Dias, C. D. S., Lage, E. M., de Oliveira, I. J. R., & Pagano, A. S. (2025). Artificial intelligence-based tools for patient support to enhance medication adherence: A focused review. *Frontiers in Digital Health*, *7*, 1523070. DOI: 10.3389/fdgth.2025.1523070

Salditt, M., Eckes, T., & Nestler, S. (2024). A tutorial introduction to heterogeneous treatment effect estimation with meta-learners. *Administration and Policy in Mental Health*, *51*(5), 650–673. DOI: 10.1007/s10488-023-01303-9

Shamanna, P., Erukulapati, R. S., Shukla, A., Shah, L., Willis, B., Thajudeen, M., & Joshi, S. (2024). One-year outcomes of a digital twin intervention for type 2 diabetes: A retrospective real-world study. *Scientific Reports*, *14*(1), 25478. DOI: 10.1038/s41598-024-76584-7

Shams, R. A., Zowghi, D., & Bano, M. (2025). AI and the quest for diversity and inclusion: A systematic literature review. *AI and Ethics*, *5*(1), 411–438. DOI: 10.1007/s43681-023-00362-w

Su, Q., Cheng, G., & Huang, J. (2023). A review of research on eligibility criteria for clinical trials. *Clinical and Experimental Medicine*, *23*(6), 1867–1879. DOI: 10.1007/s10238-022-00975-1

Teodoro, D., Naderi, N., Yazdani, A., Zhang, B., & Bornet, A. (2025). A scoping review of artificial intelligence applications in clinical trial risk assessment. *npj. Digital Medicine*, *8*(1), 486. DOI: 10.1038/s41746-025-01886-7

Twala, B. (2025). AI-driven precision diagnosis and treatment in Parkinson's disease: A comprehensive review and experimental analysis. *Frontiers in Aging Neuroscience*, *17*, 1638340. DOI: 10.3389/fnagi.2025.1638340

Unlu, O., Varugheese, M., Shin, J., Subramaniam, S. M., Stein, D. W. J., St Laurent, J. J., & Blood, A. J. (2025). Manual vs AI-assisted prescreening for trial eligibility using large language models - a randomized clinical trial. *Journal of the American Medical Association*, *333*(12), 1084–1087. DOI: 10.1001/jama.2024.28047

U.S. FDA. (2023). *U.S. Food & Drug Administration (FDA): Digital Health Technologies for Remote Data Acquisition in Clinical Investigations – Guidance for Industry, Investigators, and Other Stakeholders*. Retrieved 1 November 2025 from https://www.fda.gov/regulatory-information/search-fda-guidance-documents/digital-health-technologies-remote-data-acquisition-clinical-investigations

Vaterkowski, M., Daniel, C., La Rosa, A., Kalra, D., Jaulent, M.-C., Lame, G., & Kempf, E. (2025). Electronic health record based recruitment support systems: A scoping review to improve patient inclusion within clinical trials. *International Journal of Medical Informatics, 201*, 105900. DOI: 10.1016/j.ijmedinf.2025.105900

Voigt, I., Inojosa, H., Dillenseger, A., Haase, R., Akgün, K., & Ziemssen, T. (2021). Digital twins for multiple sclerosis. *Frontiers in Immunology, 12*, 669811. DOI: 10.3389/fimmu.2021.669811

Yingngam, B. (2025). AI in Clinical Trial Design and Patient Recruitment. In M. Lytras & S. alajlan (Eds.), *Transforming Pharmaceutical Research With Artificial Intelligence* (pp. 27-74). DOI: DOI: 10.4018/979-8-3693-6270-9.ch002

Yingngam, B., Khumsikiew, J., & Netthong, R. (2025). Digital twins for telemedicine and personalized medicine. In Iyer, S., Nayyar, A., Paul, A., & Naved, M. (Eds.), *Digital Twins for Smart Cities and Villages* (pp. 295–325). Elsevier., DOI: 10.1016/B978-0-443-28884-5.00014-2

Yingngam, B., Navabhatra, A., & Sillapapibool, P. (2024). AI-driven decision-making applications in pharmaceutical sciences. In Nguyen, T., & Vo, N. (Eds.), *Using Traditional Design Methods to Enhance AI-Driven Decision Making* (pp. 1–63)., DOI: 10.4018/979-8-3693-0639-0.ch001

Yingngam, B., & Sethabouppha, B. (2024). Advanced AI applications for drug discovery. In Shah, I., & Sial, Q. (Eds.), *Advances in Computational Intelligence for the Healthcare Industry 4.0* (pp. 42–86)., DOI: 10.4018/979-8-3693-2333-5.ch003

APPENDIX

Abbreviations

AI Artificial intelligence
AUC Area under the curve
CNN Convolutional neural network
CRF Case report form
CTMS Clinical trial management system
DCT Decentralized clinical trial
DL Deep learning
ECG Electrocardiogram
EHR Electronic health record
EMA European Medicines Agency
ePRO Electronic patient-reported outcome
FDA US Food and Drug Administration
FHIR Fast healthcare interoperability resources
FL Federated learning
GAN Generative adversarial network
GDPR General data protection regulation
GMLP Good machine learning practice
HIPAA Health Insurance Portability and Accountability Act
IoT Internet of Things
IRB Institutional review board
KPIs Key performance indicators
LIME Local interpretable model-agnostic explanations
LLM Large language model
ML Machine learning
MRI Magnetic resonance imaging
NLP Natural language processing
OMOP-CDM Observational medical outcomes partnership – common data model
PICO Population, intervention, comparison, outcome
QC Quality control
RAG Retrieval-augmented generation
RCT Randomized controlled trial
RL Reinforcement learning
SHAP Shapley additive explanations
VAE Variational autoencoder
XAI Explainable artificial intelligence

Chapter 9
Secure Smart Nutrition Systems:
AI-Powered Contextual Intelligence for Next-Gen Health and Pharmaceutical Innovation

Tulaja Saha
Amity Institute of Food Technology, Amity University, Noida, India

Samridhi Bhattacharjee
https://orcid.org/0009-0009-3642-7448
Department of Dietetics and Applied Nutrition, Amity Institute of Applied Sciences, Amity University, Kolkata, India

Khusi Thakur
Department of Dietetics and Applied Nutrition, Amity Institute of Applied Sciences, Amity University, Kolkata, India

Alifiya Akhtar
Department of Dietetics and Applied Nutrition, Amity Institute of Applied Sciences, Amity University, Kolkata, India

Joyeta Ghosh
https://orcid.org/0000-0001-9619-1793
Department of Dietetics and Applied Nutrition, Amity Institute of Applied Sciences, Amity University, Kolkata, India

ABSTRACT

Smart nutrition systems deliver personalized dietary solutions by transforming personal health management by integrating artificial intelligence, IoT, and autonomous

DOI: 10.4018/979-8-3373-5258-9.ch009

technologies. This digital evaluation system handles personal sensitive health data, influences critical dietary decisions, and interacts with broader healthcare networks, which introduces significant cyber security challenges. This chapter discusses the required need for context security framework tailored to the dynamic and personalized nature of smart nutrition technologies. It includes vulnerabilities and recent high-profile breeches. It also explores the limitation of traditional security models and importance of real-time threat detection and privacy preserving strategies.

1. INTRODUCTION

In present days Healthcare Innovation and dietary management have become digitally interconnected. Smart nutrition systems help to improve Global Health outcomes and rising burden of lifestyle related diseases. This Advanced Technological system encircles things like AI powered diet recommendation engine, IOT enabled kitchen appliances, personalized nutrition tracking platforms, autonomous male preparation systems. This new technology has an unique possibility to transform individuals ' interaction with food, manage chronic health conditions and pursue healthy lifestyles. This technology has produced possibilities of threats to cyber security which remain unexplored and unaddressed as these systems deals with sensitive health data, manages physical food preparation environment, controls critical dietary decisions and incorporate broader healthcare infrastructure. This chapter discusses the importance and lack of focus on the topic of cyber security on smart nutrition technologies scrutinizing strategic implementation of context security frameworks to protect autonomous health and dietary infrastructure against threats and ensuring functionality, accessibility and trustworthiness. Some recent occurrences have revealed this vulnerability such as the 2023 breach of NutriTech solutions' database revealing dietary profiles of over 3.2 million users (Johnson et al., 2024; Ghosh, 2023a) and 2024 Ransomware Attack on Mealsync Systems which impede meal delivery services to almost 40000 elderly and vulnerable individuals around metropolitan cities(Singh & Rodriguez, 2024). The goal of this chapter are:

- to classify and explore the unique attack surfaces prbesented by modern smart nutrition systems.
- to inspect the process of adaptation of context aware security models to highly individualised and ever changing nature of nutrition and Technologies.
- to establish a extensive security Framework which can balance a reliable defence system to individualised need immanent to dietary management technologies.

- to suggest approaches for precaution measures together with first adaptation of smart nutrition system with unwavering essential advantages to public health.

During the assessment, our purpose is to build a secure future of digital nutrition infrastructure by protecting data privacy and physical wellbeing of people depended on smart nutrition systems for everyday nutritional guidance and health management - eventually secure the safety, ethics, and equitability of smart nutrition systems across healthcare settings all over the world.

2. THREAT LANDSCAPE IN SMART NUTRITION

Smart nutrition systems are a revolutionary solution for personalized health and diet management that leverages cutting-edge technologies like the Internet of Things (IoT), artificial intelligence (AI), and mobile apps to provide personalized nutritional advice and monitoring (Smetana et al., 2021). These platforms gather and examine a large amount of individual data, such as dietary consumption, activity levels, and biometric indicators like blood glucose or heart rate, to offer personalized recommendations that can improve health outcomes (Strauss et al., 2023). Through embedding real-time data collection and analysis, intelligent nutrition systems facilitate real-time dynamic adaptation of dietary programs to enhance the efficacy and efficiency of nutrition management over static one-size-fits-all solutions (de Hoogh et al., 2021). The multidisciplinary design of these systems, incorporating nutrition science, systems biology, and behavioral sciences, enables targeted interventions that can be quantitatively optimized to benefit individual health and function (Donovan et al., 2025). The agriculture and food industry, which overlaps with intelligent nutrition through supply chain alignment, has seen a boost in ransomware assaults, which could also impact nutrition systems by making them unusable or holding important data hostage (Kulkarni et al., 2024). A case in point is the 2021 ransomware attack on JBS Foods, which closed nine US-based facilities, cost $11 million in ransom payments, and resulted in a 25% rise in meat prices, illustrating the ripple effects of such attacks on interlinked systems. In addition, denial of service (DoS) attacks can deny users access to their nutrition information and suggestions, compromising the usability and reliability of such systems (Smart Buildings). These attacks underscore the interconnectivity of smart systems wherein a vulnerability in one element, like a supply chain partner, may have deep-reaching effects across the entire ecosystem, including smart nutrition platforms.

In order to counter the varied threats smart nutrition systems are confronting, it is imperative to institute strong security protocols in all phases of system design and deployment. The use of secure coding standards, routine security audits, and keeping up with frequent software updates and patches is vital in resolving vulnerabilities (Tangari et al., 2021). User education is at the center of security improvement; through educating users on best practices, including employing robust passwords and handling app permissions with care, the security stance as a whole can be improved. In addition, the regulatory environment needs to change to adapt to the latest technology, creating definite guidelines and standards for security and privacy within personalized nutrition services (Donovan et al., 2025). International cooperation among regulatory agencies, including the European Union Data Protection Board, can facilitate secure data in partnerships and data-sharing contracts (Donovan et al., 2025). Enhancing security and privacy first allows the industry to promote trust among users, leading to increased smart nutrition system adoption and, eventually, healthier outcomes. Continuous research and coordination are required to counter the changing threat profile and ensure the secure deployment of these cutting-edge systems (Figure 1).

Figure 1. Threat Landscape and Mitigation in Smart Nutrition Systems

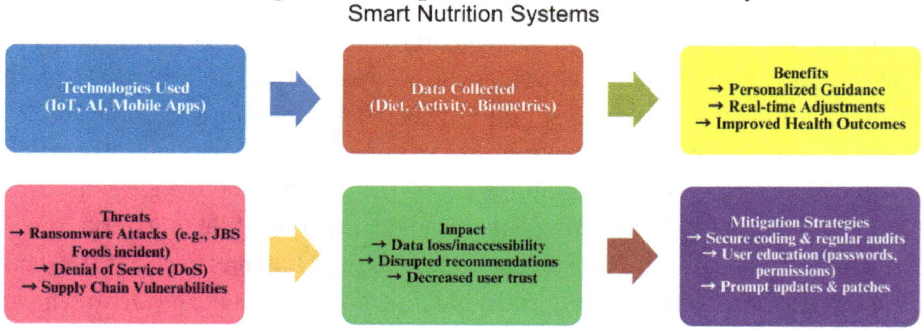

3. DATA BREACHES OF DIETARY AND HEALTH INFORMATION

Smart nutrition platforms collect extensive personal health data, making them attractive targets for cybercriminals. These breaches expose sensitive information including:

- Detailed dietary logs and consumption patterns
- Body metrics and health parameters
- Meal planning and nutritional goals
- Connected health device readings

- Personal identifiers and account information

In 2022, 2018 the nutrition tracking app MyFitnessPal experienced a follow-up breach affecting approximately 150 million users, exposing usernames, email addresses, and hashed passwords (Kessler, 2022). While dietary records were not confirmed compromised in this case, the incident highlighted the vulnerability of nutrition platforms. Similarly, in late 2023, a major breach affected NutriTrack, a popular smart nutrition service. The breach exposed the dietary information, health metrics, and personal details of over 3.2 million users. According to the company's disclosure, unauthorized access persisted for nearly three months before detection, allowing attackers to extract complete nutritional profiles and associated health data (Chen & Roberts, 2023).

Beyond specific incidents, systemic vulnerabilities in mobile health (mHealth) applications, which include nutrition apps, amplify the risk of data breaches. A comprehensive study of over 20,000 mHealth apps found that 45% relied on un-encrypted HTTP for communication, with 23% transmitting personal data such as location and passwords via these insecure channels (Iwaya et al., 2023). This exposes users to data interception risks. Additionally, 1.8% of mHealth apps were flagged as suspicious by VirusTotal, containing adware or trojans that could facilitate breaches. Another study by Alissa Knight and Approov revealed that all 30 popular mHealth apps tested were vulnerable to API attacks, enabling unauthorized access to protected health information (PHI) and personally identifiable information (PII), including social security numbers and medical results (Isibor, 2024). In particular, 50% of APIs granted permission for accessing sensitive patient information, and 100% were vulnerable to Broken Object Level Authorization (BOLA) attacks, which allowed access to unassigned patients' data. They point to the urgent need for strong security solutions to safeguard smart nutrition systems.

Ineffective authentication mechanisms like the use of weak passwords without multi-factor authentication add to weaknesses, enabling unauthorized usage of user accounts. It was established in a study that 63% of security competence is lacking among mHealth app developers, adding to such weaknesses . For nutrition apps, which keep extensive diet and health information, these vulnerabilities are serious because compromises would have important privacy intrusions and possible abuse of private health data. Smart nutrition systems present unique threats as a result of the importance of their information and possible health consequences of a breach. Data tampering is a serious issue, whereby attackers would be able to manipulate dietary information or recommendation software, causing incorrect or dangerous nutritional guidance (Joshua et al., 2022). Smart nutrition systems being linked with other healthcare devices, e.g., wearables or smart kitchen appliances, raises the prospect of ecosystem-wide attacks, where a single point of vulnerability would put the entire system at risk (Tangari et al., 2021). These interdependent systems extend the effects of breaches, which make them require thorough security measures to secure individual elements as well as the entire ecosystem.

Figure 2. Data Breaches and Security Risks in Smart Nutrition Platforms

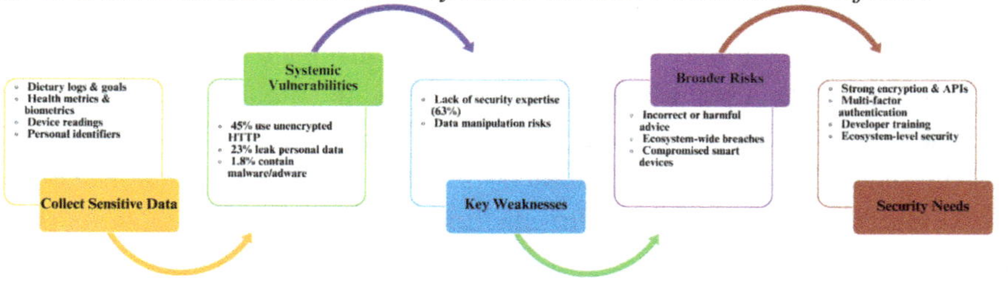

4. DEVICE SPOOFING AND UNAUTHORIZED ACCESS

Smart nutrition systems commonly consist of networked devices such as smart scales, glucose meters, and food analysers. These devices present particular security challenges: A 2023 DEF CON security conference demo saw researchers spoof a widely used smart kitchen scale, sending false weight readings to a networked nutrition app. This manipulation made the system compute wrong nutritional value, which could result in unsafe dietary choices for people with certain health conditions (Wagner et al., 2023). Researchers at Yale proved similar weaknesses in nutrition-tracking smart refrigerators. They exploited weak authentication schemes to gain unauthorized access to devices, a move that could allow attackers to alter stored food records or disrupt expiration notices (Patel et al., 2023) (Figure 2).

One of the most notable examples of such vulnerabilities includes the AEG Smart Scale PW 5653, where researchers had found weaknesses in its Bluetooth Low Energy (BLE) technology that made it susceptible to denial-of-service (DoS) and man-in-the-middle (MITM) attacks (Wang, 2024). Vulnerabilities opened the door for attackers to interfere with the functioning of the scale or intercept and alter data transmissions, virtually allowing device spoofing or unauthorized access. Continuous glucose monitors are also exposed to critical security threats due to a lack of protection. Studies have pointed out that poor security in CGMs may enable cyber attackers to gain access to confidential health information or control device functions, which may result in inaccurate readings of glucose levels that are risky for patients. Moreover, smart home gadgets, such as those that come linked with nutrition monitoring systems, have proven to possess universal security weaknesses. A research identified that 22 of the 24 smart devices, such as possible nutrition devices, had severe design deficiencies in their telemetry messaging protocols and were vulnerable to attacks that would compromise functionality or enable unauthorized access (Parihar et al., 2024). This emphasizes the clear necessity for strong security protocols to safeguard smart nutrition devices against these threats.

The consequences of device spoofing and unauthorized access in smart nutrition platforms are serious, especially for consumers who depend on accurate information for health care. For example, spoofed data from a smart scale may result in miscalculations of caloric or nutritional intake, which may result in adverse dietary choices for individuals with particular health requirements. Likewise, unauthorized access to a CGM may result in falsified glucose readouts, which may result in life-threatening complications for diabetic patients. Smart fridges, usually tied to nutrition apps for tracking inventory, have also been found susceptible. Studies have proved that poor authentication processes in smart home appliances can enable attackers to modify data or steal user credentials, further weakening the security of nutrition systems (Hammi et al., 2022). The FDA has also given warnings on Bluetooth vulnerabilities in health devices, such as glucose monitoring systems, explaining that these vulnerabilities might enable unauthorized access to crash devices or access locked functions, showing how widespread these threats. These instances show the urgent need for improved security measures to protect smart nutrition ecosystems (Figure 3).

Figure 3. Device Spoofing and Unauthorized Access in Smart Nutrition Ecosystems

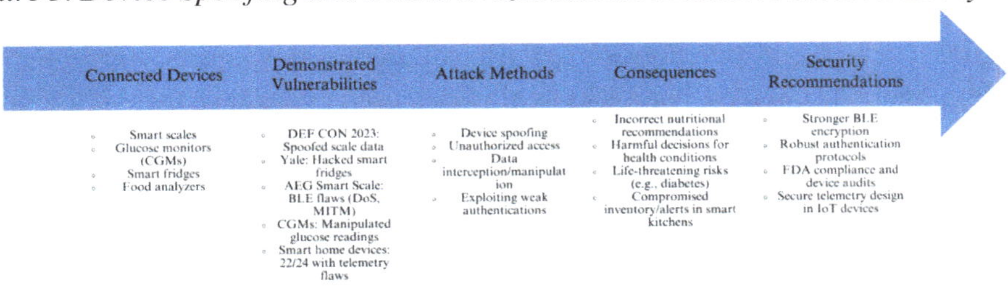

5. MANIPULATION OF NUTRITIONAL RECOMMENDATIONS

The University of Michigan's Health Security Research Group released results on AI-based nutrition services, which indicated that adversarial machine learning attacks might be used to "poison" recommendation systems. Their attack proof-of-concept induced a system to produce apparently suitable but insidiously detrimental meal plans which would worsen illnesses such as hypertension or diabetes if adopted over the long term (Ramirez et al 2024).

Adversarial machine learning (AML) encompasses methods aimed at misleading or manipulating ML models using unwanted inputs or changing training data. In intelligent nutrition systems, AML may be applied to compromise recommendation engines and create incorrect or destructive dietary recommendations. Data poisoning, for example, is injecting biased or fabricated data into the training set, leading the model to acquire wrong associations, for example, suggesting high-sodium foods for patients with hypertension (Muntzel & Drüeke, 1992). Another technique, adversarial examples, is creating inputs with carefully placed perturbations that are undetectable to humans but result in the model generating wrong outputs. For instance, making minor manipulations to reported food consumption data might cause a system to suggest inapt foods for users with allergies or diabetics. Evidence in healthcat6``re ML shows that such attacks are very effective, and it has been shown through studies that minor modifications in medical imaging or diagnostic data can result in misclassifications (Qayyum et al., 2020). These issues pinpoints the importance of strong defenses to guarantee the integrity of nutritional suggestions.

Manipulation of nutritional advice can have serious effects, especially among users with certain medical conditions who depend on reliable dietary advice. For example, a broken system could advise sugar-rich foods to a diabetic user, which could lead to life-threatening blood sugar levels, or provide high-sodium diets to patients with high blood pressure, worsening their condition (Itoh et al., 2022). In a theoretical example, an affluent attacker with economic interests in a food item may hack the algorithm of a nutrition app to push that product, biasing recommendations towards unhealthy choices. Another nagging risk is an attack on a mass scale, like a state-sponsored attack on public health through the promotion of nutritionally unsound diets to an entire population. Such manipulations may undermine confidence in smart nutrition systems and contribute to long-term health effects. The possibility of both focused and broad-based harm necessitates the utmost importance of secure AI systems in nutrition use (Mustapha).

In addition to simple data poisoning and adversarial attacks, sophisticated threats against intelligent nutrition systems are model inversion attacks and membership inference attacks. Model inversion enables the attacker to recover sensitive user information, for example, food consumption patterns or medical conditions, using the model outputs, which can result in privacy violation (Fang et al., 2024). Membership inference attacks would also allow adversaries to know if a user's information was included in the training dataset, compromising the privacy of the users. Transferability of adversarial examples between models also implies that an attack designed for one nutrition system would influence others with the same architectures, increasing the potential damage (Zhang et al 2019). Developing research also indicates the threat of backdoor attacks, where malicious attackers place covert triggers in the training data that lead the model to act maliciously under certain circumstances, like suggesting dangerous foods when certain inputs are made (Gao et al., 2020). These advanced threats necessitate sophisticated countermeasures to secure smart nutrition systems (Figure 4).

Figure 4. Manipulation of Nutritional Recommendations in Smart Nutrition Systems

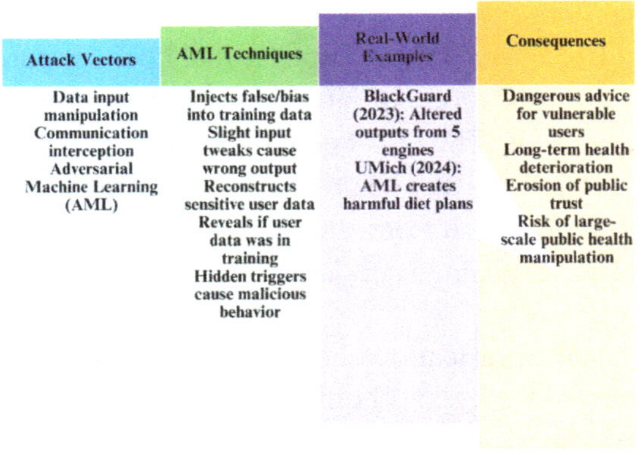

6. CYBER-PHYSICAL ATTACKS ON CONNECTED APPLIANCES

In 2023, the Cyber Physical Systems Security Coalition scientists illustrated vulnerabilities of smart cooking appliances linked to nutrition platforms. By taking advantage of vulnerabilities within a top-rated smart cooker's firmware, they were able to bypass safety features and temperature controls, posing potential fire risks. The same issues were identified with smart blenders and food processors that automatically adapt settings according to nutritional programs. Security experts showed that vulnerable devices might be able to run dangerously, destroying hardware or leading to injury .

In worst-case scenarios, cyber-physical attacks might turn kitchen appliances into weapons. A 2024 study examined the theoretical potential to hack ovens and ranges to disable safety features or manipulate gas lines to use them as makeshift explosive devices (IEDs). These attacks would be implemented through physical access during delivery or maintenance, wireless proximity attacks using Bluetooth or NFC, supply chain violations, or side-channel attacks on electromagnetic emanations (Coelho, 2021; Ghosh, 2023b). Although these are hypothetical situations, they highlight the utmost importance of secure appliances in the case of connected appliances merged with smart nutrition systems where user protection is of the highest priority. Their interconnectedness within larger ecosystems raises the risk further since one compromised device may be an entry point for purposes of entering sensitive health information or other attached devices.

The embedding of networked kitchen appliances within smart nutrition systems radically raises the risks of cyber-physical attacks. As an example, a smart scale hacked to provide false weight measurements could result in wrongly computed caloric or nutritional consumption, which could worsen ailments like diabetes or hypertension. Likewise, a hacked smart cooker that cooks according to nutritional programs can generate unsafe food, compromising the health of consumers who have certain special dietary needs. The larger ecosystem of intelligent nutrition systems, frequently involving wearables and health monitors, makes the threat environment even more challenging. A security flaw in one device has the potential to propagate throughout the network, exposing user data privacy or the overall system integrity (Yaqoob et al., 2019).

In addition, physical ramifications of these attacks go beyond health threats to encompass property damage and bodily harm. For instance, a runaway smart blender running at unsafe speeds may overheat or shatter, causing burns or cutting. The possibility of such an occurrence undermines user confidence in smart nutrition systems that depend on the transparent interconnection of connected appliances to provide dependable and safe meal advice. The absence of standardized security measures for IoT in the kitchen compounds these risks because most makers are more focused on functionality than security, making devices open to exploitation (Sahu & Mazumdar, 2024) (Figure 5).

Figure 5. Cyber-Physical Threats to Connected Appliances in Smart Nutrition Systems

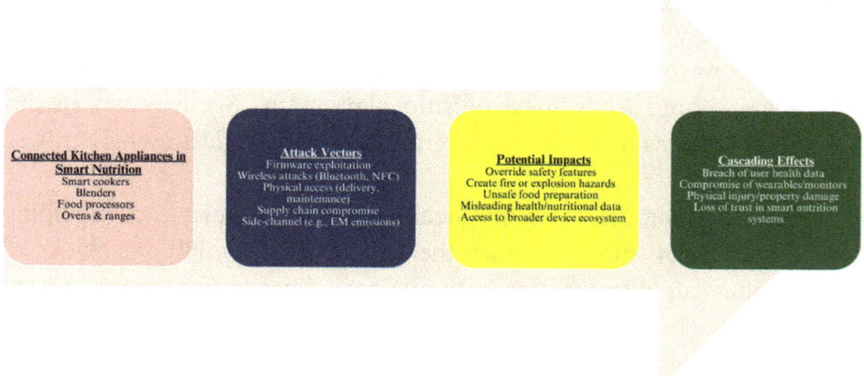

7. PRIVACY IMPLICATIONS AND DATA EXPLOITATION

Research on mobile nutrition and diet tracking applications has revealed significant privacy vulnerabilities. A 2023 study of 11 popular dietary and food timing assessment applications found that 73% (8 of 11 apps) shared user data with third-party services without maintaining transparent disclosures in their privacy policies. These applications routinely transmitted sensitive user information including complete dietary logs, health parameters, and location data to third parties. The primary stated purpose for this data sharing was to facilitate targeted advertising, though in theory such detailed dietary and health information could be leveraged for insurance underwriting decisions or employment screening (Gioia et al., 2023). Journal of Medical Internet Research released a thorough examination that illustrated how nutrition information could be utilized to make inferences about sensitive health states. Researchers were able to prove that eating habits alone were enough to predict with 78% accuracy if users had specific chronic diseases, even if those diseases were not explicitly stated (Martinez et al., 2023).

The general practice of sharing user data by nutrition apps tends to be done in a lack of transparency or consent from users, compounding privacy issues. Research suggests most health and wellness apps, as well as nutrition apps, share data with third parties for purposes other than the core activities of the app, such as advertising or analytics. For example, a study on mobile health applications revealed that 89% of them harvest personal information but just 7% clearly state their privacy policies, and as a result, users do not know how their information is utilized (Tangari et al., 2021) . Transparency can be lost this way and undermine user trust, especially when sensitive information such as dietary patterns or biometric measures is being shared. Additionally, the vulnerability of data being utilized in applications such as insurance underwriting or hiring raises ethical concerns regarding discrimination and fairness. The interdependent nature of the smart nutrition systems, which tend to integrate within other health ecosystems, further increases these risks, as one breach may open up a vast amount of personal information across ecosystems (Choudhury et al., 2024; Ghosh et al., 2022).

The capacity for making inferences about sensitive health details from diet data is a substantial privacy threat. Dietary habits have been demonstrated to indicate underlying medical conditions, including diabetes or cardiovascular disease, with high accuracy. For instance, research within the Journal of Medical Internet Research illustrated how machine learning algorithms could forecast chronic diseases from food data and emphasized potential third-party misuse. This function is especially troubling if data is released to parties such as advertisers, insurers, or employers, who might utilize deduced health information to make choices that harm users. For example, an insurer may set premiums on the basis of inferred health risk, or an employer may hire or fire on the basis of perceived health status. These activities highlight the necessity of robust data protection strategies to forestall illicit inferences and secure user privacy (Ienca et al., 2019).

In addition to privacy violations, data exploitation in smart nutrition systems also encompasses the ability for malicious tampering. An attacker might take advantage of weaknesses in data pipelines or algorithms to make changes to nutritional advice, providing nutrition information that is detrimental. For instance, through data input manipulation or communication interception, attackers may quietly alter recommendations to endorse unhealthy foods or aggravate a user's health conditions, for instance, recommending high-sugar diets for diabetic users (Spero, 2006). Interoperability with other health systems, including wearables or smart appliances in the kitchen, heightens the risk of ecosystem-level intrusions, where one vulnerability may compromise the entire system. This interconnection increases the vulnerability of data exploitation, and thus it is essential to put in place effective security measures to safeguard both data integrity and user well-being (Jaime et al., 2023). The absence of universal security protocols for use in IoT devices within nutrition systems also increases these vulnerabilities since most developers focus more on functionality than security (Figure 6).

Figure 6. Privacy and Data Exploitation Risks in Smart Nutrition Systems

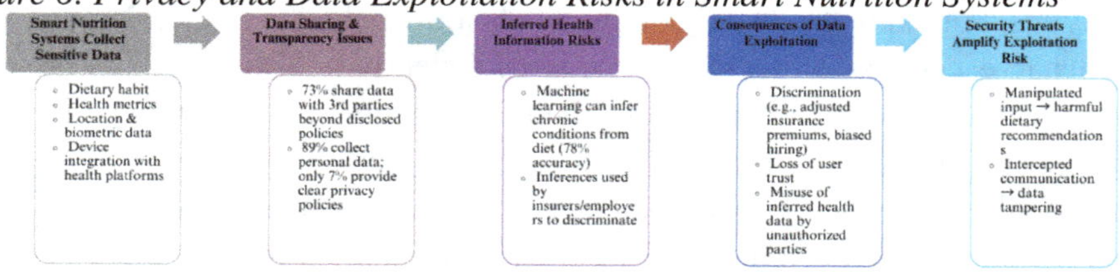

8. EMERGING THREATS IN SMART NUTRITION

As the smart nutrition ecosystem evolves, new threat vectors continue to emerge:

- Research has demonstrated how ultrasonic "dolphin attacks" using inaudible voice commands can manipulate voice-controlled devices and virtual assistants (Zhang et al., 2017). Given the increasing prevalence of voice-controlled nutrition and dietary management systems in smart kitchens and personalized nutrition platforms, these devices face similar vulnerabilities.

Such attacks could potentially be exploited to modify food orders or dietary settings without user awareness or explicit authorization (Zhang et al., 2017).

- Supply Chain Compromises: The increasing complexity of the smart nutrition ecosystem introduces supply chain risks. In late 2023, several popular nutrition applications were compromised when attackers inserted malicious code into a widely-used third-party nutritional database library. This affected over 40 applications before being detected (Cybersecurity and Infrastructure Security Agency, 2024).
- Aggregated Data Risks: As companies accumulate vast repositories of nutritional and health data, these collections become increasingly valuable targets. In 2024, a major data broker was discovered attempting to sell aggregated (though allegedly anonymized) datasets from multiple nutrition platforms. Research has repeatedly shown that such datasets can often be de-anonymized when combined with other information sources (Federal Trade Commission, 2024).

Addressing these emerging threats requires a multi-layered approach. For voice assistant vulnerabilities, developers should integrate advanced authentication mechanisms and anomaly detection systems, while manufacturers should design hardware to filter out ultrasonic frequencies. Supply chain security can be enhanced through rigorous vetting of third-party components, regular security audits, and adherence to frameworks like NIST's C-SCRM. For aggregated data risks, robust anonymization techniques, strict access controls, and transparent privacy policies are essential. Regulatory frameworks, such as the General Data Protection Regulation (GDPR) in Europe and the Health Insurance Portability and Accountability Act (HIPAA) in the U.S., provide a foundation for data protection, but specific standards for nutrition apps are needed to address their unique challenges (European Data Protection Board, 2023). User education is also critical, empowering individuals to understand the risks of data sharing and adopt secure practices, such as using strong passwords and monitoring app permissions (Figure 6).

Figure 7. Emerging Threats in Smart Nutrition Ecosystems

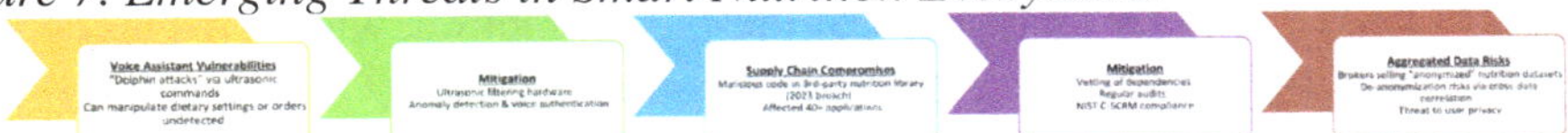
Voice Assistant Vulnerabilities
"Dolphin attacks" via ultrasonic commands
Can manipulate dietary settings or orders undetected
Mitigation
Ultrasonic filtering hardware
Anomaly detection & voice authentication
Supply Chain Compromises
Affected 40+ applications
Mitigation
Vetting of dependencies
Regular audits
NIST C-SCRM compliance
Aggregated Data Risks
Brokers selling "anonymized" nutrition datasets
correlation
Threat to user privacy

9. REGULATORY AND COMPLIANCE CHALLENGES

The EU's General Data Protection Regulation (GDPR) and the California Consumer Privacy Act (CCPA) impose significant requirements on companies handling personal health information. Several major nutrition platforms have faced regulatory action for non-compliance. In 2023, European regulators fined NutriHealth €4.3 million for improper handling of user consent and excessive data collection practices challenges (European Data Protection Board, 2023). In the healthcare context, nutrition platforms that partner with medical providers must navigate HIPAA compliance. A 2024 Office for Civil Rights investigation found multiple violations among nutrition apps claiming HIPAA compliance, including inadequate encryption, improper access controls, and insufficient audit mechanisms (Department of Health and Human Services, 2024) (Figure 7).

The General Data Protection Regulation (GDPR), in force since May 25, 2018, requires organizations processing EU residents' personal data to obtain clear consent, be transparent, and put in place strong security. In the case of smart nutrition systems, this means handling user consent for different global user populations, having data minimization in place, and having in place mechanisms for users to assert rights like access, correction, or deletion of their data. The 2022 Senseonics Inc. case shows these challenges, where insufficient technical and organizational safeguards resulted in a data breach, against GDPR Articles 5, 9, and 27 (Bertolazzi et al., 2024).

The California Consumer Privacy Act (CCPA), in effect as of January 1, 2020, provides rights to California residents to know what personal data is gathered, ask for its removal, and choose not to have it sold. Intelligent nutrition systems, which gather extensive information such as diet records and health indicators, should be transparent and offer easy methods to exercise these rights. This is difficult considering the amount of and sensitive nature of information handled, demanding the use of advanced data handling systems to monitor and act on consumer inquiries. For example, a nutrition app needs to transparently explain how dietary information is used and permit users to exclude data sharing with third parties like advertisers. Noncompliance can bring up to $7,500 fines per infraction, with consumers being able to sue for $100-$750 per record in the event of a breach (Goldman, 2021). The intersection with GDPR for consumers who are both EU residents and California residents makes it even more complicated, requiring harmonized compliance measures to cover both regulations.

For intelligent nutrition platforms that collaborate with healthcare providers or manage protected health information (PHI), they must comply with the Health Insurance Portability and Accountability Act (HIPAA). HIPAA's Privacy Rule regulates

PHI use and disclosure, whereas the Security Rule requires protection measures such as encryption, access controls, and audit controls for electronic PHI. A U.S. 2024 investigation. Department of Health and Human Services' Office for Civil Rights found several violations in nutrition apps that had indicated they were HIPAA compliant, such as poor encryption and poor access controls (Peeples, 2023). These findings verify the difficulty of ensuring that all system components, ranging from mobile apps to IoT devices such as smart scales, are compliant with HIPAA's strict standards. The integrated nature of intelligent nutrition systems, generally coupled with other health platforms, raises the potential for non-compliance, as one weak link can transgress PHI throughout the ecosystem. HIPAA violations can be fined between $100 and $50,000 per offense, up to a maximum of $1.5 million per event, highlighting financial and reputational consequences (Burks, 2024).

The international extent of smart nutrition systems requires adherence to several regulatory regimes at the same time, based on users' geographical locations. This is especially difficult for internationally operating systems since they have to deal with different requirements across jurisdictions like GDPR in the EU, CCPA in California, and others like Canada's PIPEDA or Brazil's LGPD. The interconnection of these systems with devices such as wearables and intelligent kitchen appliances only makes compliance more difficult, where a leak in one part can spill data into various platforms. The issue has been identified by research as the necessity for harmonized standards and certification procedures to meet these challenges, especially for AI-based systems that involve biomarkers and machine learning, issues of concern for user safety, security, and privacy (Shoghli et al., 2024). Additionally, the regulatory vacuum surrounding laboratory-developed tests (LDTs) used in personalized nutrition, which often lack clinical validity evidence, poses further challenges, as these tests may not fit within existing frameworks, risking misleading claims and consumer harm (Korenstein et al., 2021) (Figure 8).

Figure 8. Regulatory & Compliance Challenges in Smart Nutrition

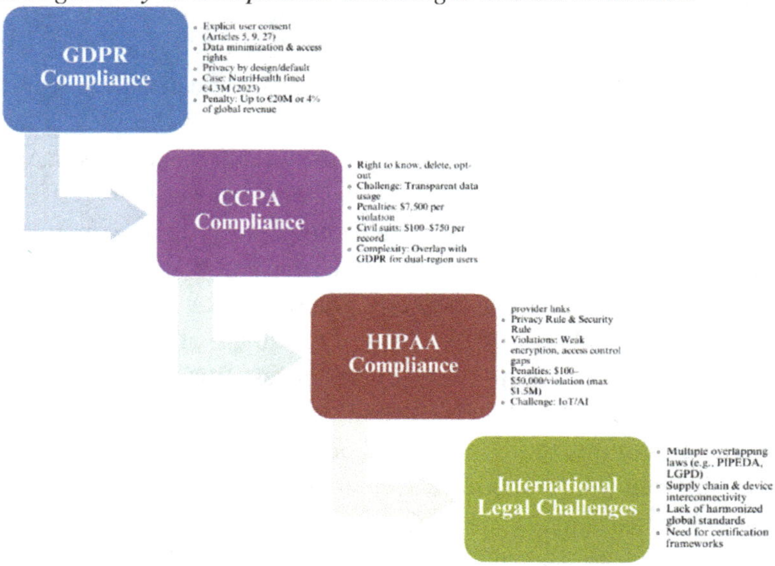

10. MITIGATION STRATEGIES

Organizations creating smart nutrition technologies can follow different measures to mitigate these risks:

Technical Safeguards

- Incorporating end-to-end encryption for every dietary and health information
- Using strong authentication methods, such as multi-factor authentication
- Creating strong API security to secure data in transit
- Conducting regular security testing and penetration testing
- Using anomaly detection to recognize abnormal patterns in recommendations or device activity

Governance Approaches

- Incorporating privacy-by-design principles during development Transparent data handling practices and clear privacy policies
- Regular compliance reviews against relevant regulations (GDPR, HIPAA, etc.)
- Implementing comprehensive data minimization strategies

- Establishing incident response procedures for potential breaches

User Empowerment

- Providing granular privacy controls for users
- Clear documentation of data usage and sharing practices
- Offering offline modes or reduced-data options
- Educating users about safe practices and potential risks

The smart nutrition landscape presents a complex array of security and privacy challenges. The increasing adoption of these technologies in healthcare and everyday life requires immediate action to fix their security weaknesses. The research and incidents show that smart nutrition systems face threats which go beyond conventional data breaches to include manipulation of health advice as well as device tampering and privacy violations. Organizations which develop these technologies need to implement security measures throughout their development process while using complete data protection strategies. People who use smart nutrition platforms need to be aware of their potential dangers while benefiting from their advantages. Nutrition technology security requires specific standards because regulatory frameworks keep evolving while addressing its unique challenges. The combination of nutritional science with technology and personal health generates highly sensitive data environments which require strategic protection methods (Figure 9).

Figure 9. Mitigation Strategies for Smart Nutrition Systems

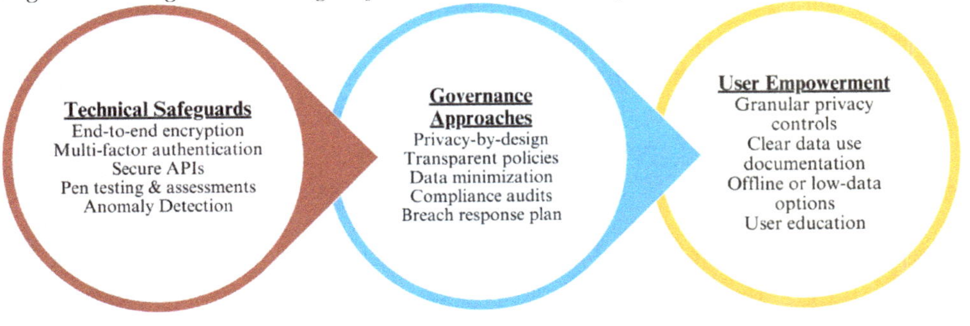

11. CONTEXT-AWARE SECURITY: CONCEPT AND RELEVANCE

11.1. What is Context-Aware Security?

Security that adapts to context represents a smart cybersecurity methodology which modifies protection measures according to environmental conditions of user systems and transactions (Perera et al.,2014). Traditional security models implement fixed rules while context-aware security examines multiple contextual elements in real-time to achieve security decisions which safeguard protection and usability. The system evaluates present contextual information to establish security measures and authentication protocols and access authorization levels in context-aware security frameworks (Hayashi et al., 2013). Security requirements differ substantially between different situations which this approach understands thus providing adaptive protection for evolving circumstances 11.2. Benefits in Adaptive and Personalized Environments

Context-aware security offers several key advantages in today's increasingly adaptive and personalized technology environments:

- Context-aware security implements adaptive authentication by reducing security friction in low-risk contexts while heightening security requirements in higher-risk situations. This approach balances user experience with security effectiveness—users experience fewer authentication interruptions during routine access (low friction) while additional authentication factors are transparently requested when risk indicators suggest potential threats (heightened security). Research demonstrates that users find this contextual approach more usable than continuous two-factor authentication while maintaining comparable security perception (Wiefling et al., 2021).
- Better Calibration of Risk Management: The security attributes can now be more tightly calibrated against the actual risk of a defined situation; this, in turn, allows for more efficient use of resources and subsequently results in less of the headache of false positives generated by static security attributes (Baracaldo et al., 2018).
- Adaptability to Change: Context-aware mechanisms adjust security controls automatically as factors about their state change. This provides continuous protection without operator input across states (Khan & Sakamura, 2015).
- Improved Behavioural Anomaly Detection: Context-aware mechanisms allow for establishing baselines based on behaviours and environments for users. As a result, context aware systems can better detect what are truly suspicious actions based on deviations to particulars that are previously defined as normal (Fridman et al., 2017).

- Efficient Resource Utilization: Systems can better allocate computing resources and security resources based on what is really required, as opposed to the worst-case or incident scenarios. This ultimately results in better execution and performance (Miettinen et al., 2018).

11.3. Key Components

11.3.1. User Context

User context encompasses personal factors that influence security needs and risk profiles:

- Age: The user's age will have differing security requirements. For example, children's apps will apply stricter controls on sharing data, while older adults may use simplified authentication methods to support their potential physical challenges .
- Health Status: Current medical circumstances also affect what security is needed in nutrition apps. A diabetic person would require a more protective barrier around their blood glucose data, and possibly dietary metrics. Compromising that info could put the user's health in serious jeopardy .
- Location: Another important variable is where a user is accessing information from. The nutrition information accessed by a user at home has different security risk factors than if accessing the same information from a café with public Wi-Fi. There are also specific regulatory compliance requirements that apply in certain locations if the user crosses jurisdictions (Bhattacharya et al., 2020).

11.3.2. Environmental Context

Environmental variables touch on the technical and temporal conditions of system use:

- Time: Activity timing may signify risk levels. Attempts made at off-hours may need more verification, whereas normal access at regular meal times may have streamlined authentication. Temporal behaviors also assist in developing baselines for regular behaviour (Zhang et al., 2019) .

11.3.3. Behavioural Context

Behavioural context leverages patterns of user interaction to establish baselines and detect anomalies:

- Usual Dietary Habits: In nutrition applications, established patterns of food logging, meal timing, ingredient preferences, and dietary restrictions are important behaviours to consider to establish and identify baselines of typical user behaviours. Deviations from these convention, such as a sudden change in caloric intake or unusual ingredient selections might signal the need for additional verification in the event the atypical behaviours take place with just one or more risk factors (Dempsey et al., 2018).
- Transaction patterns: Where nutrition application allows access to purchasing options; established patterns of ordering supplements, meal kits and/or subscriptions to services, provide important contextual information. Unusual patterns of order quantities, shipping address/locations and/or payment methods may trigger alternate verification .When the context or situational information is included, security systems in smart nutrition environments can provide smart capabilities that continuously weight protection and usability. For instance, if a user is accessing their standard meal planning functions from their home device during normal hours, the security friction may be low, but if the user wanted to change their subscription payment information, and from an unknown location, the user may face stepped-up authentication (Crossler & Bélanger, 2019). Context-aware security, in nutritional technology, is important because it enhances the ability to provide personalized access to health advice that is convenient but secure and acknowledges that the consequences of nutrition data being compromised can impact sedentary physical well-being (Figure 10).

Figure 10. Key Components of Context-Aware Security

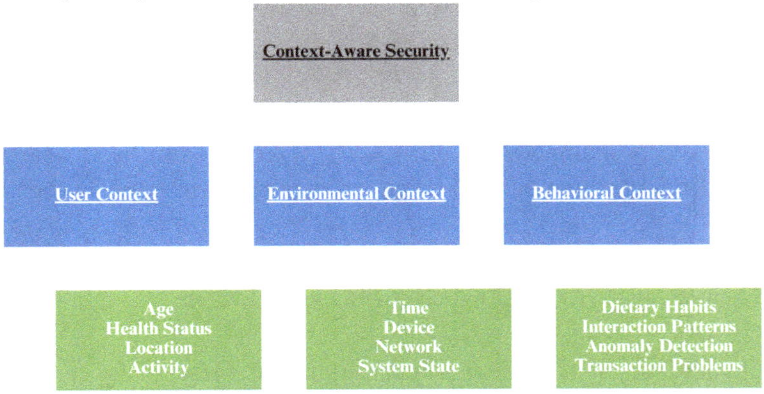

11.4. Security Architecture for Smart Nutrition Systems

11.4.1. Layered Architecture of Smart Nutrition Systems

Typically, smart nutrition systems are designed in a multi-layer architecture, creating distinct points of security threat and tailored protections, very similar to the IoT reference model. This multi-layer approach makes it possible to use defence-in-depth in a manner where security controls exist at one layer and directly complement or support another layer .

11.4.2. Perception Layer (Sensors, Wearables)

The perception layer forms the base layer of smart nutrition systems which consists of physical devices capturing both nutritional and physiological data . This layer includes:

- Wearable Devices: Smartwatches, fitness trackers, and continuous glucose monitors that track activity levels, heart rate, blood glucose, and other physiological parameters related to nutrition.
- Applications of Smart Kitchen and Environmental Sensors: Internet-connected refrigerators with food recognition cameras, smart scales, cooking devices that use temperature sensors, and food analysers that collect data on food composition and consumption .
- Food Logging Tools: Mobile applications with image recognition capabilities that identify food items and estimate nutritional content .

- Environmental Sensors: Technology that measure environmental conditions which have an impact on food safety and quality, specifically temperature and humidity sensors used in food storage .

The perception layer is especially susceptible to physical tampering, device spoofing, and sensor manipulation attacks. The threat is amplified as edge devices often possess limited computational resources to implement some level of adequate security .

11.4.3. Network Layer (Communication Protocols)

The network layer that connects perception layer devices to higher-level devices supports data transfer through diverse communication protocol usage determined by power usage, range, and data volume. Some common protocols in smart nutrition systems are:

- Personal Area Networks: Bluetooth Low Energy (BLE) and Near Field Communication (NFC) which are short-range communication used for wearables, smartphones, and local devices.
- Local Area Networks: Wi-Fi, and Ethernet connections—in residential and clinical use—provide higher-bandwidth data transfers .
- Wide Area Networks: cellular networks (4G/5G), LoRaWAN, and NB-IoT have use case where data is being transferred from a remote location to a cloud service.

Do network layer vulnerabilities include man-in- the -middle, eavesdropping, packet injection, and denial of service, many of the communication protocols in smart nutrition systems are heterogeneous, creating unique protection problems which must be addressed using a protocol specific protective method .

11.4.4. Application Layer (AI Recommendation Engines, User Interfaces)

The application layer includes software components that process, analyze, and display nutritional data to end-users, healthcare professionals, and other stakeholders . Applications, at this layer, play a critical role in the total nutrition protection framework. The significant software components of the application layer are as follows:

- Data processing systems: backend services that combine and then normalize data from diverse sources, apply data cleaning algorithms on new data, and prepare data for analysis ;
- Artificial intelligence recommendation engines: machine learning models that assess nutritional data and provide personalized dietary recommendations, meal plans, and health insights ;
- User interfaces: mobile applications, web portals, and dashboards that allow the end-user to engage with the system, see recommendations, and manage their nutritional data;
- Integration services: APIs and services that swap data with several third-party systems, such as electronic health records, fitness applications, and food delivery services .

In the application layer, many of the most common threats include (data) leakage, API abuse, injection, cross-site scripting, and poisoning of machine learning models. The myriads of potential attack vectors are created from the complexity associated with modern applications and the expansive connectivity facilitated by the cloud (Figure 11).

Figure 11. Security Architecture for Smart Nutrition Systems

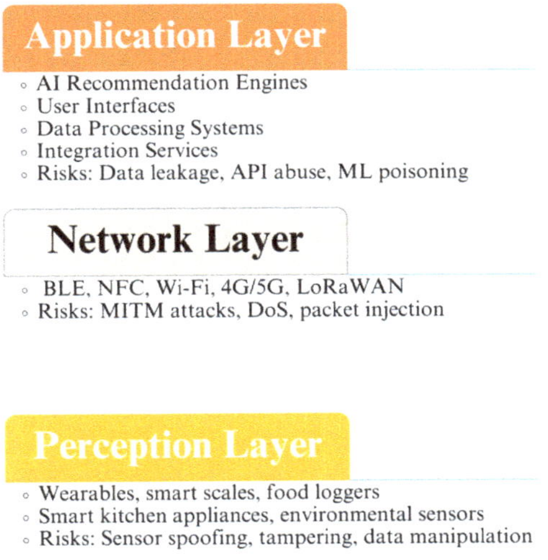

11.4.5. Context-Aware Mechanisms at Each Layer

11.4.5.1. Encryption Techniques

Encryption establishes confidentiality and integrity protections over sensitive nutritional and health data throughout the system. In terms of context-aware encryption methods, security levels can adapt in accordance with, data sensitivity, device capabilities, and environmental factors (Roy Choudhury et al., 2025).

11.4.5.2. Perception Layer Encryption

- Lightweight Symmetric Algorithms: Easy versions of AES (like AES-CCM) and specific lightweight codes such as PRESENT or SIMON give protection with minimal computational overhead (Liu et al., 2016).
- Selective Encryption: Context-aware approaches encrypt delicate parts of data at low battery levels and in limited processing capacity (Ghosh et al., 2025).

11.4.5.3. Network Layer Encryption

- Protocol-Specific Security: For protocol specific security communications, WPA3 for Wi-Fi connections, and MAC layer encryption for Bluetooth and Zigbee are needed (Granjal et al., 2015).
- Context-Adaptive Encryption: Systems which actively modify encryption parameters according to the conditions of network and delicacy of transmitted data. Such as for sensitive health metrics stronger encryption are needed and basic encryption are needed for non-identifying device status information
- End-to-End Encryption: Ensures data remains encrypted throughout transmission from perception devices to application servers, preventing exposure at intermediate network nodes

11.4.5.4. Application Layer Encryption

Comprehensive encryption stategies by higher level system protect data when at rest and during processing

- Database Encryption: Column-level and field-level encryption that safeguard subtly nutritional data and permit non-sensitive fields to ensure as a searchable entity (Samarati et al., 2010).
- Tokenization: Replacing sensitive identifiers with non-sensitive equivalents to maintain referential integrity while reducing exposure of personal information (Wang et al 2017).

- Format-Preserving Encryption: Encrypts data while maintaining its format, facilitating integration with legacy systems while providing enhanced security (Liu et al., 2016).
- Key Rotation and Management: Context-aware key lifecycle management that adjusts rotation schedules based on data sensitivity and usage patterns.

11.4.6. Authentication Protocols

Authentication protocols confirm the identity of users, devices, and services deal with smart nutrition systems. Security requirements are adjusted by the context aware authentication according to access context, balancing security with usability.

11.4.6.1. Perception Layer Authentication

The focal point of device level verification is to confirm identities for sensors and wearables:

- Device Certificates: X.509 certificates embedded during manufacturing establish device identity and enable mutual authentication with gateway devices and servers .
- Lightweight Authentication Protocols: ECC-based authentication schemes that provide sufficient security while minimizing computational demands on resource constrained devices
- Context-Based Authentication: Context based authentication encompass device location, sensor readings, and usage patterns to check device legitimacy with locating potential device spoofing or replacement (Gope & Hwang, 2016).

11.4.6.2. Application Layer Authentication

User authentications involve various factors and context analysis to make sure proper access control (Dasgupta et al., 2017):

- Multi-Factor Authentication: Combines knowledge factors (passwords), possession factors (devices), and inherence factors (biometrics) to verify user identity (Fridman et al., 2017).
- Risk-Based Authentication: Authentication requirements are modified according to contextual risk factors including location, device characteristics, and access patterns. Higher-risk context stimulates stronger authentication challenges (Fernández-Alemán et al., 2013).

11.4.7. Anomaly and Intrusion Detection

Security breaches or system malfunctions are diagnosed by anomaly detection systems. To properly differentiate among normal variations and potential threats context aware approaches built behavioural baselines and environmental norms (Ghosh, J et al., 2025).

11.4.7.1. Perception Layer Anomaly Detection

The aim of device level monitoring is to spot physical tampering, sensor manipulation, and abnormal data patterns (Diro & Chilamkurti, 2018):

- Sensor Data Analysis: Statistical methods and machine learning algorithms helps to identify physiologically impossible readings or sudden incomprehensible modifications in sensor outputs (Caviglione et al., 2016) .
- Power Consumption Monitoring: Detects unusual energy usage patterns that might indicate malware infection or hardware tampering (Seyed Farhad Aghili et al., 2019) .
- Physical Tamper Detection: Sensors and circuits that detect unauthorized physical access to device components, triggering alerts or protective measures.

11.4.7.2. Application Layer Anomaly Detection

Behavioural analysis aims to detecting doubtful user activities and application-level attacks:

- User Behaviour Analytics: User behavior analytics produce behavioural standard for every users and locate deviations specifying account compromises like unusual access patterns or unexpected feature usage (Chakraborty et al., 2018, Fridman et al., 2017).
- Data Integrity Monitoring: Check application data consistency and locate illicit changes that points to database attacks or insider threats (Diro & Chilamkurti, 2018, Ghosh et al., 2025, Ghosh J et al., 2025) .
- Context-Aware Fraud Detection: Context aware fraud detection systems inspect nutritional context by assessing potentially dubious activities like unfit dietary recommendations which points to manipulation of recommendation algorithms.

11.4.8. Trust Management and User Consent

Trust management systems initiate and continue trustworthy relationships between system components by securing proper user consent for data collection and processing.

11.4.8.1. Perception Layer Trust Management:

Device-level trust aims to assuring the integrity and reliability of data sources:

- Trust Bootstrapping: Secure device initialization procedures that establish baseline trust at deployment time through verified firmware and authenticated configuration.
- Reputation Systems: Track device reliability over time, adjusting trust levels based on historical accuracy and compliance with expected behaviour.
- Contextual Trust Evaluation: Evaluates device trustworthiness based on environmental factors, deployment location, and current operating conditions.

11.4.8.2. Network Layer Trust Management

Connection trust highlights setting up dependable communication channels and assessing peer trustworthiness:

- Trust-Based Routing: Selects communication paths based on the trustworthiness of intermediate nodes, avoiding potentially compromised network segments.
- Dynamic Trust Assessment: Continuously evaluates the trustworthiness of network connections based on observed behavior and external threat intelligence .
- Context-Aware Trust Negotiation: Adjusts trust requirements based on the sensitivity of transmitted data and current network conditions .

11.4.8.3. Application Layer Trust Management

User-centric trust emphasises on clear data practices and informed consents :

- Granular Consent Management: Allows users to provide context-specific consent for different data types and usage scenarios rather than blanket permissions .
- Dynamic Consent: Dynamic consent permit users to change consent choices time to time and introduce context-appropriate consent requests when new data types or processing activities are initiated .

- Trust Dashboards: Trust Dashboards presents clear views of nutritional data usage patterns, who obtained data and what acumen originated from it.
- Privacy Labels: Simplified privacy information that helps users understand data practices without navigating complex privacy policies (Figure 12).

Figure 12. Security Enhancements in Smart Nutrition Systems

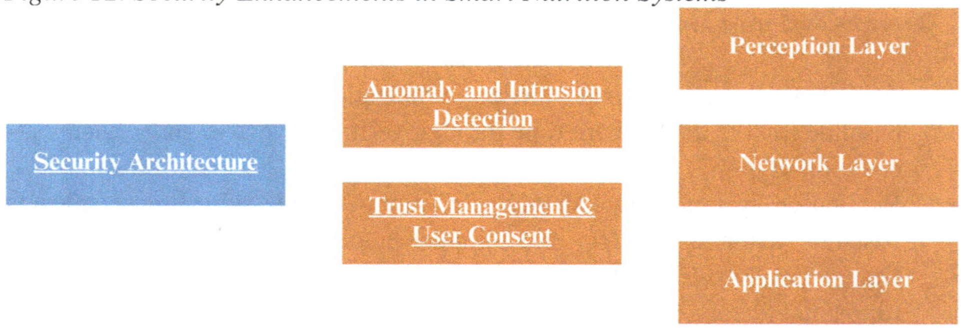

12. PRIVACY-PRESERVING DATA SHARING AND STORAGE

12.1. Context-Aware Data Sharing Models

Context-aware data sharing models alter information exposure on the basis of situational factors while adjusting usability with privacy protection. These models assesses various contextual elements to deciding proper sharing parameters .

12.2. Risk-Based Sharing

Risk-based approaches identify potential privacy harm before sharing data and accommodate protection levels correspondingly (Ghosh, J et al., 2025, Roy Choudhury et al., 2024):

- Contextual Risk Assessment: Contextual risk assessment assesses factors like recipient trustworthiness, data sensitivity, and potential for re-identification to estimate a risk score for each sharing instance .
- Adaptive Anonymization: Applies varying levels of anonymization based on assessed risk, implementing stronger protections for higher-risk sharing scenarios .

- Disclosure Limitation: Hinders the volume and detail of shared data on the basis of risk limits, potentially providing aggregated statistics rather than individual records in high-risk contexts .

12.3. Sensitivity-Based Sharing

Sensitivity-based models analyze data elements on the basis of their privacy concerns, employing proper protections to each category:

- Multi-Level Classification: classifies nutritional data into sensitivity tiers (e.g., identifying information, general dietary patterns, health conditions) with consistent protection necessities.
- Context-Aware Sensitivity Assessment: identifies that data sensitivity may change according to situational factors. For instance, meal timing information might be touchey during religious fasting periods .
- Progressive Disclosure: Appoint a gradual approach that primarily shares less sensitive information, suppling additional detail at the time of requirement and properly safeguarded.

12.4. Purpose-Based Sharing:

Purpose-based models line up data revealing with the deleberate use case, assuring that shared information is both enough and minimal for the stated purpose:

- Purpose Specification: Clearly defines and communicates the purpose for each data sharing instance, establishing boundaries for acceptable use .
- Purpose-Based Filtering: Discloses only data elements relevant to the specified purpose, withholding unrelated information even if available .
- Contextual Integrity: Assures that the flow of data ensures proper contextual norms regarding what information should be shared for proper purposes .

12.5. Role-Based and Context-Based Access Controls

Access control mechanisms regulate who can obtain nutritional data and in what situations. Context-enhanced approaches lengthen traditional role-based models by encompassing situational factors into access decisions .

12.5.1. Role-Based Access Control (RBAC)

RBAC grants permis on the basis of organizational or functional roles, clarifying management by implementing least privilege principles:

- Nutritional Role Definitions: Initiating different roles for nutritionist, personal trainer, healthcare provider, and data subject, each with forethought admittance to divergent data categories .
- Role Hierarchies: Organizes roles into hierarchical structures that reflect organizational relationships and inheritance of permissions.
- Dynamic Role Assignment: Assigns roles based on qualifications, certifications, and relationships with data subjects, ensuring appropriate access privileges.

12.5.2. Attribute-Based Access Control (ABAC)

ABAC assesses various traits of users, resources, actions, and environments to make subtle access decisions:

- User Attributes: Scrutinize traits like professional credentials, organizational affiliation, relationship to the data subject, and location when analysing access requests.
- Resource Attributes: Evaluates data characteristics including sensitivity level, collection context, age, and relevance to specific health conditions.
- Environmental Attributes: Incorporates contextual factors such as time of access, device security posture, and network characteristics into access decisions.

12.5.3. Context-Based Access Control (CBAC)

CBAC particularly highlights on situational factors which affect access appropriateness, accommodating permissions according to changing contexts (Bernabe et al., 2016):

- Spatial Context: Considers physical location when determining access rights, potentially restricting sensitive operations to secure environments like clinical settings (Bernabe et al., 2016) .
- Temporal Context: Enforces time-based restrictions such as business hours limitations or temporary elevated access during dietary emergencies .

- Purpose Context: Aligns access permissions with the declared purpose for data usage, enforcing purpose limitation principles.
- Relationship Context: analyzes the association between the data subject and the requesting party while balancing availability on the basis of professional relationship type and duration (Figure 13).

Figure 13. Privacy-Preserving Data Sharing and Access Control

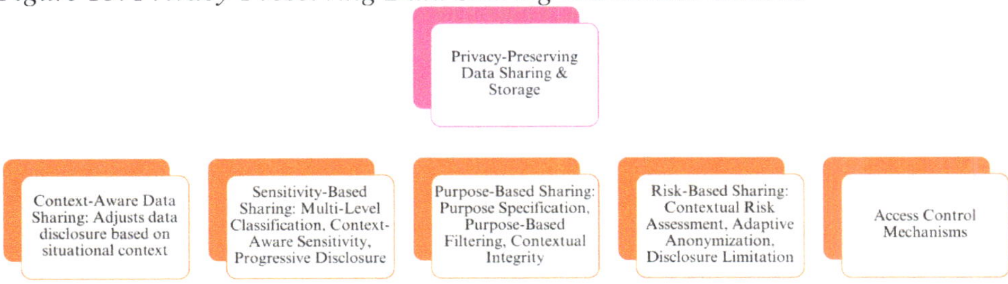

Figure 14. Advanced Privacy-Preserving Computation Techniques

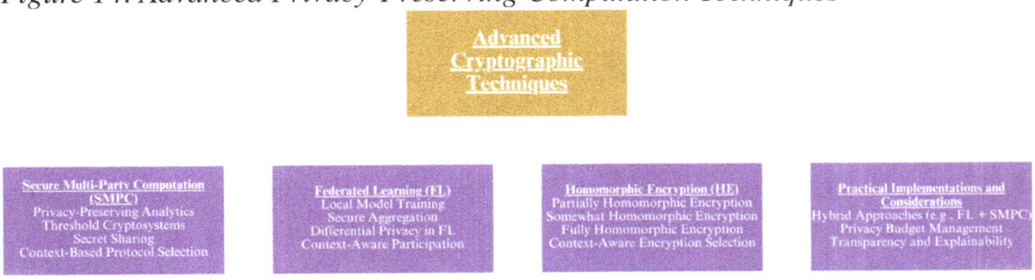

12.5.4. Adaptive Access Control

Adaptive approaches continuously re-evaluate access decisions based on changing contexts and behavioral patterns. (Hayashi, et al., 2013, Roy Choudhury et al., 2025):

- Continuous Authorization: Maintains ongoing assessment of access appropriateness throughout sessions, potentially revoking permissions if contextual factors change (Wiefling, et al., 2021).

- Risk-Adaptive Access Control: Evaluates access requests according to various risk factors, allowing entry when risk levels remain within acceptable ranges (Wiefling, et al., 2021).
- Usage Control: Extends access control beyond initial approval to govern ongoing data usage while imposing obligations and restrictions throughout the data lifecycle (Khan & Sakamura, 2015) (Figure 14).

13. SECURE MULTI-PARTY COMPUTATION, FEDERATED LEARNING, AND HOMOMORPHIC ENCRYPTION

Advanced cryptographic techniques enable privacy-preserving computation on sensitive nutritional data while preventing disclosure of underlying information (Qayyum, A et al., 2020) .

13.1. Secure Multi-Party Computation (SMPC)

SMPC protocols allow multiple parties to jointly compute functions over their inputs while protecting the privacy of those inputs from other participants (Qayyum, A et al., 2020):

- Privacy-Preserving Analytics: Enables collaborative analysis of nutritional data without parties needing to disclose their raw data, facilitating research while maintaining privacy protections (Martinez, J et al., 2023).
- Threshold Cryptosystems: Distributes trust across multiple parties, requiring collaboration to decrypt or access sensitive data (Gope & Hwang, 2016).
- Secret Sharing: Divides sensitive data into shares distributed among multiple parties, where reconstruction requires a minimum number of shares to be combined (Gope & Hwang, 2016) .
- Context-Based Protocol Selection: Selects appropriate SMPC protocols based on performance requirements, security needs, and specific computational requirements (Khan & Sakamura, 2015).

13.2. Federated Learning (FL)

Federated learning approaches enable machine learning model development across decentralized devices while keeping data locally without requiring data exchange (Qayyum, A et al .,2020):

- Local Model Training: Each participant (such as nutrition app users) trains models on their local data while sharing only model updates rather than raw nutritional or health data (Qayyum, A et al., 2020).
- Secure Aggregation: Cryptographically combines model updates from multiple participants while preventing information leakage about individual contributions (Qayyum, A et al., 2020).
- Differential Privacy in FL: Incorporates calibrated noise into model updates to provide mathematical privacy guarantees that protect against inference attacks (Fang, H et al., 2024).
- Context-Aware Participation: Enables federated learning participation based on device context, such as limiting training to devices when charging and on unmetered networks (Perera et al., 2014).

13.3. Homomorphic Encryption (HE)

Homomorphic encryption schemes allow computations to be performed on encrypted data without decryption, preserving privacy while enabling data analysis (Qayyum, A et al., 2020):

- Partially Homomorphic Encryption: Supports specific operations (such as addition or multiplication) on encrypted nutritional data, enabling selective analyses without data exposure (Qayyum, A et al., 2020).
- Somewhat Homomorphic Encryption: Allows a limited number of operations on encrypted data, balancing functionality with performance for practical nutritional analytics (Qayyum, A et al., 2020).
- Fully Homomorphic Encryption: Enables arbitrary computations on encrypted data, though with significant performance overhead that limits practical application in real-time nutrition systems (Qayyum, A et al., 2020) .
- Context-Aware Encryption Selection: Chooses appropriate homomorphic schemes based on computational requirements, performance constraints, and security needs of specific nutritional applications (Perera et al., 2014).

13.4. Practical Implementations and Considerations

Integration of these advanced techniques into smart nutrition systems requires careful consideration of performance, usability, and privacy trade-offs (Qayyum et al., 2020, Ghosh et al., 2024a, Ghosh et al., 2024b):

- Hybrid Approaches: Combines multiple privacy-preserving techniques to optimize performance while maintaining privacy protections. For example, using federated learning for model training combined with SMPC for specific sensitive calculations (Qayyum et al., 2020).

- Privacy Budget Management: Employs formal methods to track and limit privacy exposure across multiple operations and data uses, preventing privacy degradation through accumulated disclosures (Fang, H et al., 2024).
- Transparency and Explainability: Provides users with information about privacy-preserving mechanisms and their effectiveness, helping users understand how their data is protected without requiring technical expertise (Shoghli, A et al., 2024).
- Context-Aware Technique Selection: Chooses appropriate privacy-preserving methods based on data sensitivity, performance requirements, and usage context (Perera, C et al., 2014, Khan & Sakamura, 2015).

Figure 15. AI and ML-Based Behavioural Security in Smart Nutrition Systems

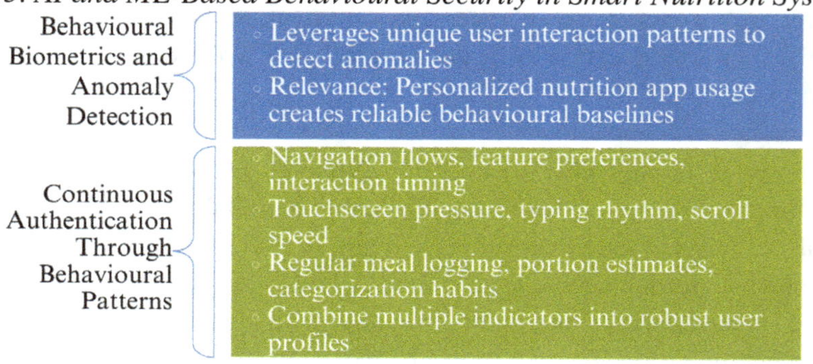

Figure 16. Dynamic Risk Assessment and Threat Prediction in Smart Nutrition Systems

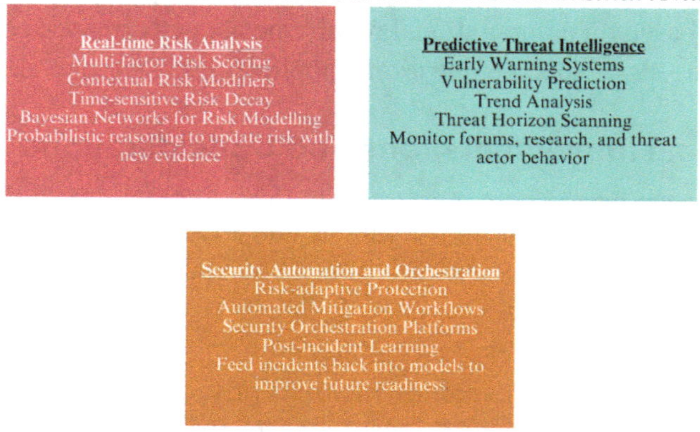

Figure 17. Adaptive Security via Reinforcement Learning in Smart Nutrition

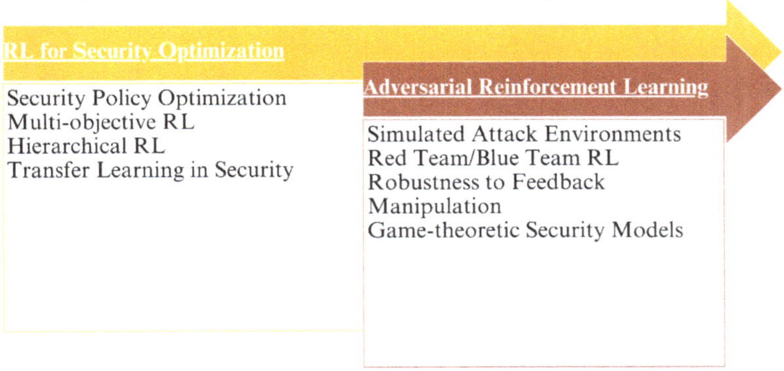

14. AI AND MACHINE LEARNING IN SECURITY

14.1. Behavioural Biometrics and Anomaly Detection (Figure 15)

Behavioural biometrics follows the distinctive methods that helps individuals to communicate with systems to provide identity and find out abnormal usage patterns pointing to security breaches .In smart nutrition systems, these methods are suitable where continuous interaction patterns can set up definite reference behavior.

14.2. Continuous Authentication Through Behavioural Patterns

Behavioural biometrics activate continuous, frictionless authentication all over the user sessions:

- Interaction Dynamics: Study of application usage patterns, with navigation flows, feature preferences, and interaction timing of nutrition applications. For instance, the way users typically log meals, search for foods and acknowledge recommendations (Fridman, L et al., 2017) .
- Usage Consistency: For individual users a stand behavior is set with the help of knowledge about regular patterns in meal logging times, portion estimation tendencies, and food categorization preferences (Acien, A., et al., 2018).

15. ANOMALY DETECTION IN NUTRITION SYSTEMS

Machine learning models can build normal behavioural patterns and flag deviations which can suggest illegitimate access or deceptive practices (Chandola, V et al., 2009):

- Contextual Anomaly Detection: Models which specify situation while assess possible abnormalities, discriminate among actual changes in behavior (for example holiday eating patterns) and doubtful deviations (Gupta et al., 2014).
- Ensemble Methods: Multiple anomaly detection techniques together can enhance accuracy of detection, reduce false positives and influence the power of different approaches (Aburomman & Reaz, 2017) (Figure 16,17).

16. ADVANCED BEHAVIOURAL ANALYSIS

Deep Learning for Behavioural Modelling: Deep neural networks enable automatic extraction of raw behavioural data and detection of subtle patterns that traditional approaches might miss. These methods have demonstrated superior performance in keystroke dynamics, gait recognition, and continuous authentication scenarios.

Transfer Learning for Limited Data Scenarios: When restricted user-specific training data is available, transfer learning techniques enable effective behavioral model establishment by applying knowledge from associated domains. This approach significantly reduces enrollment time and data collection requirements for new users.

Explainable Behavioural Analysis: Methods that provide clear explanations for distinguished anomalies while helping security professionals understand the specific behavioral deviations that triggered alerts are critical for deployment in security- sensitive applications (Gunning & Aha, 2019). XAI approaches enable security teams to validate system decisions and maintain appropriate trust in behavioral analysis systems.

Adaptive Behavioural Baselines: Continuous authentication systems evolve user behavior models to accommodate natural evolution in usage patterns while still detecting sudden suspicious changes. These adaptive systems distinguish between legitimate behavioral drift and genuinely anomalous activity (Feng et al., 2013).

17. DYNAMIC RISK ASSESSMENT AND THREAT PREDICTION

Dynamic risk assessment constantly assesses security risks according to existing situations and forecasts possible future risks before they can be exploited. These potentials are important in smart nutrition environments where threat landscapes develop quickly and possible health impacts expand the need of proactive security.

17.1. Real-Time Risk Analysis

Continuous monitoring and evaluation of security status enable adaptive security responses calibrated to current threat levels. Dynamic risk assessment combines multiple risk factors to determine appropriate security requirements for each access attempt or transaction.

- **Multi-Factor Risk Scoring:** Modern security systems employ sophisticated algorithms incorporating multiple risk indicators—including user behavior patterns, device characteristics, network conditions, and external threat intelligence feeds—to calculate dynamic risk scores for each session and transaction. These multi-factor approaches enable more nuanced risk assessments than traditional static methods.
- **Contextual Risk Modifiers:** Advanced systems modify base risk assessments based on contextual factors including access location, time of day, device security posture, network conditions, and transaction requirements. Contextual information provides granularity in risk estimation, allowing security systems to differentiate between routine and anomalous access patterns.
- **Time-Sensitive Risk Decay:** Risk assessment models increasingly incorporate temporal elements that acknowledge changing risk factor importance over time. Some risk factors naturally decay in significance (e.g., an unusual access location becomes normalized after repeated legitimate access), while others may increase in importance depending on evolving threat landscapes and organizational context.
- **Bayesian Networks for Risk Modelling:** Probabilistic frameworks using Bayesian networks provide mathematically rigorous approaches to modeling complex dependencies among multiple risk factors. These frameworks enable systems to update risk assessments dynamically as new evidence becomes available, supporting real-time decision-making (Poolsappasit et al., 2012).

17.2. Predictive Threat Intelligence

By allowing pre-emptive security measures, advanced analytics can forecast threats before their materialization and arrival:

- Early Warning Systems: Machine Learning Models can recognize the pattern which indicates upcoming attacks, like reconnaissance activities or unusual API calls that typically precede malicious actions (Shin, 2010).
- Vulnerability Prediction: Techniques that analyse code, configurations, and system architectures to predict potential security weaknesses before they can be exploited (Bozorgi, et al., 2010).
- Threat Horizon Scanning: Constant observation of security research, underground forums, and threat actor behaviours help to recognize upcoming threats which can occur to nutrition technologies (Samtani et al., 2020).

17.3. Security Automation and Orchestration

Combination of risk assessment with automated response mechanisms allows fast adaptation to changing threat conditions (Cichonski et al., 2012):

- Risk-adaptive Protection: Security controls can self-adjust according to estimated risk levels by applying more rigorous protection when needed.
- Automated Mitigation Workflows: When certain risk indicators are discovered, preset response procedures can automatically execute, decreasing time from detection to mitigation.
- Security Orchestration Platforms: These systems synchronize various security tools to execute comprehensive responses and ensure continuous protection across all system components.
- Post-incident Learning: Feedback mechanisms that analyze security incidents to improve future risk assessments and refine predictive models.

18. ADAPTIVE SECURITY MODELS USING REINFORCEMENT LEARNING

Security systems can constantly improve themselves based on previous experience and adapt to upcoming threats without specific programming through reinforcement learning (RL).In smart nutrition, this self-improving capacity is critical as novel security challenges emerge alongside evolving technologies.

18.1. Reinforcement Learning for Security Optimization

The Reinforcement Learning approach can construct security as a dynamic optimization problem where the system learns optimal protective strategies through observation and feedback

- Security Policy Optimization: RL agents learn functional security policies by experimenting with various protective actions and monitoring their impacts on security and usability
- Multi-objective Reinforcement Learning: Approaches that balance competing objectives such as security effectiveness, performance impact, and user friction (Hayes et al., 2020).
- Hierarchical Reinforcement Learning: Frameworks that break down complex security problems into manageable sub-tasks, allowing efficient learning of sophisticated strategies.
- Transfer Learning in Security Domains: Techniques that use knowledge from one context to enhance learning in a related one, boosting adaptability to new threats.

19. PRACTICAL APPLICATIONS IN SMART NUTRITION SECURITY

Reinforcement learning addresses specific security challenges within nutrition technology:

- Adaptive Authentication: RL systems that tailor authentication based on context and user behaviour, balancing usability and security.
- Dynamic Access Control: Models that update access permissions continuously based on behaviour and emerging threats.
- Anomaly Response Optimization: RL approaches that learn optimal responses to anomalies to reduce risks with minimal disruption (Folino & Sabatino, 2016).
- Security Resource Allocation: Systems that intelligently allocate limited security resources where they're most needed.

20. ADVERSARIAL ATTACKS ON NUTRITION MODELS AND COUNTER MEASURES

Nutrition systems are vulnerable to adversarial ML attacks that manipulate models to generate harmful guidance (Biggio & Roli, 2018).

20.1. Adversarial Attacks in Smart Nutrition Contexts

AI-powered nutrition systems can be targeted by various adversarial methods:

- Poisoning Attacks: Training data manipulation by attackers leading to incorrect dietary suggestions.
- Evasion Attacks: Input manipulations (e.g., altered food images) misleading nutrition analysis models
- Model Inversion and Extraction: Attackers infer sensitive data or model functionality by observing outputs.
- Backdoor Attacks: Models behave normally until secret triggers cause harmful outcomes.

20.2. Domain-Specific Vulnerabilities

Smart Nutrition Systems may suffer from domain-specific risks:

- Misidentification of allergens
- Manipulation of nutrient analysis in therapeutic diets
- Recommendation bias for commercial motives
- Undermining health goals through subtle sabotage

Figure 18. Threats & Defenses in AI-Powered Nutrition Systems

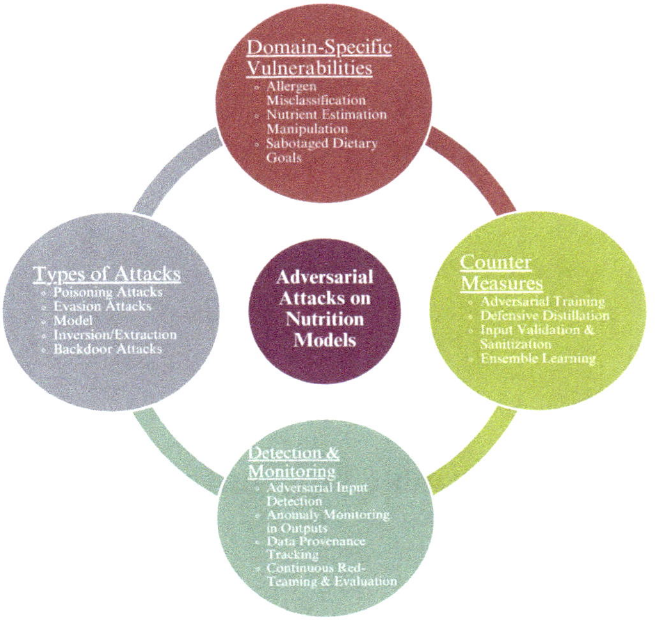
Domain-Specific Vulnerabilities
Allergen Misclassification
Nutrient Estimation Manipulation
Sabotaged Dietary Goals
Types of Attacks
Poisoning Attacks
Evasion Attacks
Model
Inversion/Extraction
Backdoor Attacks
Adversarial Attacks on Nutrition Models
Counter Measures
Adversarial Training
Defensive Distillation
Input Validation & Sanitization
Ensemble Learning
Detection & Monitoring
Adversarial Input Detection
Anomaly Monitoring in Outputs
Data Provenance Tracking
Continuous Red-Teaming & Evaluation

Figure 19. Ethical & Legal Frameworks for Smart Nutrition

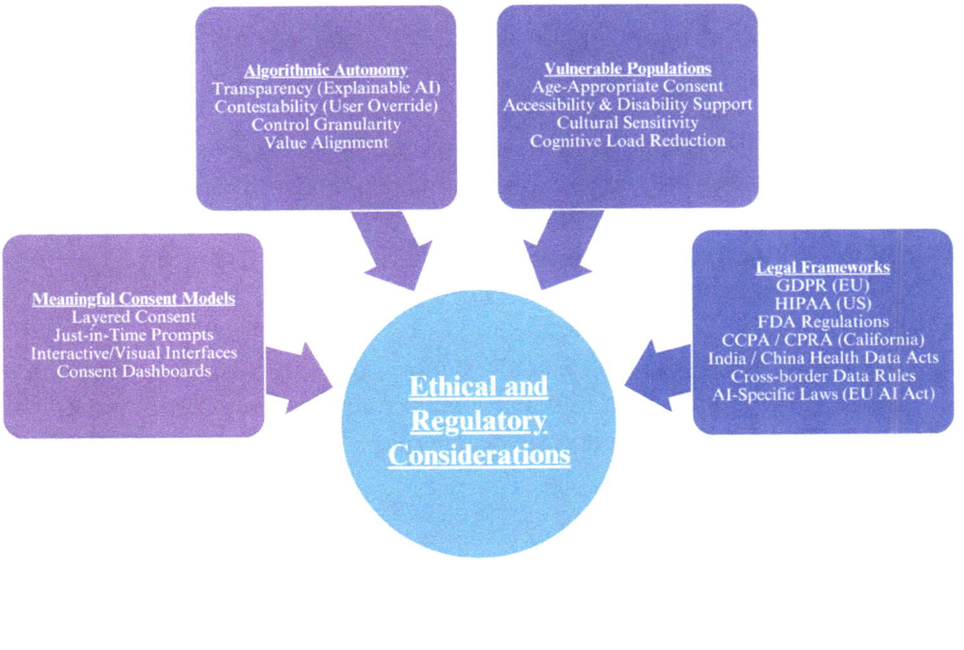

Figure 20. Ethical Dilemmas in Autonomous Dietary Decision-Making

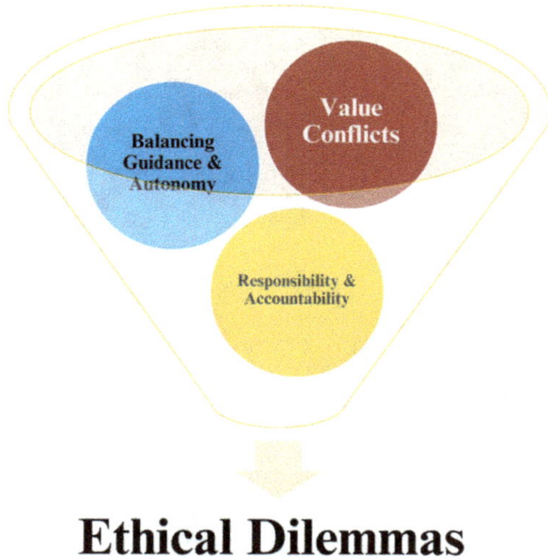

20.3. Defensive Techniques and Countermeasures

In nutritional models, adversarial influences can be lessened with the help of various approaches :

- **Adversarial Training:** Smart Nutrition systems can be more resilient in avoiding attacks on food recognition or in nutritional analysis by inserting adversarial examples to train models.
- **Defensive Distillation:** Nutrition recommendation systems can reduce vulnerabilities to adversarial examples by creating more resilient models through training with output probabilities of an earlier model.
- **Input Validation and Sanitization:** Nutrition models can detect and reject adversarial examples before they reach the model through strict input validation.
- **Ensemble Methods:** Adversarial examples can affect a single model, but when many models with different architectures are integrated together, the possibilities of any deception are decreased.

20.4. Detection and Monitoring

An additional layer of protection is provided when potential adversarial attacks on nutrition models are identified .

- **Adversarial Example Detection:** Adversarial inputs are used to review the trained neural networks and statistical methods before they can identify adversarial inputs and influence nutritional recommendations.
- **Anomaly Detection in Model Behaviour:** Adversarial manipulation or any unexpected changes in model output are detected with the help of monitoring patterns.
- **Provenance Tracking:** Tracing the origin of potential attacks and mitigating their effects are possible by recording the data lineage and model updates.
- **Continuous Model Evaluation:** Regular testing of deployed models against adversarial examples and shifting data distributions helps identify emerging vulnerabilities (Baracaldo et al., 2018) (Figure 18).

21. ETHICAL AND REGULATORY CONSIDERATIONS

21.1. Informed Consent and User Autonomy

In smart nutrition systems, ethical data practices are founded on informed consent. Users must approve how their data is collected, used, and protected. Reflective approaches are needed to handle challenges to autonomy while delivering personalized nutrition guidance (Figure 19,20).

21.2. Meaningful Consent in Complex Systems

Traditional models fail to convey the intricacies of modern nutrition systems (Beauchamp, et al 2001):

- **Layered Consent Models:** Users are allowed to access critical consent information in progressive detail layers, with full explanations provided as needed.
- **Just-in-Time Consent:** Permissions are requested when needed rather than during initial setup, offering contextual information when data is first used .
- **Interactive Consent Experiences:** Visual tools, simulations, and interactive methods are used to enhance understanding of how nutritional data will be used and secured.

- **Consent Dashboards:** Interfaces help users review and modify their consent choices while understanding their implications.

21.3. Autonomy in Algorithm-Driven Nutrition

AI plays a critical role in balancing user autonomy in dietary guidance, presenting both challenges and opportunities (Mittelstadt & Floridi, 2016):

- **Algorithmic Transparency:** Clear explanations of how nutrition recommendations are generated enable informed user decisions.
- **Contestability:** Users can question or override automated recommendations without penalty.
- **Control Granularity:** Systems should offer varying levels of automation, allowing users to choose their preferred decision-making involvement.
- **Value Alignment:** Nutrition AI should reflect and respect user values to avoid top-down imposition of external norms(Figure 21).

Figure 21. Secure-by-Design Framework for Smart Nutrition Systems

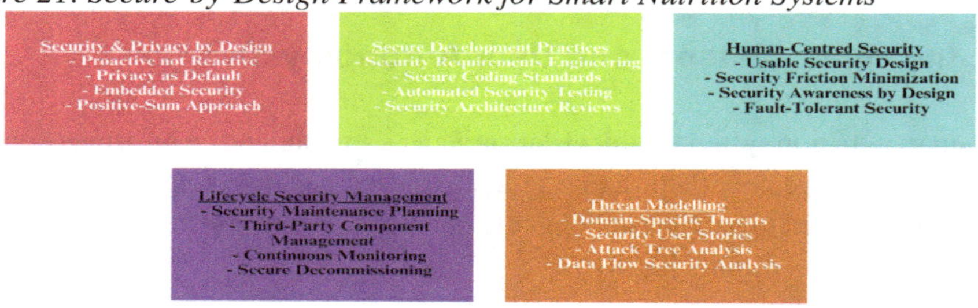

Figure 22. Nutrition Smart City Initiative in Pune, India

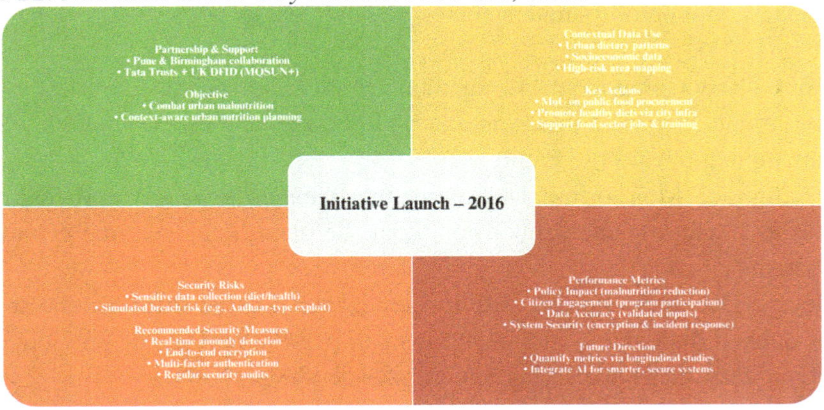
Partnership & Support
• Pune & Birmingham collaboration
• Tata Trusts + UK DFID (MQSUN+)
Objective
• Combat urban malnutrition
• Context-aware urban nutrition planning
Contextual Data Use
• Urban dietary patterns
• Socioeconomic data
• High-risk area mapping
Key Actions
• MoU on public food procurement
• Promote healthy diets via city infra
• Support food sector jobs & training
Initiative Launch – 2016
Security Risks
• Sensitive data collection (diet/health)
• Simulated breach risk (e.g., Aadhaar-type exploit)
Recommended Security Measures
• Real-time anomaly detection
• End-to-end encryption
• Multi-factor authentication
• Regular security audits
Performance Metrics
• Policy Impact (malnutrition reduction)
• Citizen Engagement (program participation)
• Data Accuracy (validated inputs)
• System Security (encryption & incident response)
Future Direction
• Quantify metrics via longitudinal studies
• Integrate AI for smarter, secure systems

Figure 23. MyFitnessPal Data Breach

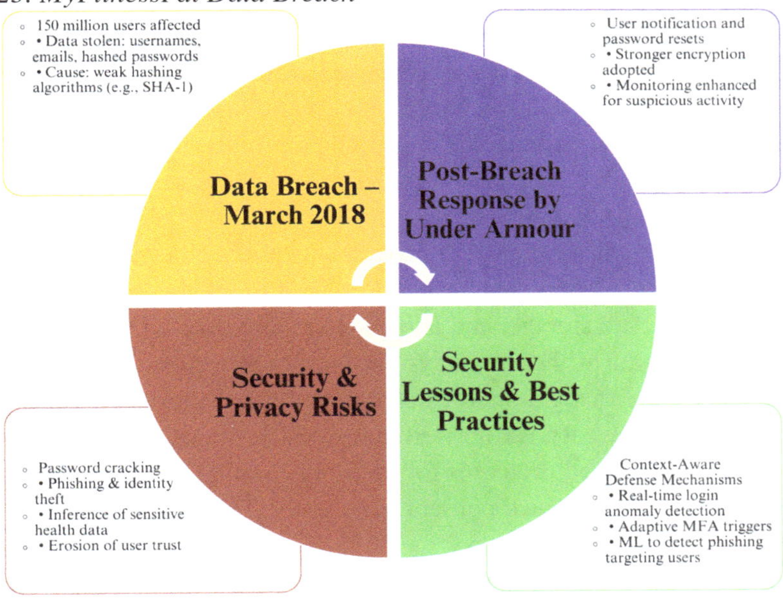

21.4. Lifecycle Security Management

Approaches that preserve security for the whole of lifespan of the system starting from formulation to retiral (Landwehr et al 1994):

- Security Maintenance Planning: Establishing processes for ongoing security updates, vulnerability management, and incident response before deployment (Figure 23).
- Third-Party Component Management: Implementing procedures for evaluating, monitoring, and updating external libraries and services integrated into nutrition applications (Figure 22) .
- Continuous Monitoring: Deploying mechanisms to detect and respond to potential security incidents throughout the operational lifetime of nutrition systems .
- Secure Decommissioning: Building mechanisms that maintain the security of deleted data and system shutdowns to prevent leakage of previous nutritional data after obsolescence (Garfinkel & Shelat, 2003).

22. FUTURE RESEARCH DIRECTIONS

The combination of smart nutrition systems with personalized medicine and genomics marks an important change in research. By using genetic data, these systems can provide personalized dietary suggestions tailored to individual traits. This approach could improve health outcomes for conditions like obesity and diabetes (Singar et al 2024). For instance, nutrigenomics reveals how genetic differences influence how the body processes nutrients, allowing for more focused interventions. However, using genomic data poses serious security risks. Genetic information is sensitive; breaches can lead to privacy violations or ethical problems, such as discrimination based on genetic traits Research highlights the need for strong encryption, secure data storage, and adherence to laws like GDPR and HIPAA to protect this information in big data analysis and personalized medicine. Additionally, it is crucial to ensure that genomic databases and smart nutrition platforms work together securely to prevent unauthorized access or data manipulation. Future studies should create standardized protocols for safely integrating genomic data to ensure ethical use and secure informed consent from users. This will help build trust and encourage broader acceptance.

Smart nutrition systems depend on collecting data from various devices and platforms, including mobile apps, wearables, smart scales, and kitchen gadgets. Achieving smooth interoperability is vital for providing accurate and timely nutritional advice, but it also brings significant security challenges. Research in IoT and healthcare underscores the need for standardized communication protocols, like HL7/FHIR, to enable secure data exchange while protecting sensitive user information. For example, securely connecting medical devices in healthcare IoT is crucial to prevent breaches and protect patient privacy. This principle also applies to smart nutrition systems (Locke et al., 2001). The variety of devices increases the risk of attacks, so it is important to implement strong security measures like encryption, authentication, and regular updates across all components. The idea of a "security and privacy nutrition label" for IoT devices suggests that manufacturers should clearly outline security features to help users make informed choices. Future research should aim to establish universal standards and frameworks that improve both interoperability and security, ensuring smart nutrition systems work effectively and safely across different devices and platforms.

Real-time context adaptation is a crucial feature for smart nutrition systems. This ability lets dietary suggestions match a user's current situation, such as physical activity, location, or emotional state. Edge computing makes this possible by processing data locally on devices or nearby servers, which reduces delays and improves responsiveness. For example, a system could use data from a fitness tracker to suggest a post-workout meal that replenishes lost nutrients . However, edge devices like wearables or smart kitchen appliances may have limited processing power and memory, making them vulnerable to cyberattacks like malware or data interception. Research stresses the importance of securing edge devices through methods like reinforcement learning for anomaly detection and secure communication protocols to safeguard data during transfer and storage (Garfinkel & Shelat, 2003).

The distributed nature of edge computing complicates security management across various devices and networks, necessitating robust security frameworks. Future studies should focus on developing solid security protocols for edge devices, including encryption, intrusion detection, and secure firmware updates. This will help protect smart nutrition systems while enabling real-time context adaptation.

Building trust and verification in smart nutrition systems is crucial for their reliability and broad acceptance. Universal frameworks can ensure that data and advice are accurate, safe, and trustworthy. Blockchain technology can create unchangeable records of food sources and nutritional content, allowing users to verify the authenticity and quality of their dietary inputs (Singar, et al 2024). Trust models for IoT devices, which are essential to smart nutrition systems, can help maintain the integrity of data collected from sensors and devices. Security frameworks like zero-trust models, which verify each transaction or access request, can protect against cyber threats. Additionally, initiatives like consumer privacy and security "nutrition labels" for smart devices can provide transparency by informing users about security features, fostering trust. Future research should concentrate on developing standardized protocols and certifications that ensure consistency and reliability across smart nutrition platforms. This will help users feel confident in the recommendations and data management practices of these systems.

Smart nutrition systems are a significant development in the way we control our health. They employ technologies such as artificial intelligence (AI), the Internet of

Things (IoT), and data analytics to provide personalized nutritional recommendations based on an individual's health parameters, eating patterns, and other parameters like location or activity level. But employing these technologies also raises several security issues, such as data compromise, device impersonation, and unauthorized data exchange. This scenario calls for the transition towards security practices that are context-sensitive. In contrast to traditional security measures based on static protection, context-aware security adapts according to users' individual circumstances and environments, e.g., the device employed or the location of the user. These adaptive security steps are crucial in safeguarding private health information in smart health systems, which extends to the case of smart nutrition platforms. For example, the 2018 MyFitnessPal data breach that compromised 150 million users highlighted the shortcomings of nutrition apps that leverage poor security controls, such as weak password encryption. Context-aware security can mitigate these risks by utilizing real-time threat detection depending on user behavior. This involves detecting suspicious login patterns and encrypting data transmission based on usage context. This methodology is crucial to avoid unauthorized access, preserve the integrity of dietary suggestions, and uphold user trust, particularly since such systems increasingly deal with more sensitive data such as genetic information or mental health information.

23. CONCLUSION

The potential of smart nutrition systems, such as real-time context adaptation and integration with personalized medicine, enhances their scope to revolutionize food management. However, these advancements must be complemented with solid security policies to shield users and adhere to legislation like the General Data Protection Regulation (GDPR) and the Health Insurance Portability and Accountability Act (HIPAA). Security-by-design principles, that combine protective elements right from the start of development, are convenient to balance this trade. Blockchain technology can be used to ensure the accuracy of data as well as tracing, exemplified in food safety systems, so that smart nutrition platforms can have secure and verifiable data streams without compromising on functionality. Such a balance is necessary so that innovation is not stifled; too tight security might hinder the evolution of features like emotion-aware nutrition advice or device integration that improve user experience. Adaptive security solutions like context-aware threat models have been shown in studies to counter evolving threats while driving innovation by reacting to the operational context of the system. Together, developers, regulators, and users must work to effectively enact these measures to maintain smart nutrition systems as revolutionary while keeping them secure. Through such cooperation, the sector can promote broader adoption while tackling privacy and security issues that have the potential to undermine user confidence.

The ultimate long-term vision for intelligent nutrition systems is to build a secure, ethical, and user-centered ecosystem that maximizes health returns while reducing risk. This involves leveraging cutting-edge technologies such as blockchain for the accuracy of data, AI for threat anticipation, and edge computing for real-time contextual adaptation to increase the resilience and capability of these systems. For example, blockchain-based platforms can create immutable histories of nutritional information, making it transparent and trustworthy, just like food traceability platforms. Furthermore, context-aware threat models intelligent enough for use in smart cyber-physical systems offer a mechanism to detect and reduce security threats on nutrition platforms by evaluating contextual information in real-time. Regulatory requirements will need to evolve further to keep up with advances in technology, enshrining precise rules that reflect the individual issues of smart nutrition systems, particularly in terms of genetic or mental health information. GDPR and HIPAA initiatives are a starting point, but distinct guidelines need to be issued for guaranteeing compliance across the globe. User education and empowerment are also central, enabling people to grasp data-sharing risks and develop secure practices such as strong password use and app permissions checking. Through embarking on this vision, intelligent nutrition systems have the ability to realize their potential to advance global health outcomes while maintaining high levels of security and ethics. Continuing research, international collaboration, and stakeholder engagement will be essential to addressing the shifting threat environment and creating a future in which these systems are both innovative and trustworthy.

REFERENCES

Aburomman, A. A., & Reaz, M. B. I. (2017). A survey of intrusion detection systems based on ensemble and hybrid classifiers. *Computers & Security, 65*, 135–152. DOI: 10.1016/j.cose.2016.11.008

Acien, A., Morales, A., Vera-Rodriguez, R., Fierrez, J., & Ortega-Garcia, J. (2018). Active detection of age groups based on touch interaction. *IET Biometrics*, *7*(5), 415–424.

Aghili, S. F., Mala, H., Shojafar, M., & Peris-Lopez, P. (2019). Lightweight three-factor authentication, access control and ownership transfer scheme for e-health systems in IoT. *Future Generation Computer Systems*.

Amin, R., Islam, S. H., Biswas, G. P., Khan, M. K., & Kumar, N. (2019). A robust and efficient bilinear pairing based mutual authentication and session key verification over insecure communication. *Multimedia Tools and Applications*, *74*(11), 3581–3605.

Baracaldo, N., Chen, B., Ludwig, H., & Safavi, J. A. (2018). Detecting poisoning attacks on machine learning in IoT environments. In *2018 IEEE International Congress on Internet of Things* (pp. 57–64).

Bernabe, J. B., Hernandez-Ramos, J. L., & Skarmeta, A. F. (2016). TACIoT: Multidimensional trust-aware access control system for the Internet of Things. *Soft Computing*, *20*(5), 1763–1779. DOI: 10.1007/s00500-015-1591-0

Bertolazzi, A., Marzęda-Młynarska, K., Kięczkowska, J., & Zanier, M. L. (2024). Datafication of care: Security and privacy issues with health technology for people with diabetes. *Societies (Basel, Switzerland)*, *14*(9), 163.

Bhattacharya, P., Tanwar, S., Shah, R., & Ladha, A. (2020). Mobile edge computing-enabled blockchain framework—A survey. In *2020 International Conference on Communication Systems & Networks* (pp. 371–376).

Biggio, B., & Roli, F. (2018). Wild patterns: Ten years after the rise of adversarial machine learning. *Pattern Recognition*, *84*, 317–331.

Bozorgi, M., Saul, L. K., Savage, S., & Voelker, G. M. (2010). Learning to classify vulnerabilities and predict exploits. In *Proceedings of the 16th ACM SIGKDD International Conference on Knowledge Discovery and Data Mining* (pp. 1058-1065).

Burks, A. (2024). *Strategies used in healthcare organizations to protect information against security breaches: A case study* (Doctoral dissertation, University of Phoenix).

Caviglione, L., Podolski, M., Mazurczyk, W., & Ianigro, M. (2016). Covert channels in personal cloud storage services: The case of Dropbox. *IEEE Transactions on Industrial Informatics*, *13*(4), 1921–1931. DOI: 10.1109/TII.2016.2607183

Chakraborty, A., Alam, M., Dey, V., Chattopadhyay, A., & Mukhopadhyay, D. (2018). Adversarial attacks and defences: A survey. *ACM Computing Surveys*, *53*(1), 20. Advance online publication. DOI: 10.1145/3357390

Chandola, V., Banerjee, A., & Kumar, V. (2009). Anomaly detection: A survey. *ACM Computing Surveys*, *41*(3), 15. Advance online publication. DOI: 10.1145/1541880.1541882

Chen, L., & Roberts, P. (2023). Analysis of the NutriTrack data breach: Timeline, impact, and lessons learned. *Journal of Digital Health Security*, *8*(2), 103–119.

Choudhury, S. R., Das, P., Koner, S., Ghosh, J., & Singh, K. (2024). Cardiovascular disease risks related to consumption of ready-to-eat food products between young adults of Kolkata, West Bengal, India. *Journal of Comprehensive Health*, *12*(1), 60.

Cichonski, P., Millar, T., Grance, T., & Scarfone, K. (2012). *Computer security incident handling guide* (NIST Special Publication 800-61 Revision 2).

Coelho, D. M. (2021). *Detection of side channel attacks at the network physical layer* (Master's thesis, Universidade de Aveiro, Portugal).

Crossler, R. E., & Bélanger, F. (2019). Why would I use location-protective settings on my smartphone? Motivating protective behaviors and the existence of the privacy knowledge-belief gap. *Information Systems Research*, *30*(3), 995–1013.

Cybersecurity and Infrastructure Security Agency. (2024). Supply chain compromise affecting nutritional database integration libraries (Alert AA24-089A). U.S. Department of Homeland Security.

Dasgupta, S., Stevens, C. F., & Navlakha, S. (2017). A neural algorithm for a fundamental computing problem. *Science*, *358*(6364), 793–796.

de Hoogh, I. M., Winters, B. L., Nieman, K. M., Bijlsma, S., Krone, T., van den Broek, T. J., Anderson, B. D., Caspers, M. P. M., Anthony, J. C., & Wopereis, S. (2021). A novel personalized systems nutrition program improves dietary patterns, lifestyle behaviors and health-related outcomes: Results from the Habit Study. *Nutrients*, *13*(6), 1763. Advance online publication. DOI: 10.3390/nu13061763

Dempsey, K., Witte, G. A., & Iorga, M. (2018). *Summary of NIST SP 800-53 revision 5, security and privacy controls for information systems and organizations*. NIST Special Publication.

Department of Health and Human Services. (2024). *OCR announces results of nutrition application HIPAA compliance investigation*. HHS Press Office.

Diro, A. A., & Chilamkurti, N. (2018). Distributed attack detection scheme using deep learning approach for Internet of Things. *Future Generation Computer Systems, 82*, 761–768. DOI: 10.1016/j.future.2017.08.043

Donovan, S. M., et al (2025). Perspective: Challenges for personalized nutrition in the current U.S. regulatory framework and future opportunities. *Advances in Nutrition*. Advance online publication. DOI: 10.1016/j.advnut.2025.100382

European Data Protection Board. (2023). *Decision regarding NutriHealth data processing practices (Case 2023-DE-17)*. EDPB Publications.

Fang, H., Qiu, Y., Yu, H., Yu, W., Kong, J., Chong, B., & Xu, K. (2024). Privacy leakage on DNNs: A survey of model inversion attacks and defenses. *arXiv*.

Federal Trade Commission. (2024). *Data broker practices in health and nutrition information marketplaces*. FTC Bureau of Consumer Protection.

Feng, H., Fawaz, M. S., & Shin, K. G. (2013). Continuous authentication for security-sensitive mobile apps. In 13th USENIX Security Symposium (USENIX Security '13) (pp. 371-386). USENIX Association.

Fernández-Alemán, J. L., Carrión Señor, I., Oliver Lozoya, P. A., & Toval, A. (2013). Security and privacy in electronic health records: A systematic literature review. *Journal of Biomedical Informatics, 46*(3), 541–562.

Folino, F., & Sabatino, P. (2016). A scalable and resilient architecture for intrusion detection based on the elastic stack. *Concurrency and Computation, 28*(7), 2009–2027.

Fridman, L., Weber, S., Greenstadt, R., & Kam, M. (2017). Active authentication on mobile devices via stylometry, application usage, web browsing, and GPS location. *IEEE Systems Journal, 11*(2), 513–521. DOI: 10.1109/JSYST.2015.2453215

Gao, Y., Doan, B. G., Zhang, Z., Ma, S., Zhang, J., Fu, A., Kim, H. (2020). Backdoor attacks and countermeasures on deep learning: A comprehensive review. *arXiv*. https://doi.org//arXiv.2007.10760DOI: 10.48550

Garfinkel, S., & Shelat, A. (2003). Remembrance of data passed: A study of disk sanitization practices. *IEEE Security and Privacy, 1*(1), 17–27.

Ghosh, J. (2023a). How evidence-based nutrition science supports nutrition communication and marketing: An Indian perspective. In Ghosh, D., Bogueva, D., & Smarta, R. (Eds.), *Nutrition science, marketing nutrition, health claims, and public policy* (pp. 71–88). Academic Press. DOI: 10.1016/B978-0-323-85615-7.00007-0

Ghosh, J. (2023b). A review on understanding the risk factors for coronary heart disease in Indian college students. *International Journal of Noncommunicable Diseases*, *8*, 117–128.

Ghosh, J., Chaudhuri, D., Saha, I., & Nag Chaudhuri, A. (2022). Association of conicity index with different cardiovascular disease risk factors among the rural elderly women of West Bengal, India. *Indian Journal of Community Medicine : Official Publication of Indian Association of Preventive & Social Medicine*, *47*, 18–22.

Ghosh, J., Choudhury, S. R., Singh, K., & Koner, S. (2024a). Application of machine learning algorithm and artificial intelligence in improving metabolic syndrome related complications: A review. *International Journal of Advancement in Life Sciences Research*, *7*(2), 41–67.

Ghosh, J., Shakil, S., Singh, K., & Mandal, S. (2024b). Depression and cognitive function in accordance with the nutritional status of elderly women residing in Rajarhat-Newtown area of Kolkata, India. *Medical Journal of Dr. D.Y. Patil Vidyapeeth*, *17*(5), 951–956. DOI: 10.4103/mjdrdypu.mjdrdypu_423_23

Ghosh, J., Taneja, J., & Kant, R. (2025). Nutritional and lifestyle predictors of rectal bleeding in functional constipation: A machine learning approach. *International Journal of Medical Informatics*, *201*, 105963. Advance online publication. DOI: 10.1016/j.ijmedinf.2025.105963

Gioia, S., Curcurullo, M., Orso, V., Avenali, M., Graffigna, G., & Canetti, M. (2023). Mobile apps for dietary and food timing assessment. *PLoS One*, *18*(8), e0288949. DOI: 10.1371/journal.pone.0288949

Goldman, E. (2021). The story of the California Consumer Privacy Act (CCPA), version 1.0. In *Research handbook on information law and governance* (pp. 300–308). Edward Elgar Publishing.

Gope, P., & Hwang, T. (2016). A realistic lightweight anonymous authentication protocol for securing real-time application data access in wireless sensor networks. *IEEE Transactions on Industrial Electronics*, *63*(11), 7124–7132.

Granjal, J., Monteiro, E., & Sá Silva, J. (2015). Security for the Internet of Things: A survey of existing protocols and open research issues. *IEEE Communications Surveys and Tutorials*, *17*(3), 1294–1312.

Gunning, D., & Aha, D. (2019). DARPA's explainable artificial intelligence program. *AI Magazine*, *40*(2), 44–58. DOI: 10.1609/aimag.v40i2.2850

Gupta, B. B., Agrawal, D. P., & Yamaguchi, S. (2014). *Handbook of research on advanced cybercrime investigation and cyberforensics*. IGI Global.

Hammi, B., Zeadally, S., Khatoun, R., & Nebhen, J. (2022). Survey on smart homes: Vulnerabilities, risks, and countermeasures. *Computers & Security, 117*, 102677.

Hayashi, E., Das, S., Amini, S., Hong, J., & Oakley, I. (2013). CASA: Context-aware scalable authentication. In *Proceedings of the Ninth Symposium on Usable Privacy and Security* (Article 3, pp. 1–10).

Hayes, D., Cappa, F., & Le-Khac, N. A. (2020). An effective approach to mobile device management: Security and privacy issues associated with mobile applications. *Digital Business, 1*(1), Article 100001.

Ienca, M., Scheibner, J., Ferretti, A., Gille, F., Amann, J., Sleigh, J., & Vayena, E. (2019). *How the General Data Protection Regulation changes the rules for scientific research: Study*. ETH Zurich.

Ishrat, M., Khan, W., & Ather, D. (n.d.). Cyber resilience in a digital world: Securing healthcare, agriculture, and food industry against emerging threats. In *Cyberology* (pp. 200–224). Chapman and Hall/CRC.

Isibor, E. (2024, July 25). Regulation of healthcare data security: Legal obligations in a digital age. *SSRN*. https://ssrn.com/abstract=4957244

Itoh, N., Tsuya, A., Togashi, H., Kimura, H., Konta, T., Nemoto, K., Yamashita, H., & Kayama, T. (2022). Increased salt intake is associated with diabetes and characteristic dietary habits: A community-based cross-sectional study in Japan. *Journal of Clinical Biochemistry and Nutrition, 71*(2), 143–150. DOI: 10.3164/jcbn.21-153

Iwaya, L. H., Babar, M. A., & Rashid, A. (2023). On the privacy of mental health apps. *Empirical Software Engineering, 28*(1), 2. Advance online publication. DOI: 10.1007/s10664-022-10236-0

Jaime, F. J., Muñoz, A., Rodríguez-Gómez, F., & Jerez-Calero, A. (2023). Strengthening privacy and data security in biomedical microelectromechanical systems by IoT communication security and protection in smart healthcare. *Sensors (Basel), 23*(21), 8944.

Johnson, K., Williams, P., & Chen, X. (2024). Anatomy of a breach: The NutriTech Solutions incident and its implications for health data security. *Cybersecurity Case Studies Quarterly, 7*(1), 48–63.

Joshua, E. S. N., Bhattacharyya, D., & Rao, N. T. (2022). Managing information security risk and Internet of Things (IoT) impact on challenges of medicinal problems with complex settings: A complete systematic approach. In *Multi-chaos, fractal and multi-fractional artificial intelligence of different complex systems* (pp. 291–310). Academic Press.

Kessler, F. (2022). MyFitnessPal breach revisited: New findings and continuing vulnerabilities. *International Journal of Information Security*, *21*(4), 378–392.

Khan, M. F., & Sakamura, K. (2015). Context-aware access control for clinical information systems. In *2015 International Conference on Innovations in Information, Embedded and Communication Systems* (pp. 1–6).

Korenstein, D., Harris, R., Elshaug, A. G., Ross, J. S., Morgan, D. J., Cooper, R. J., & Segal, J. B. (2021). To expand the evidence base about harms from tests and treatments. *Journal of General Internal Medicine, 1*, 1–6.

Kulkarni, A., Wang, Y., Gopinath, M., Sobien, D., Rahman, A., & Batarseh, F. A. (2024). A review of cybersecurity incidents in the food and agriculture sector. *arXiv*.

Landwehr, C. E., Bull, A. R., McDermott, J. P., & Choi, W. S. (1994). A taxonomy of computer program security flaws. *ACM Computing Surveys*, *26*(3), 211–254.

Liu, Q., Ma, Y., Alhussein, M., Zhang, Y., & Peng, L. (2016). Green data center with IoT sensing and cloud-assisted smart temperature control system. *Computer Networks*, *101*, 104–112. DOI: 10.1016/j.comnet.2016.01.010

Locke, C. A., & Stoll, A. L. (2001). Omega-3 fatty acids in major depression. *World Review of Nutrition and Dietetics*, *89*, 173–185. DOI: 10.1159/000059784

Martinez, J., Wong, S., & Patel, K. (2023). Inferring health conditions from dietary data: Privacy implications of nutrition tracking platforms. *Journal of Medical Internet Research*, *25*(11), e42673.

Miettinen, M., Marchal, S., Hafeez, I., Asokan, N., Sadeghi, A. R., & Tarkoma, S. (2018). IoT Sentinel: Automated device-type identification for security enforcement in IoT. In *2017 IEEE 37th International Conference on Distributed Computing Systems* (pp. 2177–2184).

Mittelstadt, B. D., & Floridi, L. (2016). The ethics of biomedical big data. In *The ethics of biomedical big data* (p. 29).

Muntzel, M., & Drüeke, T. (1992). A comprehensive review of the salt and blood pressure relationship. *American Journal of Hypertension*, *5*(4S), 1S–42S.

Mustapha, A., Mustapha, M., & Mustapha, S. (n.d.). *Harnessing artificial intelligence in personalised nutrition and microbial health: Optimising public health outcomes*. Academic Press.

Parihar, A., Prajapati, J. B., Prajapati, B. G., Trambadiya, B., Thakkar, A., & Engineer, P. (2024). Role of IoT in healthcare: Applications, security & privacy concerns. *Intelligent Pharmacy*, *2*(5), 707–714.

Patel, H., Sharma, V., & Rodriguez, T. (2023). Comprehensive risk assessment framework for integrated dietary management platforms. *Health Technology Security Journal*, *14*(2), 129–145.

Peeples, K. (2023). A sleeping giant: mHealth applications, the GDPR, and the need for federal privacy regulation in the United States. *Notre Dame Journal on Emerging Technologies*, *4*, 121.

Perera, C., Zaslavsky, A., Christen, P., & Georgakopoulos, D. (2014). Context aware computing for the Internet of Things: A survey. *IEEE Communications Surveys and Tutorials*, *16*(1), 414–454.

Poolsappasit, N., Dewri, R., & Ray, I. (2012). Dynamic security risk management using Bayesian attack graphs. *IEEE Transactions on Dependable and Secure Computing*, *9*(1), 61–74. DOI: 10.1109/TDSC.2011.34

Qayyum, A., Qadir, J., Bilal, M., & Al-Fuqaha, A. (2020). Secure and robust machine learning for healthcare: A survey. *IEEE Reviews in Biomedical Engineering*, *14*, 156–180.

Ramirez, L., Chen, W., & Thompson, S. (2024). Adversarial machine learning applied to nutritional recommendation systems. *Journal of Health Informatics and Cybersecurity*, *9*(1), 24–39.

Roy Choudhury, S., Singh, K., Koner, S., & Ghosh, J. (2025). Technology, artificial intelligence, and the era of information in healthcare and allied sciences. In *Sustainable development goals (SDG) and its intersection with health and well-being* (Chapter 16). IGI Global. DOI: 10.4018/979-8-3693-9755-8.ch016

Sahu, S. K., & Mazumdar, K. (2024). Exploring security threats and solutions techniques for Internet of Things (IoT): From vulnerabilities to vigilance. *Frontiers in Artificial Intelligence*, *7*, 1397480.

Samtani, S., Chen, H., Albanese, M., & Grisham, J. (2020). Identifying emerging hacker assets and key hackers for proactive cyber threat intelligence: A diachronic graph embedding framework. *Journal of Management Information Systems*.

Shin, D. H. (2010). The effects of trust, security, and privacy in social networking: A security-based approach to understand the pattern of adoption. *Interacting with Computers*, *22*(5), 428–439. DOI: 10.1016/j.intcom.2010.05.001

Shoghli, A., Darvish, M., & Sadeghian, Y. (2024). Balancing innovation and privacy: Ethical challenges in AI-driven healthcare. *Journal of Research in Medical Sciences : the Official Journal of Isfahan University of Medical Sciences*, *4*(1), 1–11.

Singar, S., Nagpal, R., Arjmandi, B. H., & Akhavan, N. S. (2024). Personalized Nutrition: Tailoring Dietary Recommendations through Genetic Insights. *Nutrients*, *16*(16), 2673. DOI: 10.3390/nu16162673

Singh, A., & Rodriguez, C. (2024). The MealSync ransomware attack: Impact analysis and recovery strategies in critical nutrition infrastructure. *Journal of Healthcare Security*, *8*(2), 71–89.

Smetana, S., Aganovic, K., & Heinz, V. (2021). Food supply chains as cyber-physical systems: A path for more sustainable personalized nutrition. *Food Engineering Reviews*, *13*(1), 92–103. DOI: 10.1007/s12393-020-09243-y

Spero, D. (2006). *Diabetes: Sugar-coated crisis: Who gets it, who profits, and how to stop it*. New Society Publishers.

Strauss, B., Short, S., & Lotfian, P. (2023, March 31). The evolution of personalised nutrition: Executive summary. *The Evolution of Personalised Nutrition*.

Tangari, G., Ikram, M., Sentana, I. W. B., Ijaz, K., Kaafar, M. A., & Berkovsky, S. (2021). Analyzing security issues of Android mobile health and medical applications. *Journal of the American Medical Informatics Association : JAMIA*, *28*(10), 2074–2084. DOI: 10.1093/jamia/ocab131

Wagner, M., Schmidt, J., & Torres, O. (2023). Exploiting smart kitchen scales: Implications for nutrition tracking integrity. *DEF CON 31 Conference Proceedings*.

Wang, Z. (2024). Securing Bluetooth Low Energy: A literature review. *arXiv*.

Wiefling, S., Dürmuth, M., & Lo Iacono, L. (2021). Verify it's you: How users perceive risk-based authentication. *IEEE Security and Privacy*, *19*(6), 47–57. DOI: 10.1109/MSEC.2021.3092188

Yaqoob, T., Abbas, H., & Atiquzzaman, M. (2019). Security vulnerabilities, attacks, countermeasures, and regulations of networked medical devices—A review. *IEEE Communications Surveys and Tutorials*, *21*(4), 3723–3768.

Zhang, G., Yan, C., Ji, X., Zhang, T., Zhang, T., & Xu, W. (2017). DolphinAttack: Inaudible voice commands. In *Proceedings of the 2017 ACM SIGSAC Conference on Computer and Communications Security* (pp. 103-117). ACM. DOI: 10.1145/3133956.3134052

Zhang, M., Zhang, C., Sheng, V. S., & Fuhry, D. (2019). Behaviometric: A behavior biometric user authentication approach based on machine learning techniques. In *Proceedings of the 28th ACM International Conference on Information and Knowledge Management* (pp. 2357–2360).

Chapter 10
Ethical Considerations in AI-Driven Drug Development and Pharmaceutical Industry

Yash Chandrakant Bari
https://orcid.org/0009-0007-1400-3690
Saraswathi Vidya Bhavan's College of Pharmacy, University of Mumbai, India

Mrudula Santosh Wani
https://orcid.org/0009-0001-7131-7529
Vidyalankar Institute of Technology, India

Gajanan Nagare
https://orcid.org/0000-0002-3441-2690
Vidyalankar Institute of Technology, India

Manasi Chogale
Saraswathi Vidya Bhavan's College of Pharmacy, University of Mumbai, India

Rohan Vijayanand Pai
Shobhaben Pratapbhai Patel School of Pharmacy and Technology Management, SVKM's NMIMS, India

ABSTRACT

Artificial Intelligence (AI) is revolutionizing drug development in the pharmaceutical industry by speeding up drug discovery, optimizing clinical trials and facilitating precision medicine. While these developments hold the promise of efficiency and innovation, these developments also bring intricate ethical issues. This chapter criti-

DOI: 10.4018/979-8-3373-5258-9.ch010

cally analyzes the nexus between AI and ethics within drug development, with a focus on the areas of data privacy, algorithmic bias, transparency, intellectual property, and gaps in regulations. Practical examples and case studies help us understand the implications of unregulated AI adoption. Several global and national regulatory agencies discussed along with Institutional review processes form the backbone for ethical verification and validation of results. The chapter outlines recommendations and ethical guidelines to aid responsible, explainable and collaborative AI adoption within the pharmaceutical industry. By reconciling innovation and accountability, it seeks to create a transparent and fair future for AI-driven drug development.

INTRODUCTION

Artificial Intelligence (AI) is now one of the highly emerging and most transformative technologies in the pharmaceutical industry, offering infinite opportunities to boost up the process of drug discovery, optimizing the clinical trials design, and support various initiatives (Hirani et al., luri et al., 2022). Additionally, by leveraging a few other systems like machine learning, and Natural Language Processing (NLP), an Artificial Intelligence system can analyze huge medical, pharmacological, statistical datasets, predicting different molecular interactions and also to guide decision making at various prominent stages of the drug development (Kolasa et al., 2024; Deng et al., 2022). Scientists can use special tools and computer platforms which are quite helpful in unraveling the complex protein structures and these could further add on to support the treatment planning (Noorbakhsh-Sabet et al., 2019; Savage, 2021).

In drug discovery, AI plays a critical role in target identification and molecular screening, predominantly reducing the required time and the cost associated with usual traditional laboratory experimentations (Chen et al., 2021; Alizadehsani et al., 2024). Taking an example of Atomise, which utilizes deep learning models, which helps the researchers to design or select drug candidates faster, while Insilico Medicine which principally works on Generative Adversarial Networks (GANs) to discover or create the novel compounds (Wang et al., 2022; Gao et al., 2023). Moreover, by blending the real-world data (RWD) into the AI softwares, helps a lot to provide best outcomes in patient stratification, dosage prediction and pharmacovigilance, and thus building improvement in clinical outcomes as well as trial efficiency (Hirani et al., 2024; Chen et al., 2021).

The motivation for adopting AI into pharmaceutical research is largely driven by its potential to significantly reduce the drug development time, reduction in financial risks, and enabling personalized medicines (Kolasa et al., 2024; Deng et al., 2022). Conventional drug discovery often requires a decade or more and billions of dollars before a new therapeutic product reaches to the actual market; in contrast,

AI platforms facilitate all the important aspects from preclinical to clinical stages (Kolluri et al., 2022; Alizadehsani et al., 2024).

However, with this accelerated adoption of AI, ethical challenges are also rising up. AI models can be trained on biased or incomplete datasets which unintentionally risks producing inequitable outcomes, potentially hindering drug accessibility and patient care in a negative manner (Li et al., 2023; Dara & Azarpira, 2025). The ethical background is further complicated by the concerns related to the patient's privacy, personal consent, and the use of sensitive health information of the patients (WHO, 2021; WHO, 2024).

However, regulatory frameworks such as those enforced by the regulatory agencies like FDA, EMA and CDSCO, however, are still developing and very frequently found to keep up with quick advances in AI (Gao et al., 2023; WHO,2024). In addition intellectual property rights over AI-generated molecules raise complex legal and ethical doubts. Risks related to biosecurity of generative models arise as misuse of these tools to create harmful biological information degrade the path for beneficial medical solutions. Also the models design for research in drug discovery can be intentionally used to design toxic molecules, dangerous pathogens or harmful biological agents. Even though AL technology accelerates scientific progress, it also poses serious ethical concerns if not monitored, controlled and regulated. (Savage., 2021; WHO, 2024). As a result, the AI has numerous strong promises and enormous potential for robust revolution and successful progress in the pharmaceutical sector. It also demands rigorous ethical governance and oversight to guarantee that the future innovations and development take place in a responsible manner (Li et al., 2023; WHO, 2021).

ETHICAL CHALLENGES EMERGING FROM AI APPLICATION

Application of AI in drug development and pharmaceutical research has revolutionized functions such as clinical trial optimization, patient stratification, and molecular screening. However, it has also introduced complex ethical concerns that must be handled to realize responsible, equitable, and safe innovation. The Figure 1 illustrates those concerns pictorial form. The most critical areas include data management, algorithmic fairness, explainability, and legal and regulatory concerns.

Figure 1. Various ethical and legal conundrums involved with the usage of artificial intelligence in healthcare

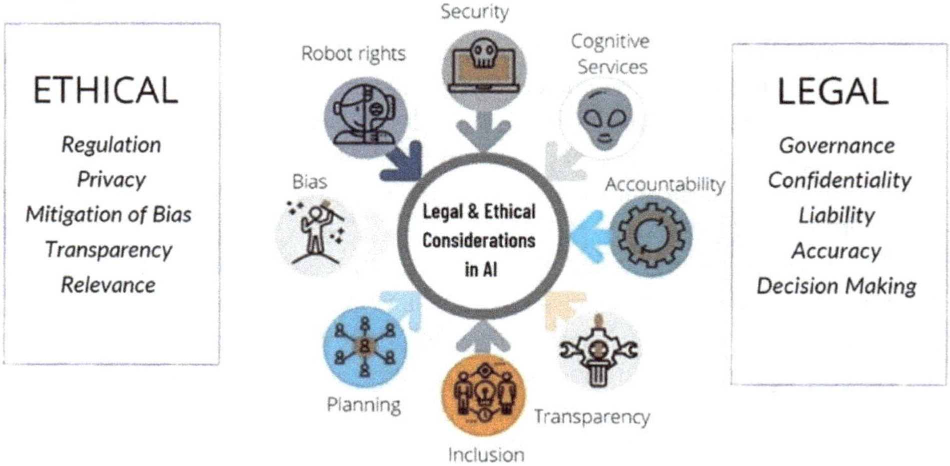

Retrieved from Naik et al., 2022.

AI based ML models highly rely on large data sets, including electronic health records (EHRs), clinical trials data, and real-world evidence, to create predictive models for drug development and patient outcomes (Li et al., 2023; WHO, 2021). While these data improve accuracy and efficiency, they also possess immense privacy, consent, and security challenges. For example, if the unencrypted patient data is used as an input for AI predictive models, the question arises on exposure of sensitive health data to discrimination or third party abuse. A classic illustration is the de-anonymization of clinical data sets, which has seen patients identified despite data protection (Dara & Azarpira, 2025). To battle such threats, organizations must possess robust cybersecurity protocols, adhere to regulations like General Data Protection Regulation (GDPR) and Health Insurance Portability and Accountability Act (HIPAA), and possess informed patient consent (Chen et al., 2021). Suggested visuals include schematic workflows of AI data pipelines that label secure vs. Insecure handling points. National Institutes of Health (NIH) Data Privacy and HIPAA Security Rule Overview are optimal reference sources for this.

AI models used in drug development are majorly dependent on the quality of the training datasets utilized. When biased or minority-underrepresented data is used to train AI models, the predictions tip the balance in the direction of some and disregard others, resulting in discriminatory treatment recommendations (Zhou & Wang, 2022; Alizadehsani et al., 2024). For instance, an AI-driven model predicting drug side effects may not work well for children or older patients if the data majority are from adults. Similarly, pharmacogenomic AI platforms can over-estimate drug efficacy among underrepresented ethnic populations participating in clinical trials. Bias is tackled with careful selection of datasets, regular monitoring of performance, and addition of multicultural patient data (Min et al., 2021). Deep learning models are part of AI algorithms, behave like "black boxes," and make interpretation more difficult for clinicians and regulators (Savage, 2021; Topol, 2019).

In drug development, AI results in advising specific patient treatment and dosage which is not clinically verified, this reduces confidence and retards it's adoption. Taking an example of an AI System suggesting personalized chemotherapy dosages without providing justification for it ; otherwise, clinicians will hesitate to adopt its recommendation (Savage, 2021; Topol, 2019).

Continuous AI deployment outpaces existing regulatory frameworks, providing an opportunity for uncertain issues of liability, intellectual property and approval standards (Gao et al., 2023; WHO, 2024). Questions of accountability come up when suggestions from AI result in adverse patient outcomes: whether the software engineer, pharma company or medical practitioner is held accountable. Intellectual property rights are also problematic, particularly for AI-generated molecular entities whose ownership and patentability remain unclear (Savage, 2021; Deng et al., 2022). AI-Specific guidelines are developed by FDA, EMA and CDSCO, but there are gaps in alignment of global norms.

Although AI makes revolutionary pharma research capabilities possible, it also needs strict ethical attention. AI-based drug development should be made secure and fair by overcoming challenges of data confidentiality, fairness in algorithms, transparency, and governance. The following case studies explain how the real pharma industry and research environments face ethical challenges.

In 2017, the collaboration of Google's DeepMind with UK's National Health service (NHS) to develop an AI tool for detecting kidney injury (Powles et al., 2017), was revealed to share 1.6 million patient records without obtaining patient consent (BBC et al., 2017). This data transfer raised serious privacy concerns and highlighted the risks of large scale EHR sharing without adequate safeguards. This case emphasizes the necessity of GDPR and HIPAA compliant frameworks and transparent consent mechanisms in pharmaceutical AI collaborations.

For providing recommendations on cancer treatment by relying on a large dataset, an IBM Watson based computer system was designed that used Artificial Intelligence (AI) to analyse large amounts of data and provide insights or recommendations (Ross et al., 2018). Clinicians reported that the system sometimes produced unsafe incorrect output, the reason behind this is the lack of explainability of AI in its decision making process, making it difficult for physicians to trust or validate outputs (Lee, 2019) The case underscores the importance of explainable AI for clinical acceptance, especially in high risk application like oncology drug protocols.

Lack of variations in clinical trial datasets has been a major challenge for numerous AI-driven drug discovery platforms. Taking an example of Cardiovascular drug trials in the U.S. have historically underrepresented women and minority groups (Singh et al., 2022). This affects the precision of AI models and results in less accurate predictions for those populations, raising fairness and equity issues (Chen et al., 2019). Propagation of inequities in drug efficacy prediction and personalized treatment recommendations caused by biased dataset can be studied through this case study.

In 2020, Insilico Medicine used AI to design a novel drug molecule for fibrosis in less than 46 days. While the breakthrough was celebrated, it also raised legal and regulatory questions: Who owns the IP of an AI-generated molecule- the algorithm's creator or the sponsoring pharmaceutical company? Moreover, existing patent systems were not fully equipped to handle AI designed compounds. This case highlights the urgent need for regulatory bodies to adapt frameworks for AI-driven innovations in pharmaceuticals.

Meanwhile AstraZeneca partnered with multiple AI startups such as BenevolentAI and Exscientia to accelerate drug discovery. Being successful in identifying new therapeutics targets, they faced major concerns in data governance (sharing of sensitive patient / genomic data across companies), explainability (ensuring regulators understand AI-Driven target identification) and compliance with evolving FDA and EMA guidance. This case is an example of how real-world industry collaborations must simultaneously address multiple ethical domains.

REGULATORY BODIES AND ETHICS OVERSIGHT ROLE

The pharmaceutical industry is the most regulated industry globally, as it directly deals with human health and safety. Regulatory Bodies serve as public health verification and validating bodies to ensure that medicines, biologics, and medical devices are safe, efficacious, and of standard quality (Sireesha & Haritha, 2024). The creation of those regulatory bodies was significantly influenced by past tragedies such as the sulfanilamide tragedy of the 1930s and the thalidomide crisis of the 1960s, which revealed the risks of open markets and initiated tougher legislation and safety standards (FDA, 2018; Gad, 2021). Ethical violations in studies, like the Tuskegee Syphilis Study, further stressed the need for robust oversight procedures to safeguard participants' welfare and rights (McNair, 2022).

Table 1. Major Pharmaceutical Regulatory Bodies Worldwide.

Region	Regulatory Bodies	Country/Area
Global	World Health Organization – Prequalification Programme (WHO)	International
North America	U.S. Food and Drug Administration (FDA)	United States
	Health Canada (HC)	Canada
Europe	European Medicines Agency (EMA)	European Union
	Medicines and Healthcare products Regulatory Agency (MHRA)	United Kingdom
	Federal Institute for Drugs and Medical Devices (BfArM)	Germany
	National Agency for the Safety of Medicines and Health Products (ANSM)	France
	Italian Medicines Agency (AIFA)	Italy
	Spanish Agency of Medicines and Medical Devices (AEMPS)	Spain
Asia	Pharmaceuticals and Medical Devices Agency (PMDA)	Japan
	National Medical Products Administration (NMPA)	China
	Central Drugs Standard Control Organization (CDSCO)	India
	Ministry of Food and Drug Safety (MFDS)	South Korea
	Department of Health – Food and Drug Administration (FDA Philippines)	Philippines
	Taiwan Food and Drug Administration (TFDA)	Taiwan
Latin America	Brazilian Health Regulatory Agency (ANVISA)	Brazil
	Federal Commission for the Protection against Sanitary Risks (COFEPRIS)	Mexico
	National Institute of Food and Drug Surveillance (INVIMA)	Colombia
	National Administration of Drugs, Foods and Medical Devices (ANMAT)	Argentina
Africa	South African Health Products Regulatory Authority (SAHPRA)	South Africa
	Pharmacy and Poisons Board (PPB)	Kenya
	National Agency for Food and Drug Administration and Control (NAFDAC)	Nigeria
	Egyptian Drug Authority (EDA)	Egypt
Oceania	Therapeutic Goods Administration (TGA)	Australia
	New Zealand Medicines and Medical Devices Safety Authority (Medsafe)	New Zealand

Regulatory agencies today act as key interfaces between scientific discovery, business interests, and patient rights. Their regulation is comprehensive across the entire life cycle of a drug, ranging from preclinical development to post-marketing surveillance, maintaining scientific stringency and ethical integrity (Khanna, 2012).

Artificial Intelligence (AI) and Machine Learning (ML) being new technologies are widely invading the pharmaceutical industry creating challenges of validation, transparency and fairness in healthcare (Gerke et al., 2020).

In India, the pharmaceutical industry is controlled under a structured framework for ensuring drug efficacy, quality, and safety. The apex body is the Central Drugs Standard Control Organization (CDSCO) supported by the Drugs Controller General of India (DCGI), state level organizations, and advisory bodies, refer Figure 2.

Figure 2. Organizational Chart of CDSCO.

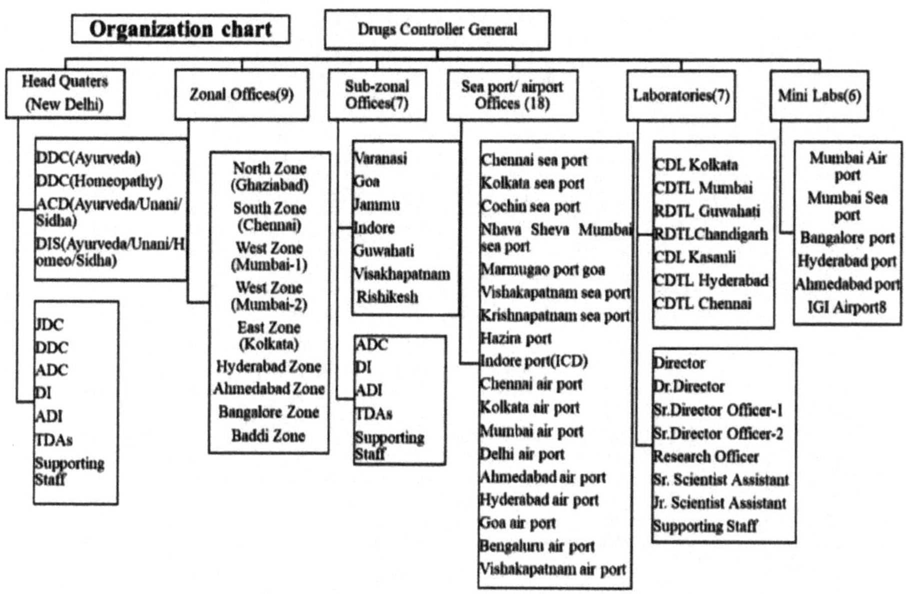

Retrieved Rupnawar, M., & Wani, P. (2024).

Role Played by FDA, CDSCO, EMA, WHO

The role of agencies like the FDA, EMA, and CDSCO has evolved from assuring the safety and effectiveness of finished drug products to regulating the integrity of the AI/ML lifecycle itself. Their regulations codify ethical ideals into implementable standards. For example, the U.S. Food and Drug Administration (FDA) has led the way in creating a regulatory avenue for AI-driven software, with a focus on Good Machine Learning Practices (GMLP) and a system for governance of pre-specified adjustments to "learning" AI systems. This directly responds to the ethical principle of safety by assuring models are strong and consistent.

Within the European Union, the European Medicines Agency (EMA) is governed by a strict legal regime set out in the General Data Protection Regulation (GDPR) and the forthcoming AI Act. The strategy of the EMA necessarily prioritizes data privacy and transparency, assuring that the processing of patient data for AI training is respectful of individual autonomy and basic rights. This makes the EMA a rights-oriented regulator, expressing the ethical principle of autonomy in terms of tangible data governance requirements.

In highly heterogeneous nations like India, the Central Drugs Standard Control Organization (CDSCO) is crucial in protecting against algorithmic bias. The ethical standard of equity and justice is at the heart of its function, for if AI models are trained on unrepresentative data, therapies may turn out to be less effective for certain ethnic groups. CDSCO's journey, encompassing the revised New Drugs and Clinical Trials Rules (2019), offers a platform for ensuring that AI-assisted drug development reaches all sections of the population.

At the International policy level, World Health Organization (WHO) plays the role of an ethical guide. Its seminal advice includes six principles at the core of AI in health, such as advancing human well-being, upholding equity, and advancing accountability. The WHO is concerned with avoiding an "AI divide" and advancing global solidarity, ensuring that benefits from AI in medicine development are shared by all countries, and not merely the richest.

The cooperative task for these regulatory agencies is to attain global standardization of standards without inhibiting innovation. Holden that while the FDA is concentrating on technical verification, the EMA on governance based on rights, and organizations such as CDSCO on contextual fairness, they are all informed by the general ethical framework provided by the WHO. The future of responsibly developed ethical AI to aid drug development relies on this multi-level watchfulness, whereby influential technologies are responsibly made and used in the interest of global public health.

Role of Institutional Review Boards (IRBs)

Institutional Review Boards (IRBs) or Ethics Committees play a crucial and knowledgeable role in order to protect active participants in research. They often go beyond standard protocol review to address new ethical issues brought by available algorithmic systems. Their duties requires to pay particular attention to assess the validity and possible biases of datasets used to train AI models, making sure algorithmic decisions are transparent and easy for patients to understand, and carefully confirming that informed consent procedures fully disclose how participant data will be used by sophisticated AI tools during the period of a trial (Vayena et al., 2018; Gerke et al., 2020; Fiske et al., 2020).

In order to preserve the values of justice and beneficence at the point of human-subject interaction, IRBs must also keep an eye out for emergent algorithmic harms in ongoing trials, such as the unjust exclusion of specific patient subgroups or skewed outcome predictions (Krittanawong et al., 2019). By guaranteeing that the ethical application of AI is continuously upheld within specific research institutions, this local oversight supports the efforts of national regulatory bodies, Figure 3 show the flow diagram of IRB review process.

Figure 3. Flow diagram of the IRB review process

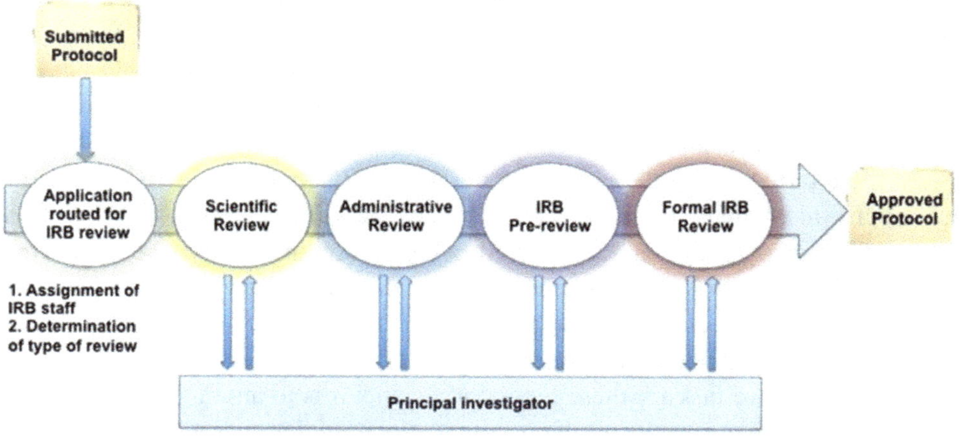

(adapted from Shoenbill et al., IRB Process Improvements, 2017).

Existing Gaps in Regulatory Practices & Role of Interdisciplinary Ethics Committees for Assessment of AI

One of the most important technological developments in pharmaceutical history is the incorporation of artificial intelligence into drug development. However, regulatory frameworks around the globe actually find it very difficult to adjust to this shift in standard perspective. Significant gaps still exist between technological capabilities and regulatory lookout, despite the outstanding efforts of organisations like the European Medicines Agency (EMA) and the U.S. Food and Drug Administration (FDA) to address AI through discussion papers and plan of action. Patient safety, data privacy, and the fair advancement of medical treatments are all severely threatened by these gaps.

The "black box" issue that many of the sophisticated AI systems, especially the seep learning models, have is the most basic hurdle. The relationship between inputs and outputs is transparent and reproducible in traditional statistical models used in drug development, but complex AI algorithms often work through layers of non-linear transformations that are difficult to understand even for the designers themselves (Vayena et al., 2018). This leads to a fundamental conflict with the regulatory requirements for comprehending the mechanism of action of a drug. Regulators face an unprecedented conundrum when an AI system predicts a patient's response or finds a novel drug target without offering a clear explanatory pathway: should they approve a therapy whose discovery rationale is statistically validated but partially opaque? This lack of transparency makes the risk-benefit analysis, which is the foundation of drug approval procedures, more difficult (Price et al., 2019). The FDA's new "Predetermined Change Control Plans" framework is a step in the right direction, but validating algorithms whose decision-making processes are not entirely explicable still presents significant methodological difficulties.

One of the challenges for regulators is when AI systems identify drug target or prediction patient response without clear explanation for the decision. Such results lack transparency resulting into complicated risk benefits evaluation in drug approvals (Price et al.,2019). Recent Predetermined Change Control Plans by FDA aims to address such issues still major challenges remain in validation of AI models over it's capability of internal interpretation. Because of variations in documentation practices, equipment sensitivity, or patient demographics, an AI model trained on academic medical centre electronic health records may not perform well when applied to community hospital populations. Worse, these biases can be self-reinforcing and multiplicative. For instance, an AI system used to recruit patients may unintentionally leave out a certain demographic groups, creating even more unrepresentative data for model training in the future (Obermeyer et al., 2019). Although the significance of representative data is acknowledged by current regulatory guidelines, they provide little in the way of useful advice on how to measure and mitigate these intricate bias pathways, particularly for models that will be used in diverse international jurisdictions.

A third regulatory challenge is the iterative nature of AI systems. Traditional drug development is usually a linear process in which, once approved, the product is essentially fixed and any modifications necessitate further applications. According to Gerke et al. (2020), artificial intelligence (AI) systems, especially those that are referred to as "continuously learning," change over time as a result of being exposed to new data. Because of this, there is regulatory ambiguity regarding what qualifies as a substantial modification that needs a new review. Should every weekly parameter update in an AI model used to predict adverse events be subject to regulatory scrutiny if it is based on fresh patient data? The pharmaceutical sector needs precise guidelines outlining the differences between routine maintenance and significant modifications to an approved product that are represented by model updates. Without this clarity, businesses risk regulatory ambiguity or lack of motivation to enhance their algorithms after approval. Through the Software Precertification Program, the FDA's Digital Health Centre of Excellence has started to address this, but this strategy is still in its infancy and has not been tried for high-risk applications such as drug development (FDA, 2021).

Data integrity and cybersecurity requirements represent a fourth gap. Artificial intelligence (AI) systems used in drug development usually need access to a large and frequently dispersed datasets, which increases the attack surfaces available to bad actors. A highly skilled attacker might introduce backdoors that cause models to fail selectively after approval or contaminate training data to influence trial results (Finlayson et al., 2019). The unique vulnerabilities of distributed AI systems that learn from multiple data sources across institutional boundaries are not specifically taken into account by the current Good Clinical Practice guidelines, despite the fact that they address data integrity in general. Specific guidelines for protecting the AI lifecycle from data gathering and model training to deployment and monitoring, must be established by regulatory frameworks. These guidelines should include various specifications for adversarial testing and robustness validation.

Lastly, there is a sizable jurisdictional disparity in the harmonisation of global regulations. Global by nature, AI-driven drug development frequently targets foreign markets and uses data from several nations. Nonetheless, different jurisdictions have quite different approaches to AI regulation. Many AI applications used in drug development would be categorised as high-risk under the European Union's AI Act, which takes a risk-based approach and imposes strict guidelines on data governance, documentation, and human oversight (European Commission, 2021). With a distinct focus on data sharing and privacy protections, China has put aggressive policies into place to hasten the adoption of AI in healthcare. For multinational pharmaceutical companies looking to develop globally applicable AI tools, these disparate approaches present difficulties. The field runs the risk of fragmenting without more international harmonisation, forcing businesses to create region-specific models that decrease efficiency.

The Role of Interdisciplinary Ethics Committees in Assessment

A supplementary oversight mechanism beyond traditional regulatory pathways is required due to the complexity and novelty of the ethical challenges presented by AI in drug development. One promising strategy for addressing the complex ethical issues that go beyond the purview of traditional regulatory review is the creation of interdisciplinary ethics committees. The committees specifically focus on algorithmic systems and their makeup, which must include knowledge of data science, computational linguistics, philosophy, law, and social sciences in addition to clinical ethics, should set them apart from traditional Institutional Review Boards (IRBs).

Conducting thorough ethical impact assessments at every level of the AI lifecycle would be the prominent objective of interdisciplinary ethics committees. Assessing the origin and methods of training data collection is the first step in this process. These committees would evaluate more general data ethics issues, as opposed to IRBs, which are mainly concerned with protecting human subjects in particular trials: For AI training, were the data sources acquired with the proper consent? Are sampling biases introduced by the data collection methods? Is it possible to implement privacy- preserving methods without sacrificing their usefulness? (Floridi and others, 2018). An ethics committee could assess whether using biobank samples obtained with broad consent for genetic research to train an AI system is in line with ethical standards and participant expectations when these samples are used for commercial drug development.

Auditing algorithmic fairness would be one of the most prominent roles of these committees. Ethics committees would very significantly investigate the performance of AI systems across different demographic subgroups, socioeconomic classes, and geographical regions, whereas regulators concentrate on validating overall performance standards. Technical expertise is highly required for complex fairness analyses that utilizes metrics such as equalized chances, predictive parity, and calibration fairness (Mehrabi et al., 2021). More importantly, ethical reasoning is required to determine which fairness definitions are most effective in specific clinical settings. For instance, to guarantee fair access to experimental treatments, an AI system that forecasts clinical trial eligibility may need to give equal opportunity across racial groups top priority, even if doing so marginally lowers overall accuracy. Such limitations on fairness could be required by ethics committees as a prerequisite for the institutional approvals.

These committees are also helpful in meeting requirements for suitable explanations and transparency. Ethics committees can make sure that developers give suitable "explanations" that are suited to various stakeholders, even though complete technical explanations might not be possible for some of the complex AI models (Arya et al., 2019). This could demand thorough documentation of the model architecture and training procedures for regulatory bodies. Case-based explanations demonstrating similar kinds of patients who benefited from the treatment could be presented to doctors thinking about implementing a therapy based on AI recommendation. Simple visualisations of how their data significantly affects recommendations may be necessary for patients. Ethics committees would assess this, and explain how well these multi-level explanations facilitate reliable and well-informed decision-making.

Another critical task is identifying societal and long term effects. Short-term advantages of AI systems are subjected to broader societal effects for patients. Taking an example of an AI model deployed to find patients with rare diseases for clinical trial recruitment, accidentally leaking the information about undiagnosed conditions may create unintentional insurance discrimination for that individual (Cohen et al., 2020). Similarly, AI systems trained to optimize the selection of clinical trial sites, may favor urban centers owing to advanced healthcare infrastructure, larger patient pools and reduced logistical challenges which collectively enhance trial efficiency. This risk in excluding the rural or un-resourced populations thereby limiting their access to innovative therapies and participation in trials, resulting in inequities across different socio-economic and geographic groups In order to identify these second-order effects and suggest mitigation strategies, ethics committees would use methods such as scenario planning and stakeholder analysis.

These committee governance structures must be structurally planned with care to guarantee their independence and efficacy. AI ethics committees may need to function at several different levels or stages, including academic medical centres, pharmaceutical companies, and independent national bodies, in contrast to institutional IRBs (Char et al., 2020). Collaboration would be important, possibly by shared databases of best practices and ethical evaluations across various institutions. Particularly when assessing AI systems created by their host institutions, committee members should have time and meaningful resources set aside for comprehensive assessments, along with clear, straightforward protocols for handling conflicts of interest.

At last, these committees need to set up continuous oversight procedures for authorized and trained AI systems. As AI tools are used in real-world situations and as social norms change, their ethical use and application might also change depending on the scenario. The identification of emergent biases, privacy issues, or unexpected consequences that were not evident during initial development would be possibly monitored and detected with ongoing working (Mittelstadt, 2019). Periodic reassessments triggered reviews and actions in response to performance alerts or adaptive oversight frameworks where the monitoring levels do vary according to the system's threats and performance history could all be part of this.

In conclusion, interdisciplinary ethical committees would offer significant relevance, moreover concentrate on justice, transparency, accountability, and society impact, while regulatory agencies primarily focus on safety and efficacy. Such committees can always assist better in ensuring that the AI-driven drug development not only results in effective therapies but also advances justice, upholds patient autonomy, and advances the basic welfare by legally addressing the ethical aspects in a development throughout the AI lifecycle.

Mechanisms for Validating AI and Model Approval

To uphold safety and efficacy along with trust, seamless validation and categorized approval of Artificial Intelligence (AI) models should be mandatory before implementing in pharmaceutical research or clinical practice. Dynamic Evolution of AI based drug development system can be achieved with continuous learning based on new data, which makes it must to have multiple layered validation framework that integrates technical, clinical and ethical considerations.

The Figure 4 depicts the multilevel validation process of AI and model approval in health. This starts with good machine learning practice (GMLP) and pre-market assessment, succeeded by clinical validation in intended trials. An AI system deployed in the market undergoes predetermined post-market surveillance and change-control plan to handle updates. Additional assurance in terms of safety, fairness and compliance can be achieved with independent auditing and third party certifications. Ultimately, sustained reliability along with performance across various clinical settings can be justified through continuous learning and real-world evidence.

Figure 4. Multi- Level Mechanisms for validating AI Model approval

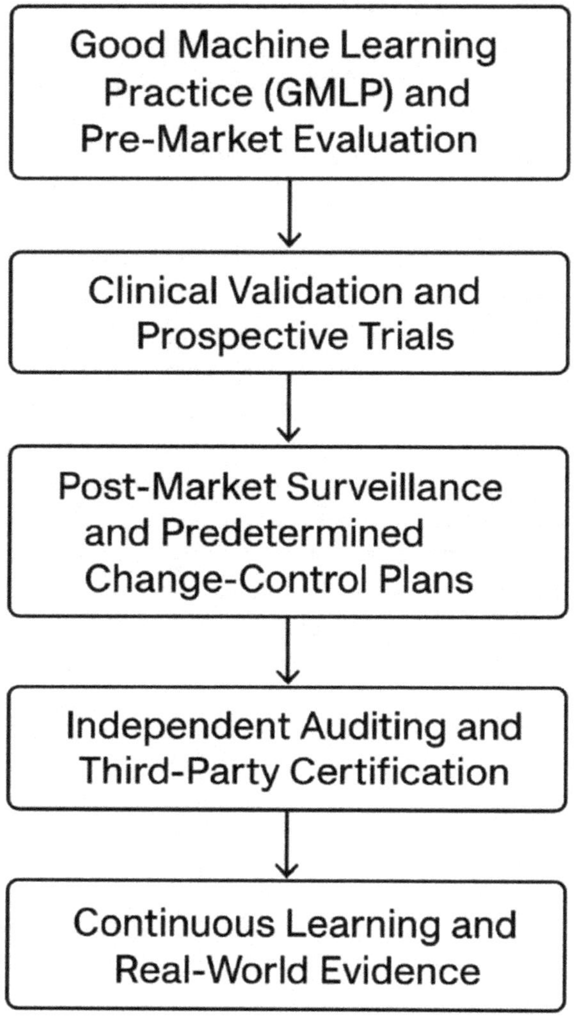

1. Good Machine Learning Practice (GMLP) and Pre-Market Evaluation

To standardize development and reduce risk, regulatory bodies such as the U.S. Food and Drug Administration (FDA) recommends adherence to Good Machine Learning Practice (GLMP). It addresses various facets critical to model reliability and safety. One of the critical elements is data provenance verification and management, whereby developers need to ensure that datasets come from verified and reliable sources—for example, an AI model projecting drug toxicity should be based on authenticated clinical trial data and not unauthenticated preclinical studies. Another essential element is the implementation of sound training and testing protocols such as cross-validation, independent test sets, and performance metrics. For instance, an artificial intelligence tool for diagnosing pneumonia from chest X-rays would have to be validated over datasets of several hospitals to allow generalizability (Alizadehsani et al., 2024). Sought as well is reproducibility documentation, made possible through "model cards" or "datasheets for datasets" that clearly specify data features, preprocessing, and algorithmic assumptions. For example, a model card could report that an AI model for predicting drug–drug interactions was trained on adult populations only and underling the importance of validation in pediatric groups (Mitchell et al., 2019). Lastly, prior to market approval, sponsors must collect and submit these records in a pre-market submission package, like a new drug application, as evidence that accuracy, sensitivity, specificity, and robustness achieve predetermined regulatory criteria (Gerke et al., 2020).

2. Clinical Validation and Prospective Trials

Technical performance alone is not enough to determine the reliability of AI systems in medicine. Future clinical validation studies are needed to ensure that an AI system not only achieves high performance in controlled settings but also enhances patient outcomes or decision quality in actual clinical practice (He et al., 2019). These studies are analogous to conventional Phase II/III drug trials but include AI-specific measures like calibration, false-positive rates, and algorithmic drift. For instance, an artificial intelligence model trained to forecast sepsis development in intensive care unit (ICU) patients would need a prospective multi-center clinical trial, wherein its forecasts are constantly benchmarked with physician judgments and real-world patient outcomes. This will make sure that the model helps lower mortality without creating too many false alarms (Wang et al., 2022). In addition, adaptive design usage provides the capability for continuous monitoring and iterative adjustment, thus keeping patient risk to a minimum while maintaining model performance in a clinically relevant fashion over time.

3. Post-Market Surveillance and Predetermined Change-Control Plans

Most AI devices are programmed to learn continuously following deployment, which renders lifecycle monitoring an integral part of regulation. To resolve this, the U.S. Food and Drug Administration (FDA) has developed the Predetermined Change Control Plan (PCCP) that enables developers to pre-determine how algorithms can be modified, the procedures for validating each modification, and what performance limits would necessitate regulatory re-review (FDA, 2021). For example, a diabetes care AI that dynamically adjusts insulin doses can refresh its predictive model weekly as it acquires new patient glucose readings. In the PCCP, developers will need to establish clear standards for acceptable accuracy; if these thresholds are violated, the update would need re-approval by the regulatory agency before deployment. Similar regulatory structures also prevail in the European Medicines Agency (EMA) under the EU Artificial Intelligence Act and in the Central Drugs Standard Control Organization (CDSCO) in India, with special focus on an international transition toward organized regulation of adaptive AI systems.

4. Independent Auditing and Third-Party Certification

Independent auditing and third-party certification offer added assurance for AI systems in healthcare. External auditors can evaluate important aspects such as fairness across demographic groups, adversarial robustness, and conformance to privacy laws such as GDPR and HIPAA (Mehrabi et al., 2021; Finlayson et al., 2019). For instance, an AI in radiology used in many hospitals could be subjected to an independent audit to ensure steady performance on images acquired through various scanners, age groups of patients, and ethnic backgrounds. Additionally, voluntary certification schemes similar to ISO 13485 for medical devices are being developed specifically for health AI with the purpose of harmonizing control and encouraging harmonized assessment practices (IMDRF, 2022).

Continuous Learning and Real-World Evidence

Validated AI models need ongoing post-market performance monitoring based on real-world evidence. Jointly agreed key performance indicators (KPIs) between developers and regulators usually consist of outcome accuracy by demographic subgroups, model drift rates, and cybersecurity incident reports (Obermeyer et al., 2019). For example, a brain hemorrhage diagnosis AI implemented in multiple hospitals can receive ongoing feedback through clinical use. Re-certification of the system on a regular basis guarantees that revisions improve the performance of detection and prevent the imposition of bias or loss of accuracy for underrepresented groups.

RECOMMENDATIONS AND ETHICAL GUIDELINES

The rapid inclusion of Artificial Intelligence (AI) into drug development and the pharmaceutical industry has evolved from conventional domains such as drug discovery and preclinical testing to clinical trial design, pharmacovigilance, and personalized medicine. While AI guarantees rapid innovation, enhances accuracy of prediction, and is economical, it also introduces complex ethical, regulatory, and societal challenges. These challenges originate from the non-transparent nature of certain AI models, risk of biased outcomes, patient privacy concerns, and the lack of harmonization among various regulatory frameworks.

Ethical considerations can be especially important in the pharmaceutical paradigm as decisions influenced by AI can have direct impact on patient safety, public health, and societal trust. For instance, a biased predictive model could unfairly and disproportionately impact certain populations, while opaque algorithms influencing clinical decisions may impair clinician accountability and patient trust (Topol, 2019; Blease et al., 2019). To resolve these concerns, a systematic set of propositions and ethical guidelines are recommended to be in place.

Such recommendations are necessary to ensure transparency and clarity in AI decision-making to cultivate trust among researchers, clinicians, regulators, patients and other stake-holders. The guidelines may ensure integration of ethical principles in the design, development, and disposition of AI systems to safeguard human welfare, privacy, and equity. Harmonization of regulatory standards aids global collaboration to ensure persistent ethical practices over different geographical locations and demographics.

The following sections outline specific guidelines and approaches under three principle areas: the development of transparent and explainable AI, the adoption of ethical AI frameworks, and the establishment of global collaborative regulations and open ethics charters. On the whole, these recommendations aim to provide an impetus to the responsible inclusion of AI in pharmaceutical innovation and research, ensuring that the resultant outputs lead to meaningful and equitable patient benefits.

Development of Transparent, Explainable AI

Transparency and precision are the key principles for the ethical use of AI in drug development and pharmaceutical research. AI models, specifically those based on complex fundamentals such as deep learning, are often regarded as "black boxes," generating predictions or recommendations without clear data. In specific circumstances, where such decisions influence patient safety, regulatory compliance, or clinical outcomes, opaque outcomes can threaten trust, hinder acceptance, and inadvertently pose severe risk to the patient's health (Doshi-Velez & Kim, 2017).

Transparency in algorithms can be imbibed, developers should document AI model architectures, training datasets, feature selection criteria, and decision rules in a systematic and accessible manner. Transparency in reporting facilitates regulatory bodies, physicians, and researchers by allowing assessment of the model's validity, limitations, and potential biases (Guidotti et al., 2018). Explainability techniques—such as attention mechanisms, SHAP (SHapley Additive exPlanations), LIME (Local Interpretable Model-agnostic Explanations), or rule-based approximations may be incorporated that allow non-technical stakeholders to easily interpret or perceive AI decisions. Explainable AI essentially allows clinicians and researchers to interpret the basis on which a model predicts a particular outcome. Such clarity is critical for trust and accountability in drug discovery, dosing algorithms, and patient stratification.

Training datasets must be closely inspected to ensure broad representation, as a biased sample results in prejudiced outcomes. For example, underrepresentation of certain demographic groups in clinical trial data of a large population may lead to incorrect predictions. Ongoing model auditing, maintaining the fairness of metrics, and implementation of corrective measures may help alleviate potential disparities (Mehrabi et al., 2021). It is equally important to ensure that the AI tools are designed such that the end-user is taken into consideration. Instead of just producing the end results, the tools must provide clear, logical and practical explanations as well. Visualization tools, decision-support dashboards, and summary reports can help stakeholders to effectively understand and interpret the complex results. Such transparent and comprehensive AI models align with upcoming regulatory expectations, like those put forth by the 'European Commission on AI ethics' and the 'FDA's guidance on AI/ML-based Software as a Medical Device (SaMD)'.

By promoting informed decision-making, encouraging regulatory compliance, and ensuring patient safety, AI models' transparency and explainability help in ethical drug development and research. Transparent AI models can be used to optimise clinical trials by explaining why a particular patient subgroup is anticipated to respond well to a medication. This allows for more real and focused enrollment choices. Similarly, interpretable AI can assist in detecting adverse drug reactions in the pharmacovigilance domain without compromising the alert's justification.

Adoption of Ethical AI Framework

The implementation of structured ethical frameworks is crucial for ensuring that AI based tools and models are deployed responsibly in drug development and the pharmaceutical industry and corroborate with regulatory requirements and societal values. While AI can potentially be used to accelerate drug development, optimize clinical trials, and personalize therapies, its influence on patient safety, data privacy, accountability, and fairness is often a point of concern (Floridi et al., 2018). A formal ethical AI guideline provides the framework that mitigate these risks while developing trust and transparency among stakeholders.

Key Recommendations

To materialize this approach, AI systems should be developed following widely recognized ethical principles, including fairness, accountability, transparency, privacy, beneficence, and non-maleficence as mentioned by Jobin et al., 2019. It is ensured that ethical considerations are considered at the very beginning of the design process rather than after the fact. Patient welfare should be the main objective of AI applications in the pharmaceutical industry. This strategy places a high priority on patient safety, promises fair access, and upholds patient autonomy. To visualize, AI models used in the estimation of drug dosing or prediction of an adverse drug event should present recommendations keeping in mind the demographic and physiological variations to avoid accidental harm to vulnerable populations.

Thorough data validation, including safe storage, confidentiality, consent management, and compliance with legal requirements like GDPR, HIPAA, etc., must be provided by ethical AI frameworks. It is necessary to have transparent policies in place for data usage and sharing so as to prevent misuse, retain public trust, and maintain compliance with global regulations. Distinct segregation of responsibilities is imperative when AI systems impact clinical or regulatory decisions. A systematic hierarchy of accountability mechanisms should be designed by organizations for developers, clinicians, and pharmaceutical companies. An appropriate framework for reporting errors, monitoring outcomes, and correcting adverse effects should be embedded into the operational plan of work. Ethical AI frameworks should integrate features such as continual monitoring, auditing, and evaluation to identify and address inadvertent outcomes. Intermittent ethical reviews, with stakeholder consultations, and impact evaluations can guarantee the alignment of AI systems with evolving societal values and regulatory requirements.

Embedment of ethical considerations into regulatory submissions can ensure approval and promote public trust. Regulatory agencies progressively emphasize the importance of developing ethical design and responsible execution of AI/ML systems in pharmaceuticals (FDA, 2021).

Employing an ethical AI framework ensures that AI-driven innovations do not compromise patient safety, aggravate prejudices, or undermine trust. For example, in drug repurposing or precision medicine, an ethical AI framework guarantees that the model recommendations are unbiased across populations and that vulnerable groups are not unwittingly excluded or harmed. Moreover, AI-driven pharmacovigilance tools aligning with ethical guidelines can identify adverse drug reactions without compromising patient privacy or autonomy.

Global Collaborative Regulations and Open Ethics Charter

Artificial intelligence in drug development is a global process, as proven by the international scope of pharmaceutical innovations and AI models. Therefore, ethical adoption and use of AI models cannot be ensured by local laws alone. Harmonization of international regulatory standards is necessary to ensure patient safety, equitable access, and responsible innovation. Establishing cooperative legal frameworks and an accessible ethics charter can give AI applications the guidance they need while fostering confidence among global stakeholders (Morley et al., 2020).

Key Recommendations

To create common standards for AI in drug development, international regulatory organizations like the FDA, EMA, PMDA, etc. must work together. International organizations can work together to prevent redundant approvals, make international research easier, and guarantee uniform safety standards for patients everywhere. As a demonstration, the International Council for Harmonization (ICH) might broaden its scope to cover AI-powered instruments in drugs surveillance and clinical trials.

A multi-stakeholder, publicly available ethics charter can offer internationally accepted guidelines for ethical AI use in medicine. As a guide for researchers, developers, and regulators alike, this charter should address issues of transparency, fairness, accountability, data protection, and bias avoidance. Open ethics charters promote compliance, ethical quandaries, and an exchange of best practices.

Significance in Pharmaceutical Applications

Global collaborative regulations and open ethics charters intend to ensure that AI-driven innovations are beneficial to humanity while trying to be least harmful. For example, a predictive AI model for adverse drug reactions used in several nations can come together to share standards for bias mitigation, data privacy, and transparency, preventing uneven safety outcomes. Similarly, open ethics charters promote transparency and trust in AI applications, enhancing broader adoption and collaboration in global drug development.

It is both strategically necessary and morally required that artificial intelligence be used ethically in drug development and the pharmaceutical sector. Impact of AI on important choices, ranging from pharmacovigilance and personalized medicine to drug discovery and clinical trial design, will grow as the technology develops, increasing both the opportunities and the risks. To preserve patient safety, public confidence, and regulatory compliance, it is crucial to make sure AI systems are open, understandable, and consistent with ethical standards.

Adopting structured ethical frameworks, grounded in fairness, accountability, and with patient-centric values, provides a roadmap for responsible AI implementation. Simultaneously, global collaboration through harmonized regulations and open-access ethical charters facilitates the steady application of ethical standards across borders, encouraging equity and trust in AI-driven pharmaceutical innovations.

In essence, the integration of AI in drug development must have a balance between technological innovation along with ethical responsibility. By adhering to these recommendations, the pharmaceutical industry can leverage AI not only to boost scientific progress but also to ensure that such progress is safe, equitable as well as aligned with societal values.

CONCLUSION

Artificial intelligence (AI) has emerged as a catalyst across the pharmaceutical value chain, enabling quicker identification of drug targets, adaptive design of clinical trials, and supporting precision-medicines strategies. The chapter has demonstrated that enabling robust discovery and development is closely entangled with profound ethical considerations. The application of huge mixed datasets also entails long-term threats of privacy violations, re-identification, and cyber-breaches, as well as the threat of biased or truncated information duplicating—and even amplifying—existing health-care disparities. Maybe equally important is the opaqueness of many deep learning architectures, its inhibiting clinical testing, making regulatory clearance more difficult, and concealing responsibility when AI-based suggestions are included in generating poor outcomes.

Good management of these technologies therefore demands a complex ethical and regulatory framework. Globally, organizations such as the U.S. Food and Drug Administration (FDA), the European Medicines Agency (EMA), the Central Drugs Standard Control Organization (CDSCO) and the World Health Organization (WHO) has begun implementation of structured principles of fairness, transparency, and beneficence into legal guidelines. Backed by this governance, institutional review boards and interdisciplinarity ethics panels provide localized monitoring of data provenance, algorithmic bias and model explainability throughout the research lifecycle.

The debate presented here emphasizes the importance of ethical incorporation of AI for drug discovery as going beyond post event compliance to designing before the fact. Model architectures that are transparent and interpretable, frequent auditing for bias, privacy-sensitive treatment of data, and express informed consent mechanisms must be seen as engineering requirements rather than aspirational safeguards. Besides, worldwide collaboration through open ethics charters, harmonized data standards, and joint post-market surveillance regimes is essential to avoid regulatory fragmentation and to attain equitable global access to AI-powered therapies.

Overall, the future of artificial intelligence-based drug discovery will be determined not by technological innovation but by industry, regulators and scientist's capacity to integrate ethical responsibility into every process of development and deployment. By establishing fairness, transparency and patient self-determination as guiding design principles, the pharmaceutical industry will be able to realize the full scientific potential of artificial intelligence while maintaining public trust and advancing global health equity.

REFERENCES

Alizadehsani, R., Oyelere, S. S., Hussain, S., Jagatheesaperumal, S. K., Calixto, R. R., Rahouti, M., & De Albuquerque, V. H. C. (2024). Explainable artificial intelligence for drug discovery and development—A comprehensive survey. *Briefings in Bioinformatics*, *25*(2), bbae101. PMID: 38493339

Arya, V., Bellamy, R. K., Chen, P. Y., Dhurandhar, A., Hind, M., Hoffman, S. C., . . . Zhang, Y. (2019). One explanation does not fit all: A toolkit and taxonomy of AI explainability techniques. arXiv preprint arXiv:1909.03012.

BBC News. (2017, July 3). Google DeepMind NHS app broke UK data law. BBC. https://www.bbc.com/news/technology-40483202

Benevolent, A. I. (2020, January 30). AstraZeneca and BenevolentAI announce collaboration to use artificial intelligence and machine learning for drug discovery. BenevolentAI. https://benevolent.com/news/astraZeneca-and-benevolentai-announce-collaboration

Blease, C., Bernstein, M. H., & Gaab, J. (2019). Artificial intelligence in medicine: Balancing innovation and accountability. *Journal of Medical Ethics*, *45*(12), 785–788.

Char, D. S., Abramoff, M. D., & Feudtner, C. (2020). Identifying ethical considerations for machine learning healthcare applications. *The American Journal of Bioethics*, *20*(11), 7–17. PMID: 33103967

Chen, I. Y., Szolovits, P., & Ghassemi, M. (2019). Can AI help reduce disparities in general medical and mental health care? *AMA Journal of Ethics*, *21*(2), 167–179. DOI: 10.1001/amajethics.2019.167 PMID: 30794127

Chen, Z., Liu, X., Hogan, W., Shenkman, E., & Bian, J. (2021). Applications of artificial intelligence in drug development using real-world data. *Drug Discovery Today*, *26*(5), 1256–1264. DOI: 10.1016/j.drudis.2020.12.013 PMID: 33358699

Cohen, I. G., Evgeniou, T., Gerke, S., & Minssen, T. (2020). The European artificial intelligence strategy: Implications and challenges for digital health. *The Lancet. Digital Health*, *2*(7), e376–e377. PMID: 33328096

Dara, M., & Azarpira, N. (2025). Ethical considerations emerge from artificial intelligence (AI) in biotechnology. *Avicenna Journal of Medical Biotechnology*, *17*(1), 80–81. DOI: 10.18502/ajmb.v17i1.17680 PMID: 40094090

Deng, J., Yang, Z., Ojima, I., Samaras, D., & Wang, F. (2022). Artificial intelligence in drug discovery: Applications and techniques. *Briefings in Bioinformatics*, *23*(1), bbab430. PMID: 34734228

Doshi-Velez, F., & Kim, B. (2017). Towards a rigorous science of interpretable machine learning. arXiv:1702.08608.

European Commission. (2021). Proposal for a regulation of the European Parliament and of the Council laying down harmonised rules on artificial intelligence.

European Medicines Agency. (2020). EMA big data steering group: Workplan 2020-2022.

European Union. (2016). Regulation (EU) 2016/679 of the European Parliament and of the Council of 27 April 2016 on the protection of natural persons with regard to the processing of personal data and on the free movement of such data (General Data Protection Regulation). Official Journal of the European Union, L 119/1.

European Union. (2021). Proposal for a regulation of the European Parliament and of the Council laying down harmonised rules on artificial intelligence (Artificial Intelligence Act). COM(2021) 206 final.

FDA. (2021). Artificial intelligence/machine learning (AI/ML)-based software as a medical device (SaMD) action plan.

Finlayson, S. G., Bowers, J. D., Ito, J., Zittrain, J. L., Beam, A. L., & Kohane, I. S. (2019). Adversarial attacks on medical machine learning. *Science*, *363*(6433), 1287–1289. DOI: 10.1126/science.aaw4399 PMID: 30898923

Fiske, A., Henningsen, P., & Buyx, A. (2020). Your robot therapist will see you now: Ethical implications of embodied artificial intelligence in psychiatry, psychology, and psychotherapy. *Journal of Medical Internet Research*, *22*(5), e13216. PMID: 31094356

Floridi, L., Cowls, J., Beltrametti, M., Chatila, R., Chazerand, P., Dignum, V., & Vayena, E. (2018). AI4People—An ethical framework for a good AI society: Opportunities, risks, principles, and recommendations. *Minds and Machines*, *28*(4), 689–707. PMID: 30930541

Food and Drug Administration. (2018). FDA's evolution: A brief history of the regulation of drugs and biologics. U.S. Food and Drug Administration. https://www.fda.gov

Food and Drug Administration. (2021). Artificial intelligence/machine learning (AI/ML)-based software as a medical device action plan. https://www.fda.gov/media/145022/download

Gad, S. C. (2021). *Drug safety evaluation* (4th ed.). John Wiley & Sons.

Gao, Y., Gao, H., Xiao, H., & Yao, F. (2023). Vaccine supply chain coordination using blockchain and artificial intelligence technologies. *Computers & Industrial Engineering, 175*, 108885. PMID: 36505091

Gao, Z., Deng, J., & Liang, H. (2023). Legal challenges of AI in drug discovery and development. *Journal of Law and the Biosciences, 10*(1), lsad005. Advance online publication. DOI: 10.1093/jlb/lsad005 PMID: 36938304

Gerke, S., Minssen, T., & Cohen, G. (2020). Ethical and legal challenges of artificial intelligence-driven healthcare. In Bohr, A., & Memarzadeh, K. (Eds.), *Artificial intelligence in healthcare* (pp. 295–336). Academic Press., DOI: 10.1016/B978-0-12-818438-7.00012-5

Government of India. (2019). New drugs and clinical trials rules, 2019. The Gazette of India.

Guidotti, R., Monreale, A., Ruggieri, S., Turini, F., Giannotti, F., & Pedreschi, D. (2018). A survey of methods for explaining black box models. *ACM Computing Surveys, 51*(5), 1–42.

He, J., Baxter, S. L., Xu, J., Xu, J., Zhou, X., & Zhang, K. (2019). The practical implementation of artificial intelligence technologies in medicine. *Nature Medicine, 25*(1), 30–36. DOI: 10.1038/s41591-018-0307-0 PMID: 30617336

Hirani, R., Noruzi, K., Khuram, H., Hussaini, A. S., Aifuwa, E. I., Ely, K. E., Lewis, J. M., Gabr, A. E., Smiley, A., Tiwari, R. K., & Etienne, M. (2024). Artificial intelligence and healthcare: A journey through history, present innovations, and future possibilities. *Life (Chicago, Ill.), 14*(5), 557. DOI: 10.3390/life14050557 PMID: 38792579

Insilico Medicine. (2025, June 3). Insilico Medicine announces Nature Medicine publication of Phase IIa results evaluating Rentosertib, the novel TNIK inhibitor for idiopathic pulmonary fibrosis discovered and designed with a pioneering AI approach https://www.biospace.com/press-releases/insilico-medicine-announces-nature-medicine-publication-of-phase-iia-results-evaluating-rentosertib

International Medical Device Regulators Forum. (2022). AI and machine learning medical devices: Regulatory considerations. https://www.imdrf.org

Jobin, A., Ienca, M., & Vayena, E. (2019). The global landscape of AI ethics guidelines. *Nature Machine Intelligence*, *1*(9), 389–399.

Kapur, S., Chen, H., & Saxena, N. (2021). Reducing racial bias in AI models for clinical use requires a top-down intervention. *Nature Machine Intelligence*, *3*, 893–898. DOI: 10.1038/s42256-021-00362-7

Khanna, I. (2012). Drug discovery in pharmaceutical industry: Productivity challenges and trends. *Drug Discovery Today*, *17*(19–20), 1088–1102. DOI: 10.1016/j.drudis.2012.05.007 PMID: 22627006

Kolasa, K., Admassu, B., Hołownia-Voloskova, M., Kędzior, K. J., Poirrier, J. E., & Perni, S. (2024). Systematic reviews of machine learning in healthcare: A literature review. *Expert Review of Pharmacoeconomics & Outcomes Research*, *24*(1), 63–115. PMID: 37955147

Kolluri, S., Lin, J., Liu, R., Zhang, Y., & Zhang, W. (2022). Machine learning and artificial intelligence in pharmaceutical research and development: A review. *The AAPS Journal*, *24*(1). Advance online publication. DOI: 10.1208/s12248-021-00644-3 PMID: 34984579

Krittanawong, C., Johnson, K. W., Rosenson, R. S., Wang, Z., Aydar, M., Baber, U., Min, J. K., Tang, W. H. W., & Halperin, J. L. (2019). Artificial intelligence in precision cardiovascular medicine. *Journal of the American College of Cardiology*, *69*(21), 2657–2664. PMID: 28545640

Lee, D. (2019). Case study: IBM Watson Health and the challenge of AI in medicine. *Journal of the American Medical Informatics Association : JAMIA*, *26*(11), 1618–1622. DOI: 10.1093/jamia/ocz143

Li, F., Ruijs, N., & Lu, Y. (2023). Ethics & AI: A systematic review on ethical concerns and related strategies for designing with AI in healthcare. *AI*, *4*(1), 28–53. DOI: 10.3390/ai4010003

Mak, K. K., & Pichika, M. R. (2019). Artificial intelligence in drug development: Present status and future prospects. *Drug Discovery Today*, *24*(3), 773–780. DOI: 10.1016/j.drudis.2018.11.014 PMID: 30472429

Mak, K. K., Pichika, M. R., & Sun, J. (2022). Artificial intelligence in drug development: A systematic review. *Drug Discovery Today*, *27*(5), 1407–1415.

McNair, L. (2022). Ethical and regulatory oversight of clinical research: The role of the Institutional Review Board. *Experimental Biology and Medicine*, *247*(7), 561–566. DOI: 10.1177/15353702221083314 PMID: 35172623

Mehrabi, N., Morstatter, F., Saxena, N., Lerman, K., & Galstyan, A. (2021). A survey on bias and fairness in machine learning. *ACM Computing Surveys*, *54*(6), 1–35. DOI: 10.1145/3457607

Min, S., Lee, B., & Yoon, S. (2021). Deep learning in bioinformatics. *Briefings in Bioinformatics*, *22*(2), 125–144. PMID: 27473064

Mitchell, M., Wu, S., Zaldivar, A., Barnes, P., Vasserman, L., Hutchinson, B., & Gebru, T. (2019). Model cards for model reporting. *Proceedings of the Conference on Fairness, Accountability, and Transparency*, 220–229. https://doi.org/DOI: 10.1145/3287560.3287596

Morley, J., Machado, C. C. V., Burr, C., Cowls, J., Joshi, I., Taddeo, M., & Floridi, L. (2020). The ethics of AI in health care: A mapping review. *Social Science & Medicine*, *260*, 113172. PMID: 32702587

Naik, N., Hameed, B. M. Z., Shetty, D. K., Swain, D., Shah, M., Paul, R., Aggarwal, K., Ibrahim, S., Patil, V., Smriti, K., Shetty, S., Rai, B. P., Chlosta, P., & Somani, B. K. (2022). Legal and ethical consideration in artificial intelligence in healthcare: Who takes responsibility? *Frontiers in Surgery*, *9*, 862322. DOI: 10.3389/fsurg.2022.862322 PMID: 35360424

Noorbakhsh-Sabet, N., Zand, R., Zhang, Y., & Abedi, V. (2019). Artificial intelligence transforms the future of health care. *The American Journal of Medicine*, *132*(7), 795–801. DOI: 10.1016/j.amjmed.2019.01.017 PMID: 30710543

Obermeyer, Z., Powers, B., Vogeli, C., & Mullainathan, S. (2019). Dissecting racial bias in an algorithm used to manage the health of populations. *Science*, *366*(6464), 447–453. PMID: 31649194

OECD. (2019). Recommendation of the Council on Artificial Intelligence. OECD/LEGAL/0449.

Patel, V. L., Shortliffe, E. H., Stefanelli, M., Szolovits, P., Berthold, M. R., Bellazzi, R., & Abu-Hanna, A. (2019). Watson for Oncology and beyond: How machine learning and artificial intelligence can improve healthcare. *Journal of Clinical Oncology*, *37*(15, suppl), 8527. DOI: 10.1200/JCO.2017.35.15_suppl.8527

Powles, J., & Hodson, H. (1765-1766). (Price, W. N., Gerke, S., & Cohen, I. G. (2019). Potential liability for physicians using artificial intelligence. *Journal of the American Medical Association*, *322*(18).

Powles, J., & Hodson, H. (2017). Google DeepMind and healthcare in an age of algorithms. *Health and Technology*, *7*(4), 351–367. DOI: 10.1007/s12553-017-0179-1 PMID: 29308344

Rajkomar, A., Hardt, M., Howell, M. D., Corrado, G., & Chin, M. H. (2018). Ensuring fairness in machine learning to advance health equity. *Annals of Internal Medicine*, *169*(12), 866–872. PMID: 30508424

Ross, C., & Swetlitz, I. (2018, July 25). IBM pitched its Watson supercomputer as a revolution in cancer care. It's nowhere close. STAT. https://www.statnews.com/2018/07/25/ibm-watson-recommended-unsafe-incorrect-treatments

Rupnawar, M., & Wani, P. (2024). Pharmaceutical Regulatory Affairs: An Overview of Global Regulatory Frameworks and Emerging Trends. International Journal of Scientific Research and Technology.

Savage, N. (2021). Tapping into the drug discovery potential of AI. Nature. https://www.nature.com/articles/d43747-021-00045-7

Savage, N. (2021). Drugs by AI: Making new medicines in days. *Nature*, *595*(7867), S12–S14. DOI: 10.1038/d41586-021-02212-5

Shoenbill, K., Song, Y., Cobb, N. L., Drezner, M. K., & Mendonça, E. A. (2017). IRB process improvements: A machine learning analysis. *Journal of Clinical and Translational Science*, *1*(3), 176–183. DOI: 10.1017/cts.2016.25 PMID: 29082031

Singh, A., Attwood, S., & Wilkinson, P. (2022). Inclusion of under-represented racial and ethnic groups in cardiovascular clinical trials. *Journal of the American Heart Association*, *11*(14), e024706. DOI: 10.1161/JAHA.121.024706

Sireesha, B., & Haritha, S. (2024). A review on regulatory affairs and regulatory requirements for new drug approval. *International Journal of Health Care and Biological Sciences*, *3*(1), 22–28.

Strickland, E. (2019). IBM Watson, heal thyself: How IBM overpromised and underdelivered on AI health care. *IEEE Spectrum*, *56*(4), 24–31. https://spectrum.ieee.org/ibm-watson

Topol, E. J. (2019). High-performance medicine: The convergence of human and artificial intelligence. *Nature Medicine*, *25*(1), 44–56. PMID: 30617339

Topol, E. J. (2019). High-performance medicine: The convergence of human and artificial intelligence. *Nature Medicine*, *25*, 44–56. PMID: 30617339

U.S. Food and Drug Administration. (2021). *Artificial intelligence/machine learning (AI/ML)-based software as a medical device (SaMD) action plan*. U.S. Department of Health and Human Services.

U.S. Food and Drug Administration. (2023). *Using AI/ML in the development of drug and biological products: Discussion paper and request for feedback*. U.S. Department of Health and Human Services.

Vayena, E., Blasimme, A., & Cohen, I. G. (2018). Machine learning in medicine: Addressing ethical challenges. *PLoS Medicine*, *15*(11), e1002689. PMID: 30399149

Wang, Z., Gao, C., Glass, L. M., & Sun, J. (2022). Artificial intelligence for in silico clinical trials: A review. arXiv preprint arXiv:2209.09023.

Wang, Z., Gao, C., Glass, L. M., & Sun, J. (2022). Artificial intelligence for in silico clinical trials: A review. arXiv preprint arXiv:2209.09023.

WHO. (2021). Ethics and governance of artificial intelligence for health. World Health Organization. https://www.who.int/publications/i/item/9789240029200

WHO. (2024). Benefits and risks of using artificial intelligence for pharmaceutical development and delivery. World Health Organization. https://www.who.int/publications/i/item/9789240088108

World Health Organization. (2021). Ethics and governance of artificial intelligence for health: WHO guidance.

World Health Organization. (2023). Regulatory system strengthening for medical products: Why it matters. 93. Xu, J., Hagler, A., & Feher, M. (2021). AI in pharmaceutical research: from molecule design to clinical trial simulation. *Frontiers in Pharmacology*, *12*, 700680.

Zhavoronkov, A., Ivanenkov, Y. A., & Aliper, A.. (2019). Deep learning enables rapid identification of potent DDR1 kinase inhibitors. *Nature Biotechnology*, *37*(9), 1038–1040. DOI: 10.1038/s41587-019-0224-x PMID: 31477924

Zhavoronkov, A., Ivanenkov, Y. A., Aliper, A., Veselov, M. S., Aladinskiy, V. A., Aladinskaya, A. V., & Aspuru-Guzik, A. (2019). Deep learning enables rapid identification of potent DDR1 kinase inhibitors. *Nature Biotechnology*, *37*(9), 1038–1040. DOI: 10.1038/s41587-019-0224-x PMID: 31477924

Zhou, Y., & Wang, F. (2022). Explainable AI in healthcare and drug discovery: Trends and challenges. *Trends in Pharmacological Sciences*, *43*(6), 457–469. PMID: 35469690

KEY TERMS AND DEFINITIONS

Algorithm Bias: A systematic error within AI systems tht occurs when algorithms are trained on incomplete or skewed datasets, leading to unfair or discriminatory outcomes.

Artificial Intelligence (AI): A field of computer science focused on developing systems that can perform tasks typically requiring human intelligence,such as learning, reasoning and problem solving.

Central Drugs Standard Control Organization (CDSCO): India's national regulatory authority overseeing the approval, quality and safety of drugs, medical devices, and clinical research.

Data Privacy: The protection of personal and sensitive health information from unauthorized access or misuse, ensuring compliance with ethical and legal standards.

Drug Development: A Structured process involving preclinical studies, clinical trials and regulatory approval aimed at confirming the safety, efficacy and quality of new drugs before public use.

Ethical AI: The application of artificial Intelligence in ways that uphold moral principles such as fairness accountability, privacy, transparency and respect for human rights.

European Medicine Agency (EMA): The regulatory body of the European Union that evaluates and supervises medicinal products to ensure they are safe, effective and of high quality.

Explainable AI: AI System designed to make their decision-making processes transparent and understandable to users, clinicians and regulators.

Food and Drug Administration (FDA): The U.S. government agency that regulates drugs, biologics and medical devices, ensuring their safety, efficacy and ethical compliance.

Good Machine Learning Practice (GMLP): A set of standardized practices for designing, training, validating and maintaining reliable and safe machine learning models used in healthcare and pharmaceuticals.

Institutional Review Board (IRB): An ethics committee responsible for protecting humans research participants by reviewing and approving study protocols ensuring informed consent and ethical compliance.

Machine Learning (ML): A subset of AI that enables computer systems to automatically learn and improve from data, enhancing prediction and decision making without explicit programming.

Real World Data (RWD): Health-related information collected outside controlled clinical trials, such as from electroic health records or patient registries used to assess drug safety and performance.

World Health Organization (WHO): A global public health body that provides international guidance and ethical frameworks for AI, healthcare and pharmaceutical governance.

Compilation of References

Abbas, M. K. G., Rassam, A., Karamshahi, F., Abunora, R., & Abouseada, M. (2024). The role of AI in drug discovery. *ChemBioChem*, *25*(14), e202300816. PMID: 38735845

Abed, A. H. (2025). Artificial intelligence-driven pharmaceutical research: a comprehensive analysis of applications and challenges. *Journal of computers and digital business, 4*(1), 37-44.

Abo El-Enen, M., Saad, S., & Nazmy, T. (2025). A survey on retrieval-augmentation generation (RAG) models for healthcare applications. *Neural Computing & Applications*, *37*, 28191–28267. DOI: 10.1007/s00521-025-11666-9

Abramson, J., Adler, J., Dunger, J., Evans, R., Green, T., Pritzel, A., Ronneberger, O., Willmore, L., Ballard, A. J., & Bambrick, J. (2024). Accurate structure prediction of biomolecular interactions with AlphaFold 3. *Nature*, *630*(8016), 493–500. PMID: 38718835

Aburomman, A. A., & Reaz, M. B. I. (2017). A survey of intrusion detection systems based on ensemble and hybrid classifiers. *Computers & Security*, *65*, 135–152. DOI: 10.1016/j.cose.2016.11.008

Achtyes, E. D., Hopkins, S. C., Dedic, N., Dworak, H., Zeni, C., & Koblan, K. (2023). Ulotaront: Review of preliminary evidence for the efficacy and safety of a TAAR1 agonist in schizophrenia. *European Archives of Psychiatry and Clinical Neuroscience*, *273*(7), 1543–1556. PMID: 37165101

Acien, A., Morales, A., Vera-Rodriguez, R., Fierrez, J., & Ortega-Garcia, J. (2018). Active detection of age groups based on touch interaction. *IET Biometrics*, *7*(5), 415–424.

Actionable absolute risk prediction of atherosclerotic cardiovascular disease based on the UK Biobank. (2025, July 2). *UK Biobank.* https://www.ukbiobank.ac.uk/publications/actionable-absolute-risk-prediction-of-atherosclerotic-cardiovascular-disease-based-on-the-uk-biobank/

Adamo, R. G., van der Pol, C. B., Alabousi, M., Lam, E., Salameh, J.-P., Abedrabbo, N., Lerner, E., Naringrekar, H., Bashir, M. R., Costa, A. F., Osman, H., Ansari, D., Levis, B., Polikoff, A., Furlan, A., Tang, A., Kierans, A. S., Singal, A. G., Arvind, A., & McInnes, M. D. F. (2025). Diagnostic Performance of CT/MRI LI-RADS Version 2018 Major Feature Combinations: Individual Participant Data Meta-Analysis. *Radiology, 315*(3), e243450. DOI: 10.1148/radiol.243450

Adebanjo, E. A., Bakare, K. M., Matthew, U. O., Fatai, L. O., & Precious, A. U. (2023). Therapeutic approaches to immunotherapy-induced chronic inflammatory diseases. *HAFED POLY Journal of Science. Management and Technology, 5*(2), 144–159.

Afzal, M., Sah, A. K., Agarwal, S., Tanzeel, A., Elshaikh, R. H., Alobeidli, F. A., & Choudhary, A. (2024). Advancements in the treatment of autoimmune diseases: Integrating artificial intelligence for personalized medicine. *Trends in Immunotherapy, 8*(2), 8970.

Agatonovic-Kustrin, S., & Beresford, R. (2000). Basic concepts of artificial neural network (ANN) modeling and its application in pharmaceutical research. *Journal of Pharmaceutical and Biomedical Analysis, 22*(5), 717–727. DOI: 10.1016/s0731-7085(99)00272-1 PMID: 10815714

Aghili, S. F., Mala, H., Shojafar, M., & Peris-Lopez, P. (2019). Lightweight three-factor authentication, access control and ownership transfer scheme for e-health systems in IoT. *Future Generation Computer Systems.*

Ahmad, F. (2025). Optimizing Treatment: The Role of Pharmacology, Genomics, and AI in Improving Patient Outcomes. *Drug Development Research, 86*(3), e70093. PMID: 40285487

Ahmad, F., Dwivedi, S., Khan, Z. H., & Mittal, N. (2025). Advancing green artificial intelligence: strategies for a sustainable future. In *Energy Efficient Algorithms and Green Data Centers for Sustainable Computing* (pp. 291–322). IGI Global Scientific Publishing.

Ahmad, H. A., East, J. E., Panaccione, R., Travis, S., Canavan, J. B., Usiskin, K., & Byrne, M. F. (2023). Artificial intelligence in inflammatory bowel disease: Implications for clinical practice and future directions. *Intestinal Research, 21*(3), 283–294.

Ahmed, M., Maldonado, A. M., & Durrant, J. D. (2023). From byte to bench to bedside: Molecular dynamics simulations and drug discovery. *BMC Biology*, *21*(1), 299. PMID: 38155355

Ahmed, Z. (2022). Precision medicine with multi-omics strategies, deep phenotyping, and predictive analysis. *Progress in Molecular Biology and Translational Science*, *190*(1), 101–125. DOI: 10.1016/bs.pmbts.2022.02.002

Akbarialiabad, H., Pasdar, A., Murrell, D. F., Mostafavi, M., Shakil, F., Safaee, E., . . . Grada, A. (2025). Enhancing randomized clinical trials with digital twins. *npj Systems Biology and Applications*, *11*(1), 110. DOI: PMID: 41044102DOI: 10.1038/s41540-025-00592-0

Akhi, S. S., Hussain, A. H., Islam, S., Hasan, M. N., & Islam, M. M. (2023). Artificial intelligence–enhanced quantum computing for medical simulations: Accelerating drug discovery, protein folding, and personalized healthcare with performance optimization and predictive accuracy. *World Journal of Advanced Research and Review*, *18*(01), 1328–1335.

Akhmedov, M., Arribas, A., Montemanni, R., Bertoni, F., & Kwee, I. (2017). Omicsnet: Integration of multi-omics data using path analysis in multilayer networks. *BioRxiv*, 238766.

Al Zo'ubi, M. (2025). Review of 2024 publications on the applications of artificial intelligence in rheumatology. *Clinical Rheumatology*, *44*(4), 1427–1438. *Scopus*. Advance online publication. DOI: 10.1007/s10067-025-07382-3

Alagendran, S., Archunan, G., Prabhu, S. V., Orozco, B. E., & Guzman, R. G. (2010). Biochemical evaluation in human saliva with special reference to ovulation detection. *Indian Journal of Dental Research*, *21*, 165–168.

Albahri, O. S., Zaidan, A. A., Albahri, A. S., Zaidan, B. B., Abdulkareem, K. H., Al-Qaysi, Z. T., Alamoodi, A. H., Aleesa, A. M., Chyad, M. A., Alesa, R. M., Kem, L. C., Lakulu, M. M., Ibrahim, A. B., & Rashid, N. A. (2020). Systematic review of artificial intelligence techniques in the detection and classification of COVID-19 medical images in terms of evaluation and benchmarking: Taxonomy analysis, challenges, future solutions and methodological aspects. *Journal of Infection and Public Health*, *13*(10), 1381–1396. DOI: 10.1016/j.jiph.2020.06.028 PMID: 32646771

Alekseenko, J., Stieltjes, B., Bach, M., Boerries, M., Opitz, O., Karargyris, A., & Padoy, N. (2024). Clinnova federated learning proof of concept: key takeaways from a cross-border collaboration. *arXiv preprint arXiv:2410.02443*.

Alex, H. (2024). Enhancing drug safety: AIs role in pharmacovigilance and adverse event reporting. *International Research Journal of Innovations in Engineering and Technology*, *8*(9), 194–197.

Alfaddagh, A., Martin, S. S., Leucker, T. M., Michos, E. D., Blaha, M. J., Lowenstein, C. J., Jones, S. R., & Toth, P. P. (2020). Inflammation and cardiovascular disease: From mechanisms to therapeutics. *American Journal of Preventive Cardiology*, *4*, 100130. DOI: 10.1016/j.ajpc.2020.100130

Alfa, R., Considine, T., Virani, S., Pfeiffer, M., Donato, A., Dickerson, D., Shuster, D., Ellis, J., Rushton, K., & Wei, H. (2024). Clinical pharmacology and tolerability of REC-994, a redox-cycling nitroxide compound, in randomized phase 1 dose-finding studies. *Pharmacology Research & Perspectives*, *12*(3), e1200. PMID: 38655895

Alfonso-González, L., Fernández, F. J., & Vega, M. C. (2025). Systems immunology: When systems biology meets immunology. *Frontiers in Immunology*, *16*, 1630488.

Algarvio, R. C., Conceição, J., Rodrigues, P. P., Ribeiro, I., & Ferreira-da-Silva, R. (2025). Artificial intelligence in pharmacovigilance: A narrative review and practical experience with an expert-defined Bayesian network tool. *International Journal of Clinical Pharmacy*, *47*, 932–944.

Alicic, R. Z., Neumiller, J. J., & Tuttle, K. R. (2025). Combination therapy: An upcoming paradigm to improve kidney and cardiovascular outcomes in chronic kidney disease. *Nephrology, Dialysis, Transplantation*, *40*(Supplement_1), i3–i17. DOI: 10.1093/ndt/gfae212

Ali, M., Naeem, F., Tariq, M., & Kaddoum, G. (2022). Federated learning for privacy preservation in smart healthcare systems: A comprehensive survey. *IEEE Journal of Biomedical and Health Informatics*, *27*(2), 778–789.

Alimguzhin, V., Mancini, T., Massini, A., Sinisi, S., & Tronci, E. (2020). In silico clinical trials through AI and statistical model checking. [). CEUR-WS.]. *CEUR Workshop Proceedings*, *2509*, 17–22.

Ali, N., Hanif, N., Khan, H. A., Waseem, M. A., Saeed, A., Zakir, S., & Saleem, A. (2025). Deep learning and artificial intelligence for drug discovery, application, challenge, and future perspectives. *Discover Applied Sciences*, *7*(6), 533. DOI: 10.1007/s42452-025-06991-6

Alizadehsani, R., Oyelere, S. S., Hussain, S., Jagatheesaperumal, S. K., Calixto, R. R., Rahouti, M., & De Albuquerque, V. H. C. (2024). Explainable artificial intelligence for drug discovery and development—A comprehensive survey. *Briefings in Bioinformatics*, *25*(2), bbae101. PMID: 38493339

Al-Maini, M., Maindarkar, M., Kitas, G. D., Khanna, N. N., Misra, D. P., Johri, A. M., Mantella, L., Agarwal, V., Sharma, A., Singh, I. M., Tsoulfas, G., Laird, J. R., Faa, G., Teji, J., Turk, M., Viskovic, K., Ruzsa, Z., Mavrogeni, S., Rathore, V., & Suri, J. S. (2023). Artificial intelligence-based preventive, personalized and precision medicine for cardiovascular disease/stroke risk assessment in rheumatoid arthritis patients: A narrative review. *Rheumatology International*, *43*(11), 1965–1982. DOI: 10.1007/s00296-023-05415-1

Alsabah, M., Naser, M. A., Albahri, A. S., Albahri, O. S., Alamoodi, A. H., Abdulhussain, S. H., & Alzubaidi, L. (2025). A comprehensive review on key technologies toward smart healthcare systems based IoT: Technical aspects, challenges and future directions. *Artificial Intelligence Review*, *58*(11), 343. DOI: 10.1007/s10462-025-11342-3

Alshehade, S. A., Al Zarzour, R. H., Bitar, A. N., Alshehadeh, A. R., Tamilwanan, S., & Safni, S. (2026). Ethical Considerations in the Application of Artificial Intelligence in the Pharmaceutical Industry. In Alshehadeh A.R., El-Qirem I.A., & Ghaleb Awad Elrefae G.A. (Eds.), *Lect. Notes Networks Syst.: Vol. 1503 LNNS* (pp. 326–335). Springer Science and Business Media Deutschland GmbH; Scopus. https://doi.org/DOI: 10.1007/978-3-031-96631-6_32

Alzoubi, Y. I., & Mishra, A. (2024). Green artificial intelligence initiatives: Potentials and challenges. *Journal of Cleaner Production*, *468*, 143090.

Amin, R., Islam, S. H., Biswas, G. P., Khan, M. K., & Kumar, N. (2019). A robust and efficient bilinear pairing based mutual authentication and session key verification over insecure communication. *Multimedia Tools and Applications*, *74*(11), 3581–3605.

Amorim, A. M., Piochi, L. F., Gaspar, A. T., Preto, A. J., Rosário-Ferreira, N., & Moreira, I. S. (2024). Advancing drug safety in drug development: Bridging computational predictions for enhanced toxicity prediction. *Chemical Research in Toxicology*, *37*(6), 827–849. PMID: 38758610

Anderson, B., Lyons, M., Henao-Tamayo, M. I., Juarrero, M. G., & Robertson, G. (2020). Improving the computational reproducibility of immunological research. *The Journal of Immunology : Official Journal of the American Association of Immunologists*, *204*(1, Supplement), 222–225.

Anderson, N., & Smith, R. (2024). Rethinking the Three Rs: Growing momentum toward a new gold standard in Australian research. *Alternatives to Laboratory Animals*, *52*(4), 224–231.

Angello, N. H., Friday, D. M., Hwang, C., Yi, S., Cheng, A. H., Torres-Flores, T. C., Jira, E. R., Wang, W., Aspuru-Guzik, A., & Burke, M. D. (2024). Closed-loop transfer enables artificial intelligence to yield chemical knowledge. *Nature*, *633*(8029), 351–358. PMID: 39198655

Angello, N., Friday, D., Hwang, C., Yi, S., Cheng, A., Torres-Flores, T., Jira, E., Wang, W., Aspuru-Guzik, A., Burke, M., Schroeder, C., Diao, Y., & Jackson, N. (2023). *Closed-Loop Transfer Enables AI to Yield Chemical Knowledge*. https://doi.org/DOI: 10.26434/chemrxiv-2023-jqbqt

Angoulvant, D., Amarenco, P., Bastien, A., Bechet, E., Boccara, F., Boissel, J. P., & Steg, P. G. (2023). Design of a knowledge-based mechanistic model of atherosclerotic cardiovascular disease for in silico trials. *European Heart Journal*, *44*(Supplement_2), ehad655–2944.

Arango-Argoty, G., Bikiel, D. E., Sun, G. J., Kipkogei, E., Smith, K. M., Carrasco Pro, S., & Jacob, E. (2025). AI-driven predictive biomarker discovery with contrastive learning to improve clinical trial outcomes. *Cancer Cell*, *43*(5), 875–890. e878. DOI: 10.1016/j.ccell.2025.03.029

Arnold, N., Lechner, K., Waldeyer, C., Shapiro, M. D., & Koenig, W. (2021). Inflammation and Cardiovascular Disease: The Future. *European Cardiology Review*, *16*, e20. DOI: 10.15420/ecr.2020.50

Arrell, D. K., & Terzic, A. (2010). Network systems biology for drug discovery. *Clinical Pharmacology and Therapeutics*, *88*(1), 120–125.

Artrith, N., Butler, K. T., Coudert, F.-X., Han, S., Isayev, O., Jain, A., & Walsh, A. (2021). Best practices in machine learning for chemistry. *Nature Chemistry*, *13*(6), 505–508. PMID: 34059804

Arumugam, V. A., Thangavelu, S., Fathah, Z., Ravindran, P., Sanjeev, A. M. A., Babu, S., Arun, M., Mohd. Iqbal, Y., Khan, S., Ruchi, T., Megha Katare, P., Ranjit, S., Chandra, R., & Dhama, K. (2020). COVID-19 and the world with co-morbidities of heart disease, hypertension and diabetes. *Journal of Pure & Applied Microbiology*, *14*(3), 1623–1638.

Arus-Pous, J., Awale, M., Probst, D., & Reymond, J. L. (2019). Exploring Chemical Space with Machine Learning. *Chimia*, *73*(12), 1018–1023. DOI: 10.2533/chimia.2019.1018 PMID: 31883554

Arús-Pous, J., Johansson, S. V., Prykhodko, O., Bjerrum, E. J., Tyrchan, C., Reymond, J. L., Chen, H., & Engkvist, O. (2019). Randomized SMILES strings improve the quality of molecular generative models. *Journal of Cheminformatics*, *11*(1). Advance online publication. DOI: 10.1186/s13321-019-0393-0 PMID: 33430971

Arús-Pous, J., Patronov, A., Bjerrum, E. J., Tyrchan, C., Reymond, J. L., Chen, H., & Engkvist, O. (2020). SMILES-based deep generative scaffold decorator for de-novo drug design. *Journal of Cheminformatics*, *12*(1). Advance online publication. DOI: 10.1186/s13321-020-00441-8 PMID: 33431013

Arya, V., Bellamy, R. K., Chen, P. Y., Dhurandhar, A., Hind, M., Hoffman, S. C., . . . Zhang, Y. (2019). One explanation does not fit all: A toolkit and taxonomy of AI explainability techniques. arXiv preprint arXiv:1909.03012.

Asediya, V. S., Anjaria, P. A., Mathakiya, R. A., Koringa, P. G., Nayak, J. B., Bisht, D., & Desai, D. N. (2024). Vaccine development using artificial intelligence and machine learning: A review. *International Journal of Biological Macromolecules*, *282*, 136643.

Ashish, V. (2017). Attention is all you need. *Advances in Neural Information Processing Systems*, *30*, I.

Ashraf, F. B., Zhang, Z., Paco, K., Mendivil, M. P., Lay, J. A., Ray, A., & Lonardi, S. (2024). A large language model guides the affinity maturation of variant antibodies generated by combinatorial optimization. *bioRxiv*, 2024.

Askin, S., Burkhalter, D., Calado, G., & El Dakrouni, S. (2023). Artificial Intelligence Applied to clinical trials: Opportunities and challenges. *Health and Technology*, *13*(2), 203–213. DOI: 10.1007/s12553-023-00738-2 PMID: 36923325

Askr, H., Elgeldawi, E., Aboul Ella, H., Elshaier, Y. A. M. M., Gomaa, M. M., & Hassanien, A. E. (2023). Deep learning in drug discovery: An integrative review and future challenges. *Artificial Intelligence Review*, *56*(7), 5975–6037. DOI: 10.1007/s10462-022-10306-1 PMID: 36415536

Asti, G., Apellaniz, P. A., Carota, L., Casadei, F., Piscia, D., Delleani, M., & Álvarez Garcia, F. (2025). Development, implementation, and validation of an open-source federated learning platform to accelerate innovation and boost personalized medicine in rare and ultra-rare haematological diseases: an initiative by GenoMed4All Consortium. medRxiv, 2025-08.

Atanasov, A. G., Zotchev, S. B., & Dirsch, V. M., International Natural Product Sciences, T., & Supuran, C. T. (2021). Natural products in drug discovery: Advances and opportunities. *Nature Reviews. Drug Discovery*, *20*(3), 200–216. DOI: 10.1038/s41573-020-00114-z PMID: 33510482

Athieniti, E., & Spyrou, G. M. (2023). A guide to multi-omics data collection and integration for translational medicine. *Computational and Structural Biotechnology Journal*, *21*, 134–149. DOI: 10.1016/j.csbj.2022.11.050

Athira, R. K., Kripamol, R., Anju, M. S., Maya, B., Pai, R. R., Ajit, S., & Kasoju, N. (2022). Alternatives to animal testing: concepts, state of art, and regulations. *Biomedical product and materials evaluation*, 501-529.

Auger, S. D., & Scott, G. (2025). Machine learning detects hidden treatment response patterns only in the presence of comprehensive clinical phenotyping. *PLoS One*, *20*(10), e0334858.

Avey, S., Chatterjee, M., Manyakov, N. V., Cooper, P., Sabins, N., Mosca, K., & Pandis, I. (2024). Using a wearable patch to develop a digital monitoring biomarker of inflammation in response to LPS challenge. *Clinical and Translational Science*, *17*(2), e13734.

Awan, R. E., Zainab, S., Yousuf, F. J., & Mughal, S. (2024). AI-driven drug discovery: Exploring Abaucin as a promising treatment against multidrug-resistant Acinetobacter baumannii. *Health Science Reports*, *7*(6), e2150. PMID: 38841115

Azmal, M., Paul, J. K., Shohan, M. N. H., Haque, A. N. M. S. N. B., Mrinmoy, M., Talukder, O. F., & Ghosh, A. (2025). Evaluating computational and experimental approaches in early-stage Alzheimer's drug discovery: A systematic review. *Journal of Computer-Aided Molecular Design*, *39*(1), 27. DOI: 10.1007/s10822-025-00610-7

Badhe, P. (2025). A multi-omics and network biology case study of CLIC1 using AI generated prompts. https://doi.org/DOI: 10.20944/preprints202509.2223.v1

Bagane, M., & Jorgewad, D. R. (2024). From AI labs to clinics: A review of 21st-century drug candidates powered by artificial intelligence. *International Journal for Research in Applied Science and Engineering Technology*, *12*, 1419–1428.

Bai, C., Wu, L., Li, R., Cao, Y., He, S., & Bo, X. (2025). Machine Learning-Enabled Drug-Induced Toxicity Prediction. *Advancement of Science*, *12*(16), 2413405. PMID: 39899688

Bakchi, B., Krishna, A. D., Sreecharan, E., Ganesh, V. B. J., Niharika, M., Maharshi, S., Puttagunta, S. B., Sigalapalli, D. K., Bhandare, R. R., & Shaik, A. B. (2022). An overview on applications of SwissADME web tool in the design and development of anticancer, antitubercular and antimicrobial agents: A medicinal chemist's perspective. *Journal of Molecular Structure*, *1259*, 132712.

Baldan-Martin, M., Azkargorta, M., Aransay, A., Gil-Redondo, R., Moreno-Indias, I., & Iloro, I., & * Authors share co-senior authorship. (2025). OP04 multi-omics biomarkers for predicting therapeutic efficacy in inflammatory bowel disease: Advancing towards tailored treatments. *Journal of Crohn's and Colitis*, *19*(Supplement_1), i7–i8.

Baltrusaitis, T., Ahuja, C., & Morency, L. P. (2019). Multimodal Machine Learning: A Survey and Taxonomy. *IEEE Transactions on Pattern Analysis and Machine Intelligence*, *41*(2), 423–443. DOI: 10.1109/TPAMI.2018.2798607 PMID: 29994351

Baracaldo, N., Chen, B., Ludwig, H., & Safavi, J. A. (2018). Detecting poisoning attacks on machine learning in IoT environments. In *2018 IEEE International Congress on Internet of Things* (pp. 57–64).

Barbarroja, N., López-Medina, C., Escudero-Contreras, A., & Arias-de la Rosa, I. (2024). Clinical and molecular insights into cardiovascular disease in psoriatic patients and the potential protective role of apremilast. *Frontiers in Immunology*, *15*, 1459185. DOI: 10.3389/fimmu.2024.1459185

Barcelos, M. P., & de Paula da Silva, C. H. T. (2024). The Role of Artificial Intelligence in the Discovery of New Drugs. In *Eng. Mater.: Vol. Part F3949* (pp. 353–370). Springer Science and Business Media Deutschland GmbH; Scopus. https://doi.org/DOI: 10.1007/978-3-031-75984-0_14

Barker, R. (2010). A flexible blueprint for the future of drug development. *Lancet*, *375*(9712), 357–359. DOI: 10.1016/S0140-6736(10)60141-9

Barua, R. (2024). The emerging role of artificial intelligence in organ-on-a-chip (ooac) biomedical devices. In *Reshaping Healthcare with Cutting-Edge Biomedical Advancements* (pp. 369–381). IGI Global Scientific Publishing.

Basha, S. A., & Hanirex, D. K. (2024). Artificial intelligence in immunology: predictive models for immune system disorders. In *2024 Global Conference on Communications and Information Technologies (GCCIT)* (pp. 1-6). IEEE.

Bauer, A., Sappler, N., von Stülpnagel, L., Klemm, M., Schreinlechner, M., Wenner, F., Schier, J., Al Tawil, A., Dolejsi, T., & Krasniqi, A. (2022). Telemedical cardiac risk assessment by implantable cardiac monitors in patients after myocardial infarction with autonomic dysfunction (SMART-MI-DZHK9): A prospective investigator-initiated, randomised, multicentre, open-label, diagnostic trial. *The Lancet. Digital Health*, *4*(2), e105–e116. PMID: 35090674

Bauman, K. D., Butler, K. S., Moore, B. S., & Chekan, J. R. (2021). Genome mining methods to discover bioactive natural products. *Natural Product Reports*, *38*(11), 2100–2129. DOI: 10.1039/d1np00032b PMID: 34734626

BBC News. (2017, July 3). Google DeepMind NHS app broke UK data law. BBC. https://www.bbc.com/news/technology-40483202

Beasley, J. M. T., Schatz, K., Ding, E., DeLuca, M., Zaid, N. A., Tucker, N. N., & Muratov, E. N. (2025). TARRAGON: Therapeutic target applicability ranking and retrieval-augmented generation over networks. bioRxiv, 2025-04.

Bellucci, M., Delestre, N., Malandain, N., & Zanni-Merk, C. (2021). Towards a terminology for a fully contextualized XAI. *Procedia Computer Science*, *192*, 241–250.

Benevolent, A. I. (2020, January 30). AstraZeneca and BenevolentAI announce collaboration to use artificial intelligence and machine learning for drug discovery. BenevolentAI. https://benevolent.com/news/astraZeneca-and-benevolentai-announce-collaboration

Ben-Israel, D., Jacobs, W. B., Casha, S., Lang, S., Ryu, W. H. A., de Lotbiniere-Bassett, M., & Cadotte, D. W. (2020). The impact of machine learning on patient care: A systematic review. *Artificial Intelligence in Medicine*, *103*, 101785. DOI: 10.1016/j.artmed.2019.101785 PMID: 32143792

Benjamin, K., Bhandari, A., Kepple, J. D., Qi, R., Shang, Z., Xing, Y., An, Y., Zhang, N., Hou, Y., Crockford, T. L., McCallion, O., Issa, F., Hester, J., Tillmann, U., Harrington, H. A., & Bull, K. R. (2024). Multiscale topology classifies cells in subcellular spatial transcriptomics. *Nature*, *630*(8018), 943–949. DOI: 10.1038/s41586-024-07563-1

Benson, M. (2023). Digital twins for predictive, preventive personalized, and participatory treatment of immune-mediated diseases. *Arteriosclerosis, Thrombosis, and Vascular Biology*, *43*(3), 410–416.

Berdiugina, O. V. (2025). Usage of artificial intelligence capabilities in immunology: From literature review to statistical processing and analysis of obtained data. *Russian Journal of Immunology*, *28*(3), 355–362.

Bernabe, J. B., Hernandez-Ramos, J. L., & Skarmeta, A. F. (2016). TACIoT: Multidimensional trust-aware access control system for the Internet of Things. *Soft Computing*, *20*(5), 1763–1779. DOI: 10.1007/s00500-015-1591-0

Bertolazzi, A., Marzęda-Młynarska, K., Kięczkowska, J., & Zanier, M. L. (2024). Datafication of care: Security and privacy issues with health technology for people with diabetes. *Societies (Basel, Switzerland)*, *14*(9), 163.

Bhatia, N., Khan, M. M. U., & Arora, S. (2024). The Role of Artificial Intelligence in Revolutionizing Pharmacological Research. *Current Pharmacology Reports*, *10*(6), 323–329.

Bhat, S., Palepu, K., Hong, L., Mao, J., Ye, T., Iyer, R., & Chatterjee, P. (2025). De novo design of peptide binders to conformationally diverse targets with contrastive language modelling. *Science Advances*, *11*(4), eadr8638.

Bhattacharjee, A., Kumar, A., Ojha, P. K., & Kar, S. (2025). Artificial intelligence to predict inhibitors of drug-metabolizing enzymes and transporters for safer drug design. *Expert Opinion on Drug Discovery*, *20*(5), 621–641. PMID: 40241626

Bhattacharya, P., Tanwar, S., Shah, R., & Ladha, A. (2020). Mobile edge computing-enabled blockchain framework—A survey. In *2020 International Conference on Communication Systems & Networks* (pp. 371–376).

Bhatt, P., Singh, S., Kumar, V., Nagarajan, K., Mishra, S. K., Dixit, P. K., & Kumar, S. (2024). Artificial intelligence in pharmaceutical industry: Revolutionizing drug development and delivery. *Current Artificial Intelligence*, *2*(1), E051223224198.

Bhotla, H. K., Balasubramanian, B., Meyyazhagan, A., Pushparaj, K., & Easwaran, M., Pappusamy, Alwin Robert, A., Arumugam, V.A. Tsibizova, V., Msaad Alfalih, A. Aljowaie, R.M., Saravanan, M., & Di Renzo, G. C. (2021). Opportunistic mycoses in COVID-19 patients/survivors: Epidemic inside a pandemic. *Journal of Infection and Public Health*, *14*(11), 1720–1726.

Biggio, B., & Roli, F. (2018). Wild patterns: Ten years after the rise of adversarial machine learning. *Pattern Recognition*, *84*, 317–331.

Bijral, R. K., Singh, I., Manhas, J., & Sharma, V. (2022). Exploring artificial intelligence in drug discovery: A comprehensive review. *Archives of Computational Methods in Engineering*, *29*(4), 2513–2529.

Bikou, A. G., Deligianni, E., Dermiki-Gkana, F., Liappas, N., Teriús-Padrón, J. G., Beltrán Jaunsarás, M. E., & Kontogiorgis, C. (2024). Improving participant recruitment in clinical trials: Comparative analysis of innovative digital platforms. *Journal of Medical Internet Research*, *26*, e60504. DOI: 10.2196/60504

Bindu, C. H., Babu, R., Bhimana, S., Babu, M. K., Devadas, C., & Jalaiah, M. (2025). Revolutionizing pharmaceutical sciences: a comprehensive review of artificial intelligence's impact on drug discovery and development. *Genomics-Driven Drug Discovery Through Pharmacogenomics*, 217-246.

Björnsson, B., Borrebaeck, C., Elander, N., Gasslander, T., Gawel, D. R., Gustafsson, M., Jörnsten, R., Lee, E. J., Li, X., & Lilja, S. (2019). Digital twins to personalize medicine. *Genome Medicine, 12*(1), 4. PMID: 31892363

Blanco-Gonzalez, A., Cabezon, A., Seco-Gonzalez, A., Conde-Torres, D., Antelo-Riveiro, P., Pineiro, A., & Garcia-Fandino, R. (2023). The Role of AI in Drug Discovery: Challenges, Opportunities, and Strategies. *Pharmaceuticals (Basel, Switzerland), 16*(6). Advance online publication. DOI: 10.3390/ph16060891 PMID: 37375838

Blease, C., Bernstein, M. H., & Gaab, J. (2019). Artificial intelligence in medicine: Balancing innovation and accountability. *Journal of Medical Ethics, 45*(12), 785–788.

Bogatu, A., Wysocka, M., Wysocki, O., Butterworth, H., Landers, D., Kilgour, E., & Freitas, A. (2022). Metareview-informed explainable cytokine storm detection during CAR-T cell therapy. *arXiv preprint arXiv:2206.10612.*

Boldini, D., Grisoni, F., Kuhn, D., Friedrich, L., & Sieber, S. A. (2023). Practical guidelines for the use of gradient boosting for molecular property prediction. *Journal of Cheminformatics, 15*(1), 73. PMID: 37641120

Bordukova, M., Makarov, N., Rodriguez-Esteban, R., Schmich, F., & Menden, M. P. (2024). Generative artificial intelligence empowers digital twins in drug discovery and clinical trials. *Expert Opinion on Drug Discovery, 19*(1), 33–42. DOI: 10.1080/17460441.2023.2273839

Bothwell, L. E., Avorn, J., Khan, N. F., & Kesselheim, A. S. (2018). Adaptive design clinical trials: A review of the literature and ClinicalTrials.gov. *BMJ Open, 8*(2), e018320. DOI: 10.1136/bmjopen-2017-018320

Boyko, M., Beliaeva, A., Kornilov, D., Bernstein, A., & Sharaev, M. (2025). impuTMAE: Multi-modal transformer with masked pre-training for missing modalities imputation in cancer survival prediction. *arXiv preprint arXiv:2508.09195.*

Bozorgi, M., Saul, L. K., Savage, S., & Voelker, G. M. (2010). Learning to classify vulnerabilities and predict exploits. In *Proceedings of the 16th ACM SIGKDD International Conference on Knowledge Discovery and Data Mining* (pp. 1058-1065).

Braga, D. M., & Rawal, B. (2025). Harnessing AI and Quantum Computing for Revolutionizing Drug Discovery and Approval Processes: Case Example for Collagen Toxicity. *JMIR Bioinformatics and Biotechnology*, *6*(1), e69800. PMID: 41342151

Brand, D., Singh, J. A., McKay, A. G. N., Cengiz, N., & Moodley, K. (2022). Data sharing governance in sub-Saharan Africa during public health emergencies: Gaps and guidance. *South African Journal of Science*, *118*(11-12).

Briefing, L. B. Early evidence and emerging trends: How AI is shaping drug discovery and clinical development.

Burks, A. (2024). *Strategies used in healthcare organizations to protect information against security breaches: A case study* (Doctoral dissertation, University of Phoenix).

Busuioc, M. (2022). AI algorithmic oversight: new frontiers in regulation. In *Handbook of regulatory authorities* (pp. 470–486). Edward Elgar Publishing.

Cai, C., Wu, Q., Luo, Y., Ma, H., Shen, J., Zhang, Y., Yang, L., Chen, Y., Wen, Z., & Wang, Q. (2017). In silico prediction of ROCK II inhibitors by different classification approaches. *Molecular Diversity*, *21*(4), 791–807. DOI: 10.1007/s11030-017-9772-5 PMID: 28770474

Cai, C., Xu, L., Fang, J., Dai, Z., Wu, Q., Liu, X., Wang, Q., Fang, J., Liu, A. L., & Du, G. H. (2021). In Silico Prediction and Bioactivity Evaluation of Chemical Ingredients Against Influenza A Virus From Isatis tinctoria L. *Frontiers in Pharmacology*, *12*, 755396. DOI: 10.3389/fphar.2021.755396 PMID: 34950027

Cai, Y., Zeng, M., & Chen, Y. Z. (2021). The pharmacological mechanism of Huashi Baidu Formula for the treatment of COVID-19 by combined network pharmacology and molecular docking. *Annals of Palliative Medicine*, *10*(4), 3864–3895. DOI: 10.21037/apm-20-1759 PMID: 33691446

Calderaro, J., Seraphin, T. P., Luedde, T., & Simon, T. G. (2022). Artificial intelligence for the prevention and clinical management of hepatocellular carcinoma. *Journal of Hepatology*, *76*(6), 1348–1361. DOI: 10.1016/j.jhep.2022.01.014 PMID: 35589255

Campos, R. (2024). Hybrid Quantum-Classical Algorithms. *arXiv preprint arXiv:2406.12371*.

Cañete, P. F., & Tuong, Z. K. (2024). Embracing computational immunology. *Immunology and Cell Biology*, *102*(8), 663.

Cannarozzi, A. L., Latiano, A., Massimino, L., Bossa, F., Giuliani, F., Riva, M., & Palmieri, O. (2024). Inflammatory bowel disease genomics, transcriptomics, proteomics and metagenomics meet artificial intelligence. *United European Gastroenterology Journal*, *12*(10), 1461–1480.

Cano-Gamez, E., Burnham, K. L., Goh, C., Allcock, A., Malick, Z. H., Overend, L., & Goh, C. (2022). An immune dysfunction score for stratification of patients with acute infection based on whole-blood gene expression. *Science Translational Medicine*, *14*(669), eabq4433.

Canuel, V., Rance, B., Avillach, P., Degoulet, P., & Burgun, A. (2015). Translational research platforms integrating clinical and omics data: A review of publicly available solutions. *Briefings in Bioinformatics*, *16*(2), 280–290. DOI: 10.1093/bib/bbu006

Cao, H., Liu, Z., Lu, X., Yao, Y., & Li, Y. (2023). Instructmol: Multi-modal integration for building a versatile and reliable molecular assistant in drug discovery. *arXiv preprint arXiv:2311.16208.*

Cao, C., Zhao, W., Guo, J., Wang, Z., Lu, A., & Liang, C. (2025). Leveraging artificial intelligence and machine learning for unraveling pathogenesis and advancing precision medicine in autoimmune diseases. *The Innovation Medicine*, *3*(3), 100154–1.

Capodice, J. L., & Chubak, B. M. (2021). Traditional Chinese herbal medicine-potential therapeutic application for the treatment of COVID-19. *Chinese Medicine*, *16*(1), 24. DOI: 10.1186/s13020-020-00419-6 PMID: 33618736

Cardiovascular diseases (CVDs). (n.d.). Retrieved August 27, 2025, from https://www.who.int/news-room/fact-sheets/detail/cardiovascular-diseases-(cvds)

Caviglione, L., Podolski, M., Mazurczyk, W., & Ianigro, M. (2016). Covert channels in personal cloud storage services: The case of Dropbox. *IEEE Transactions on Industrial Informatics*, *13*(4), 1921–1931. DOI: 10.1109/TII.2016.2607183

Cearns, M., Amare, A. T., Schubert, K. O., Thalamuthu, A., Frank, J., & Streit, F.Major Depressive Disorder Working Group of the Psychiatric Genomics Consortium. (2022). Using polygenic scores and clinical data for bipolar disorder patient stratification and lithium response prediction: Machine learning approach. *The British Journal of Psychiatry*, *220*(4), 219–228.

Ceron-Carrasco, J. P. (2022). When Virtual Screening Yields Inactive Drugs: Dealing with False Theoretical Friends. *ChemMedChem*, *17*(16), e202200278. DOI: 10.1002/cmdc.202200278 PMID: 35726731

Chaiburi, C., & Yingngam, B. (2025). Digital twin technology fundamentals. In Iyer, S., Nayyar, A., Paul, A., & Naved, M. (Eds.), *Digital Twins for Smart Cities and Villages* (pp. 1–35). Elsevier., DOI: 10.1016/B978-0-443-28884-5.00001-4

Chakraborty, A., Alam, M., Dey, V., Chattopadhyay, A., & Mukhopadhyay, D. (2018). Adversarial attacks and defences: A survey. *ACM Computing Surveys*, *53*(1), 20. Advance online publication. DOI: 10.1145/3357390

Chan, A. C. (2008). A golden era of opportunity in immunotherapy discovery and development. *Immunological Reviews*, *223*(1), 5–6.

Chandola, V., Banerjee, A., & Kumar, V. (2009). Anomaly detection: A survey. *ACM Computing Surveys*, *41*(3), 15. Advance online publication. DOI: 10.1145/1541880.1541882

Chaparro-Cárdenas, S. L., Ramirez-Bautista, J.-A., Terven, J., Córdova-Esparza, D.-M., Romero-Gonzalez, J.-A., Ramírez-Pedraza, A., & Chavez-Urbiola, E. A. (2025). A Technological Review of Digital Twins and Artificial Intelligence for Personalized and Predictive Healthcare. *Health Care*, *13*(14), 1763. DOI: 10.3390/healthcare13141763

Char, D. S., Abramoff, M. D., & Feudtner, C. (2020). Identifying ethical considerations for machine learning healthcare applications. *The American Journal of Bioethics*, *20*(11), 7–17. PMID: 33103967

Chatterjee, A., Paul, S., Bisht, B., Bhattacharya, S., Sivasubramaniam, S., & Paul, M. K. (2022). Advances in targeting the WNT/β-catenin signaling pathway in cancer. *Drug Discovery Today*, *27*(1), 82–101. PMID: 34252612

Chatzianastasis, M., Burns, R., Costa, H., Rabinowitz, M., & Zhang, F. (2025). Abstract B056: Deep Antigen Sets, a new deep-learning framework, enables in vivo modelling of patient neoantigens for effective targeted immunotherapy design. *Clinical Cancer Research*, *31*(13, Supplement), B056–B056.

Chavda, V. P., Anand, K., & Apostolopoulos, V. (2023). *Bioinformatics Tools for Pharmaceutical Drug Product Development*. John Wiley & Sons.

Chen, T., & Guestrin, C. (2016). Xgboost: A scalable tree boosting system. Proceedings of the 22nd acm sigkdd international conference on knowledge discovery and data mining, Chithrananda, S., Grand, G., & Ramsundar, B. (2020). ChemBERTa: large-scale self-supervised pretraining for molecular property prediction. *arXiv preprint arXiv:2010.09885*.

Chen, A.-T., Zhang, Y., & Zhang, J. (2025). Artificial intelligence in cardiac metabolism: The next frontier in cardiovascular health. *Metabolism and Target Organ Damage, 5*(1). *Scopus*. Advance online publication. DOI: 10.20517/mtod.2024.82

Chen, B., Khodadoust, M. S., Olsson, N., Wagar, L. E., Fast, E., Liu, C. L., Muftuoglu, Y., Sworder, B. J., Diehn, M., & Levy, R. (2019). Predicting HLA class II antigen presentation through integrated deep learning. *Nature Biotechnology*, *37*(11), 1332–1343. PMID: 31611695

Cheng, F., Kovacs, I. A., & Barabasi, A. L. (2019). Network-based prediction of drug combinations. *Nature Communications*, *10*(1), 1197. DOI: 10.1038/s41467-019-09186-x PMID: 30867426

Cheng, J., Liang, T., Xie, X. Q., Feng, Z., & Meng, L. (2024). A new era of antibody discovery: An in-depth review of AI-driven approaches. *Drug Discovery Today*, *29*(6), 103984.

Chen, H. Y., Lin, Y. H., Hu, S., Yang, S. H., Chen, J. L., & Chen, Y. C. (2015). Identifying chinese herbal medicine network for eczema: Implications from a nationwide prescription database. *Evidence-Based Complementary and Alternative Medicine : eCAM*, *347164*. Advance online publication. DOI: 10.1155/2015/347164 PMID: 25685167

Chen, H., Cheng, F., & Li, J. (2020). iDrug: Integration of drug repositioning and drug-target prediction via cross-network embedding. *PLoS Computational Biology*, *16*(7), e1008040.

Chen, H., Engkvist, O., Wang, Y., Olivecrona, M., & Blaschke, T. (2018). The rise of deep learning in drug discovery. *Drug Discovery Today*, *23*(6), 1241–1250. DOI: 10.1016/j.drudis.2018.01.039 PMID: 29366762

Chen, H., & He, Y. (2022). Machine Learning Approaches in Traditional Chinese Medicine: A Systematic Review. *The American Journal of Chinese Medicine*, *50*(1), 91–131. DOI: 10.1142/S0192415X22500045 PMID: 34931589

Chen, I. Y., Szolovits, P., & Ghassemi, M. (2019). Can AI help reduce disparities in general medical and mental health care? *AMA Journal of Ethics*, *21*(2), 167–179. DOI: 10.1001/amajethics.2019.167 PMID: 30794127

Chen, J., Liu, H., Cui, X., Li, Z., & Chen, H.-F. (2022). RNA-specific force field optimization with CMAP and reweighting. *Journal of Chemical Information and Modeling*, *62*(2), 372–385. PMID: 35021622

Chen, L. T., Quinn, Z., Dumas, M., Peng, C., Hong, L., Lopez-Gonzalez, M., & Chatterjee, P. (2025). Target sequence-conditioned design of peptide binders using masked language modelling. *Nature Biotechnology*, •••, 1–9.

Chen, L., Deng, H., Cui, H., Fang, J., Zuo, Z., Deng, J., Li, Y., Wang, X., & Zhao, L. (2017). Inflammatory responses and inflammation-associated diseases in organs. *Oncotarget*, *9*(6), 7204–7218. DOI: 10.18632/oncotarget.23208

Chen, L., & Roberts, P. (2023). Analysis of the NutriTrack data breach: Timeline, impact, and lessons learned. *Journal of Digital Health Security*, *8*(2), 103–119.

Chen, L., Zhang, C., Niu, R., Xiong, S., He, J., Wang, Y., & Feng, R. (2025). Multi-omics biomarkers for predicting efficacy of biologic and small-molecule therapies in adults with inflammatory bowel disease: A systematic review. *United European Gastroenterology Journal*, *13*(4), 517–530.

Chen, S., Li, T., Yang, L., Zhai, F., Jiang, X., Xiang, R., & Ling, G. (2022). Artificial intelligence-driven prediction of multiple drug interactions. *Briefings in Bioinformatics*, *23*(6), bbac427. Advance online publication. DOI: 10.1093/bib/bbac427

Chen, W., Liu, X., Zhang, S., & Chen, S. (2023). Artificial intelligence for drug discovery: Resources, methods, and applications. *Molecular Therapy. Nucleic Acids*, *31*, 691–702. DOI: 10.1016/j.omtn.2023.02.019 PMID: 36923950

Chen, X., Haddish-Berhane, N., Moore, P., Clark, T., Yang, Y., Li, H., & Barletta, F. (2016). Mechanistic projection of first-in-human dose for bispecific immunomodulatory P-Cadherin LP-DART: An integrated PK/PD modelling approach. *Clinical Pharmacology and Therapeutics*, *100*(3), 232–241.

Chen, Y., Guo, X., Pan, Y., Xia, Y., & Yuan, Y. (2023b). Dynamic feature splicing for few-shot rare disease diagnosis. *Medical Image Analysis*, *90*, 102959.

Chen, Y., & Zhang, L. (2022). How much can deep learning improve prediction of the responses to drugs in cancer cell lines? *Briefings in Bioinformatics*, *23*(1). Advance online publication. DOI: 10.1093/bib/bbab378 PMID: 34529029

Chen, Z., Liu, X., Hogan, W., Shenkman, E., & Bian, J. (2021). Applications of artificial intelligence in drug development using real-world data. *Drug Discovery Today*, *26*(5), 1256–1264. DOI: 10.1016/j.drudis.2020.12.013 PMID: 33358699

Chinedu-Nzereogu, O. P., Olorunfemi, V. O., Osifeso, J. O., & John, T. (2025). Computational immunogenomics: Leveraging AI to uncover novel biomarkers for disease diagnosis and therapy. *International Journal of Life Science Research Archive*, *9*(1), 102–119.

Chodankar, D., Raval, T. K., & Jeyaraj, J. (2024). The role of remote data capture, wearables, and digital biomarkers in decentralized clinical trials. *Perspectives in Clinical Research*, *15*(1), 38–41. DOI: 10.4103/picr.picr_219_22

Choi, H., Kang, E., Song, D., & Jung, G. (2025). Integrating Multimodal Data with Large Foundation Models in Healthcare. https://doi.org/DOI: 10.20944/preprints202508.0498.v1

Cho, J., Xu, Q., Wong, C. H., & Lo, A. W. (2025). Predicting clinical trial duration via statistical and machine learning models. *Contemporary Clinical Trials Communications*, *45*, 101473. DOI: 10.1016/j.conctc.2025.101473

Choudhury, S. R., Das, P., Koner, S., Ghosh, J., & Singh, K. (2024). Cardiovascular disease risks related to consumption of ready-to-eat food products between young adults of Kolkata, West Bengal, India. *Journal of Comprehensive Health*, *12*(1), 60.

Chu, H., Moon, S., Park, J., Bak, S., Ko, Y., & Youn, B. Y. (2022). The Use of Artificial Intelligence in Complementary and Alternative Medicine: A Systematic Scoping Review. *Frontiers in Pharmacology*, *13*, 826044. DOI: 10.3389/fphar.2022.826044 PMID: 35431917

Chun, M. (2023). *How artificial intelligence is revolutionizing drug discovery. Bill of Health*. Harvard Law School.

Cichońska, A., Ravikumar, B., & Rahman, R. (2024). AI for targeted polypharmacology: The next frontier in drug discovery. *Current Opinion in Structural Biology*, *84*, 102771.

Cichonski, P., Millar, T., Grance, T., & Scarfone, K. (2012). *Computer security incident handling guide* (NIST Special Publication 800-61 Revision 2).

Clemm, C., Stobbe, L., Wimalawarne, K., & Druschke, J. (2024). Towards green AI: Current status and future research. In *2024 Electronics Goes Green 2024+(EGG)* (pp. 1-11). IEEE.

Coelho, D. M. (2021). *Detection of side channel attacks at the network physical layer* (Master's thesis, Universidade de Aveiro, Portugal).

Cohen, I. G., Evgeniou, T., Gerke, S., & Minssen, T. (2020). The European artificial intelligence strategy: Implications and challenges for digital health. *The Lancet. Digital Health*, *2*(7), e376–e377. PMID: 33328096

Colombo, S., Beck-Broichsitter, M., Botker, J. P., Malmsten, M., Rantanen, J., & Bohr, A. (2018). Transforming nanomedicine manufacturing toward Quality by Design and microfluidics. *Advanced Drug Delivery Reviews*, *128*, 115–131. DOI: 10.1016/j.addr.2018.04.004 PMID: 29626549

Conde, G. D., Qaiser, T., Wu, E., Andrea, C. E. D., Shields, J., Artzi, R., & Reischl, J. (2024). Immunotherapy efficacy prediction in cancer: an artificial intelligence approach with unannotated H&E whole-slide images. medRxiv, 2024-02.

Cong, Y., Han, X., Wang, Y., Chen, Z., Lu, Y., Liu, T., & Zhang, X. (2020). Drug toxicity evaluation based on organ-on-a-chip technology: A review. *Micromachines*, *11*(4), 381.

Conrad, S., Auth, P., Masselter, T., & Speck, T. (2025). Lowering the Entrance Hurdle for Lab Automation: An Artificial Intelligence-Supported, Interactive Robotic arm for automated, repeated testing procedures. *Advanced Intelligent Systems*, •••, 2401086.

Correll, C. U., Abi-Dargham, A., & Howes, O. (2022). Emerging treatments in schizophrenia. *The Journal of Clinical Psychiatry*, *83*(1), 39683. PMID: 35172048

Cowen-Rivers, A. I., Gorinski, P. J., Sootla, A., Khan, A., Furui, L., Wang, J., & Ammar, H. B. (2022). Structured q-learning for antibody design. *arXiv preprint arXiv:2209.04698.*

Cozac, R., Hasic, H., Choong, J. J., Richard, V., Beheshti, L., Froehlich, C., Koyama, T., Matsumoto, S., Kojima, R., Iwata, H., Hasegawa, A., Otsuka, T., & Okuno, Y. (2025). kMoL: An open-source machine and federated learning library for drug discovery. *Journal of Cheminformatics*, *17*(1). Advance online publication. DOI: 10.1186/s13321-025-00967-9 PMID: 40001146

Creemers, J. H., Ankan, A., Roes, K. C., Schröder, G., Mehra, N., Figdor, C. G., & Textor, J. (2023). In silico cancer immunotherapy trials uncover the consequences of therapy-specific response patterns for clinical trial design and outcome. *Nature Communications*, *14*(1), 2348.

Cremonesi, F., Vesin, M., Cansiz, S., Bouillard, Y., Balelli, I., Innocenti, L., & Lorenzi, M. (2025). Fed-biomed: Open, transparent and trusted federated learning for real-world healthcare applications. In *Federated Learning Systems: Towards Privacy-Preserving Distributed AI* (pp. 19–41). Springer Nature Switzerland.

Crossler, R. E., & Bélanger, F. (2019). Why would I use location-protective settings on my smartphone? Motivating protective behaviors and the existence of the privacy knowledge-belief gap. *Information Systems Research*, *30*(3), 995–1013.

Cuccarese, M. F., Earnshaw, B. A., Heiser, K., Fogelson, B., Davis, C. T., McLean, P. F., & Gibson, C. C. (2020). Functional immune mapping with deep-learning enabled phenomics applied to immunomodulatory and COVID-19 drug discovery. Biorxiv, 2020-08.

Cucu, I. (2022). Signalling pathways in inflammation and cardiovascular diseases: An update of therapeutic strategies. *Immuno*, *2*(4), 630–650.

Culver, A., Stayrook, K., Comerota, M., Oblak, A., & Burris, T. (2025). Animal models for development of anti-obesity drugs in the age of GLP-1 agents. *Expert Opinion on Drug Discovery*, *20*(7), 913–925. DOI: 10.1080/17460441.2025.2507766

Curion, F., & Theis, F. J. (2024). Machine learning integrative approaches to advance computational immunology. *Genome Medicine*, *16*(1), 80.

Cybersecurity and Infrastructure Security Agency. (2024). Supply chain compromise affecting nutritional database integration libraries (Alert AA24-089A). U.S. Department of Homeland Security.

D'Silva, S., Rajadhyaksha, S. B., & Singh, M. (2019). *Immune dysregulation in MDS: the role of cytokines and immune cells. Recent Developments in Myelodysplastic Syndromes*. IntechOpen.

da Silva, B. M., Ascher, D. B., Geard, N., & Pires, D. E. (2023). AI driven B-cell immunotherapy design. *arXiv preprint arXiv:2309.01122*.

Dağlarli, E. (2020). Explainable artificial intelligence (xAI) approaches and deep meta-learning models. In *Advances and applications in deep learning*. IntechOpen.

Daly, B., Brawley, O. W., Gospodarowicz, M. K., Olopade, O. I., Fashoyin-Aje, L., Smart, V. W., & Li, B. T. (2024). Remote monitoring and data collection for decentralized clinical trials. *JAMA Network Open*, *7*(4), e246228–e246228. DOI: 10.1001/jamanetworkopen.2024.6228

Daniore, P., Nittas, V., Haag, C., Bernard, J., Gonzenbach, R., & von Wyl, V. (2024). From wearable sensor data to digital biomarker development: Ten lessons learned and a framework proposal. *NPJ Digital Medicine*, *7*(1), 161.

Dankar, F. K., Gergely, M., & Dankar, S. K. (2019). Informed Consent in Biomedical Research. *Computational and Structural Biotechnology Journal*, *17*, 463–474. DOI: 10.1016/j.csbj.2019.03.010

Dara, M., & Azarpira, N. (2025). Ethical considerations emerge from artificial intelligence (ai) in biotechnology. *Avicenna Journal of Medical Biotechnology*, *17*(1), 80.

Dara, M., & Azarpira, N. (2025). Ethical considerations emerge from artificial intelligence (AI) in biotechnology. *Avicenna Journal of Medical Biotechnology, 17*(1), 80–81. DOI: 10.18502/ajmb.v17i1.17680 PMID: 40094090

Dara, S., Dhamercherla, S., Jadav, S. S., Babu, C. M., & Ahsan, M. J. (2022). Machine Learning in Drug Discovery: A Review. *Artificial Intelligence Review, 55*(3), 1947–1999. DOI: 10.1007/s10462-021-10058-4 PMID: 34393317

Dasgupta, S., Stevens, C. F., & Navlakha, S. (2017). A neural algorithm for a fundamental computing problem. *Science, 358*(6364), 793–796.

Das, U. (2025). Generative AI for drug discovery and protein design: The next frontier in AI-driven molecular science. *Medicine in Drug Discovery*, •••, 100213.

Das, U. (2025). Transforming precision medicine through generative AI: Advanced architectures and tailored therapeutic design for patient-specific drug discovery. *ChemistrySelect, 10*(36), e02448.

David, L., Thakkar, A., Mercado, R., & Engkvist, O. (2020). Molecular representations in AI-driven drug discovery: a review and practical guide. In *Journal of Cheminformatics* (Vol. 12, Issue 1). BioMed Central Ltd. https://doi.org/DOI: 10.1186/s13321-020-00460-5

David, B. G. (2024). Artificial intelligence in predicting adaptive immune responses. *INOSR EXPERIMENTAL SCIENCES Учредители: International Digital Organization for Scientific Research, 14*(2), 17–22.

Davidson, L., & Boland, M. R. (2020). Enabling pregnant women and their physicians to make informed medication decisions using artificial intelligence. *Journal of Pharmacokinetics and Pharmacodynamics, 47*(4), 305–318. DOI: 10.1007/s10928-020-09685-1

Dawuti, A., Sun, S., Wang, R., Gong, D., Liu, R., Kong, D., Yuan, T., Zhou, J., Lu, Y., Wang, S., Du, G., & Fang, L. (2023). Salvianolic acid A alleviates heart failure with preserved ejection fraction via regulating TLR/Myd88/TRAF/NF-κB and p38MAPK/CREB signaling pathways. *Biomedicine & Pharmacotherapy = Biomedecine & Pharmacotherapie, 168*, 115837. https://doi.org/DOI: 10.1016/j.biopha.2023.115837

de Anda-Jáuregui, G., Guo, K., McGregor, B. A., & Hur, J. (2018). Exploration of the anti-inflammatory drug space through network pharmacology: Applications for drug repurposing. *Frontiers in Physiology, 9*, 151.

De Cao, N., & Kipf, T. (2018). MolGAN: An implicit generative model for small molecular graphs. *arXiv preprint arXiv:1805.11973.*

de Hoogh, I. M., Winters, B. L., Nieman, K. M., Bijlsma, S., Krone, T., van den Broek, T. J., Anderson, B. D., Caspers, M. P. M., Anthony, J. C., & Wopereis, S. (2021). A novel personalized systems nutrition program improves dietary patterns, lifestyle behaviors and health-related outcomes: Results from the Habit Study. *Nutrients*, *13*(6), 1763. Advance online publication. DOI: 10.3390/nu13061763

de Thé, F. X. B., Baudier, C., Pereira, R. A., Lefebvre, C., & Moingeon, P.Patrimony Working Group. (2023). Transforming drug discovery with a high-throughput AI-powered platform: A 5-year experience with Patrimony. *Drug Discovery Today*, *28*(11), 103772.

De Vivo, M., Masetti, M., Bottegoni, G., & Cavalli, A. (2016). Role of molecular dynamics and related methods in drug discovery. *Journal of Medicinal Chemistry*, *59*(9), 4035–4061. PMID: 26807648

Dedic, N., Jones, P. G., Hopkins, S. C., Lew, R., Shao, L., Campbell, J. E., Spear, K. L., Large, T. H., Campbell, U. C., & Hanania, T. (2019). SEP-363856, a novel psychotropic agent with a unique, non-D2 receptor mechanism of action. *The Journal of Pharmacology and Experimental Therapeutics*, *371*(1), 1–14. PMID: 31371483

Dempsey, K., Witte, G. A., & Iorga, M. (2018). *Summary of NIST SP 800-53 revision 5, security and privacy controls for information systems and organizations*. NIST Special Publication.

Deng, J., Yang, Z., Ojima, I., Samaras, D., & Wang, F. (2022). Artificial intelligence in drug discovery: Applications and techniques. *Briefings in Bioinformatics*, *23*(1). PMID: 34734228

Department of Health and Human Services. (2024). *OCR announces results of nutrition application HIPAA compliance investigation*. HHS Press Office.

Dermawan, D., & Alotaiq, N. (2025). From Lab to Clinic: How Artificial Intelligence (AI) Is Reshaping Drug Discovery Timelines and Industry Outcomes. *Pharmaceuticals*, *18*(7), 981. PMID: 40732273

DesRochers, N., Renaud, J. B., Tanney, J. B., Ibrahim, A., Yeung, K. K.-C., & Sumarah, M. W. (2023). Non-targeted Screening of Natural Products from 288 Fungal Endophytes from Canadian Fruit Crops. *ACS Omega*, *8*(27), 24561–24572. PMID: 37457466

Dev Sharma, P., Alhudhaibi, A. M., Al Noman, A., Abdallah, E. M., Taha, T. H., & Sharma, H. (2025). Systems biology-driven discovery of host-targeted therapeutics for oropouche virus: Integrating network pharmacology, molecular docking, and drug repurposing. *Pharmaceuticals*, *18*(5), 613. PMID: 40430433

Devaprasad, A., Radstake, T. R., & Pandit, A. (2021). Integration of immunome with disease-gene network reveals common cellular mechanisms between IMIDs and drug repurposing strategies. *Frontiers in Immunology*, *12*, 669400.

Dhillon, B. K., Smith, M., Baghela, A., Lee, A. H., & Hancock, R. E. (2020). Systems biology approaches to understanding the human immune system. *Frontiers in Immunology*, *11*, 1683.

Dhudum, R., Ganeshpurkar, A., & Pawar, A. (2024). Revolutionizing drug discovery: A comprehensive review of AI applications. *Drugs and Drug Candidates*, *3*(1), 148–171.

DiMasi, J. A., Grabowski, H. G., & Hansen, R. W. (2016). Innovation in the pharmaceutical industry: New estimates of R&D costs. *Journal of Health Economics*, *47*, 20–33. PMID: 26928437

Dimitrov, D. V. (2014). Systems patientomics: The virtual in-silico patient. *New Horizons in Translational Medicine*, *2*(1), 1–4.

Ding, K., Zhou, M., Metaxas, D. N., & Zhang, S. (2023). Pathology-and-genomics multimodal transformer for survival outcome prediction. In *International Conference on Medical Image Computing and Computer-Assisted Intervention* (pp. 622-631). Cham: Springer Nature Switzerland.

Diro, A. A., & Chilamkurti, N. (2018). Distributed attack detection scheme using deep learning approach for Internet of Things. *Future Generation Computer Systems*, *82*, 761–768. DOI: 10.1016/j.future.2017.08.043

Dixit, S., Kumar, A., Srinivasan, K., Vincent, P. D. R., & Ramu Krishnan, N. (2024). Advancing genome editing with artificial intelligence: Opportunities, challenges, and future directions. *Frontiers in Bioengineering and Biotechnology*, *11*, 1335901.

Doneva, N., Doytchinova, I., & Dimitrov, I. (2021). Predicting immunogenicity risk in biopharmaceuticals. *Symmetry*, *13*(3), 388.

Dong, J., Cao, D. S., Miao, H. Y., Liu, S., Deng, B. C., Yun, Y. H., Wang, N. N., Lu, A. P., & Zeng, W. Bin, & Chen, A. F. (2015). ChemDes: An integrated web-based platform for molecular descriptor and fingerprint computation. *Journal of Cheminformatics*, *7*(1). Advance online publication. DOI: 10.1186/s13321-015-0109-z PMID: 26664458

Dong, S., Nessler, I., Kopp, A., Rubahamya, B., & Thurber, G. M. (2022). Predictive simulations in preclinical oncology to guide the translation of biologics. *Frontiers in Pharmacology*, *13*, 836925.

Donovan, S. M., et al (2025). Perspective: Challenges for personalized nutrition in the current U.S. regulatory framework and future opportunities. *Advances in Nutrition*. Advance online publication. DOI: 10.1016/j.advnut.2025.100382

Doshi-Velez, F., & Kim, B. (2017). Towards a rigorous science of interpretable machine learning. arXiv:1702.08608.

Dounas, A., Cotet, T. S., & Yermanos, A. (2024). Learning immune receptor representations with protein language models. *arXiv preprint arXiv:2402.03823*.

Dubey, A. (2020). Showcasing the Impact of Machine Learning in Healthcare. *Bioinformatics & Proteomics Open Access Journal*, *4*(1). Advance online publication. DOI: 10.23880/bpoj-16000131

Durso-Finley, J., Barile, B., Falet, J. P., Arnold, D. L., Pawlowski, N., & Arbel, T. (2024). Probabilistic temporal prediction of continuous disease trajectories and treatment effects using neural SDEs. In *International Conference on Medical Image Computing and Computer-Assisted Intervention* (pp. 400-410). Cham: Springer Nature Switzerland.

Du, Z., Huang, D., Shi, P., Dong, Z., Wang, X., Li, M., Chen, W., Zhang, F., & Sun, L. (2022). Integrated Chemical Interpretation and Network Pharmacology Analysis to Reveal the Anti-Liver Fibrosis Effect of Penthorum chinense. *Frontiers in Pharmacology*, *13*, 788388. DOI: 10.3389/fphar.2022.788388 PMID: 35721129

Eftimie, R., Mavrodin, A., & Bordas, S. P. (2023). From digital control to digital twins in medicine: A brief review and future perspectives. *Advances in Applied Mechanics*, *56*, 323–368.

El Belghiti, I., Hammani, O., Moustaoui, F., Aghrouch, M., Lemkhente, Z., Boubrik, F., & Belmouden, A. (2025). Halicin: A New Approach to Antibacterial Therapy, a Promising Avenue for the Post-Antibiotic Era. *Antibiotics (Basel, Switzerland)*, *14*(7), 698. PMID: 40723999

Elemam, N. M., Talaat, I. M., Elmeligy, O. A. A., & Hundt, J. E. (2025). Cellular and molecular regulators in non-neoplastic immune-mediated diseases. *Frontiers in Immunology*, *16*, 1694308.

ElShal, S., Tranchevent, L. C., Sifrim, A., Ardeshirdavani, A., Davis, J., & Moreau, Y. (2016). Beegle: From literature mining to disease-gene discovery. *Nucleic Acids Research*, *44*(2), e18–e18.

EMA. (2023). *European Medicines Agency (EMA): Reflection paper on the use of artificial intelligence in the lifecycle of medicines*. Retrieved 1 November 2023 from https://www.ema.europa.eu/en/documents/scientific-guideline/reflection-paper-use-artificial-intelligence-ai-medicinal-product-lifecycle_en.pdf

Enni, M. A., & Maraj, M. A. A. (2022). In silico drug repurposing for inflammatory diseases: A systematic review of molecular docking and virtual screening studies. *American Journal of Advanced Technology and Engineering Solutions*, *2*(04), 35–64.

Entzeroth, M., Flotow, H., & Condron, P. (2009). Overview of high-throughput screening. In *Current Protocols in Pharmacology* (Issue SUPPL. 44). https://doi.org/DOI: 10.1002/0471141755.ph0904s44

Erhard, A., Poulsen Nautrup, H., Meth, M., Postler, L., Stricker, R., Stadler, M., Negnevitsky, V., Ringbauer, M., Schindler, P., & Briegel, H. J. (2021). Entangling logical qubits with lattice surgery. *Nature*, *589*(7841), 220–224. PMID: 33442044

Ernst, D. (2023). *Disappointing Results for Ulotaront in Two Phase 3 Schizophrenia Trials. Neurology Advisor*. NA-NA.

Eslami, M., Fadaee Dowlat, B., Yaghmayee, S., Habibian, A., Keshavarzi, S., Oksenych, V., & Naderian, R. (2025). Next-generation vaccine platforms: Integrating synthetic biology, nanotechnology, and systems immunology for improved immunogenicity. *Vaccines*, *13*(6), 588.

European Commission. (2021). Proposal for a regulation of the European Parliament and of the Council laying down harmonised rules on artificial intelligence.

European Data Protection Board. (2023). *Decision regarding NutriHealth data processing practices (Case 2023-DE-17)*. EDPB Publications.

European Medicines Agency. (2020). EMA big data steering group: Workplan 2020-2022.

European Union. (2016). Regulation (EU) 2016/679 of the European Parliament and of the Council of 27 April 2016 on the protection of natural persons with regard to the processing of personal data and on the free movement of such data (General Data Protection Regulation). Official Journal of the European Union, L 119/1.

European Union. (2021). Proposal for a regulation of the European Parliament and of the Council laying down harmonised rules on artificial intelligence (Artificial Intelligence Act). COM(2021) 206 final.

Exscientia—Exscientia Reports Topline Data From EXS-21546 Phase 1a Study Demonstrating Targeted A2A Receptor Signaling Inhibition in Healthy Volunteers. (n.d.). Retrieved August 27, 2025, from https://investors.exscientia.ai/press-releases/press-release-details/2022/Exscientia-Reports-Topline-Data-From-EXS-21546-Phase-1a-Study-Demonstrating-Targeted-A2A-Receptor-Signaling-Inhibition-in-Healthy-Volunteers/default.aspx

Fang, H., Qiu, Y., Yu, H., Yu, W., Kong, J., Chong, B., & Xu, K. (2024). Privacy leakage on DNNs: A survey of model inversion attacks and defenses. *arXiv*.

Fang, J., Cai, C., Chai, Y., Zhou, J., Huang, Y., Gao, L., Wang, Q., & Cheng, F. (2019). Quantitative and systems pharmacology 4. Network-based analysis of drug pleiotropy on coronary artery disease. *European Journal of Medicinal Chemistry*, *161*, 192–204. DOI: 10.1016/j.ejmech.2018.10.020 PMID: 30359818

Fang, J., Liu, C., Wang, Q., Lin, P., & Cheng, F. (2018). In silico polypharmacology of natural products. *Briefings in Bioinformatics*, *19*(6), 1153–1171. DOI: 10.1093/bib/bbx045 PMID: 28460068

Fang, R., Zhou, R., Ju, D., Li, M., Wang, H., Pan, L., Wang, X., Han, M., & Yu, Y. (2024). Zhen-wu-tang protects against myocardial fibrosis by inhibiting M1 macrophage polarization via the TLR4/NF-κB pathway. *Phytomedicine*, *130*, 155719. DOI: 10.1016/j.phymed.2024.155719

Fan, X., Fang, S., Li, Z., Ji, H., Yue, M., Li, J., & Ren, X. (2025). ICVAE: Interpretable conditional variational autoencoder for de novo molecular design. *International Journal of Molecular Sciences*, *26*(9), 3980. PMID: 40362221

Fatima, G., Siddiqui, Z., & Parvez, S. (2024). AI and precision medicine: paving the way for future treatment. https://doi.org/DOI: 10.20944/preprints202412.0036.v1

Fausch, I., Zeyer-Iyengar, D., Morales, R. M. C., Elger, B., Enzmann, V., & Früh, A. (2025). exploring alternatives to animal testing: scientific, legal and ethical challenges in developing novel alternative methods with a focus on organoids as potential NAMs. *LEOH-Journal of Animal Law, Ethics and One Health*, 81-99.

FDA. (2021). Artificial intelligence/machine learning (AI/ML)-based software as a medical device (SaMD) action plan.

Federal Trade Commission. (2024). *Data broker practices in health and nutrition information marketplaces*. FTC Bureau of Consumer Protection.

Feng, H., Fawaz, M. S., & Shin, K. G. (2013). Continuous authentication for security-sensitive mobile apps. In 13th USENIX Security Symposium (USENIX Security '13) (pp. 371-386). USENIX Association.

Feng, C., Zhou, S., Qu, Y., Wang, Q., Bao, S., Li, Y., & Yang, T. (2021). Overview of Artificial Intelligence Applications in Chinese Medicine Therapy. *Evidence-Based Complementary and Alternative Medicine : eCAM, 6678958*. Advance online publication. DOI: 10.1155/2021/6678958 PMID: 33815559

Fernández-Alemán, J. L., Carrión Señor, I., Oliver Lozoya, P. A., & Toval, A. (2013). Security and privacy in electronic health records: A systematic literature review. *Journal of Biomedical Informatics*, *46*(3), 541–562.

Fernandez, M. M., Motrich, R. D., Ostrowski, M., & De Marzi, M. (2024). Immune system disorders: From molecular mechanisms to clinical implications. *Frontiers in Immunology*, *15*, 1498830.

Ferreira, F. J. N., & Carneiro, A. S. (2025). AI-driven drug discovery: A comprehensive review. *ACS Omega*, *10*(23), 23889–23903. DOI: 10.1021/acsomega.5c00549

Ferreira, F. J., & Carneiro, A. S. (2025). AI-Driven Drug Discovery: A Comprehensive Review. *ACS Omega*. PMID: 40547666

Ferroni, J. M., & Parenti, P. (2024). Ethical and regulatory challenges of Artificial Intelligence in medical research: reflections on intelligent regulation. *Binational Brazil-Argentina Journal: Dialogue between sciences, 14* (02), 103-119.

Fialková, V., Zhao, J., Papadopoulos, K., Engkvist, O., Bjerrum, E. J., Kogej, T., & Patronov, A. (2021). LibINVENT: Reaction-based generative scaffold decoration for in silico library design. *Journal of Chemical Information and Modeling*, *62*(9), 2046–2063. PMID: 34460269

Finlayson, S. G., Bowers, J. D., Ito, J., Zittrain, J. L., Beam, A. L., & Kohane, I. S. (2019). Adversarial attacks on medical machine learning. *Science*, *363*(6433), 1287–1289. DOI: 10.1126/science.aaw4399 PMID: 30898923

Fiske, A., Henningsen, P., & Buyx, A. (2020). Your robot therapist will see you now: Ethical implications of embodied artificial intelligence in psychiatry, psychology, and psychotherapy. *Journal of Medical Internet Research*, *22*(5), e13216. PMID: 31094356

Fleming, N. (2018). How artificial intelligence is changing drug discovery. *Nature*, *557*(7707), S55–S57. DOI: 10.1038/d41586-018-05267-x PMID: 29849160

Flores, J. E., Claborne, D. M., Weller, Z. D., Webb-Robertson, B.-J. M., Waters, K. M., & Bramer, L. M. (2023). Missing data in multi-omics integration: Recent advances through artificial intelligence. *Frontiers in Artificial Intelligence*, *6*, 1098308. PMID: 36844425

Floridi, L., Cowls, J., Beltrametti, M., Chatila, R., Chazerand, P., Dignum, V., & Vayena, E. (2018). AI4People—An ethical framework for a good AI society: Opportunities, risks, principles, and recommendations. *Minds and Machines*, *28*(4), 689–707. PMID: 30930541

Fokunang, C. N., Ndikum, V., Tabi, O. Y., Jiofack, R. B., Ngameni, B., Guedje, N. M., Tembe-Fokunang, E. A., Tomkins, P., Barkwan, S., Kechia, F., Asongalem, E., Ngoupayou, J., Torimiro, N. J., Gonsu, K. H., Sielinou, V., Ngadjui, B. T., Angwafor, F.III, Nkongmeneck, A., Abena, O. M., & Kamsu, K. (2011). Traditional medicine: Past, present and future research and development prospects and integration in the National Health System of Cameroon. *African Journal of Traditional, Complementary, and Alternative Medicines : AJTCAM*, *8*(3), 284–295. DOI: 10.4314/ajtcam.v8i3.65276 PMID: 22468007

Folasole, A., Eshua, P. E., & Elesho, O. E. (2025). Modelling spatiotemporal immune dynamics in inflammatory diseases using integrative multi-modal analytics and high-dimensional longitudinal datasets. *World Journal of Biology Pharmacy and Health Sciences*, *23*(2), 196–218.

Folino, F., & Sabatino, P. (2016). A scalable and resilient architecture for intrusion detection based on the elastic stack. *Concurrency and Computation*, *28*(7), 2009–2027.

Food and Drug Administration. (2018). FDA's evolution: A brief history of the regulation of drugs and biologics. U.S. Food and Drug Administration. https://www.fda.gov

Food and Drug Administration. (2021). Artificial intelligence/machine learning (AI/ML)-based software as a medical device action plan. https://www.fda.gov/media/145022/download

Foroughi, M., Torabinejad, M., Angelov, N., Ojcius, D. M., Parang, K., Ravnan, M., & Lam, J. (2025). Bridging oral and systemic health: Exploring pathogenesis, biomarkers, and diagnostic innovations in periodontal disease. *Infection*. Advance online publication. DOI: 10.1007/s15010-025-02568-y

Frąk, W., Wojtasińska, A., Lisińska, W., Młynarska, E., Franczyk, B., & Rysz, J. (2022). Pathophysiology of Cardiovascular Diseases: New Insights into Molecular Mechanisms of Atherosclerosis, Arterial Hypertension, and Coronary Artery Disease. *Biomedicines*, *10*(8), 1938. DOI: 10.3390/biomedicines10081938

Frattini, E., Faustini, G., Lopez, G., Carsana, E. V., Tosi, M., Trezzi, I., Magni, M., Soldà, G., Straniero, L., Facchi, D., Samarani, M., Martá-Ariza, M., De Luca, C. M. G., Vezzoli, E., Pittaro, A., Stepanyan, A., Silipigni, R., Rosety, I., Schwamborn, J. C., & Di Fonzo, A. (2025). Lewy pathology formation in patient-derived GBA1 Parkinson's disease midbrain organoids. *Brain, 148*(4), 1242–1257. DOI: 10.1093/brain/awae365

Fridman, L., Weber, S., Greenstadt, R., & Kam, M. (2017). Active authentication on mobile devices via stylometry, application usage, web browsing, and GPS location. *IEEE Systems Journal, 11*(2), 513–521. DOI: 10.1109/JSYST.2015.2453215

Fu, X., Mervin, L. H., Li, X., Yu, H., Li, J., Mohamad Zobir, S. Z., Zoufir, A., Zhou, Y., Song, Y., Wang, Z., & Bender, A. (2017). Toward Understanding the Cold, Hot, and Neutral Nature of Chinese Medicines Using in Silico Mode-of-Action Analysis. *Journal of Chemical Information and Modeling, 57*(3), 468–483. DOI: 10.1021/acs.jcim.6b00725 PMID: 28257573

Gadade, D. D., Kulkarni, D. A., Raj, R., Patil, S. G., & Modi, A. (2024). Pushing Boundaries: The Landscape of AI-Driven Drug Discovery and Development with Insights Into Regulatory Aspects. In *Artificial Intelligence and Machine Learning in Drug Design and Development* (pp. 533–561). wiley; Scopus. https://doi.org/DOI: 10.1002/9781394234196.ch17

Gad, S. C. (2021). *Drug safety evaluation* (4th ed.). John Wiley & Sons.

Gallone, G., Bruno, F., D'Ascenzo, F., & Ferrari, G. M. D. (2022). What will we ask to artificial intelligence for cardiovascular medicine in the next decade? *Minerva Cardiology and Angiology, 70*(1), 92–101.

Gallo, P. (2006). Executive summary of the PhRMA working group on adaptive designs in clinical drug development. *Journal of Biopharmaceutical Statistics, 16*, 275–283. PMID: 16724485

Galvin, J. E., Cummings, J. L., Benea, M. L., de Moor, C., Allegri, R. F., Atri, A., Chertkow, H., Paquet, C., Porter, V. R., Ritchie, C. W., Sikkes, S. A. M., Smith, M. R., Grassi, C. M., & Rubino, I. (2024). Generating real-world evidence in Alzheimer's disease: Considerations for establishing a core dataset. *Alzheimer's & Dementia, 20*(6), 4331–4341. DOI: 10.1002/alz.13785

Gantla, M. R., Tsigelny, I. F., & Kouznetsova, V. L. (2023). Repurposing of drugs for combined treatment of COVID-19 cytokine storm using machine learning. *Medicine in Drug Discovery, 17*, 100148.

Gan, X., Shu, Z., Wang, X., Yan, D., Li, J., Ofaim, S., Albert, R., Li, X., Liu, B., Zhou, X., & Barabasi, A. L. (2023). Network medicine framework reveals generic herb-symptom effectiveness of traditional Chinese medicine. *Science Advances*, *9*(43), eadh0215. Advance online publication. DOI: 10.1126/sciadv.adh0215 PMID: 37889962

Gao, J., Hu, J., Liu, L., Xue, Y., Zhu, K., Zhang, X., & Fang, X. (2024). Precise antigen-antibody structure predictions enhance antibody development with HelixFold-multimer. *arXiv preprint arXiv:2412.09826*.

Gao, Y., Doan, B. G., Zhang, Z., Ma, S., Zhang, J., Fu, A., Kim, H. (2020). Backdoor attacks and countermeasures on deep learning: A comprehensive review. *arXiv*. https://doi.org//arXiv.2007.10760DOI: 10.48550

Gao, B., Qiang, B., Tan, H., Ren, M., Jia, Y., Lu, M., Liu, J., Ma, W., & Lan, Y. (2023). *DrugCLIP: Contrastive Protein-Molecule Representation Learning for Virtual Screening*. https://arxiv.org/abs/2310.06367

Gao, Y., Gao, H., Xiao, H., & Yao, F. (2023). Vaccine supply chain coordination using blockchain and artificial intelligence technologies. *Computers & Industrial Engineering*, *175*, 108885. PMID: 36505091

Gao, Z., Deng, J., & Liang, H. (2023). Legal challenges of AI in drug discovery and development. *Journal of Law and the Biosciences*, *10*(1), lsad005. Advance online publication. DOI: 10.1093/jlb/lsad005 PMID: 36938304

Gardiner, L. J., Carrieri, A. P., Bingham, K., Macluskie, G., Bunton, D., McNeil, M., & Pyzer-Knapp, E. O. (2022). Combining explainable machine learning, demographic and multi-omic data to inform precision medicine strategies for inflammatory bowel disease. *PLoS One*, *17*(2), e0263248.

Garfinkel, S., & Shelat, A. (2003). Remembrance of data passed: A study of disk sanitization practices. *IEEE Security and Privacy*, *1*(1), 17–27.

Garrido-Trigo, A., Corraliza, A. M., Veny, M., Dotti, I., Melón-Ardanaz, E., Rill, A., & Salas, A. (2023). Macrophage and neutrophil heterogeneity at single-cell spatial resolution in human inflammatory bowel disease. *Nature Communications*, *14*(1), 4506.

Gerke, S., Minssen, T., & Cohen, G. (2020). Ethical and legal challenges of artificial intelligence-driven healthcare. In Bohr, A., & Memarzadeh, K. (Eds.), *Artificial intelligence in healthcare* (pp. 295–336). Academic Press., DOI: 10.1016/B978-0-12-818438-7.00012-5

Ghasemi, F., Mehridehnavi, A., Perez-Garrido, A., & Perez-Sanchez, H. (2018). Neural network and deep-learning algorithms used in QSAR studies: Merits and drawbacks. *Drug Discovery Today*, *23*(10), 1784–1790. DOI: 10.1016/j.drudis.2018.06.016 PMID: 29936244

Ghazi Vakili, M., Gorgulla, C., Snider, J., Nigam, A., Bezrukov, D., Varoli, D., Aliper, A., Polykovsky, D., Padmanabha Das, K. M., & Cox Iii, H. (2025). Quantum-computing-enhanced algorithm unveils potential KRAS inhibitors. *Nature Biotechnology*, •••, 1–6. PMID: 39843581

Gholap, A. D., Uddin, M. J., Faiyazuddin, M., Omri, A., Gowri, S., & Khalid, M. (2024). Advances in artificial intelligence in drug delivery and development: A comprehensive review. *Computers in Biology and Medicine*, •••, 108702. PMID: 38878397

Ghosh, J. (2023a). How evidence-based nutrition science supports nutrition communication and marketing: An Indian perspective. In Ghosh, D., Bogueva, D., & Smarta, R. (Eds.), *Nutrition science, marketing nutrition, health claims, and public policy* (pp. 71–88). Academic Press. DOI: 10.1016/B978-0-323-85615-7.00007-0

Ghosh, J. (2023b). A review on understanding the risk factors for coronary heart disease in Indian college students. *International Journal of Noncommunicable Diseases*, *8*, 117–128.

Ghosh, J., Chaudhuri, D., Saha, I., & Nag Chaudhuri, A. (2022). Association of conicity index with different cardiovascular disease risk factors among the rural elderly women of West Bengal, India. *Indian Journal of Community Medicine : Official Publication of Indian Association of Preventive & Social Medicine*, *47*, 18–22.

Ghosh, J., Choudhury, S. R., Singh, K., & Koner, S. (2024a). Application of machine learning algorithm and artificial intelligence in improving metabolic syndrome related complications: A review. *International Journal of Advancement in Life Sciences Research*, *7*(2), 41–67.

Ghosh, J., Shakil, S., Singh, K., & Mandal, S. (2024b). Depression and cognitive function in accordance with the nutritional status of elderly women residing in Rajarhat-Newtown area of Kolkata, India. *Medical Journal of Dr. D.Y. Patil Vidyapeeth*, *17*(5), 951–956. DOI: 10.4103/mjdrdypu.mjdrdypu_423_23

Ghosh, J., Taneja, J., & Kant, R. (2025). Nutritional and lifestyle predictors of rectal bleeding in functional constipation: A machine learning approach. *International Journal of Medical Informatics*, *201*, 105963. Advance online publication. DOI: 10.1016/j.ijmedinf.2025.105963

Ghosh, P., Muhasina, K., Swaroop, A. K., Esakkimuthukumar, M., Singh, R. P., Singh, R., Justin, A., Selvaraj, J., & Basavan, D. (2024). Artificial Intelligence in Drug Research—A New Wave of Innovation in Drug Discovery. In *Computational Approaches in Biomaterials and Biomedical Engineering Applications* (pp. 162–188). CRC Press.

Ghule, P. J., Kale, P. A., & Kale, S. P. (2024). Ai-enhanced drug discovery and pharmaceutical development. *Futuristic Trends in Pharmacy & Nursing. IIP: Chikkamagaluru, India, 3*, 254–267.

Giannini, N., Gadducci, G., Fuentes, T., Gonnelli, A., Di Martino, F., Puccini, P., Naso, M., Pasqualetti, F., Capaccioli, S., & Paiar, F. (2024). Electron FLASH radiotherapy in vivo studies. A systematic review. *Frontiers in Oncology, 14*, 1373453. DOI: 10.3389/fonc.2024.1373453

Gioia, S., Curcurullo, M., Orso, V., Avenali, M., Graffigna, G., & Canetti, M. (2023). Mobile apps for dietary and food timing assessment. *PLoS One, 18*(8), e0288949. DOI: 10.1371/journal.pone.0288949

Giriprasath, K. S., Pandiyarajan, P., Santhosh, C., Aneesh, K., & Vasanth, R. (2024). Revolutionizing drug development: navigating the convergence of artificial intelligence and pharmaceutical innovation. In *Analyzing Explainable AI in Healthcare and the Pharmaceutical Industry* (pp. 154–180). IGI Global Scientific Publishing.

Goertzel, B. (2014). Artificial general intelligence: Concept, state of the art, and future prospects. *Journal of Artificial General Intelligence, 5*(1), 1.

Goh, G. B., Siegel, C., Vishnu, A., Hodas, N. O., & Baker, N. (2017). *Chemception: A Deep Neural Network with Minimal Chemistry Knowledge Matches the Performance of Expert-developed QSAR/QSPR Models.*

Goldberg Jana, M., Amin Nivee, P., Zachariah Krista, A., & Bhatt Ami, B. (2024). The introduction of AI into decentralized clinical trials. *JACC Advances, 3*(8), 101094. DOI: 10.1016/j.jacadv.2024.101094

Goldman, E. (2021). The story of the California Consumer Privacy Act (CCPA), version 1.0. In *Research handbook on information law and governance* (pp. 300–308). Edward Elgar Publishing.

Gomase, V. S., Ghatule, A. P., Sharma, R., & Dhamane, S. P. (2025). Quantum computing in drug discovery techniques, challenges, and emerging opportunities. *Current Drug Discovery Technologies.*

Gomez-Bombarelli, R., Wei, J. N., Duvenaud, D., Hernandez-Lobato, J. M., Sanchez-Lengeling, B., Sheberla, D., Aguilera-Iparraguirre, J., Hirzel, T. D., Adams, R. P., & Aspuru-Guzik, A. (2018). Automatic Chemical Design Using a Data-Driven Continuous Representation of Molecules. *ACS Central Science*, *4*(2), 268–276. DOI: 10.1021/acscentsci.7b00572 PMID: 29532027

Gómez-Bombarelli, R., Wei, J. N., Duvenaud, D., Hernández-Lobato, J. M., Sánchez-Lengeling, B., Sheberla, D., Aguilera-Iparraguirre, J., Hirzel, T. D., Adams, R. P., & Aspuru-Guzik, A. (2018). Automatic chemical design using a data-driven continuous representation of molecules. *ACS Central Science*, *4*(2), 268–276. PMID: 29532027

Goncharov, L., Suominen, H., & Cook, M. (2022). Dynamic consent and personalised medicine. *The Medical Journal of Australia*, *216*(11), 547–549. DOI: 10.5694/mja2.51555

Gong, D., Arbesfeld-Qiu, J. M., Perrault, E., Bae, J. W., & Hwang, W. L. (2024). Spatial oncology: Translating contextual biology to the clinic. *Cancer Cell*, *42*(10), 1653–1675. DOI: 10.1016/j.ccell.2024.09.001

Gonzalez-Garcia, I., Irurzun-Arana, I., Ruiz-Cerda, L., Hu, C., Zhou, H., Vermeulen, A., & Gomez-Mantilla, J. D. (2015). Building an inflammatory bowel disease network, a systems pharmacology approach. In *6th American conference on Pharmacometrics (ACoP-6)* (Vol. 42, No. suppl. 1, pp. S83-S84).

Gope, P., & Hwang, T. (2016). A realistic lightweight anonymous authentication protocol for securing real-time application data access in wireless sensor networks. *IEEE Transactions on Industrial Electronics*, *63*(11), 7124–7132.

Gopsill, J., Johns, G., & Hicks, B. (2021). Quantum combinatorial design. *Proceedings of the design society, 1*, 2511-2520.

Gorgulla, C. (2024). Structure-based ultra-large virtual screenings. *Computational Drug Discovery: Methods and Applications*, *2*, 441–470.

Goryanin, I., Goryanin, I., & Demin, O. (2025). Revolutionizing drug discovery: Integrating artificial intelligence with quantitative systems pharmacology. *Drug Discovery Today*, •••, 104448.

Government of India. (2019). New drugs and clinical trials rules, 2019. The Gazette of India.

Gow, S., Niranjan, M., Kanza, S., & Frey, J. G. (2022). A review of reinforcement learning in chemistry. In *Digital Discovery* (Vol. 1, Issue 5, pp. 551–567). Royal Society of Chemistry. https://doi.org/DOI: 10.1039/d2dd00047d

Granjal, J., Monteiro, E., & Sá Silva, J. (2015). Security for the Internet of Things: A survey of existing protocols and open research issues. *IEEE Communications Surveys and Tutorials*, *17*(3), 1294–1312.

Gray, I. D., Kross, A. R., Renfrew, M. E., & Wood, P. (2019). Precision Medicine in Lifestyle Medicine: The Way of the Future? *American Journal of Lifestyle Medicine*, *14*(2), 169–186. DOI: 10.1177/1559827619834527

GREGORY, B. (2020). A Molecule Designed By AI Exhibits' Druglike'Qualities. Wired. In.

Guan, J., Yao, L., Chung, C. R., Xie, P., Zhang, Y., Deng, J., & Lee, T. Y. (2023). Predicting anti-inflammatory peptides by ensemble machine learning and deep learning. *Journal of Chemical Information and Modeling*, *63*(24), 7886–7898.

Guan, X., Li, H., Zhang, L., & Zhi, H. (2025). Mechanisms of mitochondrial damage-associated molecular patterns associated with inflammatory response in cardiovascular diseases. *Inflammation Research*, *74*(1), 18. DOI: 10.1007/s00011-025-01993-x

Guedj, M., Swindle, J., Hamon, A., Hubert, S., Desvaux, E., Laplume, J., & Moingeon, P. (2022). Industrializing AI-powered drug discovery: Lessons learned from the patrimony computing platform. *Expert Opinion on Drug Discovery*, *17*(8), 815–824.

Guerreschi, G. G., & Smelyanskiy, M. (2017). Practical optimization for hybrid quantum-classical algorithms. *arXiv preprint arXiv:1701.01450.*

Guerrisi, A., Miseo, L., Falcone, I., Messina, C., Ungania, S., Elia, F., Desiderio, F., Valenti, F., Cantisani, V., Soriani, A., & Caterino, M. (2024). Quantitative ultrasound radiomics analysis to evaluate lymph nodes in patients with cancer: A systematic review. *Ultraschall in Der Medizin (Stuttgart, Germany: 1980), 45*(6), 586–596. https://doi.org/DOI: 10.1055/a-2275-8342

Guidotti, R., Monreale, A., Ruggieri, S., Turini, F., Giannotti, F., & Pedreschi, D. (2018). A survey of methods for explaining black box models. *ACM Computing Surveys*, *51*(5), 1–42.

Gundappa, M., Arumugam, V. A., Hsieh, H. L., Balasubramanian, B., & Shanmugam, V. (2022). Expression of tissue factor and TF-mediated integrin regulation in HTR-8/SVneo trophoblast cells. *Journal of Reproductive Immunology*, *150*, 103473.

Gunning, D., & Aha, D. (2019). DARPA's explainable artificial intelligence program. *AI Magazine*, *40*(2), 44–58. DOI: 10.1609/aimag.v40i2.2850

Guo, Z., Wang, Y., Liu, L., Sun, S., Feng, B., & Zhao, X. (2021). Siamese network-based few-shot learning for classification of human peripheral blood leukocyte. In *2021 IEEE 4th International Conference on Electronic Information and Communication Technology (ICEICT)* (pp. 818-822). IEEE.

Guo, S., Guan, J., & Zhou, S. (2024). Diffusing on two levels and optimizing for multiple properties: A novel approach to generating molecules with desirable properties. *IEEE/ACM Transactions on Computational Biology and Bioinformatics*.

Guo, Y., Ren, X., Chen, Y. X., & Wang, T. J. (2019). Artificial Intelligence Meets Chinese Medicine. *Chinese Journal of Integrative Medicine*, *25*(9), 648–653. DOI: 10.1007/s11655-019-3169-5 PMID: 31650485

Gupta, U., Pranav, A., Kohli, A., Ghosh, S., & Singh, D. (2024). The contribution of artificial intelligence to drug discovery: Current progress and prospects for the future. *Microbial Data Intelligence and Computational Techniques for Sustainable Computing*, 1-23.

Gupta, U., Pranav, A., Kohli, A., Ghosh, S., & Singh, D. (2024). The contribution of artificial intelligence to drug discovery: Current progress and prospects for the future. *Microbial data intelligence and computational techniques for sustainable computing, 47*, 1-23.

Gupta, A. K., & Raghavachari, K. (2022). Three-Dimensional Convolutional Neural Networks Utilizing Molecular Topological Features for Accurate Atomization Energy Predictions. *Journal of Chemical Theory and Computation*, *18*(4), 2132–2143. DOI: 10.1021/acs.jctc.1c00504 PMID: 35226496

Gupta, A., Müller, A. T., Huisman, B. J. H., Fuchs, J. A., Schneider, P., & Schneider, G. (2018). Generative Recurrent Networks for De Novo Drug Design. *Molecular Informatics*, *37*(1). Advance online publication. DOI: 10.1002/minf.201700111 PMID: 29095571

Gupta, A., Müller, A. T., Huisman, B. J., Fuchs, J. A., Schneider, P., & Schneider, G. (2018). Generative recurrent networks for de novo drug design. *Molecular Informatics*, *37*(1-2), 1700111.

Gupta, B. B., Agrawal, D. P., & Yamaguchi, S. (2014). *Handbook of research on advanced cybercrime investigation and cyberforensics*. IGI Global.

Gupta, D., Sudhakar, R., Mujawar, S. S., Kadam, R., Patil, V., Kumar, A., & Gupta, K. (2026). The potential of generative AI in drug development. In *Applications of Artificial Intelligence in Pharmaceuticals* (pp. 125–156). IGI Global Scientific Publishing.

Gupta, P., Singh, A., & Mukherjee, D. (2025). Artificial intelligence based in silico clinical trials for vaccines. https://doi.org/DOI: 10.26434/chemrxiv-2025-3nh8w

Gurard-Levin, Z. A., Scholle, M. D., Eisenberg, A. H., & Mrksich, M. (2011). High-throughput screening of small molecule libraries using SAMDI mass spectrometry. *ACS Combinatorial Science*, *13*(4), 347–350. DOI: 10.1021/co2000373 PMID: 21639106

Gu, X., Aranganathan, A., & Tiwary, P. (2024). Empowering AlphaFold2 for protein conformation selective drug discovery with AlphaFold2-RAVE. *eLife*, *13*, RP99702.

Hafez Ghoran, S., Abdjan, M. I., Kristanti, A. N., & Aminah, N. S. (2025). Insights into *in vitro* and *in silico* studies of α-glucosidase inhibitors isolated from the leaves of *Grewia optiva* (Malvaceae). *International Journal of Biological Macromolecules*, *287*, 138590. PMID: 39667462

Hafez Ghoran, S., Babaei, E., Rezaei Seresht, H., & Karimzadeh, Z. (2019). Cytotoxic constituents and molecular docking study of the active triterpenoids from *Tripleurospermum disciforme* (CA Mey.) Schultz-Bip. *Jundishapur Journal of Natural Pharmaceutical Products*, *15*(2), e65760. https://doi.org/https://doi.org/10.5812/jjnpp.65760

Hafez Ghoran, S., Firuzi, O., Pirhadi, S., Khattab, O. M., El-Seedi, H. R., & Jassbi, A. R. (2023). Sappanin-type homoisoflavonoids from *Scilla bisotunensis* Speta.: Cytotoxicity, molecular docking, and chemotaxonomic significance. *Journal of Molecular Structure*, *1273*, 134326.

Hafez Ghoran, S., Yousuf, M., Zafar, H., Abdjan, M. I., & Ayatollahi, S. A., Atia-tul-Wahab, Aminah, N. S., Kristanti, A. N., Aziz-ur-Rehman, & Choudhary, M. I. (2025). In vitro, in silico, and STD-NMR studies of flavonoids from *Hypericum helianthemoides* (Spach) Boiss. against Leishmania major pteridine reductase 1 (Lm PTR1). *Journal of Biomolecular Structure & Dynamics*, *43*(12), 6366–6380. PMID: 40025779

Hafez-Ghoran, S., Sajid, M., Abdjan, M. I., Teia, F. K. F., Siddiqui, H., Sanjaya, G. M., Ridassepri, A. F., Nadeem, F., Ayatollahi, S. A., & Choudhary, M. I. (2025). New methyl and ethyl gallate esters linked chlorinated benzoyl derivatives as anti-*Candida* albicans agents: Isolation, semi-synthesis, *in vitro* and *in silico* studies. *Chemistry & Biodiversity*, •••, 202500153. PMID: 40234190

Hafez-Ghoran, S., Wang, W., & Sang, S. (2025). Insights into phenolamides in whole grain barley: Chemical profile and their levels in barley-based products. *Journal of Agricultural and Food Chemistry*, *73*(35), 21905–21919. PMID: 40828649

Haggenmüller, S., Maron, R. C., Hekler, A., Utikal, J. S., Barata, C., Barnhill, R. L., Beltraminelli, H., Berking, C., Betz-Stablein, B., Blum, A., Braun, S. A., Carr, R., Combalia, M., Fernandez-Figueras, M.-T., Ferrara, G., Fraitag, S., French, L. E., Gellrich, F. F., Ghoreschi, K., … Brinker, T. J. (2021). Skin cancer classification via convolutional neural networks: Systematic review of studies involving human experts. *European Journal of Cancer (Oxford, England: 1990), 156*, 202–216. https://doi.org/DOI: 10.1016/j.ejca.2021.06.049

Haghighatlari, M., Marze, N., Seward, R., Ciarla, A., Hindin, R., Calderini, J., & Tourdot, S. (2025). HLAIIPred: Cross-attention mechanism for modelling the interaction of HLA class Ii molecules with peptides. *Communications Biology*, *8*(1), 1133.

Hähnel, M. (2025). Ethical challenges and solutions in AI-driven medical data management: A focus on distributed machine learning. *Discover Artificial Intelligence*, *5*(1), 53.

Halpin, H. (2007). Reinventing Technology: Artificial Intelligence from the Top of a Sycamore Tree. *CONSTITUENT IMAGINATION*, 155.

Hamano, H., Tanaka, Y., & Zamami, Y. (2025). An integrative drug discovery strategy using real-world data, in silico modelling, and network pharmacology. *Nihon yakurigaku zasshi. Folia pharmacologica Japonica, 160*(5), 352-359.

Hameed, P. N., Verspoor, K., Kusljic, S., & Halgamuge, S. (2018). A two-tiered unsupervised clustering approach for drug repositioning through heterogeneous data integration. *BMC Bioinformatics*, *19*(1). Advance online publication. DOI: 10.1186/s12859-018-2123-4 PMID: 29642848

Hamelin, B., Rowe, P., Molony, C., Kruger, M., LoCasale, R., Khan, A. H., & Jacob, D. (2022). Immunolab: Combining targeted real-world data with advanced analytics to generate evidence at scale in immunology. *Frontiers in Allergy*, *3*, 951795.

Hammi, B., Zeadally, S., Khatoun, R., & Nebhen, J. (2022). Survey on smart homes: Vulnerabilities, risks, and countermeasures. *Computers & Security*, *117*, 102677.

Han, L., Sayyid, Z. N., & Altman, R. B. (2021). Modelling drug response using network-based personalized treatment prediction (NetPTP) with applications to inflammatory bowel disease. *PLoS Computational Biology*, *17*(2), e1008631.

Hansen, K., Biegler, F., Ramakrishnan, R., Pronobis, W., von Lilienfeld, O. A., Muller, K. R., & Tkatchenko, A. (2015). Machine Learning Predictions of Molecular Properties: Accurate Many-Body Potentials and Nonlocality in Chemical Space. *The Journal of Physical Chemistry Letters*, *6*(12), 2326–2331. DOI: 10.1021/acs.jpclett.5b00831 PMID: 26113956

Harding, J. J., Telli, M., Munster, P., Voss, M. H., Infante, J. R., DeMichele, A., Dunphy, M., Le, M. H., Molineaux, C., & Orford, K. (2021). A phase I dose-escalation and expansion study of telaglenastat in patients with advanced or metastatic solid tumors. *Clinical Cancer Research, 27*(18), 4994–5003. PMID: 34285061

Hassabis, D. (2022). Alphafold reveals the structure of the protein universe. *URL https://www. deepmind. com/blog/alphafold-reveals-the-structure-of-the-protein-universe, 2.*

Hassan, B. A. R., & Mohammed, A. H. (2024). Utilizing artificial intelligence in the development of medicinal drugs: Practical applications. *Journal of Innovations in Medical Research, 3*(1), 22–25.

Hassan, M., Awan, F. M., Naz, A., deAndrés-Galiana, E. J., Alvarez, O., Cernea, A., Fernández-Brillet, L., Fernández-Martínez, J. L., & Kloczkowski, A. (2022). Innovations in Genomics and Big Data Analytics for Personalized Medicine and Health Care: A Review. *International Journal of Molecular Sciences, 23*(9), 4645. DOI: 10.3390/ijms23094645

Hassanzadeh, P., Atyabi, F., & Dinarvand, R. (2019). The significance of artificial intelligence in drug delivery system design. *Advanced Drug Delivery Reviews, 151-152*, 169–190. DOI: 10.1016/j.addr.2019.05.001 PMID: 31071378

Hayashi, E., Das, S., Amini, S., Hong, J., & Oakley, I. (2013). CASA: Context-aware scalable authentication. In *Proceedings of the Ninth Symposium on Usable Privacy and Security* (Article 3, pp. 1–10).

Hayes, D., Cappa, F., & Le-Khac, N. A. (2020). An effective approach to mobile device management: Security and privacy issues associated with mobile applications. *Digital Business, 1*(1), Article 100001.

Health, C. for D. and R. (2025). Artificial Intelligence in Software as a Medical Device. *FDA*. https://www.fda.gov/medical-devices/software-medical-device-samd/artificial-intelligence-software-medical-device

Hefti, F. F. (2008). Requirements for a lead compound to become a clinical candidate. *BMC Neuroscience, 9*(S3), S7. DOI: 10.1186/1471-2202-9-S3-S7

He, J., Baxter, S. L., Xu, J., Xu, J., Zhou, X., & Zhang, K. (2019). The practical implementation of artificial intelligence technologies in medicine. *Nature Medicine, 25*(1), 30–36. DOI: 10.1038/s41591-018-0307-0 PMID: 30617336

Henna, S. (2021). Modelling human innate immune response using graph neural networks. *IEEE Access : Practical Innovations, Open Solutions, 9*, 167117–167127.

Hervella, A. S., Rouco, J., Novo, J., & Ortega, M. (2022). Multimodal image encoding pre-training for diabetic retinopathy grading. *Computers in Biology and Medicine*, *143*, 105302. PMID: 35219187

Hickey, S. L., McKim, A., Mancuso, C. A., & Krishnan, A. (2022). A network-based drug repurposing approach identifies new treatment opportunities for the systemic chronic inflammation underlying multiple complex diseases. *Frontiers in Pharmacology*, *13*, 995459.

Hinkson, I. V., Madej, B., & Stahlberg, E. A. (2020). Accelerating Therapeutics for Opportunities in Medicine: A Paradigm Shift in Drug Discovery. *Frontiers in Pharmacology*, *11*, 770. DOI: 10.3389/fphar.2020.00770

Hirani, R., Noruzi, K., Khuram, H., Hussaini, A. S., Aifuwa, E. I., Ely, K. E., Lewis, J. M., Gabr, A. E., Smiley, A., Tiwari, R. K., & Etienne, M. (2024). Artificial intelligence and healthcare: A journey through history, present innovations, and future possibilities. *Life (Chicago, Ill.)*, *14*(5), 557. DOI: 10.3390/life14050557 PMID: 38792579

Hoces, D., Miguens Blanco, J., & Hernández-López, R. A. (2023). A synthetic biology approach to engineering circuits in immune cells. *Immunological Reviews*, *320*(1), 120–137.

Hong, N., Jiang, D., Wang, Z., Sun, H., Luo, H., Bao, L., & Hou, T. (2024). TransfIGN: a structure-based deep learning method for modelling the interaction between HLA-A* 02: 01 and antigen peptides. *Journal of Chemical Information and Modeling*, *64*(13), 5016–5027.

Hou, J., Kouznetsova, V. L., & Tsigelny, I. F. (2022). Calming the storm: Identifying multi-cytokine inhibiting drugs with machine learning for COVID-19 induced cytokine storms. *Microbiology & Infectious Diseases (Wilmington, Del.)*, *6*(1), 1–7.

Houssein, E. H., Gamal, A. M., Younis, E. M. G., & Mohamed, E. (2025). Explainable artificial intelligence for medical imaging systems using deep learning: A comprehensive review. *Cluster Computing*, *28*(7), 469. DOI: 10.1007/s10586-025-05281-5

Hou, X., Yang, F., Liu, W., Fu, Z., Chen, L., Li, Z., & Cao, G. (2015). Signalling pathways that facilitate chronic inflammation-induced carcinogenesis. *Journal of Cellular Signaling*, *1*, 9.

Huang, Q., He, Y., & Liu, K. (2025). Antibody immunogenicity prediction and optimization with ImmunoSeq. bioRxiv, 2025-08.

Huang, D., Ye, X., & Sakurai, T. (2024). Multi-party collaborative drug discovery via federated learning. *Computers in Biology and Medicine*, *171*, 108181. PMID: 38428094

Huang, D., Ye, X., Zhang, Y., & Sakurai, T. (2023). Collaborative analysis for drug discovery by federated learning on non-IID data. *Methods (San Diego, Calif.)*, *219*, 1–7. PMID: 37689121

Huang, J., Tao, G., Liu, J., Cai, J., Huang, Z., & Chen, J. X. (2020). Current Prevention of COVID-19: Natural Products and Herbal Medicine. *Frontiers in Pharmacology*, *11*, 588508. DOI: 10.3389/fphar.2020.588508 PMID: 33178026

Huang, K., Chandak, P., Wang, Q., Havaldar, S., Vaid, A., Leskovec, J., & Zitnik, M. (2024). A foundation model for clinician-centered drug repurposing. *Nature Medicine*, *30*(12), 3601–3613.

Huang, R., Sun, Y., Liu, R., Zhu, B., Zhang, H., & Wu, H. (2024). ZeXieYin formula alleviates atherosclerosis by inhibiting the MAPK/NF-κB signaling pathway in APOE-/- mice to attenuate vascular inflammation and increase plaque stability. *Journal of Ethnopharmacology*, *327*, 117969. DOI: 10.1016/j.jep.2024.117969

Huang, Y., Fang, J., Lu, W., Wang, Z., Wang, Q., Hou, Y., Jiang, X., Reizes, O., Lathia, J., Nussinov, R., Eng, C., & Cheng, F. (2019). A Systems Pharmacology Approach Uncovers Wogonoside as an Angiogenesis Inhibitor of Triple-Negative Breast Cancer by Targeting Hedgehog Signaling. *Cell Chemical Biology*, *26*(8), 1143–1158 e1146. DOI: 10.1016/j.chembiol.2019.05.004 PMID: 31178408

Hughes, J. P., Rees, S. S., Kalindjian, S. B., & Philpott, K. L. (2011). Principles of early drug discovery. In *British Journal of Pharmacology* (Vol. 162, Issue 6, pp. 1239–1249). https://doi.org/DOI: 10.1111/j.1476-5381.2010.01127.x

Hu, K., Gong, S., Zhang, Q., Seng, C., Xia, M., & Jiang, S. (2024). An overview of implementing security and privacy in federated learning. *Artificial Intelligence Review*, *57*(8), 204. DOI: 10.1007/s10462-024-10846-8

Huo, C., Nguyen, Q. N., Alishir, A., Ra, M.-J., Jung, S.-M., Yu, J.-N., Gwon, H.-J., Kang, K. S., & Kim, K. H. (2023). Global Natural Products Social (GNPS)-based molecular-networking-guided isolation of phenolic compounds from *Ginkgo biloba* fruits and the identification of estrogenic phenolic glycosides. *Plants*, *12*(23), 3970. PMID: 38068607

Hu, X. (2025). AI CAR Loop 1.0: A modular AI-driven platform for accelerated CAR-T therapy development, illustrated with CLDN18. 2-positive gastric cancer. https://doi.org/DOI: 10.21203/rs.3.rs-7350290/v1

Iacucci, M., & Santacroce, G. (2024). Multi-OMICs orchestration enabled by artificial intelligence in inflammatory bowel disease: An exciting future. *United European Gastroenterology Journal*, *12*(10), 1350.

Ienca, M., Scheibner, J., Ferretti, A., Gille, F., Amann, J., Sleigh, J., & Vayena, E. (2019). *How the General Data Protection Regulation changes the rules for scientific research: Study*. ETH Zurich.

Iivanainen, S., Ekstrom, J., Virtanen, H., Kataja, V. V., & Koivunen, J. P. (2021). Electronic patient-reported outcomes and machine learning in predicting immune-related adverse events of immune checkpoint inhibitor therapies. *BMC Medical Informatics and Decision Making*, *21*(1), 205.

Imetkul, I., Kallow, Z. S., Edrees, A. E., Akram, S. A., Sabah, A., & Zhumagaliuly, A. (2025). Understanding the immunopathogenesis of autoimmune disorders: A comprehensive review. *Trends in Immunotherapy*, *9*(3), 47–60.

Inc, L. P. (2025). *Lantern Pharma Secures EU Patent Allowance for LP-284, Bolstering Global IP Position for AI-Developed Cancer Therapy*. Lantern Pharma Inc.

Insilico Medicine. (2025, June 3). Insilico Medicine announces Nature Medicine publication of Phase IIa results evaluating Rentosertib, the novel TNIK inhibitor for idiopathic pulmonary fibrosis discovered and designed with a pioneering AI approach https://www.biospace.com/press-releases/insilico-medicine-announces-nature-medicine-publication-of-phase-iia-results-evaluating-rentosertib

International Medical Device Regulators Forum. (2022). AI and machine learning medical devices: Regulatory considerations. https://www.imdrf.org

Ioachimescu, O. C., & Shaker, R. (2025). Translational science and related disciplines. *Journal of Investigative Medicine*, *73*(1), 3–26. DOI: 10.1177/10815589241283515

Ishrat, M., Khan, W., & Ather, D. (n.d.). Cyber resilience in a digital world: Securing healthcare, agriculture, and food industry against emerging threats. In *Cyberology* (pp. 200–224). Chapman and Hall/CRC.

Isibor, E. (2024, July 25). Regulation of healthcare data security: Legal obligations in a digital age. *SSRN*. https://ssrn.com/abstract=4957244

Islas-Avila, A. L., Martinez-Rebollar, A., Castrejon-Salgado, R., Avila-Jimenez, L., Estrada-Esquivel, H., & Sanchez-Gutierrez, A. F. (2025). Classification of generalized anxiety through life history strategies with random forest and explainable machine learning. In *Mexican International Conference on Artificial Intelligence* (pp. 115-128). Cham: Springer Nature Switzerland.

Ismail, S., & Barakat, K. (2025). Neoantigen mRNA cancer vaccines: how deep learning is advancing design and breaking barriers. https://doi.org/DOI: 10.5772/intechopen.1011567

Itoh, N., Tsuya, A., Togashi, H., Kimura, H., Konta, T., Nemoto, K., Yamashita, H., & Kayama, T. (2022). Increased salt intake is associated with diabetes and characteristic dietary habits: A community-based cross-sectional study in Japan. *Journal of Clinical Biochemistry and Nutrition*, *71*(2), 143–150. DOI: 10.3164/jcbn.21-153

Ivanenkov, Y. A., Polykovskiy, D., Bezrukov, D., Zagribelnyy, B., Aladinskiy, V., Kamya, P., Aliper, A., Ren, F., & Zhavoronkov, A. (2023). Chemistry42: An AI-driven platform for molecular design and optimization. *Journal of Chemical Information and Modeling*, *63*(3), 695–701. PMID: 36728505

Iwaya, L. H., Babar, M. A., & Rashid, A. (2023). On the privacy of mental health apps. *Empirical Software Engineering*, *28*(1), 2. Advance online publication. DOI: 10.1007/s10664-022-10236-0

Jabarulla, M. Y., & Lee, H. N. (2021). A blockchain and artificial intelligence-based, patient-centric healthcare system for combating the COVID-19 pandemic: Opportunities and applications. []. Mdpi.]. *Health Care*, *9*(8), 1019.

Jaime, F. J., Muñoz, A., Rodríguez-Gómez, F., & Jerez-Calero, A. (2023). Strengthening privacy and data security in biomedical microelectromechanical systems by IoT communication security and protection in smart healthcare. *Sensors (Basel)*, *23*(21), 8944.

Jain, N., Nagaich, U., Pandey, M., Chellappan, D. K., & Dua, K. (2022). Predictive genomic tools in disease stratification and targeted prevention: A recent update in personalized therapy advancements. *The EPMA Journal*, *13*(4), 561–580. DOI: 10.1007/s13167-022-00304-2

Jaiswal, Y., Liang, Z., & Zhao, Z. (2016). Botanical drugs in Ayurveda and Traditional Chinese Medicine. *Journal of Ethnopharmacology*, *194*, 245–259. DOI: 10.1016/j.jep.2016.06.052 PMID: 27394388

Jalal, S., Nicolaou, S., & Parker, W. (2019). Artificial Intelligence, Radiology, and the Way Forward. *Canadian Association of Radiologists Journal*, *70*(1), 10–12. DOI: 10.1016/j.carj.2018.09.004 PMID: 30691556

Jang, H. Y., Song, J., Kim, J. H., Lee, H., Kim, I. W., Moon, B., & Oh, J. M. (2022). Machine learning-based quantitative prediction of drug exposure in drug-drug interactions using drug label information. *NPJ Digital Medicine*, *5*(1), 88. DOI: 10.1038/s41746-022-00639-0 PMID: 35817846

Jarab, A. S., Abu Heshmeh, S. R., & Al Meslamani, A. Z. (2024). Bridging the gap: The future of biosimilars regulations. *Human Vaccines & Immunotherapeutics*, *20*(1), 2362450.

Jarallah, S. J., Almughem, F. A., Alhumaid, N. K., Fayez, N. A., Alradwan, I., Al-sulami, K. A., & Alshehri, A. A. (2025). Artificial intelligence revolution in drug discovery: A paradigm shift in pharmaceutical innovation. *International Journal of Pharmaceutics*, •••, 125789.

Jayatunga, K. P. M., Ayers, M., Bruens, L., Jayanth, D., & Meier, C. (2024). How successful are AI-discovered drugs in clinical trials? A first analysis and emerging lessons. In *Drug Discovery Today* (Vol. 29, Issue 6). Elsevier Ltd. https://doi.org/ DOI: 10.1016/j.drudis.2024.104009

Jeddi, Z., & Bohr, A. (2020). Remote patient monitoring using artificial intelligence. In *Artificial Intelligence in Healthcare* (pp. 203–234). Elsevier., DOI: 10.1016/ B978-0-12-818438-7.00009-5

Jemielita, T. O., & Mehrotra, D. V. (2019). PRISM: patient response identifiers for stratified medicine. *arXiv preprint arXiv:1912.03337.*

Jiang, J., Chen, S., Tsou, T., McGinnis, C. S., Khazaei, T., Zhu, Q., & Thomson, M. (2022). Therapeutic algebra of immunomodulatory drug responses at single-cell resolution. *arXiv preprint arXiv:2208.10661.*

Jiang, D. (2025). Optimizing drug synthesis driven by artificial intelligence. *Theoretical and Natural Science*, *131*, 80–87.

Jiang, D., Wu, Z., Hsieh, C. Y., Chen, G., Liao, B., Wang, Z., Shen, C., Cao, D., Wu, J., & Hou, T. (2021). Could graph neural networks learn better molecular representation for drug discovery? A comparison study of descriptor-based and graph-based models. *Journal of Cheminformatics*, *13*(1). Advance online publication. DOI: 10.1186/s13321-020-00479-8 PMID: 33597034

Jiang, T., Gradus, J. L., & Rosellini, A. J. (2020). Supervised Machine Learning: A Brief Primer. *Behavior Therapy*, *51*(5), 675–687. DOI: 10.1016/j.beth.2020.05.002 PMID: 32800297

Jiang, X., Lu, L., Li, J., Jiang, J., Zhang, J., Zhou, S., & Bai, R. (2024). Synthetically feasible De Novo molecular design of leads based on a reinforcement learning model: AI-assisted discovery of an Anti-IBD lead targeting CXCR4. *Journal of Medicinal Chemistry*, *67*(12), 10057–10075.

Jia, Z.-C., Yang, X., Wu, Y.-K., Li, M., Das, D., Chen, M.-X., & Wu, J. (2024). The Art of Finding the Right Drug Target: Emerging Methods and Strategies. *Pharmacological Reviews*, *76*(5), 896–914. DOI: 10.1124/pharmrev.123.001028

Ji, B., Wang, X., Wang, X., Xu, L., & Peng, S. (2024). scDCA: Deciphering the dominant cell communication assembly of downstream functional events from single-cell RNA-seq data. *Briefings in Bioinformatics*, *26*(1), bbae663.

Jiménez-Luna, J., Grisoni, F., Weskamp, N., & Schneider, G. (2021). Artificial intelligence in drug discovery: Recent advances and future perspectives. *Expert Opinion on Drug Discovery*, *16*(9), 949–959. PMID: 33779453

Jobin, A., Ienca, M., & Vayena, E. (2019). The global landscape of AI ethics guidelines. *Nature Machine Intelligence*, *1*(9), 389–399.

Johnson, K., Williams, P., & Chen, X. (2024). Anatomy of a breach: The NutriTech Solutions incident and its implications for health data security. *Cybersecurity Case Studies Quarterly*, *7*(1), 48–63.

Johnson, M., Albizri, A., & Simsek, S. (2022). Artificial intelligence in healthcare operations to enhance treatment outcomes: A framework to predict lung cancer prognosis. *Annals of Operations Research*, *308*(1–2), 275–305. DOI: 10.1007/s10479-020-03872-6

Jokinen, E., Dumitrescu, A., Huuhtanen, J., Gligorijević, V., Mustjoki, S., Bonneau, R., & Lähdesmäki, H. (2023). TCRconv: Predicting recognition between T cell receptors and epitopes using contextualized motifs. *Bioinformatics (Oxford, England)*, *39*(1), btac788.

Jordan, M. I. (2019). Artificial Intelligence—The Revolution Hasn't Happened Yet. *Harvard Data Science Review*. Advance online publication. DOI: 10.1162/99608f92.f06c6e61

Joshi, R. P., & Kumar, N. (2021). Artificial intelligence for autonomous molecular design: A perspective. In *Molecules* (Vol. 26, Issue 22). MDPI. https://doi.org/DOI: 10.3390/molecules26226761

Joshi, C., Chaudhari, A., Joshi, C., Joshi, M., & Bagatharia, S. (2022). Repurposing of the herbal formulations: Molecular docking and molecular dynamics simulation studies to validate the efficacy of phytocompounds against SARS-CoV-2 proteins. *Journal of Biomolecular Structure & Dynamics*, *40*(18), 8405–8419. DOI: 10.1080/07391102.2021.1922095 PMID: 33988079

Joshi, R. P., & Kumar, N. (2021). Artificial intelligence for autonomous molecular design: A perspective. *Molecules (Basel, Switzerland)*, *26*(22), 6761.

Joshua, E. S. N., Bhattacharyya, D., & Rao, N. T. (2022). Managing information security risk and Internet of Things (IoT) impact on challenges of medicinal problems with complex settings: A complete systematic approach. In *Multi-chaos, fractal and multi-fractional artificial intelligence of different complex systems* (pp. 291–310). Academic Press.

Jurisica, I. (2024). Explainable biology for improved therapies in precision medicine: AI is not enough. *Best Practice & Research. Clinical Rheumatology*, *38*(4), 102006. DOI: 10.1016/j.berh.2024.102006

Kalil, A. C., Patterson, T. F., Mehta, A. K., Tomashek, K. M., Wolfe, C. R., Ghazaryan, V., Marconi, V. C., Ruiz-Palacios, G. M., Hsieh, L., & Kline, S. (2021). Baricitinib plus remdesivir for hospitalized adults with Covid-19. *The New England Journal of Medicine*, *384*(9), 795–807. PMID: 33306283

Kamuntavičius, G., Prat, A., Paquet, T., Bastas, O., Aty, H. A., Sun, Q., & Norvaišas, P. (2024). Accelerated hit identification with target evaluation, deep learning and automated labs: Prospective validation in IRAK1. *Journal of Cheminformatics*, *16*(1), 127.

Kamya, P., Ozerov, I. V., Pun, F. W., Tretina, K., Fokina, T., Chen, S., Naumov, V., Long, X., Lin, S., & Korzinkin, M. (2024). PandaOmics: An AI-driven platform for therapeutic target and biomarker discovery. *Journal of Chemical Information and Modeling*, *64*(10), 3961–3969. PMID: 38404138

Kandregula, N. (2025). Accelerating drug discovery with generative AI: Aa paradigm shift in pharmaceutical innovation and development.

Kanthi, Y., de la Zerda, A., & Smith, B. R. (2020). Nanotherapeutic Shots through the Heart of Plaque. *ACS Nano*, *14*(2), 1236–1242. DOI: 10.1021/acsnano.0c00245

Kant, S., Deepika, & Roy, S. (2025). Artificial intelligence in drug discovery and development: Transforming challenges into opportunities. *Discover Pharmaceutical Sciences*, *1*(1), 7.

Kany, S., Vollrath, J. T., & Relja, B. (2019). Cytokines in Inflammatory Disease. *International Journal of Molecular Sciences*, *20*(23), 6008. DOI: 10.3390/ijms20236008

Kapoor, G., Prakash, S., Jaiswal, V., & Singh, A. K. (2025). Chronic inflammation and cancer: Key pathways and targeted therapies. *Cancer Investigation*, *43*(1), 1–23.

Kapur, S., Chen, H., & Saxena, N. (2021). Reducing racial bias in AI models for clinical use requires a top-down intervention. *Nature Machine Intelligence*, *3*, 893–898. DOI: 10.1038/s42256-021-00362-7

Kapustina, O., Burmakina, P., Gubina, N., Serov, N., & Vinogradov, V. (2024). User-friendly and industry-integrated AI for medicinal chemists and pharmaceuticals. *Artificial Intelligence Chemistry.*, •••, 100072.

Karger, E., & Kureljusic, M. (2022). Using artificial intelligence for drug discovery: A bibliometric study and future research agenda. *Pharmaceuticals*, *15*(12), 1492. PMID: 36558943

Katkar, G. D., Sayed, I., Anandachar, M. S., Castillo, V., Vidales, E., Toobian, D., & Ghosh, P. (2021). AI-guided use of balanced peroxisome proliferator-activated receptor a/g dual agonist finetunes macrophage responses in inflammatory bowel disease. *The Journal of Immunology : Official Journal of the American Association of Immunologists*, *206*(1, Supplement), 109–01.

Katsoulakis, E., Wang, Q., Wu, H., Shahriyari, L., Fletcher, R., Liu, J., & Deng, J. (2024). Digital twins for health: A scoping review. *npj. Digital Medicine*, *7*(1), 77. DOI: 10.1038/s41746-024-01073-0

Kaur, S., & Sharma, H. (2025). Causal representation learning for predicting autoimmune disease progression from longitudinal multimodal clinical data. *13*, 150010-150027. *IEEE Access.*

Kaur, R., Bhardwaj, A., & Gupta, S. (2023). Cancer treatment therapies: Traditional to modern approaches to combat cancers. *Molecular Biology Reports*, *50*(11), 9663–9676. DOI: 10.1007/s11033-023-08809-3

Kaur, S., & Sharma, H. (2025). Causal representation learning for predicting autoimmune disease progression from longitudinal multimodal clinical data. *IEEE Access : Practical Innovations, Open Solutions*, *13*, 150010–150027.

Kengkanna, A., & Ohue, M. (2024). Enhancing property and activity prediction and interpretation using multiple molecular graph representations with MMGX. *Communications Chemistry*, *7*(1). Advance online publication. DOI: 10.1038/s42004-024-01155-w PMID: 38580841

Kessler, F. (2022). MyFitnessPal breach revisited: New findings and continuing vulnerabilities. *International Journal of Information Security*, *21*(4), 378–392.

Khan, M. F., & Sakamura, K. (2015). Context-aware access control for clinical information systems. In *2015 International Conference on Innovations in Information, Embedded and Communication Systems* (pp. 1–6).

Khanna, I. (2012). Drug discovery in pharmaceutical industry: Productivity challenges and trends. *Drug Discovery Today*, *17*(19–20), 1088–1102. DOI: 10.1016/j.drudis.2012.05.007 PMID: 22627006

Khan, S. R., Al Rijjal, D., Piro, A., & Wheeler, M. B. (2021). Integration of AI and traditional medicine in drug discovery. *Drug Discovery Today*, *26*(4), 982–992. DOI: 10.1016/j.drudis.2021.01.008 PMID: 33476566

Khan, S. R., Manialawy, Y., Wheeler, M. B., & Cox, B. J. (2019). Unbiased data analytic strategies to improve biomarker discovery in precision medicine. *Drug Discovery Today*, *24*(9), 1735–1748. DOI: 10.1016/j.drudis.2019.05.018 PMID: 31158511

Khater, T., Alkhatib, S. A., AlShehhi, A., Pitsalidis, C., Pappa, A. M., Ngo, S. T., & Truong, V. K. (2025). Generative artificial intelligence based models optimization towards molecule design enhancement. *Journal of Cheminformatics*, *17*(1), 116.

Khurana, D., Koli, A., Khatter, K., & Singh, S. (2023). Natural language processing: State of the art, current trends and challenges. *Multimedia Tools and Applications*, *82*(3), 3713–3744. DOI: 10.1007/s11042-022-13428-4 PMID: 35855771

Kidd, B. A., & Dudley, J. T. (2015). Systems immunology. In *Translational Immunology: Mechanisms and Pharmacologic Approaches* (pp. 4-32). Academia Press.

Kiessling, P., & Kuppe, C. (2024). Spatial multi-omics: Novel tools to study the complexity of cardiovascular diseases. *Genome Medicine*, *16*(1), 14. DOI: 10.1186/s13073-024-01282-y

Kim, J., Ryu, S., Park, H., & Seok, C. (2025). SHARP: generating synthesizable molecules via fragment-based hierarchical action-space reinforcement learning for pareto optimization. bioRxiv, 2025-07.

Kim, E., Choi, A. S., & Nam, H. (2019). Drug repositioning of herbal compounds via a machine-learning approach. *BMC Bioinformatics*, *20*(Suppl 10), 247. DOI: 10.1186/s12859-019-2811-8 PMID: 31138103

Kim, H. Y., Kim, H. R., & Lee, S. H. (2014). Advances in systems biology approaches for autoimmune diseases. *Immune Network*, *14*(2), 73–80.

Kim, H., Kim, E., Lee, I., Bae, B., Park, M., & Nam, H. (2020). Artificial Intelligence in Drug Discovery: A Comprehensive Review of Data-driven and Machine Learning Approaches. *Biotechnology and Bioprocess Engineering; BBE*, *25*(6), 895–930. DOI: 10.1007/s12257-020-0049-y PMID: 33437151

Kingham, R., Klasa, G., & Carver, K. H. (2010). Key regulatory guidelines for the development of biologics in the United States and Europe. *Pharmaceutical Sciences Encyclopedia: Drug Discovery, Development, and Manufacturing*, 1-36.

Kitani, T., Maddipatla, S. C., Madupuri, R., Baraniuk, J. N., Greco, C., Hartman, J., & Vasudevan, S. (2020). In search of newer targets for IBD: a systems and a network medicine approach. *arXiv preprint arXiv:2006.04181*.

Kitchen, D. B., Decornez, H., Furr, J. R., & Bajorath, J. (2004). Docking and scoring in virtual screening for drug discovery: Methods and applications. *Nature Reviews. Drug Discovery*, *3*(11), 935–949. DOI: 10.1038/nrd1549

Kleeberger, J. A. (2025). Virtual patients in clinical trials for drug development: A narrative review. *Cureus*, *17*(6), e85380. DOI: 10.7759/cureus.85380

Klee, E. W., Cousin, M. A., Pinto, E., Vairo, F., Morales-Rosado, J. A., Macke, E. L., Jenkinson, W. G., Ferrer, A., Schultz-Rogers, L. E., Olson, R. J., Oliver, G. R., Sigafoos, A. N., Schwab, T. L., Zimmermann, M. T., Urrutia, R. A., Kaiwar, C., Gupta, A., Blackburn, P. R., Boczek, N. J., & Lazaridis, K. N. (2021). Impact of integrated translational research on clinical exome sequencing. *Genetics in Medicine: Official Journal of the American College of Medical Genetics*, *23*(3), 498–507. DOI: 10.1038/s41436-020-01005-9

Klopp-Schulze, L., Shaw, J. V., Dong, J. Q., Khandelwal, A., Vazquez-Mateo, C., & Goteti, K. (2022). Applying modeling and simulations for rational dose selection of novel toll-like receptor 7/8 inhibitor enpatoran for indications of high medical need. *Clinical Pharmacology and Therapeutics*, *112*(2), 297–306. PMID: 35390178

Kolasa, K., Admassu, B., Hołownia-Voloskova, M., Kędzior, K. J., Poirrier, J. E., & Perni, S. (2024). Systematic reviews of machine learning in healthcare: A literature review. *Expert Review of Pharmacoeconomics & Outcomes Research*, *24*(1), 63–115. PMID: 37955147

Kolbinger, F. R., Veldhuizen, G. P., Zhu, J., Truhn, D., & Kather, J. N. (2024). Reporting guidelines in medical artificial intelligence: A systematic review and meta-analysis. *Communications Medicine*, *4*(1), 71. DOI: 10.1038/s43856-024-00492-0

Kolluri, S., Lin, J., Liu, R., Zhang, Y., & Zhang, W. (2022). Machine learning and artificial intelligence in pharmaceutical research and development: A review. *The AAPS Journal*, *24*(1). Advance online publication. DOI: 10.1208/s12248-021-00644-3 PMID: 34984579

Komi, L. S., Mustapha, A. Y., Forkuo, A. Y., & Osamika, D. (2025). Reviewing pharmacovigilance strategies using real-world data for drug safety monitoring and management. *International Journal of Scientific Research in Computer Science. Engineering and Information Technology*, *11*(2), 3771–3779.

Korenstein, D., Harris, R., Elshaug, A. G., Ross, J. S., Morgan, D. J., Cooper, R. J., & Segal, J. B. (2021). To expand the evidence base about harms from tests and treatments. *Journal of General Internal Medicine, 1*, 1–6.

Koscher, B. A., Canty, R. B., McDonald, M. A., Greenman, K. P., McGill, C. J., Bilodeau, C. L., & Jensen, K. F. (2023). Autonomous, multiproperty-driven molecular discovery: From predictions to measurements and back. *Science*, *382*(6677), eadi1407.

Koul, P., & Koul, I. B. (2025). Applications of artificial intelligence and robotics in pharmaceutical sciences: advancing drug discovery, personalized medicine, and pharmaceutical manufacturing. *Tropical Journal of Pharmaceutical and Life Sciences, 12*(2), 01-21.

Koutsoukas, A., Monaghan, K. J., Li, X., & Huan, J. (2017). Deep-learning: Investigating deep neural networks hyper-parameters and comparison of performance to shallow methods for modeling bioactivity data. *Journal of Cheminformatics*, *9*(1), 42. DOI: 10.1186/s13321-017-0226-y PMID: 29086090

Krishnan, K., Chugh, A., Rajaram, R., Sridharan, S., Setlur, A. S., Uttarkar, A., & Niranjan, V. (2025). Computational modelling and optimization of peptide-based CAR-T cell receptors targeting CD19 for enhanced efficacy and minimized toxicity. https://doi.org/DOI: 10.21203/rs.3.rs-6115435/v2

Krittanawong, C., Johnson, K. W., Rosenson, R. S., Wang, Z., Aydar, M., Baber, U., Min, J. K., Tang, W. H. W., & Halperin, J. L. (2019). Artificial intelligence in precision cardiovascular medicine. *Journal of the American College of Cardiology*, *69*(21), 2657–2664. PMID: 28545640

Krittanawong, C., Zhang, H., Wang, Z., Aydar, M., & Kitai, T. (2017). Artificial Intelligence in Precision Cardiovascular Medicine. *Journal of the American College of Cardiology*, *69*(21), 2657–2664. DOI: 10.1016/j.jacc.2017.03.571

Kuang, Z., Thomson, J., Caldwell, M., Peissig, P., Stewart, R., & Page, D. (2016). Computational drug repositioning using continuous self-controlled case series. In *Proceedings of the 22nd ACM SIGKDD international conference on knowledge discovery and data mining* (pp. 491-500).

Kuchi Bhotla, H., Kaul, T., Balasubramanian, B., Easwaran, M., Arumugam, V. A., Pappusamy, M., Muthupandian, S., & Meyyazhagan, A. (2020). Platelets to surrogate lung inflammation in COVID-19 patients. *Medical Hypotheses*, *143*, 110098.

Kulkarni, A., Wang, Y., Gopinath, M., Sobien, D., Rahman, A., & Batarseh, F. A. (2024). A review of cybersecurity incidents in the food and agriculture sector. *arXiv*.

Kumar, M. A., & Sisir, A. T. (2025). Generative Ai: A new paradigm for antibody design and development. *Journal of Advances in Computational Sciences and Information Technology*, *13*(1), 37.

Kumar, R. (2025). AI-generated drug innovations and indian patent law: legal challenges and ethical responses. *Preprints*. https://doi.org/DOI: 10.20944/preprints202506.1166.v1

Kurji, C. N. Transforming drug discovery with AI and computational biophysics.

Kushwaha, V., Prabha, A., Sharma, V., Devi, A., Ramniwas, S., Sharma, A., & Kaur, D. (2024). Immunoinformatics: computational keys to immune system secrets. *Bioinformatics: Drug Discovery*, 123.

Laigle, L., Chadli, L., & Moingeon, P. (2023). Biomarker-driven development of new therapies for autoimmune diseases: Current status and future promises. *Expert Review of Clinical Immunology*, *19*(3), 305–314.

Lai, X., Wang, X., Hu, Y., Su, S., Li, W., & Li, S. (2020). Editorial: Network Pharmacology and Traditional Medicine. *Frontiers in Pharmacology*, *11*, 1194. DOI: 10.3389/fphar.2020.01194 PMID: 32848794

Landais, P., Gueguen, S., Clement, A., & Amselem, S., & RaDiCo Program. (2025). The RaDiCo information system for rare disease cohorts. *Orphanet Journal of Rare Diseases*, *20*(1), 166. DOI: 10.1186/s13023-025-03629-z

Landwehr, C. E., Bull, A. R., McDermott, J. P., & Choi, W. S. (1994). A taxonomy of computer program security flaws. *ACM Computing Surveys*, *26*(3), 211–254.

Laubenbacher, R., Niarakis, A., Helikar, T., An, G., Shapiro, B., Malik-Sheriff, R. S., & Glazier, J. A. (2022). Building digital twins of the human immune system: Toward a roadmap. *NPJ Digital Medicine*, *5*(1), 64.

Laude, M. C., Lebras, L., Sesques, P., Ghesquieres, H., Favre, S., Bouabdallah, K., Croizier, C., Guieze, R., Drieu La Rochelle, L., & Gyan, E. (2021). First-line treatment of double-hit and triple-hit lymphomas: Survival and tolerance data from a retrospective multicenter French study. *American Journal of Hematology*, *96*(3), 302–311. PMID: 33306213

Laurentino Schwabe, D. The METRIC-framework for assessing data quality for trustworthy AI in medicine: a systematic review.

Lavecchia, A. (2025). Explainable artificial intelligence in drug discovery: Bridging predictive power and mechanistic insight. *Wiley Interdisciplinary Reviews. Computational Molecular Science*, *15*(5), e70049.

Lax, T., Fallach, N., Stemmer, E., Shrem, G., & Salmon-Divon, M. (2025). Early risk prediction for biologic therapy in psoriasis using machine learning models based on routine health records. *Journal of Clinical Medicine*, *14*(18), 6421.

Lee, D. (2019). Case study: IBM Watson Health and the challenge of AI in medicine. *Journal of the American Medical Informatics Association : JAMIA*, *26*(11), 1618–1622. DOI: 10.1093/jamia/ocz143

Lee, J., Yoon, W., Kim, S., Kim, D., Kim, S., So, C. H., & Kang, J. (2020). BioBERT: A pre-trained biomedical language representation model for biomedical text mining. *Bioinformatics (Oxford, England)*, *36*(4), 1234–1240. PMID: 31501885

Lee, K., Mai, Y., Liu, Z., Raja, K., Jun, T., Ma, M., & Wang, X. (2024). CriteriaMapper: Establishing the automatic identification of clinical trial cohorts from electronic health records by matching normalized eligibility criteria and patient clinical characteristics. *Scientific Reports*, *14*(1), 25387. DOI: 10.1038/s41598-024-77447-x

Lee, S. I., & Topol, E. J. (2024). The clinical potential of counterfactual AI models. *Lancet*, *403*(10428), 717.

Lee, T. H., Liu, P. S., Wang, S. J., Tsai, M. M., Shanmugam, V., & Hsieh, H. L. (2021). Bradykinin, as a reprogramming factor, induces transdifferentiation of brain astrocytes into neuron-like cells. *Biomedicines*, *9*(8), 923.

Lee, W. Y., Lee, C. Y., Kim, Y. S., & Kim, C. E. (2019). The Methodological Trends of Traditional Herbal Medicine Employing Network Pharmacology. *Biomolecules*, *9*(8). Advance online publication. DOI: 10.3390/biom9080362 PMID: 31412658

Lee, Y., Min, J., Kim, S., Park, W., Ko, J., & Jeon, N. L. (2025). Recapitulating the cancer-immunity cycle on a chip. *Advanced Healthcare Materials*, *14*(1), 2401927.

Lee, Y., Xu, Y., Gao, P., & Chen, J. (2024). Tenet: Triple-enhancement based graph neural network for cell-cell interaction network reconstruction from spatial transcriptomics. *Journal of Molecular Biology*, *436*(9), 168543.

Lee, Y.-Y., Guler, M., Chigumba, D. N., Wang, S., Mittal, N., Miller, C., Krummenacher, B., Liu, H., Cao, L., & Kannan, A. (2023). HypoRiPPAtlas as an Atlas of hypothetical natural products for mass spectrometry database search. *Nature Communications*, *14*(1), 4219. PMID: 37452020

Leung, H., Duan, C., Gou, W., Chen, J., Xin, Y., Zheng, Z., & Zhavoronkov, A. (2025). Advancing target discovery through disease-specific integration of multimodal target identification models and comprehensive target benchmarking system. bioRxiv, 2025-08.

Li, Y., Zhang, C., Zhang, X., & Zhang, Y. (2024b). TCRfinder: Improved TCR virtual screening for novel antigenic peptides with tailored language models. bioRxiv, 2024-06.

Liebman, M. (2022). The role of artificial intelligence in drug discovery and development. *Chemistry International*, *44*(1), 16–19.

Li, F., Ruijs, N., & Lu, Y. (2023). Ethics & AI: A systematic review on ethical concerns and related strategies for designing with AI in healthcare. *AI*, *4*(1), 28–53. DOI: 10.3390/ai4010003

Lin, Z., Akin, H., Rao, R., Hie, B., Zhu, Z., Lu, W., Smetanin, N., Verkuil, R., Kabeli, O., & Shmueli, Y. (2023). Evolutionary-scale prediction of atomic-level protein structure with a language model. *science, 379*(6637), 1123-1130.

Lin, A., Wang, Z., Jiang, A., Chen, L., Qi, C., Zhu, L., & Luo, P. (2025). Large language models in clinical trials: Applications, technical advances, and future directions. *BMC Medicine*, *23*(1), 563. DOI: 10.1186/s12916-025-04348-9

Lindsey, M. L., Brunt, K. R., Kirk, J. A., Kleinbongard, P., Calvert, J. W., de Castro Brás, L. E., DeLeon-Pennell, K. Y., Del Re, D. P., Frangogiannis, N. G., Frantz, S., Gumina, R. J., Halade, G. V., Jones, S. P., Ritchie, R. H., Spinale, F. G., Thorp, E. B., Ripplinger, C. M., & Kassiri, Z. (2021). Guidelines for in vivo mouse models of myocardial infarction. *American Journal of Physiology. Heart and Circulatory Physiology*, *321*(6), H1056–H1073. DOI: 10.1152/ajpheart.00459.2021

Lindsley, C. W. (2014). *New statistics on the cost of new drug development and the trouble with CNS drugs* (Vol. 5). ACS Publications.

Lin, J., Zhu, S., Yin, M., Xue, H., Liu, L., Liu, X., & Zhu, J. (2024). Few-shot learning for the classification of intestinal tuberculosis and Crohn's disease on endoscopic images: A novel learn-to-learn framework. *Heliyon*, *10*(4).

Lin, K., Wang, A., Zhai, C., Zhao, Y., Hu, H., Huang, D., Zhai, Q., Yan, Y., & Ge, J. (2025). Semaglutide protects against diabetes-associated cardiac inflammation via Sirt3-dependent RKIP pathway. *British Journal of Pharmacology*, *182*(7), 1561–1581. DOI: 10.1111/bph.17327

Lin, M., Guo, J., Gu, Z., Tang, W., Tao, H., You, S., Jia, D., Sun, Y., & Jia, P. (2025). Machine learning and multi-omics integration: Advancing cardiovascular translational research and clinical practice. *Journal of Translational Medicine*, *23*(1), 388. DOI: 10.1186/s12967-025-06425-2

Lin, T.-Y., & Chou, L.-C. (2025). A systematic review of artificial intelligence applications and methodological advances in patent analysis. *World Patent Information, 82*, 102383.

Lin, Y. C., Huang, W. T., Ou, S. C., Hung, H. H., Cheng, W. Z., Lin, S. S., Lin, H. J., & Huang, S. T. (2019). Neural network analysis of Chinese herbal medicine prescriptions for patients with colorectal cancer. *Complementary Therapies in Medicine, 42*, 279–285. DOI: 10.1016/j.ctim.2018.12.001 PMID: 30670255

Lin, Z., & Chou, W.-C. (2022). Machine Learning and Artificial Intelligence in Toxicological Sciences. *Toxicological Sciences, 189*(1), 7–19. DOI: 10.1093/toxsci/kfac075

Lionta, E., Spyrou, G. K., Vassilatis, D., & Cournia, Z. (2014). Structure-based virtual screening for drug discovery: Principles, applications and recent advances. *Current Topics in Medicinal Chemistry, 14*(16), 1923–1938. PMID: 25262799

Li, S., Zhu, P., Cai, G., Li, J., Huang, T., & Tang, W. (2023). Application of machine learning models in predicting insomnia severity: An integrative approach with constitution of traditional Chinese medicine. *Frontiers in Medicine, 10*, 1292761. DOI: 10.3389/fmed.2023.1292761 PMID: 37928471

Li, T., Chen, X., & Tong, W. (2024). Bridging organ transcriptomics for advancing multiple organ toxicity assessment with a generative AI approach. *NPJ Digital Medicine, 7*(1), 310.

Liu, C., Wang, Y., Zhou, L., Cai, F., Tang, X., Wang, L., & Zhang, X. (2025). Exploration of potential biomarkers and immune cell infiltration characteristics for peripheral atherosclerosis in sjögren's syndrome based on comprehensive bioinformatics analysis and machine learning. *Frontiers in Genetics, 16*, 1546315. DOI: 10.3389/fgene.2025.1546315

Liu, G. P., Yan, J. J., Wang, Y. Q., Zheng, W., Zhong, T., Lu, X., & Qian, P. (2014). Deep learning based syndrome diagnosis of chronic gastritis. *Computational and Mathematical Methods in Medicine, 938350*. Advance online publication. DOI: 10.1155/2014/938350 PMID: 24734118

Liu, G., Catacutan, D. B., Rathod, K., Swanson, K., Jin, W., Mohammed, J. C., Chiappino-Pepe, A., Syed, S. A., Fragis, M., & Rachwalski, K. (2023). Deep learning-guided discovery of an antibiotic targeting Acinetobacter baumannii. *Nature Chemical Biology, 19*(11), 1342–1350. PMID: 37231267

Liu, H., Wang, Y., Huang, Y., Xiong, D., Shen, J., Siqueiros, L., & Daar, E. S. (2022). Ingestible sensor system for measuring, monitoring and enhancing adherence to antiretroviral therapy: An open-label, usual care-controlled, randomized trial. *EBioMedicine*, *86*, 104330. DOI: 10.1016/j.ebiom.2022.104330

Liu, M., Yue, Y., Chen, X., Xian, K., Dong, C., Shi, M., Xiong, H., Tian, K., Li, Y., Zhang, Q. C., & He, A. (2025). Genome-coverage single-cell histone modifications for embryo lineage tracing. *Nature*, *640*(8059), 828–839. DOI: 10.1038/s41586-025-08656-1

Liu, Q., Ma, Y., Alhussein, M., Zhang, Y., & Peng, L. (2016). Green data center with IoT sensing and cloud-assisted smart temperature control system. *Computer Networks*, *101*, 104–112. DOI: 10.1016/j.comnet.2016.01.010

Liu, W., Puri, A., Fu, D., Chen, L., Wang, C., Kellis, M., & Yang, J. (2024). Dissecting the tumor microenvironment in response to immune checkpoint inhibitors via single-cell and spatial transcriptomics. *Clinical & Experimental Metastasis*, *41*(4), 313–332.

Liu, X., Zhang, J., Wang, X., Teng, M., Wang, G., & Zhou, X. (2025a). Application of artificial intelligence large language models in drug target discovery. *Frontiers in Pharmacology*, *16*, 1597351.

Liu, X., Zhu, F., & Ma, H, X., Shi, Z., Y Yang, S., Q Wei, Y., & Z Chen, Y. (2013). Predicting targeted polypharmacology for drug repositioning and multi-target drug discovery. *Current Medicinal Chemistry*, *20*(13), 1646–1661.

Liu, Y. T., Zhang, L. L., Jiang, Z. Y., Tian, X. S., Li, P. L., Wu, P. H., & Sun, C. (2025b). Applications of artificial intelligence in biotech drug discovery and product development. *MedComm*, *6*(8), e70317.

Li, W., Wang, H., Zhao, J., Xia, J., & Sun, X. (2024a). scHyper: Reconstructing cell–cell communication through hypergraph neural networks. *Briefings in Bioinformatics*, *25*(5), bbae436.

Li, X., Ren, J., Zhang, W., Zhang, Z., Yu, J., Wu, J., Sun, H., Zhou, S., Yan, K., Yan, X., & Wang, W. (2022). LTM-TCM: A comprehensive database for the linking of Traditional Chinese Medicine with modern medicine at molecular and phenotypic levels. *Pharmacological Research*, *178*, 106185. DOI: 10.1016/j.phrs.2022.106185 PMID: 35306140

Li, Y. X., Zhong, Z., Zhang, W. P., & Qian, P. Y. (2018). Discovery of cationic nonribosomal peptides as Gram-negative antibiotics through global genome mining. *Nature Communications*, *9*(1), 3273. DOI: 10.1038/s41467-018-05781-6 PMID: 30115920

Li, Y., Liu, B., Deng, J., Guo, Y., & Du, H. (2024). Image-based molecular representation learning for drug development: A survey. *Briefings in Bioinformatics*, *25*(4). Advance online publication. DOI: 10.1093/bib/bbae294 PMID: 38920347

Li, Y., Peng, H., Zhao, H., Han, X., Zhang, P., Ning, J., & Hao, F. (2025). A novel approach for antibody affinity maturation using AI-driven mutation prediction. *Cancer Research*, *85*(8, Supplement_1), 5679–5679.

Li, Y., Wu, F., Ge, W., Zhang, Y., Hu, Y., Zhao, L., Gou, W., Shi, J., Ni, Y., Li, L., Fu, W., Lin, X., Yu, Y., Han, Z., Chen, C., Xu, R., Zhang, S., Zhou, L., Pan, G., & Luo, D. (2024). Risk stratification of papillary thyroid cancers using multidimensional machine learning. *International Journal of Surgery (London, England)*, *110*(1), 372–384. DOI: 10.1097/JS9.0000000000000814

Lo, Y.-C., Ren, G., Honda, H., & Davis, L. K. (2020). Artificial Intelligence-Based Drug Design and Discovery. In *Cheminformatics and its Applications*. IntechOpen. https://doi.org/DOI: 10.5772/intechopen.89012

Locke, C. A., & Stoll, A. L. (2001). Omega-3 fatty acids in major depression. *World Review of Nutrition and Dietetics*, *89*, 173–185. DOI: 10.1159/000059784

Long, A., Kleiner, A., & Looney, R. J. (2023). Immune dysregulation. *The Journal of Allergy and Clinical Immunology*, *151*(1), 70–80.

Lopez-Perez, L., Merino, B., Rujas, M., Maccaro, A., Guillén, S., Pecchia, L., & Fico, G. (2024). Regulatory frameworks and validation strategies for advancing artificial intelligence in healthcare. In *European Medical and Biological Engineering Conference* (pp. 260-265). Cham: Springer Nature Switzerland.

Lotter, W., Kreiman, G., & Cox, D. (2020). A neural network trained for prediction mimics diverse features of biological neurons and perception. *Nature Machine Intelligence*, *2*(4), 210–219. DOI: 10.1038/s42256-020-0170-9 PMID: 34291193

Lu, M., Covert, I., White, N. J., & Lee, S. I. (2024). CODE-XAI: construing and deciphering treatment effects via explainable ai using real-world data. medRxiv, 2024-09.

Lubitz, S. A., Faranesh, A. Z., Selvaggi, C., Atlas, S. J., McManus, D. D., Singer, D. E., & Foulkes, A. S. (2022). Detection of atrial fibrillation in a large population using wearable devices: The fitbit heart study. *Circulation*, *146*(19), 1415–1424. DOI: 10.1161/circulationaha.122.060291

Lund, B., Orhan, Z., Mannuru, N. R., Bevara, R. V. K., Porter, B., Vinaih, M. K., & Bhaskara, P. (2025). Standards, frameworks, and legislation for artificial intelligence (AI) transparency. *AI and Ethics*, •••, 1–17.

Lu, T., Zhang, Z., Zhu, J., Wang, Y., Jiang, P., Xiao, X., & Wang, T. (2021). Deep learning-based prediction of the T cell receptor–antigen binding specificity. *Nature Machine Intelligence*, *3*(10), 864–875.

Lutgens, E., Atzler, D., Döring, Y., Duchene, J., Steffens, S., & Weber, C. (2019). Immunotherapy for cardiovascular disease. *European Heart Journal*, *40*(48), 3937–3946. DOI: 10.1093/eurheartj/ehz283

Lu, X., Ma, W., Fan, B., Li, P., Gao, J., Liu, Q., Hu, C., Li, Y., Yao, M., Ning, H., & Xing, L. (2021). Integrating Network Pharmacology, Transcriptome and Artificial Intelligence for Investigating Into the Effect and Mechanism of Ning Fei Ping Xue Decoction Against the Acute Respiratory Distress Syndrome. *Frontiers in Pharmacology*, *12*, 731377. DOI: 10.3389/fphar.2021.731377 PMID: 34803679

Lyne, P. D. (2002). Structure-based virtual screening: An overview. *Drug Discovery Today*, *7*(20), 1047–1055. PMID: 12546894

Lynn, L. A. (2019). Artificial intelligence systems for complex decision-making in acute care medicine: A review. *Patient Safety in Surgery*, *13*, 6. DOI: 10.1186/s13037-019-0188-2 PMID: 30733829

Madathil, N. T., Dankar, F. K., Gergely, M., Belkacem, A. N., & Alrabaee, S. (2025). Revolutionizing healthcare data analytics with federated learning: A comprehensive survey of applications, systems, and future directions. *Computational and Structural Biotechnology Journal*, *28*, 217–238. DOI: 10.1016/j.csbj.2025.06.009

Madrid-Paredes, A., Martín, J., & Márquez, A. (2022). -Omic approaches and treatment response in rheumatoid arthritis. *Pharmaceutics*, *14*(8), 1648.

Madugula, S. S., John, L., Nagamani, S., Gaur, A. S., Poroikov, V. V., & Sastry, G. N. (2021). Molecular descriptor analysis of approved drugs using unsupervised learning for drug repurposing. *Computers in Biology and Medicine*, *138*, 104856. DOI: 10.1016/J.COMPBIOMED.2021.104856 PMID: 34555571

Mahmoud, A., & Awad, W. A. (2025). AI-driven laboratory automation: transforming experimental phases of drug discovery. In *The Role of Artificial Intelligence in Advancing Applied Life Sciences* (pp. 361–378). IGI Global Scientific Publishing.

Maia, E. H. B., Assis, L. C., de Oliveira, T. A., da Silva, A. M., & Taranto, A. G. (2020). Structure-Based Virtual Screening: From Classical to Artificial Intelligence. In *Frontiers in Chemistry* (Vol. 8). Frontiers Media S.A. https://doi.org/DOI: 10.3389/fchem.2020.00343

Ma, J., Wang, S., Zhao, C., Yan, X., Ren, Q., Dong, Z., & Liu, S. (2023). Computer-aided discovery of potent broad-spectrum vaccine adjuvants. *Angewandte Chemie International Edition*, *62*(18), e202301059.

Mak, K. K., Wong, Y. H., & Pichika, M. R. (2024). Artificial intelligence in drug discovery and development. *Drug discovery and evaluation: safety and pharmacokinetic assays*, 1461-1498.

Mak, K.-K., Wong, Y.-H., & Pichika, M. R. (2024). Artificial intelligence in drug discovery and development. *Drug discovery and evaluation: safety and pharmacokinetic assays*, 1461-1498.

Mak, K. K., Pichika, M. R., & Sun, J. (2022). Artificial intelligence in drug development: A systematic review. *Drug Discovery Today*, *27*(5), 1407–1415.

Mak, K.-K., & Pichika, M. R. (2019). Artificial intelligence in drug development: Present status and future prospects. *Drug Discovery Today*, *24*(3), 773–780. PMID: 30472429

Makutam, V., Achanti, S., & Doostan, M. (2024). Integration of artificial intelligence in adaptive trial designs: Enhancing efficiency and patientcentric outcomes. *International Journal of Advanced Research*, *12*(205215), 1021474.

Malani, M., Kasturi, A., Moinul, M., Gayen, S., Hota, C., & Nirmal, J. (2023). Role of artificial intelligence in the toxicity prediction of drugs. In *Biomedical Applications and Toxicity of Nanomaterials* (pp. 589–636). Springer Nature Singapore.

Malheiro, V., Santos, B., Figueiras, A., & Mascarenhas-Melo, F. (2025). The Potential of Artificial Intelligence in Pharmaceutical Innovation: From Drug Discovery to Clinical Trials. *Pharmaceuticals*, *18*(6), 788. PMID: 40573185

Mallesh, N., Zhao, M., Meintker, L., Höllein, A., Elsner, F., Lüling, H., Haferlach, T., Kern, W., Westermann, J., & Brossart, P. (2021). Knowledge transfer to enhance the performance of deep learning models for automated classification of B cell neoplasms. *Patterns (New York, N.Y.)*, *2*(10). PMID: 34693376

Mandlik, M. R., Pathan, N. H., & Mahanor, P. B. (2024). INTEGRATING ARTIFICIAL INTELLIGENCE INTO DRUG DEVELOPMENT AND MANUFACTURING: ADVANCEMENTS AND CHALLENGES.

Mane, D. V., Deshmukh, A. N., Ambare, R. H., Solankar, A. A., & Madane, C. S. (2024). AI in autoimmune diseases: Transforming diagnosis and treatment. *Journal of Pharmaceutical and Biological Sciences*, *12*(2), 109–118.

Man, J. P., Koole, M. A. C., Meregalli, P. G., Handoko, M. L., Stienen, S., de Lange, F. J., Winter, M. M., Schijven, M. P., Kok, W. E. M., Kuipers, D. I., van der Harst, P., Asselbergs, F. W., Zwinderman, A. H., Dijkgraaf, M. G. W., Chamuleau, S. A. J., & Schuuring, M. J. (2024). Digital consults in heart failure care: A randomized controlled trial. *Nature Medicine*, *30*(10), 2907–2913. DOI: 10.1038/s41591-024-03238-6

Mao, J., Wang, J., Zeb, A., Cho, K. H., Jin, H., Kim, J., Lee, O., Wang, Y., & No, K. T. (2024). Transformer-Based Molecular Generative Model for Antiviral Drug Design. *Journal of Chemical Information and Modeling*, *64*(7), 2733–2745. DOI: 10.1021/acs.jcim.3c00536 PMID: 37366644

Mariam, Z., Niazi, S. K., & Magoola, M. (2024). Unlocking the future of drug development: Generative AI, digital twins, and beyond. *BioMedInformatics*, *4*(2), 1441–1456.

Marinov, T. M., Abu-Shmais, A. A., Janke, A. K., & Georgiev, I. S. (2024). Design of antigen-specific antibody CDRH3 sequences using AI and germline-based templates. *bioRxiv*.

Marques, L., Costa, B., Pereira, M., Silva, A., Santos, J., Saldanha, L., & Vale, N. (2024). Advancing precision medicine: A review of innovative in silico approaches for drug development, clinical pharmacology and personalized healthcare. *Pharmaceutics*, *16*(3), 332. PMID: 38543226

Martinelli, C., Repetto, M., & Curigliano, G. (2024). Artificial intelligence in small-molecule drug discovery. In *Artificial Intelligence for Medicine* (pp. 37–45). Academic Press.

Martinez, J., Wong, S., & Patel, K. (2023). Inferring health conditions from dietary data: Privacy implications of nutrition tracking platforms. *Journal of Medical Internet Research*, *25*(11), e42673.

März, J. W., Baumgartner, M., Blau, N., & Biller-Andorno, N. (2025). Digital twins for children with rare diseases: An exploration of the legal and ethical issues. *Ethics and Information Technology*, *27*(3), 44. DOI: 10.1007/s10676-025-09848-z

Mathew, A., Amudha, P., & Sivakumari, S. (2021). Deep learning techniques: an overview. *Advanced Machine Learning Technologies and Applications: Proceedings of AMLTA 2020*, 599–608.

Maxwell, G., & MacKay, C. (2008). Application of a systems biology approach to skin allergy risk assessment. *Alternatives to Laboratory Animals*, *36*(5), 521–556.

Mayr, A., Klambauer, G., Unterthiner, T., & Hochreiter, S. (2016). DeepTox: Toxicity prediction using deep learning. *Frontiers in Environmental Science*, *3*, 80.

Mayrink, N. N. V., Alcoforado, L., Chioro, A., Fernandes, F., Lima, T. S., Camargo, E. B., & Valentim, R. A. M. (2022). Translational research in health technologies: A scoping review. *Frontiers in Digital Health*, *4*, 957367. DOI: 10.3389/fdgth.2022.957367

Mbituyimana, B., Bukatuka, C. F., Qi, F., Ma, G., Shi, Z., & Yang, G. (2023). Microneedle-mediated drug delivery for scar prevention and treatment. *Drug Discovery Today*, *28*(11), 103801. PMID: 37858631

McCloskey, K., Sigel, E. A., Kearnes, S., Xue, L., Tian, X., Moccia, D., Gikunju, D., Bazzaz, S., Chan, B., & Clark, M. A. (2020). Machine learning on DNA-encoded libraries: A new paradigm for hit finding. *Journal of Medicinal Chemistry*, *63*(16), 8857–8866. PMID: 32525674

McCulloch, C. A., Downey, G. P., & El-Gabalawy, H. (2006). Signalling platforms that modulate the inflammatory response: New targets for drug development. *Nature Reviews. Drug Discovery*, *5*(10), 864–876.

McNair, L. (2022). Ethical and regulatory oversight of clinical research: The role of the Institutional Review Board. *Experimental Biology and Medicine*, *247*(7), 561–566. DOI: 10.1177/15353702221083314 PMID: 35172623

Medabalimi, V. (2024). Gradient oriented active learning for candidate drug design. bioRxiv, 2024-07.

Medicine, I. (2025, March 7). *Insilico Medicine's AI-driven drug Rentosertib receives official generic name*. News-Medical. https://www.news-medical.net/news/20250307/Insilico-Medicines-AI-driven-drug-Rentosertib-receives-official-generic-name.aspx

Mega Vascular Cognitive Impairment and Dementia (MEGAVCID) consortium. (2024). A genome-wide association meta-analysis of all-cause and vascular dementia. *Alzheimer's & Dementia*, *20*(9), 5973–5995. DOI: 10.1002/alz.14115

Mehrabi, N., Morstatter, F., Saxena, N., Lerman, K., & Galstyan, A. (2021). A survey on bias and fairness in machine learning. *ACM Computing Surveys*, *54*(6), 1–35. DOI: 10.1145/3457607

Mehta, P. (2025). System: A Delicate Balance. *Cell Death Regulation in Pathology*, 201.

Menard, P., & Bott, G. J. (2025). Artificial intelligence misuse and concern for information privacy: New construct validation and future directions. *Information Systems Journal, 35*(1), 322–367.

Mendolia, I., Contino, S., Perricone, U., Ardizzone, E., & Pirrone, R. (2020). Convolutional architectures for virtual screening. *BMC Bioinformatics, 21*. Advance online publication. DOI: 10.1186/s12859-020-03645-9 PMID: 32938359

Mennella, C., Maniscalco, U., De Pietro, G., & Esposito, M. (2024). Ethical and regulatory challenges of AI technologies in healthcare: A narrative review. *Heliyon, 10*(4). PMID: 38384518

Merk, D., Friedrich, L., Grisoni, F., & Schneider, G. (2018). De novo design of bioactive small molecules by artificial intelligence. *Molecular Informatics, 37*(1-2), 1700153.

Merk, D., Friedrich, L., Grisoni, F., & Schneider, G. (2018). De Novo Design of Bioactive Small Molecules by Artificial Intelligence. *Molecular Informatics, 37*(1-2). Advance online publication. DOI: 10.1002/minf.201700153 PMID: 29319225

Mesko, B. (2017). *The role of artificial intelligence in precision medicine* (Vol. 2). Taylor & Francis.

Mettleq, A. S. A., Akkila, A. N., Alkahlout, M. A., ALmurshidi, S. H., Abu-Nasser, B. S., & Abu-Naser, S. S. (2024). Revolutionizing Drug Discovery: The Role of Artificial Intelligence in Accelerating Pharmaceutical Innovation.

Meyyazhagan, A., Balasubramanian, B., Easwaran, M., Alagamuthu, K. K., Shanmugam, S., Kuchi Bhotla, H., Pappusamy, M., Arumugam, V. A., Thangaraj, A., Kaul, T., Keshavarao, S., & Cacabelos, R. (2020). Biomarker study of the biological parameter and neurotransmitter levels in autistics. *Molecular and Cellular Biochemistry, 474*(1-2), 277–284.

Meyyazhagan, A., Pushparaj, K., Balasubramanian, B., Kuchi Bhotla, H., Pappusamy, M., Arumugam, V. A., Easwaran, M., Pottail, L., Mani, P., Tsibizova, V., & Di Renzo, G. C. (2022). COVID-19 in pregnant women and children: Insights on clinical manifestations, complexities, and pathogenesis. *International Journal of Gynaecology and Obstetrics: the Official Organ of the International Federation of Gynaecology and Obstetrics, 156*(2), 216–224.

Midani, W., Ouarda, W., & Ayed, M. B. (2023). DeepArr: An investigative tool for arrhythmia detection using a contextual deep neural network from electrocardiograms (ECG) signals. *Biomedical Signal Processing and Control, 85*, 104954. DOI: 10.1016/j.bspc.2023.104954

Miettinen, M., Marchal, S., Hafeez, I., Asokan, N., Sadeghi, A. R., & Tarkoma, S. (2018). IoT Sentinel: Automated device-type identification for security enforcement in IoT. In *2017 IEEE 37th International Conference on Distributed Computing Systems* (pp. 2177–2184).

Miller, M. I., Shih, L. C., & Kolachalama, V. B. (2023). Machine learning in clinical trials: A primer with applications to neurology. *Neurotherapeutics; the Journal of the American Society for Experimental NeuroTherapeutics*, *20*(4), 1066–1080. DOI: 10.1007/s13311-023-01384-2

Min, S., Lee, B., & Yoon, S. (2021). Deep learning in bioinformatics. *Briefings in Bioinformatics*, *22*(2), 125–144. PMID: 27473064

Mirakhori, F., & Niazi, S. K. (2025). Harnessing the AI/ML in drug and biological products discovery and development: The regulatory perspective. *Pharmaceuticals*, *18*(1), 47. PMID: 39861110

Mirakhori, F., & Niazi, S. K. (2025). Harnessing the AI/ML in Drug and Biological Products Discovery and Development: The Regulatory Perspective. *Pharmaceuticals*, *18*(1), 47. PMID: 39861110

Mirakhori, F., & Niazi, S. K. (2025). Harnessing the AI/ML in Drug and Biological Products Discovery and Development: The Regulatory Perspective. *Pharmaceuticals*, *18*(1). *Scopus*. Advance online publication. DOI: 10.3390/ph18010047

Mishra, T., Wang, M., Metwally, A. A., Bogu, G. K., Brooks, A. W., Bahmani, A., & Snyder, M. P. (2020). Presymptomatic detection of COVID-19 from smartwatch data. *Nature Biomedical Engineering*, *4*(12), 1208–1220. DOI: 10.1038/s41551-020-00640-6

Mitchell, M., Wu, S., Zaldivar, A., Barnes, P., Vasserman, L., Hutchinson, B., & Gebru, T. (2019). Model cards for model reporting. *Proceedings of the Conference on Fairness, Accountability, and Transparency*, 220–229. https://doi.org/DOI: 10.1145/3287560.3287596

Mittelstadt, B. D., & Floridi, L. (2016). The ethics of biomedical big data. In *The ethics of biomedical big data* (p. 29).

Moen, E., Bannon, D., Kudo, T., Graf, W., Covert, M., & Van Valen, D. (2019). Deep learning for cellular image analysis. *Nature Methods*, *16*(12), 1233–1246. PMID: 31133758

Mohammad, A. A. S., Mohammad, S. I. S., Al Oraini, B., Vasudevan, A., Hindieh, A., Altarawneh, A., & Ali, I. (2025). Strategies for applying interpretable and explainable AI in real world IoT applications. *Discover Internet of Things*, *5*(1), 71. DOI: 10.1007/s43926-025-00155-z

Mohanraj, K., Karthikeyan, B. S., Vivek-Ananth, R. P., Chand, R. P. B., Aparna, S. R., Mangalapandi, P., & Samal, A. (2018). IMPPAT: A curated database of Indian Medicinal Plants, Phytochemistry And Therapeutics. *Scientific Reports*, *8*(1), 4329. DOI: 10.1038/s41598-018-22631-z PMID: 29531263

Mohd, Y., Balasubramanian, B., Meyyazhagan, A., Kuchi Bhotla, H., Shanmugam, S.K., Ramesh Kumar, M.K., Pappusamy, M., Alagamuthu, K.K., Keshavarao, S., & Arumugam, V.A. (2021). Extricating the association between the prognostic factors of colorectal cancer. *J Gastrointest Cancer, 52*(3), 022-1028.

Mohd, Y., Kumar, P., Kuchi Bhotla, H., Meyyazhagan, A., Balasubramanian, B., Ramesh Kumar, M. K., Pappusamy, M., Alagamuthu, K. K., Orlacchio, A., Keshavarao, S., Sampathkumar, P., & Arumugam, V. A. (2021). Transmission jeopardy of adenomatosis polyposis coli and methylenetetrahydrofolate reductase in colorectal cancer. *Journal of the Renin-Angiotensin-Aldosterone System : JRAAS*, *2021*, 2021.

Mohsen, F., Ali, H., El Hajj, N., & Shah, Z. (2022). Artificial intelligence-based methods for fusion of electronic health records and imaging data. *Scientific Reports*, *12*(1), 17981. DOI: 10.1038/s41598-022-22514-4

Mohsen, F., Al-Saadi, B., Abdi, N., Khan, S., & Shah, Z. (2023). Artificial Intelligence-Based Methods for Precision Cardiovascular Medicine. *Journal of Personalized Medicine*, *13*(8), 1268. DOI: 10.3390/jpm13081268

Moingeon, P., Garbay, C., Dahan, M., Fermont, I., Benmakhlouf, A., Gouyette, A., & Saint-Pierre, A. (2024). The revolution of AI in drug development. *Medecine Sciences. Ms*, *40*(4), 369–376.

Moise, L., Marcello, A., Tassone, R., Cousens, L., Martin, W., & De Groot, A. S. (2013). Building better biotherapeutics and vaccines by design: EpiVax, Inc., an immunology company. *Rhode Island Medical Journal*, *1*(96), 19–21.

Momtazmanesh, S., Nowroozi, A., & Rezaei, N. (2022). Artificial Intelligence in Rheumatoid Arthritis: Current Status and Future Perspectives: A State-of-the-Art Review. *Rheumatology and Therapy*, *9*(5), 1249–1304. DOI: 10.1007/s40744-022-00475-4

Monga, A., Jain, K., Popli, H., Telgote, P., Kaur, G., Rizwani, F., & Tuli, H. S. (2025). Organs-on-chips: Revolutionizing biomedical research. *Biophysica*, *5*(3), 38.

Montgomery, R. M. (2024). Molecular mechanisms of chronic stress in immune dysregulation: From cytokine networks to clinical manifestations. *Wired Neurosci, 1*, 24–53.

Moon, S., Zhung, W., Yang, S., Lim, J., & Kim, W. Y. (2022). PIGNet: A physics-informed deep learning model toward generalized drug-target interaction predictions. *Chemical Science (Cambridge), 13*(13), 3661–3673. DOI: 10.1039/d1sc06946b PMID: 35432900

Morley, J., Machado, C. C. V., Burr, C., Cowls, J., Joshi, I., Taddeo, M., & Floridi, L. (2020). The ethics of AI in health care: A mapping review. *Social Science & Medicine, 260*, 113172. PMID: 32702587

Morsink, M. A., Willemen, N. G., Leijten, J., Bansal, R., & Shin, S. R. (2020). Immune organs and immune cells on a chip: An overview of biomedical applications. *Micromachines, 11*(9), 849.

Mortadha, M. M. (2024). GRNIX: A graph neural network framework for explainable gene regulatory network inference in autoimmune diseases using XAI. bioRxiv, 2024-11.

Mottaghi-Dastjerdi, N., & Soltany-Rezaee-Rad, M. (2024). Advancements and Applications of Artificial Intelligence in Pharmaceutical Sciences: A Comprehensive Review. *Iranian Journal of Pharmaceutical Research : IJPR, 23*(1), e150510. PMID: 39895671

Moulange, R., Langenkamp, M., Alexanian, T., Curtis, S., & Livingston, M. (2023). Towards responsible governance of biological design tools. *arXiv preprint arXiv:2311.15936.*

Muhammad, U., Uzairu, A., & Ebuka Arthur, D. (2018). Review on: Quantitative structure activity relationship (QSAR) modeling. *Journal of Analytical & Pharmaceutical Research, 7*(2). Advance online publication. DOI: 10.15406/japlr.2018.07.00232

Muller, S. H., van Thiel, G. J., Mostert, M., & van Delden, J. J. (2023). Dynamic consent, communication and return of results in large-scale health data reuse: Survey of public preferences. *Digital Health, 9*, 20552076231190997. DOI: 10.1177/20552076231190997

Mun, S. J., Ryu, J.-S., Lee, M.-O., Son, Y. S., Oh, S. J., Cho, H.-S., Son, M.-Y., Kim, D.-S., Kim, S. J., Yoo, H. J., Lee, H.-J., Kim, J., Jung, C.-R., Chung, K.-S., & Son, M. J. (2019). Generation of expandable human pluripotent stem cell-derived hepatocyte-like liver organoids. *Journal of Hepatology, 71*(5), 970–985. DOI: 10.1016/j.jhep.2019.06.030

Muntzel, M., & Drüeke, T. (1992). A comprehensive review of the salt and blood pressure relationship. *American Journal of Hypertension, 5*(4S), 1S–42S.

Murmu, A., & Győrffy, B. (2024). Artificial intelligence methods available for cancer research. *Frontiers of Medicine, 18*(5), 778–797. DOI: 10.1007/s11684-024-1085-3

Murugan, A., Nair, S. A. H., & Kumar, K. P. S. (2019). Detection of Skin Cancer Using SVM, Random Forest and kNN Classifiers. *Journal of Medical Systems, 43*(8), 269. DOI: 10.1007/s10916-019-1400-8 PMID: 31273532

Musnier, A., Dumet, C., Mitra, S., Verdier, A., Keskes, R., Chassine, A., & Poupon, A. (2024). Applying artificial intelligence to accelerate and de-risk antibody discovery. *Frontiers in Drug Discovery, 4*, 1339697.

Mustapha, A., Mustapha, M., & Mustapha, S. (n.d.). *Harnessing artificial intelligence in personalised nutrition and microbial health: Optimising public health outcomes*. Academic Press.

Mutha, R. E., Bagul, V. S., Tade, R. S., & Vinchurkar, K. (2024). An Overview of Artificial Intelligence (AI) In Drug Delivery and Development. *AI Innovations in Drug Delivery and Pharmaceutical Sciences; Advancing Therapy through. Technology*, •••, 1–27.

Muvva, S. (2021). Ethical AI and responsible data engineering: A framework for bias mitigation and privacy preservation in large-scale data pipelines. *International Journal of Scientific Research in Engineering and Management, 5*(09).

Nada, H., Gul, A. R., Elkamhawy, A., Kim, S., Kim, M., Choi, Y., Park, T. J., & Lee, K. (2023). Machine learning-based approach to developing potent EGFR inhibitors for breast cancer— Design, synthesis, and in vitro evaluation. *ACS Omega, 8*(35), 31784–31800. PMID: 37692247

Naderian, M., Hafez Ghoran, S., Abdjan, M. I., Sabahi, Z., Moein, S., Jassbi, A. R., & Moein, M. (2025). A new labdane diterpenoid, in vitro and in silico cytotoxicity, and protease inhibitory effects of phytochemicals from Juniperus polycarpos K. Koch leaves. *Natural Product Research, 39*(11), 3053–3064. PMID: 38501578

Nag, S., Baidya, A. T., Mandal, A., Mathew, A. T., Das, B., Devi, B., & Kumar, R. (2022). Deep learning tools for advancing drug discovery and development. *3 Biotech, 12*(5), 110.

Naik, N., Hameed, B. M. Z., Shetty, D. K., Swain, D., Shah, M., Paul, R., Aggarwal, K., Ibrahim, S., Patil, V., Smriti, K., Shetty, S., Rai, B. P., Chlosta, P., & Somani, B. K. (2022). Legal and ethical consideration in artificial intelligence in healthcare: Who takes responsibility? *Frontiers in Surgery*, *9*, 862322. DOI: 10.3389/fsurg.2022.862322 PMID: 35360424

Nair, S. (2025). Explainable AI in Gxp validation: Balancing automation, traceability, and regulatory trust in the pharmaceutical industry. *Clinical Medicine and Health Research Journal*, *5*(05), 1430–1442.

Narang, V., Decraene, J., Wong, S. Y., Aiswarya, B. S., Wasem, A. R., Leong, S. R., & Gouaillard, A. (2012). Systems immunology: A survey of modelling formalisms, applications and simulation tools. *Immunologic Research*, *53*(1), 251–265.

Nashwan, A. J., & Rao, A. G. (2024). Integrating Traditional Chinese Medicine and Artificial Intelligence for insomnia: A promising frontier. *Brain Behavior and Immunity Integrative*, *7*, 100071.

Nayarisseri, A., Khandelwal, R., Tanwar, P., Madhavi, M., Sharma, D., Thakur, G., Speck-Planche, A., & Singh, S. K. (2021). Artificial Intelligence, Big Data and Machine Learning Approaches in Precision Medicine & Drug Discovery. *Current Drug Targets*, *22*(6), 631–655. DOI: 10.2174/1389450122999210104205732 PMID: 33397265

Nelson, K., Fuster, V., & Ridker, P. M. (2023). Low-Dose Colchicine for Secondary Prevention of Coronary Artery Disease: JACC Review Topic of the Week. *Journal of the American College of Cardiology*, *82*(7), 648–660. DOI: 10.1016/j.jacc.2023.05.055

Nematov, D., & Raufov, I. (2025). The bright future of materials science with ai: self-driving laboratories and closed-loop discovery. *Preprints*. https://doi.org/DOI: 10.20944/preprints202509.1369.v1

Nguyen, T., Le, H., Quinn, T. P., Nguyen, T., Le, T. D., & Venkatesh, S. (2020). *GraphDTA: predicting drug-target binding affinity with graph neural networks*. https://doi.org/DOI: 10.5281/zenodo.3603523

Nhat Phuong, D., Flower, D. R., Chattopadhyay, S., & Chattopadhyay, A. K. (2023). Towards Effective Consensus Scoring in Structure-Based Virtual Screening. *Interdisciplinary Sciences, Computational Life Sciences*, *15*(1), 131–145. DOI: 10.1007/s12539-022-00546-8 PMID: 36550341

Niarakis, A., Laubenbacher, R., An, G., Ilan, Y., Fisher, J., Flobak, Å., & Glazier, J. A. (2024). Immune digital twins for complex human pathologies: Applications, limitations, and challenges. *NPJ Systems Biology and Applications*, *10*(1), 141.

Niazi, S. K., & Mariam, Z. (2023). *Recent Advances in Machine Learning-Based Chemoinformatics: A Comprehensive Review*. https://doi.org/DOI: 10.20944/preprints202306.0803.v1

Nieto, P., Elosua-Bayes, M., Trincado, J. L., Marchese, D., Massoni-Badosa, R., Salvany, M., & Heyn, H. (2021). A single-cell tumor immune atlas for precision oncology. *Genome Research*, *31*(10), 1913–1926.

Nikolakis, D., Garantziotis, P., Sentis, G., Fanouriakis, A., Bertsias, G., Frangou, E., & Boumpas, D. T. (2023). Restoration of aberrant gene expression of monocytes in systemic lupus erythematosus via a combined transcriptome-reversal and network-based drug repurposing strategy. *BMC Genomics*, *24*(1), 207.

Nishan, M. N. H. (2025). AI-powered drug discovery for neglected diseases: Accelerating public health solutions in the developing world. *Journal of Global Health*, *15*, 03002.

Noor, N. M., Daperno, M., de Laffolie, J., Mookhoek, A., Sinonquel, P., Kopylov, U., & Baumgart, D. C. (2025). Results of the 9th scientific workshop of the european crohn's and colitis organisation (ECCO): artificial intelligence in IBD: regulatory and methodological considerations. *Journal of Crohn's and Colitis*, jjaf136.

Noorbakhsh-Sabet, N., Zand, R., Zhang, Y., & Abedi, V. (2019). Artificial intelligence transforms the future of health care. *The American Journal of Medicine*, *132*(7), 795–801. DOI: 10.1016/j.amjmed.2019.01.017 PMID: 30710543

Noor, F., Asif, M., Ashfaq, U. A., & Qasim, M., & Tahir ul Qamar, M. (2023). Machine learning for synergistic network pharmacology: A comprehensive overview. *Briefings in Bioinformatics*, *24*(3), bbad120.

Noriega, H. A., & Wang, X. S. (2025). AI-driven innovation in antibody-drug conjugate design. *Frontiers in Drug Discovery*, *5*, 1628789.

Nosrati, H., & Nosrati, M. (2023). Artificial intelligence in regenerative medicine: Applications and implications. *Biomimetics*, *8*(5), 442. PMID: 37754193

O'Neill, L. A. (2006). Targeting signal transduction as a strategy to treat inflammatory diseases. *Nature Reviews. Drug Discovery*, *5*(7), 549–563.

Obermeyer, Z., Powers, B., Vogeli, C., & Mullainathan, S. (2019). Dissecting racial bias in an algorithm used to manage the health of populations. *Science*, *366*(6464), 447–453. PMID: 31649194

Ocana, A., Pandiella, A., Privat, C., Bravo, I., Luengo-Oroz, M., Amir, E., & Gyorffy, B. (2025). Integrating artificial intelligence in drug discovery and early drug development: a transformative approach. In *Biomarker Research* (Vol. 13, Issue 1). BioMed Central Ltd. https://doi.org/DOI: 10.1186/s40364-025-00758-2

Ocana, A., Pandiella, A., Privat, C., Bravo, I., Luengo-Oroz, M., Amir, E., & Gyorffy, B. (2025). Integrating artificial intelligence in drug discovery and early drug development: A transformative approach. *Biomarker Research*, *13*(1), 45. PMID: 40087789

Ocana, A., Pandiella, A., Siu, L. L., & Tannock, I. F. (2011). Preclinical development of molecular-targeted agents for cancer. *Nature Reviews. Clinical Oncology*, *8*(4), 200–209. DOI: 10.1038/nrclinonc.2010.194

Occhipinti, A., Verma, S., & Angione, C. (2024). Mechanism-aware and multimodal AI: Beyond model-agnostic interpretation. *Trends in Cell Biology*, *34*(2), 85–89.

OECD. (2019). Recommendation of the Council on Artificial Intelligence. OECD/LEGAL/0449.

Ogut, E. (2025). Artificial Intelligence in Clinical Medicine: Challenges Across Diagnostic Imaging, Clinical Decision Support, Surgery, Pathology, and Drug Discovery. *Clinics and Practice*, *15*(9), 169. PMID: 41002784

Okpete, U. E., & Byeon, H. (2025). Explainable artificial intelligence for personalized management of inflammatory bowel disease: A minireview of recent advances. *World Journal of Gastroenterology*, *31*(35), 111033.

Oktem, E. K., & Yazar, M. (2022). Drug repositioning identifies six drug candidates for systemic autoimmune diseases by integrative analyses of transcriptomes from scleroderma, systemic lupus erythematosus, and Sjogren's syndrome. *OMICS: A Journal of Integrative Biology*, *26*(12), 683–693.

Olawade, D. B., Clement David-Olawade, A., Adereni, T., Egbon, E., Teke, J., & Boussios, S. (2025). Integrating AI into cancer immunotherapy—A narrative review of current applications and future directions. *Diseases (Basel, Switzerland)*, *13*(1), 24.

Olawade, D. B., Fidelis, S. C., Marinze, S., Egbon, E., Osunmakinde, A., & Osborne, A. (2026). Artificial intelligence in clinical trials: A comprehensive review of opportunities, challenges, and future directions. *International Journal of Medical Informatics*, *206*, 106141. DOI: 10.1016/j.ijmedinf.2025.106141

Olawade, D. B., Teke, J., Fapohunda, O., Weerasinghe, K., Usman, S. O., Ige, A. O., & David-Olawade, A. C. (2024). Leveraging artificial intelligence in vaccine development: A narrative review. *Journal of Microbiological Methods*, *224*, 106998.

Omarov, M., Zhang, L., Jorshery, S. D., Malik, R., Das, B., Bellomo, T. R., Mansmann, U., Menten, M. J., Natarajan, P., Dichgans, M., Raghu, V. K., Anderson, C. D., & Georgakis, M. K. (2024). Deep Learning-Based Detection of Carotid Plaques Informs Cardiovascular Risk Prediction and Reveals Genetic Drivers of Atherosclerosis. *medRxiv*, 2024.10.17.24315675. https://doi.org/DOI: 10.1101/2024.10.17.24315675

Omolayo, O., Aduloju, T. D., Okare, B. P., & Taiwo, A. E. (2022). Digital twin frameworks for simulating multiscale patient physiology in precision oncology: A review of real-time data assimilation, predictive tumor modelling, and clinical decision interfaces. *International Journal of Multidisciplinary Futuristic Development*, *3*(1), 1–8.

Onódi, Z., Koch, S., Rubinstein, J., Ferdinandy, P., & Varga, Z. V. (2023). Drug repurposing for cardiovascular diseases: New targets and indications for probenecid. *British Journal of Pharmacology*, *180*(6), 685–700. DOI: 10.1111/bph.16001

Ooka, T. (2025). The Era of Preemptive Medicine: Developing Medical Digital Twins through Omics, IoT, and AI Integration. *JMA Journal*, *8*(1), 1–10. DOI: 10.31662/jmaj.2024-0213

Ooms, F. (2000). Molecular modeling and computer aided drug design. Examples of their applications in medicinal chemistry. *Current Medicinal Chemistry*, *7*(2), 141–158. PMID: 10637360

Orlando, G., Molon, B., Viola, A., Alaibac, M., Angioni, R., & Piaserico, S. (2022). Psoriasis and cardiovascular diseases: An immune-mediated cross talk? *Frontiers in Immunology*, *13*, 868277.

Ouedraogo, G., Alépée, N., Tan, B., & Roper, C. S. (2025). A call to action: Advancing new approach methodologies (NAMs) in regulatory toxicology through a unified framework for validation and acceptance. *Regulatory Toxicology and Pharmacology*, *162*, 105904.

Ou-Yang, S.-s., Lu, J.-y., Kong, X.-q., Liang, Z.-j., Luo, C., & Jiang, H. (2012). Computational drug discovery. *Acta Pharmacologica Sinica*, *33*(9), 1131–1140. PMID: 22922346

Ozdemir, Z., & Keles, H. Y., & ozgur Tanriover, O. (2025). Meta-transfer derm-diagnosis: Exploring few-shot learning and transfer learning for skin disease classification in long-tail distribution. *IEEE Journal of Biomedical and Health Informatics*. Advance online publication. DOI: 10.1109/JBHI.2025.3615479

Öztürk, H., Özgür, A., & Ozkirimli, E. (2018). DeepDTA: Deep drug-target binding affinity prediction. *Bioinformatics (Oxford, England)*, *34*(17), i821–i829. DOI: 10.1093/bioinformatics/bty593 PMID: 30423097

Pala, L., Pagan, E., Sala, I., Oriecuia, C., Oliari, M., De Pas, T., Specchia, C., Cocorocchio, E., Zattarin, E., Rossi, G., Catania, C., Ceresoli, G. L., Laszlo, D., Canzian, J., Valenzi, E., Viale, G., Gelber, R. D., Mantovani, A., Bagnardi, V., & Conforti, F. (2024). Outcomes of patients with advanced solid tumors who discontinued immune-checkpoint inhibitors: A systematic review and meta-analysis. *EClinicalMedicine*, *73*, 102681. DOI: 10.1016/j.eclinm.2024.102681

Palshikar, M. G., Min, X., Crystal, A., Meng, J., Hilchey, S. P., Zand, M. S., & Thakar, J. (2023). Executable network models of integrated multiomics data. *Journal of Proteome Research*, *22*(5), 1546–1556.

Pan, Y., Ren, H., Lan, L., Li, Y., & Huang, T. (2023). Review of Predicting Synergistic Drug Combinations. In *Life* (Vol. 13, Issue 9). Multidisciplinary Digital Publishing Institute (MDPI). https://doi.org/DOI: 10.3390/life13091878

Panda, P. K., & Ghosh, S. (2025). Ethical use of AI in infectious diagnostic decision and therapeutic stewardship. *IDCases*, •••, 02356.

Panda, P., & Mohapatra, R. (2024). Revolutionizing Patient Safety: Machine Learning and AI for the Early Detection of Adverse Drug Reactions and Drug-Induced Toxicity. *Current Artificial Intelligence*, *02*, e29503752308394. DOI: 10.2174/01 29503752308394241013165241

Panda, P., & Mohapatra, R. (2024). *Revolutionizing Patient Safety: Machine Learning and AI for the Early Detection of Adverse Drug Reactions and Drug-Induced Toxicity*. Current Artificial Intelligence.

Pandey, D. R., Dash, S. S., & Mishra, A. (2024). Advances of AI-driven drug design and discovery in pharmaceuticals-review. *Integrative Biomedical Research*, *8*(1), 1–10.

Papagiannopoulos, O. D., Papaloukas, C., & Fotiadis, D. I. (2023). Deep learning for biomarkers discovery in auto-inflammatory disorders. In *2023 IEEE EMBS Special Topic Conference on Data Science and Engineering in Healthcare, Medicine and Biology* (pp. 87-88). IEEE.

Papanastasiou, G., Scutari, M., Tachdjian, R., Hernandez-Trujillo, V., Raasch, J., Billmeyer, K., & Ivanov, V. (2024). Causal modelling in large-scale data to improve identification of adults at risk for combined and common variable immunodeficiencies. medRxiv, 2024-08.

Pappachan, P., Moslehpour, M., Bansal, R., & Rahaman, M. (2024). Transparency and accountability. In *Challenges in large language model development and AI ethics* (pp. 178–211). IGI Global Scientific Publishing.

Paranitharan, N., Kataria, S., Arumugam, V. A., Hsieh, H., Muthukrishnan, S., & Velayuthaprabhu, S. (2025). Integrin α1 upregulation by tf:fviia complex promotes cervical cancer migration through par2-dependent mek1/2 activation. *Biochemical and Biophysical Research Communications*, *742*, 151151.

Parekh, A.-D. E., & Shaikh, O. A., Simran, Manan, S., & Hasibuzzaman, Md. Al. (2023). Artificial intelligence (AI) in personalized medicine: AI-generated personalized therapy regimens based on genetic and medical history: short communication. *Annals of Medicine and Surgery (London)*, *85*(11), 5831–5833. DOI: 10.1097/ms9.0000000000001320 PMID: 37915639

Parihar, A., Prajapati, J. B., Prajapati, B. G., Trambadiya, B., Thakkar, A., & Engineer, P. (2024). Role of IoT in healthcare: Applications, security & privacy concerns. *Intelligent Pharmacy*, *2*(5), 707–714.

Park, N., & Lee, J. H. (2025). A systematic multi-LLM AI framework for immunotherapy biomarker discovery and target identification. bioRxiv, 2025-06.

Parker, C. G., & Pratt, M. R. (2020). Click Chemistry in Proteomic Investigations. *Cell*, *180*(4), 605–632. DOI: 10.1016/j.cell.2020.01.025

Park, M. (2024). Improving the diagnosis of systemic lupus erythematosus with machine learning algorithms based on real-world data. *Mathematics*, *12*(18), 2849.

Park, M., Kim, M. H., Park, S. Y., Choi, I., & Kim, C. E. (2022). Individualized Diagnosis and Prescription in Traditional Medicine: Decision-Making Process Analysis and Machine Learning-Based Analysis Tool Development. *The American Journal of Chinese Medicine*, *50*(7), 1827–1844. DOI: 10.1142/S0192415X2250077X PMID: 36056467

Park, Y. J., & Bae, M. H. (2025). Screening and diagnosis of atrial fibrillation usinwearable devices. *The Korean Journal of Internal Medicine*, *40*(1), 7–14. DOI: 10.3904/kjim.2023.521

Park, Y., & Nycklemoe, S. (2025). MARGO: Machine learning-assisted adaptive randomization for group sequential trials based on overlap weights. *Statistics in Medicine*, *44*(15-17), e70158. DOI: 10.1002/sim.70158

Parsaei, M., Arvin, A., Taebi, M., Seyedmirzaei, H., Cattarinussi, G., Sambataro, F., Pigoni, A., Brambilla, P., & Delvecchio, G. (2024). Machine Learning for prediction of violent behaviors in schizophrenia spectrum disorders: A systematic review. *Frontiers in Psychiatry*, *15*, 1384828. DOI: 10.3389/fpsyt.2024.1384828

Pasas-Farmer, S., & Jain, R. (2025). From discovery to delivery: Governance of AI in the pharmaceutical industry. *Green Analytical Chemistry, 13. Scopus.* Advance online publication. DOI: 10.1016/j.greeac.2025.100268

Patel, D. D., Pathak, R. S., Patel, K. S., Bhatt, H. G., & Patel, P. K. (2025). The Future of Medicine: AI and ML Driven Drug Discovery Advancements. *Current Topics in Medicinal Chemistry*. PMID: 40207759

Patel, H., Sharma, V., & Rodriguez, T. (2023). Comprehensive risk assessment framework for integrated dietary management platforms. *Health Technology Security Journal*, *14*(2), 129–145.

Patel, V. L., Shortliffe, E. H., Stefanelli, M., Szolovits, P., Berthold, M. R., Bellazzi, R., & Abu-Hanna, A. (2019). Watson for Oncology and beyond: How machine learning and artificial intelligence can improve healthcare. *Journal of Clinical Oncology*, *37*(15, suppl), 8527. DOI: 10.1200/JCO.2017.35.15_suppl.8527

Patel, V., & Shah, M. (2022). Artificial intelligence and machine learning in drug discovery and development. *Intelligent Medicine*, *2*(3), 134–140.

Patil, D. (2024). Explainable Artificial Intelligence (XAI): enhancing transparency and trust in machine learning models. *Available at SSRN* 5057400. http://dx.doi.org/ DOI: 10.2139/ssrn.5057400

Patil, S. P., Fattakhova, E., Hofer, J., Oravic, M., Bender, A., Brearey, J., & Smith, Z. (2022). Machine-learning guided discovery of bioactive inhibitors of PD1-PDL1 interaction. *Pharmaceuticals*, *15*(5), 613.

Patne, A. Y., Dhulipala, S. M., Lawless, W., Prakash, S., Mohapatra, S. S., & Mohapatra, S. (2024). Drug discovery in the age of artificial intelligence: Transformative target-based approaches. *International Journal of Molecular Sciences*, *25*(22), 12233.

Paul, A., Al-Bahrani, R., Agrawal, A., Jha, D., Liao, W.-K., & Choudhary, A. (2018). *CheMixNet: Mixed DNN Architectures for Predicting Chemical Properties using Multiple Molecular Representations*. https://github.com/paularindam/CheMixNet

Paul, D., Sanap, G., Shenoy, S., Kalyane, D., Kalia, K., & Tekade, R. K. (2021). Artificial intelligence in drug discovery and development. *Drug Discovery Today, 26*(1), 80–93. DOI: 10.1016/j.drudis.2020.10.010 PMID: 33099022

Paul, S. M., Mytelka, D. S., Dunwiddie, C. T., Persinger, C. C., Munos, B. H., Lindborg, S. R., & Schacht, A. L. (2010). How to improve R&D productivity: The pharmaceutical industry's grand challenge. *Nature Reviews. Drug Discovery, 9*(3), 203–214. DOI: 10.1038/nrd3078

Pawar, V., Patil, A., Tamboli, F., Gaikwad, D., Mali, D., & Shinde, A. (2021). Harnessing the power of AI in pharmacokinetics and pharmacodynamics: A comprehensive review. *AAPS PharmSciTech, 14*(2), 426–439.

Pedroso, A. F., & Khera, R. (2025). Leveraging AI-enhanced digital health with consumer devices for scalable cardiovascular screening, prediction, and monitoring. *npj Cardiovascular Health, 2*(1), 34. DOI: PMID: 40620667DOI: 10.1038/s44325-025-00071-9

Peeples, K. (2023). A sleeping giant: mHealth applications, the GDPR, and the need for federal privacy regulation in the United States. *Notre Dame Journal on Emerging Technologies, 4*, 121.

Peng, L., Wang, L., Chen, L., & Shen, Z. (2025). Machine learning-driven prediction models for brodalumab therapeutic effect and response speed in plaque psoriasis. *Psoriasis: Targets and Therapy*, 429-442.

Peng, J., Jury, E. C., Dönnes, P., & Ciurtin, C. (2021). Machine learning techniques for personalised medicine approaches in immune-mediated chronic inflammatory diseases: Applications and challenges. *Frontiers in Pharmacology, 12*, 720694.

Pennisi, M., Salanitri, F. P., Bellitto, G., Casella, B., Aldinucci, M., Palazzo, S., & Spampinato, C. (2024). FedER: Federated learning through experience replay and privacy-preserving data synthesis. *Computer Vision and Image Understanding, 238*, 103882.

Perera, C., Zaslavsky, A., Christen, P., & Georgakopoulos, D. (2014). Context aware computing for the Internet of Things: A survey. *IEEE Communications Surveys and Tutorials, 16*(1), 414–454.

Perez, M. V., Mahaffey, K. W., Hedlin, H., Rumsfeld, J. S., Garcia, A., Ferris, T., & Turakhia, M. P. (2019). Large-scale assessment of a smartwatch to identify atrial fibrillation. *The New England Journal of Medicine, 381*(20), 1909–1917. DOI: 10.1056/NEJMoa1901183

Peters, R., Rhrissorrakrai, K., Parthasarathy, P. B., Ratner, V., Gujarati, T. P., Tolunay, M., & Alban, T. J. (2025). Quantum convolutional HLA immunogenic peptide prediction (Q-CHIPP): next-generation neoantigen prediction with quantum neural networks. bioRxiv, 2025-07.

Petrovsky, N., & Brusic, V. (2002). Computational immunology: The coming of age. *Immunology and Cell Biology*, *80*(3), 248–254.

Pettinati, M. J., Lajevardi-Khosh, A., Rajput, K. S., Majmudar, M., & Selvaraj, N. (2022). Towards remote continuous monitoring of cytokine release syndrome. In *2022 44th Annual International Conference of the IEEE Engineering in Medicine & Biology Society (EMBC)* (pp. 966-970). IEEE.

Pfortmueller, C. A., Meisel, C., Fux, M., & Schefold, J. C. (2017). Assessment of immune organ dysfunction in critical illness: Utility of innate immune response markers. *Intensive Care Medicine Experimental*, *5*(1), 49. DOI: 10.1186/s40635-017-0163-0

Philippidis, A. (2022). Double dare: exscientia expands AI platform into antibody design: British pioneer of data-driven drug discovery eyes doubling the number of potential druggable sites, as well as a future move into more complex biologics. *GEN Edge*, *4*(1), 896–902.

Philippidis, A. (2023). BMS Collaboration Paying Off for Exscientia: AI drug developer designs EXS4318, the I&I small molecule that has entered Phase I trials overseen by pharma giant in up-to-$1.3 B+ partnership. *GEN Edge*, *5*(1), 147–150.

Philippidis, A. (2025). Healx Candidate, SpringWorks Therapy Expand NF1 Treatment Options: Healx doses first patient in Phase II trial of HLX-1502 for neurofibromatosis type 1, while SpringWorks wins FDA approval for Gomekli, first drug designed to treat the disease in adults and children. *GEN Edge*, *7*(1), 136–141.

Pierini, E., Mazza, L., Petti, M., & Tieri, P. (2024). Exploring drug repurposing success stories through a network-based approach: insights from a case study. In *2024 IEEE International Conference on Bioinformatics and Biomedicine (BIBM)* (pp. 6959-6964). IEEE.

Poddar, A., & Rao, S. R. (2024). Evolving intellectual property landscape for AI-driven innovations in the biomedical sector: Opportunities in stable IP regime for shared success. *Frontiers in Artificial Intelligence*, *7*, 1372161.

Poh, M. Z., Battisti, A. J., Cheng, L. F., Lin, J., Patwardhan, A., Venkataraman, G. S., & Ghanbari, H. (2023). Validation of a deep learning algorithm for continuous, real-time detection of atrial fibrillation using a wrist-worn device in an ambulatory environment. *Journal of the American Heart Association*, *12*(19), e030543. DOI: 10.1161/jaha.123.030543

Poolsappasit, N., Dewri, R., & Ray, I. (2012). Dynamic security risk management using Bayesian attack graphs. *IEEE Transactions on Dependable and Secure Computing*, *9*(1), 61–74. DOI: 10.1109/TDSC.2011.34

Popova, M., Isayev, O., & Tropsha, A. (2018). Deep reinforcement learning for de novo drug design. *Science Advances*, *4*(7), eaap7885. PMID: 30050984

Porcari, S., Benech, N., Valles-Colomer, M., Segata, N., Gasbarrini, A., Cammarota, G., Sokol, H., & Ianiro, G. (2023). Key determinants of success in fecal microbiota transplantation: From microbiome to clinic. *Cell Host & Microbe*, *31*(5), 712–733. DOI: 10.1016/j.chom.2023.03.020

Porter, T. M., Andersen, K. M., Paez, W., Corr, P., & Figueiredo, S. (2025). Acceptance and Utilization of Real-World Evidence among Cancer Care Physicians in the USA: A National Survey. *Pharmaceutical Medicine*, *39*(6), 453–463. DOI: 10.1007/s40290-025-00586-7

Powles, J., & Hodson, H. (1765-1766). (Price, W. N., Gerke, S., & Cohen, I. G. (2019). Potential liability for physicians using artificial intelligence. *Journal of the American Medical Association*, *322*(18).

Powles, J., & Hodson, H. (2017). Google DeepMind and healthcare in an age of algorithms. *Health and Technology*, *7*(4), 351–367. DOI: 10.1007/s12553-017-0179-1 PMID: 29308344

Prashar, A., Singh, M., Sharma, S., Kuna, S. S., Putha, S., Gudekota, S., . . . Joshi, R. (2026). AI-driven multi-omics analysis for personalized healthcare. In: Goar, V., Gajrani, J., Yousuf, M. A., R. s. Tavares, J. M. (eds) Proceedings of International Conference on Computational Complexity and Intelligent Algorithms. IC3IA 2025. Algorithms for Intelligent Systems. Springer, Singapore. DOI: DOI: 10.1007/978-981-96-7473-2_21

Proietti, M., Ragno, A., La Rosa, B., Ragno, R., & Capobianco, R. (2024). Explainable AI in drug discovery: Self-interpretable graph neural network for molecular property prediction using concept whitening. *Machine Learning*, *113*(4), 2013–2044. DOI: 10.1007/s10994-023-06369-y

Puentes-Osorio, Y., Amariles, P., Calleja, M. Á., Merino, V., Díaz-Coronado, J. C., & Taborda, D. (2021). Potential clinical biomarkers in rheumatoid arthritis with an omic approach. *Auto-Immunity Highlights*, *12*(1), 9.

Puniya, B. L., Bessell, B., Zhao, Z., Loecker, J., Aghamiri, S. S., Mohanty, S., & Helikar, T. (2023). A computational pipeline for drug discovery in immunometabolism against autoimmune diseases. *The Journal of Immunology : Official Journal of the American Association of Immunologists*, *210*(Supplement_1), 85–15.

Pushpakom, S., Iorio, F., Eyers, P. A., Escott, K. J., Hopper, S., Wells, A., Doig, A., Guilliams, T., Latimer, J., McNamee, C., Norris, A., Sanseau, P., Cavalla, D., & Pirmohamed, M. (2019). Drug repurposing: Progress, challenges and recommendations. *Nature Reviews. Drug Discovery*, *18*(1), 41–58. DOI: 10.1038/nrd.2018.168 PMID: 30310233

Pushparaj, K., Kuchi Bhotla, H., Arumugam, V. A., Pappusamy, M., Easwaran, M., Liu, W. C., Issara, U., Rengasamy, K. R. R., Meyyazhagan, A., & Balasubramanian, B. (2022). Mucormycosis (black fungus) ensuing COVID-19 and comorbidity meets - magnifying global pandemic grieve and catastrophe begins. *The Science of the Total Environment*, *805*, 150355.

Qadri, Y. A., Shaikh, S., Ahmad, K., Choi, I., Kim, S. W., & Vasilakos, A. V. (2025). Explainable artificial intelligence: A perspective on drug discovery. *Pharmaceutics*, *17*(9), 1119.

Qayyum, A., Qadir, J., Bilal, M., & Al-Fuqaha, A. (2020). Secure and robust machine learning for healthcare: A survey. *IEEE Reviews in Biomedical Engineering*, *14*, 156–180.

Qian, L., Lu, X., Haris, P., Zhu, J., Li, S., & Yang, Y. (2024). A Survey of Artificial Intelligence Methods for Clinical Trial Outcome Prediction. *ChemRxiv*. https://doi.org/DOI: 10.26434/chemrxiv-2024-08t4w

Qian, L., Lu, X., Haris, P., Zhu, J., Li, S., & Yang, Y. (2025). Enhancing clinical trial outcome prediction with artificial intelligence: A systematic review. *Drug Discovery Today*, *30*(4), 104332. DOI: 10.1016/j.drudis.2025.104332

Qiu, S., Zhao, S., & Yang, A. (2023). DLTKcat: Deep learning-based prediction of temperature-dependent enzyme turnover rates. *Briefings in Bioinformatics*, *25*(1). PMID: 38189538

Qu, Y., Siegler, E., Cheng, C., Liu, J., Cinay, G., Bagrodia, N., & Wang, P. (2019). Engineering CAR-expressing natural killer cells with cytokine signalling and synthetic switch for an off-the-shelf cell-based cancer immunotherapy. *MRS Communications*, *9*(2), 433–440.

Ragoza, M., Hochuli, J., Idrobo, E., Sunseri, J., & Koes, D. R. (2017). Protein–ligand scoring with convolutional neural networks. *Journal of Chemical Information and Modeling*, *57*(4), 942–957. PMID: 28368587

Raikar, G. V. S., Raikar, A. S., & Somnache, S. N. (2023). Advancements in artificial intelligence and machine learning in revolutionising biomarker discovery. *Brazilian Journal of Pharmaceutical Sciences*, *59*, e23146.

Rajchenberg, D., Hess, R., Lins, M., Manor, A., Degany, O., & Shoenfeld, Y. (2025). Challenges, limitations, and ethical considerations of AI in immunology and healthcare. In *AI-Assisted Computational Approaches for Immunological Disorders* (pp. 393–426). IGI Global Scientific Publishing.

Rajkomar, A., Hardt, M., Howell, M. D., Corrado, G., & Chin, M. H. (2018). Ensuring fairness in machine learning to advance health equity. *Annals of Internal Medicine*, *169*(12), 866–872. PMID: 30508424

Raman, R., Pattnaik, D., Lathabai, H. H., Kumar, C., Govindan, K., & Nedungadi, P. (2024). Green and sustainable AI research: An integrated thematic and topic modelling analysis. *Journal of Big Data*, *11*(1), 1–28.

Ramirez, L., Chen, W., & Thompson, S. (2024). Adversarial machine learning applied to nutritional recommendation systems. *Journal of Health Informatics and Cybersecurity*, *9*(1), 24–39.

Ramya, S., Poornima, P., Jananisri, A., Geofferina, I. P., Bavyataa, V., Divya, M., Priyanga, P., Vadivukarasi, J., Sujitha, S., Elamathi, S., Anand, A. V., & Balamuralikrishnan, B. (2023). Role of hormones and the potential impact of multiple stresses on infertility. *Stresses*, *3*(2), 454–474.

Ran, Y., Su, W., Gao, F., Ding, Z., Yang, S., Ye, L., Chen, X., Tian, G., Xi, J., & Liu, Z. (2021). Curcumin Ameliorates White Matter Injury after Ischemic Stroke by Inhibiting Microglia/Macrophage Pyroptosis through NF-κB Suppression and NLRP3 Inflammasome Inhibition. *Oxidative Medicine and Cellular Longevity*, *1552127*. Advance online publication. DOI: 10.1155/2021/1552127

Rao, I. (2023). NovoMol: Recurrent Neural Network for Orally Bioavailable Drug Design and Validation on PDGFR {\alpha} Receptor. *arXiv preprint arXiv:2312.01527.*

Rappaport, N., Nogal, B., Perrott, K., Domina, V., Hood, L., & Price, N. D. (2026). Early detection of wellness-to-disease transitions in the AI era: Implications for pharmacology and toxicology. *Annual Review of Pharmacology and Toxicology*, •••, 66.

Ratwani, R. M., Sutton, K., & Galarraga, J. E. (2024). Addressing AI algorithmic bias in health care. *Journal of the American Medical Association, 332*(13), 1051–1052.

Reis, Z. S. N., Pereira, G. M. V., Dias, C. D. S., Lage, E. M., de Oliveira, I. J. R., & Pagano, A. S. (2025). Artificial intelligence-based tools for patient support to enhance medication adherence: A focused review. *Frontiers in Digital Health, 7*, 1523070. DOI: 10.3389/fdgth.2025.1523070

Ren, F., Aliper, A., Chen, J., Zhao, H., Rao, S., Kuppe, C., Ozerov, I. V., Zhang, M., Witte, K., & Kruse, C. (2025). A small-molecule TNIK inhibitor targets fibrosis in preclinical and clinical models. *Nature Biotechnology, 43*(1), 63–75. PMID: 38459338

Ren, F., Ding, X., Zheng, M., Korzinkin, M., Cai, X., Zhu, W., Mantsyzov, A., Aliper, A., Aladinskiy, V., & Cao, Z. (2023). AlphaFold accelerates artificial intelligence powered drug discovery: Efficient discovery of a novel CDK20 small molecule inhibitor. *Chemical Science (Cambridge), 14*(6), 1443–1452. PMID: 36794205

Ren, F., Ding, X., Zheng, M., Korzinkin, M., Cai, X., Zhu, W., Mantsyzov, A., Aliper, A., Aladinskiy, V., Cao, Z., Kong, S., Long, X., Liu, B. H. M., Liu, Y., Naumov, V., Shneyderman, A., Ozerov, I. V., Wang, J., Pun, F. W., & Zhavoronkov, A. (2022). *AlphaFold Accelerates Artificial Intelligence Powered Drug Discovery: Efficient Discovery of a Novel Cyclin-dependent Kinase 20 (CDK20) Small Molecule Inhibitor*. https://arxiv.org/abs/2201.09647

Ren, X., Shao, X. X., Li, X. X., Jia, X. H., Song, T., Zhou, W. Y., Wang, P., Li, Y., Wang, X. L., Cui, Q. H., Qiu, P. J., Zhao, Y. G., Li, X. B., Zhang, F. C., Li, Z. Y., Zhong, Y., Wang, Z. G., & Fu, X. J. (2020). Identifying potential treatments of COVID-19 from Traditional Chinese Medicine (TCM) by using a data-driven approach. *Journal of Ethnopharmacology, 258*, 112932. DOI: 10.1016/j.jep.2020.112932 PMID: 32376368

Ren, Y., Pieper, A. A., & Cheng, F. (2025). Utilization of precision medicine digital twins for drug discovery in Alzheimer's disease. *Neurotherapeutics; the Journal of the American Society for Experimental NeuroTherapeutics*, •••, 00553.

Rhie, A., McCarthy, S. A., Fedrigo, O., Damas, J., Formenti, G., Koren, S., Uliano-Silva, M., Chow, W., Fungtammasan, A., Kim, J., Lee, C., Ko, B. J., Chaisson, M., Gedman, G. L., Cantin, L. J., Thibaud-Nissen, F., Haggerty, L., Bista, I., Smith, M., & Jarvis, E. D. (2021). Towards complete and error-free genome assemblies of all vertebrate species. *Nature*, *592*(7856), 737–746. DOI: 10.1038/s41586-021-03451-0

Richardson, S., Hirsch, J. S., Narasimhan, M., Crawford, J. M., McGinn, T., Davidson, K. W., Barnaby, D. P., Becker, L. B., Chelico, J. D., & Cohen, S. L. (2020). Presenting characteristics, comorbidities, and outcomes among 5700 patients hospitalized with COVID-19 in the New York City area. *Journal of the American Medical Association*, *323*(20), 2052–2059. PMID: 32320003

Robert, K., Kaium, O., & Alasa, L. (2025). Generative AI and pharmaceutical innovation: Accelerating drug discovery with deep learning and predictive analytics. *International Journal of Multidisciplinary Evolutionary Research*, *6*(2), 44–52.

Rood, J. E., Hupalowska, A., & Regev, A. (2024). Toward a foundation model of causal cell and tissue biology with a perturbation cell and tissue atlas. *Cell*, *187*(17), 4520–4545.

Ross, C., & Swetlitz, I. (2018, July 25). IBM pitched its Watson supercomputer as a revolution in cancer care. It's nowhere close. STAT. https://www.statnews.com/2018/07/25/ibm-watson-recommended-unsafe-incorrect-treatments

Rossier, J. S., Baranek, S., Morier, P., Vollet, C., Vulliet, F., De Chastonay, Y., & Reymond, F. (2008). GRAVI: Robotized microfluidics for fast and automated immunoassays in low volume. *JALA: Journal of the Association for Laboratory Automation*, *13*(6), 322–329.

Roth, H. R., Xu, Z., Chen, C., Xu, D., Dogra, P., Flores, M., & Feng, A. (2025). Overview of real-world applications of federated learning with NVIDIA FLARE. *Journal of Biopharmaceutical Statistics*, •••, 1–11.

Rovenchak, A., & Druchok, M. (2024). Machine learning-assisted search for novel coagulants: When machine learning can be efficient even if data availability is low. *Journal of Computational Chemistry*, *45*(13), 937–952. PMID: 38174834

Roy Choudhury, S., Singh, K., Koner, S., & Ghosh, J. (2025). Technology, artificial intelligence, and the era of information in healthcare and allied sciences. In *Sustainable development goals (SDG) and its intersection with health and well-being* (Chapter 16). IGI Global. DOI: 10.4018/979-8-3693-9755-8.ch016

Roybal, K. T., & Lim, W. A. (2017). Synthetic immunology: Hacking immune cells to expand their therapeutic capabilities. *Annual Review of Immunology*, *35*(1), 229–253.

Ru, J., Li, P., Wang, J., Zhou, W., Li, B., Huang, C., Li, P., Guo, Z., Tao, W., Yang, Y., Xu, X., Li, Y., Wang, Y., & Yang, L. (2014). TCMSP: A database of systems pharmacology for drug discovery from herbal medicines. *Journal of Cheminformatics*, *6*, 13. DOI: 10.1186/1758-2946-6-13 PMID: 24735618

Rupnawar, M., & Wani, P. (2024). Pharmaceutical Regulatory Affairs: An Overview of Global Regulatory Frameworks and Emerging Trends. International Journal of Scientific Research and Technology.

Rustandi, T., Prihandiwati, E., Nugroho, F., Hayati, F., Afriani, N., Alfian, R., Aisyah, N., Niah, R., Rahim, A., & As-Shiddiq, H. (2023). Application of artificial intelligence in the development of Jamu "traditional Indonesian medicine" as a more effective drug. *Frontiers in Artificial Intelligence*, *6*, 1274975. DOI: 10.3389/frai.2023.1274975 PMID: 38028667

Saboya-Galindo, P., Cifuentes-González, C., Rojas-Carabali, W., Mejía-Salgado, G., Le Tong, Y., Putera, I., Song, X. Y. R., Walter, C. F. Y., Shengjuan, Z., Chan, R., La Distia Nora, R., Biswas, J., Gangaputra, S., Pulido, J. S., Kempen, J. H., Nguyen, Q. D., de-la-Torre, A., Gupta, V., Rosenbaum, J. T., … REVISE-IUSG study group. (2025). Clinical trials and quasi-experimental studies in the treatment of noninfectious retinal vasculitis: A systematic review from the International Uveitis Study Group (IUSG) Retinal Vasculitis Study (ReViSe) - Report 4. *Survey of Ophthalmology*, S0039-6257(25)00173-0. https://doi.org/DOI: 10.1016/j.survophthal.2025.09.013

Sabry, Z., Arora, H. S., Chandrasekaran, S., & Wang, Z. (2025). AI-driven drug discovery and repurposing using multi-omics for myocardial infarction and heart failure. *Exploration of Medicine, 6. Scopus.* Advance online publication. DOI: 10.37349/emed.2025.1001340

Sadée, C., Testa, S., Barba, T., Hartmann, K., Schuessler, M., Thieme, A., Church, G. M., Okoye, I., Hernandez-Boussard, T., Hood, L., Shmulevich, I., Kuhl, E., & Gevaert, O. (2025). Medical digital twins: Enabling precision medicine and medical artificial intelligence. *The Lancet. Digital Health*, *7*(7), 100864. DOI: 10.1016/j.landig.2025.02.004

Sadybekov, A. V., & Katritch, V. (2023). Computational approaches streamlining drug discovery. *Nature*, *616*(7958), 673–685. DOI: 10.1038/s41586-023-05905-z PMID: 37100941

Saeed, A., & Alajlan, S. A. (2025). The Dawn of AI in Pharmaceutical Research: AI Transforming Pharma-Ethics, Trials, and Beyond. In *Transforming Pharmaceutical Research With Artificial Intelligence* (pp. 1–26). IGI Global; Scopus. https://doi.org/DOI: 10.4018/979-8-3693-6270-9.ch001

Sahoo, D., Swanson, L., Sayed, I. M., Katkar, G. D., Ibeawuchi, S. R., Mittal, Y., & Ghosh, P. (2021). Artificial intelligence guided discovery of a barrier-protective therapy in inflammatory bowel disease. *Nature Communications*, *12*(1), 4246.

Sahu, S. K., & Mazumdar, K. (2024). Exploring security threats and solutions techniques for Internet of Things (IoT): From vulnerabilities to vigilance. *Frontiers in Artificial Intelligence*, *7*, 1397480.

Saikia, S., & Bordoloi, M. (2019). Molecular Docking: Challenges, Advances and its Use in Drug Discovery Perspective. *Current Drug Targets*, *20*(5), 501–521. DOI: 10.2174/1389450119666181022153016 PMID: 30360733

Saini, J. P. S., Thakur, A., & Yadav, D. (2025). AI-driven innovations in pharmaceuticals: optimizing drug discovery and industry operations. In *RSC Pharmaceutics* (Vol. 2, Issue 3, pp. 437–454). Royal Society of Chemistry. https://doi.org/DOI: 10.1039/d4pm00323c

Sakhamuri, M. R., Henna, S., Creedon, L., & Meehan, K. (2023). graph modelling and graph-attention neural network for immune response prediction. In *2023 34th Irish Signals and Systems Conference (ISSC)* (pp. 1-6). IEEE.

Salditt, M., Eckes, T., & Nestler, S. (2024). A tutorial introduction to heterogeneous treatment effect estimation with meta-learners. *Administration and Policy in Mental Health*, *51*(5), 650–673. DOI: 10.1007/s10488-023-01303-9

Saldivar-Gonzalez, F. I., Aldas-Bulos, V. D., Medina-Franco, J. L., & Plisson, F. (2022). Natural product drug discovery in the artificial intelligence era. *Chemical Science (Cambridge)*, *13*(6), 1526–1546. DOI: 10.1039/d1sc04471k PMID: 35282622

Saleem, R. (2025). Revolutionizing Pharmaceutical Engineering: A Deep Dive Into AI- Driven Drug Discovery and Development. In *Transforming Pharmaceutical Research With Artificial Intelligence* (pp. 113–139). IGI Global; Scopus. https://doi.org/DOI: 10.4018/979-8-3693-6270-9.ch004

Samant, T. S., Mangal, N., Lukacova, V., & Schmidt, S. (2015). Quantitative clinical pharmacology for size and age scaling in pediatric drug development: A systematic review. *Journal of Clinical Pharmacology*, *55*(11), 1207–1217. DOI: 10.1002/jcph.555

Sampathi, S., & Bhatia, N. (2024). AI-Enabled Models in the Restoration of Drug Efficacy and Drug Design. In *Biosystems, Biomedical & Drug Delivery Systems: Characterization, Restoration and Optimization* (pp. 83–103). Springer Nature Singapore.

Sampene, A. K., & Nyirenda, F. (2024). Evaluating the effect of artificial intelligence on pharmaceutical product and drug discovery in China. *Future Journal of Pharmaceutical Sciences*, *10*(1). Advance online publication. DOI: 10.1186/s43094-024-00632-2

Samtani, S., Chen, H., Albanese, M., & Grisham, J. (2020). Identifying emerging hacker assets and key hackers for proactive cyber threat intelligence: A diachronic graph embedding framework. *Journal of Management Information Systems*.

Sanches, P. H. G., de Melo, N. C., Porcari, A. M., & de Carvalho, L. M. (2024). Integrating molecular perspectives: Strategies for comprehensive multi-omics integrative data analysis and machine learning applications in transcriptomics, proteomics, and metabolomics. *Biology (Basel)*, *13*(11), 848.

Sangeetha, T., Anand, A. V., & Begum, T. N. (2022). Assessment of inter-relationship between anemia and COPD in accordance with altitude. *The Open Respiratory Medicine Journal*, *16*, e187430642206270.

Sangeetha, T., Nargis Begum, T., Balamuralikrishnan, B., Arun, M., Rengasamy, K. R. R., Senthilkumar, N., Velayuthaprabhu, S., Saradhadevi, M., Sampathkumar, P., & Vijaya Anand, A. (2022). Influence of SERPINA1 gene polymorphisms on anemia and chronic obstructive pulmonary disease. *Journal of the Renin-Angiotensin-Aldosterone System : JRAAS*, *2022*, 2022.

Sarapultsev, A., Gusev, E., Hu, D., & Komelkova, M. (2025). Experimental PTSD Models in Zebrafish: A Systematic Review of Behavioral, Neurochemical, and Molecular Outcomes. *Biology (Basel)*, *14*(5), 456. DOI: 10.3390/biology14050456

Sathyanarayanan, A., Mueller, T. T., Ali Moni, M., & Schueler, K., ECNP TWG Network members, Baune, B. T., Lio, P., Mehta, D., Baune, B. T., Dierssen, M., Ebert, B., Fabbri, C., Fusar-Poli, P., Gennarelli, M., Harmer, C., Howes, O. D., Janzing, J. G. E., Lio, P., Maron, E., … Xicota, L. (2023). Multi-omics data integration methods and their applications in psychiatric disorders. *European Neuropsychopharmacology: The Journal of the European College of Neuropsychopharmacology*, *69*, 26–46. DOI: 10.1016/j.euroneuro.2023.01.001

Savage, N. (2021). Tapping into the drug discovery potential of AI. Nature. https://www.nature.com/articles/d43747-021-00045-7

Savage, N. (2021). Drugs by AI: Making new medicines in days. *Nature*, *595*(7867), S12–S14. DOI: 10.1038/d41586-021-02212-5

Savira, F., Magaye, R., Liew, D., Reid, C., Kelly, D. J., Kompa, A. R., Sangaralingham, S. J., Burnett, J. C., Kaye, D., & Wang, B. H. (2020). Cardiorenal syndrome: Multi-organ dysfunction involving the heart, kidney and vasculature. *British Journal of Pharmacology*, *177*(13), 2906–2922. DOI: 10.1111/bph.15065

Scannell, J. W., Blanckley, A., Boldon, H., & Warrington, B. (2012). Diagnosing the decline in pharmaceutical R&D efficiency. *Nature Reviews. Drug Discovery*, *11*(3), 191–200. PMID: 22378269

Schneider, M., Radoux, C. J., Hercules, A., Ochoa, D., Dunham, I., Zalmas, L.-P., Hessler, G., Ruf, S., Shanmugasundaram, V., Hann, M. M., Thomas, P. J., Queisser, M. A., Benowitz, A. B., Brown, K., & Leach, A. R. (2021). The PROTACtable genome. *Nature Reviews. Drug Discovery*, *20*(10), 789–797. DOI: 10.1038/s41573-021-00245-x

Schneider, P., Walters, W. P., Plowright, A. T., Sieroka, N., Listgarten, J., Goodnow, R. A.Jr, Fisher, J., Jansen, J. M., Duca, J. S., Rush, T. S., Zentgraf, M., Hill, J. E., Krutoholow, E., Kohler, M., Blaney, J., Funatsu, K., Luebkemann, C., & Schneider, G. (2020). Rethinking drug design in the artificial intelligence era. *Nature Reviews. Drug Discovery*, *19*(5), 353–364. DOI: 10.1038/s41573-019-0050-3 PMID: 31801986

Schöler, D., Kostev, K., Peters, M., Zamfir, C., Wolk, A., Roderburg, C., & Loosen, S. H. (2022). Machine learning can predict the probability of biologic therapy in patients with Inflammatory Bowel Disease. *Journal of Clinical Medicine*, *11*(15), 4586.

Schork, N. J. (2019). Artificial Intelligence and Personalized Medicine. In Von Hoff, D. D., & Han, H. (Eds.), *Precision Medicine in Cancer Therapy* (Vol. 178, pp. 265–283). Springer International Publishing., DOI: 10.1007/978-3-030-16391-4_11

Schultz, M. B., Vera, D., & Sinclair, D. A. (2020). Can artificial intelligence identify effective COVID-19 therapies? *EMBO Molecular Medicine*, *12*(8), e12817.

Schwam, E. M., Nicholas, T., Chew, R., Billing, C. B., Davidson, W., Ambrose, D., & Altstiel, L. D. (2014). A multicenter, double-blind, placebo-controlled trial of the PDE9A inhibitor, PF-04447943, in Alzheimer's disease. *Current Alzheimer Research*, *11*(5), 413–421. PMID: 24801218

Sedeeq, F. S., & Arman, P. (2025). Human-centric AI governance: An adaptive public international law framework for ethical and inclusive AI regulation in public health. *The Journal of Law, Medicine & Ethics*, •••, 1–12.

Seetharam, K., Kagiyama, N., & Sengupta, P. P. (2019). Application of mobile health, telemedicine and artificial intelligence to echocardiography. *Echo Research and Practice*, *6*(2), R41–R52. DOI: 10.1530/ERP-18-0081 PMID: 30844756

Seijas-Bellido, J. A., Samanta, B., Valadez-Villalobos, K., Gallardo, J. J., Navas, J., Balestra, S. R., Madero Castro, R. M. a., Vicent-Luna, J. M., Tao, S., & Toroker, M. C. (2022). Transferable classical force field for pure and mixed metal halide perovskites parameterized from first-principles. *Journal of Chemical Information and Modeling*, *62*(24), 6423–6435. PMID: 35576452

Sejnowski, T. J. (2020). The unreasonable effectiveness of deep learning in artificial intelligence. *Proceedings of the National Academy of Sciences of the United States of America*, *117*(48), 30033–30038. DOI: 10.1073/pnas.1907373117 PMID: 31992643

Sekaran, S. D., Manikam, R., Thergerajan, G., Prasad, H., Alagar, M., & Tan, C. K. (2025). The role of personalized precision medicine in enhancing diagnostic accuracy and clinical outcomes. *Advances in Biomedical and Health Sciences*, *4*(2), 52–60.

Sen, S., & Kilic, K. D. (2025). Digital twins in medicine, AI-driven personalized healthcare, and predictive analytics. In *AI-Powered Digital Twins for Predictive Healthcare: Creating Virtual Replicas of Humans* (pp. 359-396). IGI Global Scientific Publishing.

Senior, A. W., Evans, R., Jumper, J., Kirkpatrick, J., Sifre, L., Green, T., Qin, C., Žídek, A., Nelson, A. W., & Bridgland, A. (2020). Improved protein structure prediction using potentials from deep learning. *Nature*, *577*(7792), 706–710. PMID: 31942072

Serrano, D. R., Luciano, F. C., Anaya, B. J., Ongoren, B., Kara, A., Molina, G., Ramirez, B. I., Sánchez-Guirales, S. A., Simon, J. A., Tomietto, G., Rapti, C., Ruiz, H. K., Rawat, S., Kumar, D., & Lalatsa, A. (2024). Artificial Intelligence (AI) Applications in Drug Discovery and Drug Delivery: Revolutionizing Personalized Medicine. In *Pharmaceutics* (Vol. 16, Issue 10). Multidisciplinary Digital Publishing Institute (MDPI). https://doi.org/DOI: 10.3390/pharmaceutics16101328

Serrano, D. R., Luciano, F. C., Anaya, B. J., Ongoren, B., Kara, A., Molina, G., Ramirez, B. I., Sánchez-Guirales, S. A., Simon, J. A., & Tomietto, G. (2024). Artificial intelligence (AI) applications in drug discovery and drug delivery: Revolutionizing personalized medicine. *Pharmaceutics*, *16*(10), 1328. PMID: 39458657

Shafik, W. (2025). Ethical considerations in automated healthcare. In *Next-Generation Therapeutics Using Internet of Things and Machine Learning* (pp. 315–338). IGI Global Scientific Publishing.

Shah, D. K., Al Qaraghuli, F., & Zhang, W. (2020). PK/PD-driven starting and effective human dose determination for immuno-oncology drugs. In *Identification and Quantification of Drugs, Metabolites, Drug Metabolizing Enzymes, and Transporters* (pp. 657-667). Elsevier.

Shahid, S., Maity, D., & Chakrabarty, S. (2025). MTAN-ADMET: A multi-task adaptive neural network for efficient and accurate prediction of ADMET properties. *ChemRxiv*. http://dx.doi.org/DOI: 10.26434/chemrxiv-2025-zhrsk

Shahzadi, M., Rafique, H., Waheed, A., Naz, H., Waheed, A., Zokirova, F. R., & Khan, H. (2024). Artificial intelligence for chimeric antigen receptor-based therapies: A comprehensive review of current applications and future perspectives. *Therapeutic Advances in Vaccines and Immunotherapy*, *12*, 25151355241305856.

Shaki, F., Amirkhanloo, M., & Chahardori, M. (2024). The Future and Application of Artificial Intelligence in Toxicology. *Asia Pacific Journal of Medical Toxicology*, *13*(1).

Shamanna, P., Erukulapati, R. S., Shukla, A., Shah, L., Willis, B., Thajudeen, M., & Joshi, S. (2024). One-year outcomes of a digital twin intervention for type 2 diabetes: A retrospective real-world study. *Scientific Reports*, *14*(1), 25478. DOI: 10.1038/s41598-024-76584-7

Shameer, K., Readhead, B., & Dudley, J. T. (2015). Computational and experimental advances in drug repositioning for accelerated therapeutic stratification. *Current Topics in Medicinal Chemistry*, *15*(1), 5–20. DOI: 10.2174/15680266156661501 12103510 PMID: 25579574

Shamim, M. A., Shamim, M. A., Arora, P., & Dwivedi, P. (2024). Artificial intelligence and big data for pharmacovigilance and patient safety. *Journal of Medicine, Surgery, and Public Health*, *3*, 100139. DOI: 10.1016/j.glmedi.2024.100139

Shams, R. A., Zowghi, D., & Bano, M. (2025). AI and the quest for diversity and inclusion: A systematic literature review. *AI and Ethics*, *5*(1), 411–438. DOI: 10.1007/s43681-023-00362-w

Shanehsazzadeh, A., Bachas, S., McPartlon, M., Kasun, G., Sutton, J. M., Steiger, A. K., & Meier, J. (2023). Unlocking de novo antibody design with generative artificial intelligence. BioRxiv, 2023-01.

Shanker, V. R., Bruun, T. U., Hie, B. L., & Kim, P. S. (2024). Unsupervised evolution of protein and antibody complexes with a structure-informed language model. *Science*, *385*(6704), 46–53.

Shanmugam, R., Thangavelu, S., Fathah, Z., Yatoo, M. I., Tiwari, R., Pandey, M. K., Dhama, J., Chandra, R., Malik, Y. S., Dhama, K., Sah, R., Chaicumpa, W., Shanmugam, V., & Arumugam, V. A. (2020). SARS-CoV-2 / COVID-19 pandemic – an update. *Journal of Experimental Biology and Agricultural Sciences, 8*(Special Issue 1), S219-S245.

Shao, J., Meng, Y., Yuan, K., Wu, Q., Zhu, S., Li, Y., Wu, P., Zheng, J., & Shi, H. (2023). RU.521 mitigates subarachnoid hemorrhage-induced brain injury via regulating microglial polarization and neuroinflammation mediated by the cGAS/STING/NF-κB pathway. *Cell Communication and Signaling : CCS, 21*(1), 264. DOI: 10.1186/s12964-023-01274-2

Sharma, S., Chaubey, A., Pathan, M. N., & Tyagi, S. (2024). AI-powered virtual screening for drug discovery: Methods and challenges. *International Journal of Pharmacy and Pharmaceutical Sciences, 6*(2), 157–164. DOI: 10.33545/26647222.2024.v6.i2b.136

Sharma, V., & McNeill, J. H. (2009). To scale or not to scale: The principles of dose extrapolation. *British Journal of Pharmacology, 157*(6), 907–921. DOI: 10.1111/j.1476-5381.2009.00267.x PMID: 19508398

Sheller, M. J., Edwards, B., Reina, G. A., Martin, J., Pati, S., Kotrotsou, A., & Bakas, S. (2020). Federated learning in medicine: Facilitating multi-institutional collaborations without sharing patient data. *Scientific Reports, 10*(1), 12598.

Shen, R., & Zhang, Y. (2025). Relationship between amino acid metabolism and inflammation in coronary heart disease [Review]. *International Journal of Molecular Medicine, 56*(2), 120. DOI: 10.3892/ijmm.2025.5561

Shen, Y., Yang, R., Zhou, R., Lu, W., Li, L., Niu, Z., Chen, M., Wang, J., Wang, Y., Fang, L., & Du, G. (2021). Xiaoxuming Decoction Regulates Vascular Function by Modulating G Protein-Coupled Receptors: A Molecular Docking Study. *BioMed Research International, 5575443*. Advance online publication. DOI: 10.1155/2021/5575443 PMID: 34195269

Shi, C., Gao, T., Lyu, W., Qiang, B., Chen, Y., Chen, Q., & Liu, Z. (2024). Deep-Learning-Driven Discovery of SN3–1, a Potent NLRP3 Inhibitor with Therapeutic Potential for Inflammatory Diseases. *Journal of Medicinal Chemistry, 67*(19), 17833–17854.

Shi, J., Wei, X., Xun, Z., Ding, X., Liu, Y., Liu, L., & Ye, Y. (2024). The web-based portal SpatialTME integrates histological images with single-cell and spatial transcriptomics to explore the tumor microenvironment. *Cancer Research, 84*(8), 1210–1220.

Shin, D. H. (2010). The effects of trust, security, and privacy in social networking: A security-based approach to understand the pattern of adoption. *Interacting with Computers*, *22*(5), 428–439. DOI: 10.1016/j.intcom.2010.05.001

Shoenbill, K., Song, Y., Cobb, N. L., Drezner, M. K., & Mendonça, E. A. (2017). IRB process improvements: A machine learning analysis. *Journal of Clinical and Translational Science*, *1*(3), 176–183. DOI: 10.1017/cts.2016.25 PMID: 29082031

Shoghli, A., Darvish, M., & Sadeghian, Y. (2024). Balancing innovation and privacy: Ethical challenges in AI-driven healthcare. *Journal of Research in Medical Sciences : the Official Journal of Isfahan University of Medical Sciences*, *4*(1), 1–11.

Shraim, R., Mooney, B., Conkrite, K. L., Hamilton, A. K., Morin, G. B., Sorensen, P. H., & Sacan, A. (2025). ImmunoTar—Integrative prioritization of cell surface targets for cancer immunotherapy. *Bioinformatics (Oxford, England)*, *41*(3), btaf060.

Sidhom, J. W., Oliveira, G., Ross-MacDonald, P., Wind-Rotolo, M., Wu, C. J., Pardoll, D. M., & Baras, A. S. (2022). Deep learning reveals predictive sequence concepts within immune repertoires to immunotherapy. *Science Advances*, *8*(37), eabq5089.

Silverman, A. L., Shung, D., Stidham, R. W., Kochhar, G. S., & Iacucci, M. (2025). How artificial intelligence will transform clinical care, research, and trials for inflammatory bowel disease. *Clinical Gastroenterology and Hepatology*, *23*(3), 428–439.

Singar, S., Nagpal, R., Arjmandi, B. H., & Akhavan, N. S. (2024). Personalized Nutrition: Tailoring Dietary Recommendations through Genetic Insights. *Nutrients*, *16*(16), 2673. DOI: 10.3390/nu16162673

Singh, A. V., & Negi, A. (2019). Towards better drug repositioning using joint learning. In *2019 IEEE 16th India Council International Conference (INDICON)* (pp. 1-4). IEEE.

Singh, K., Gupta, A., Siddiqui, I., Sinha, A., Patwa, M. K., & Singh, U. (2025). Rational design of anti-inflammatory therapeutics. *Computational Methods for Rational Drug Design*, 389-402.

Singh, A. (2024). Artificial intelligence for drug repurposing against infectious diseases. *Artificial Intelligence Chemistry.*, *2*(2), 100071. DOI: 10.1016/j.aichem.2024.100071

Singh, A., Attwood, S., & Wilkinson, P. (2022). Inclusion of under-represented racial and ethnic groups in cardiovascular clinical trials. *Journal of the American Heart Association*, *11*(14), e024706. DOI: 10.1161/JAHA.121.024706

Singh, A., & Rodriguez, C. (2024). The MealSync ransomware attack: Impact analysis and recovery strategies in critical nutrition infrastructure. *Journal of Healthcare Security*, *8*(2), 71–89.

Singh, B., Crasto, M., Ravi, K., & Singh, S. (2024). *Pharmaceutical advances: Integrating artificial intelligence in QSAR, combinatorial and green chemistry practices*. Intelligent Pharmacy.

Singh, R., Zhou, K., & Auclair, J. R. (2025). Reimagining drug regulation in the age of AI: A framework for the AI-enabled Ecosystem for Therapeutics. *Frontiers in Medicine*, *12*. Advance online publication. DOI: 10.3389/fmed.2025.1679611

Singh, S., Gupta, H., Sharma, P., & Sahi, S. (2024). Advances in Artificial Intelligence (AI)-assisted approaches in drug screening. *Artificial Intelligence Chemistry.*, *2*(1), 100039. DOI: 10.1016/j.aichem.2023.100039

Singh, S., Shingatgeri, V., & Srivastava, P. (2024). Revolutionizing new drug discovery: Harnessing AI and machine learning to overcome traditional challenges and accelerate targeted therapies. *Artificial Intelligence in Health*, *2*(2), 29–40.

Sinha, S., McLaren, E., Mullick, M., Penrose, H. M., Tindle, C., Singh, S., & Ghosh, P. (2025). FORWARD: A data-driven framework for network-based target prioritization in drug discovery. bioRxiv, 2024-07.

Sireesha, B., & Haritha, S. (2024). A review on regulatory affairs and regulatory requirements for new drug approval. *International Journal of Health Care and Biological Sciences*, *3*(1), 22–28.

Sirén, J., & Paten, B. (2022). GBZ file format for pangenome graphs. *Bioinformatics (Oxford, England)*, *38*(22), 5012–5018. PMID: 36179091

Smetana, S., Aganovic, K., & Heinz, V. (2021). Food supply chains as cyber-physical systems: A path for more sustainable personalized nutrition. *Food Engineering Reviews*, *13*(1), 92–103. DOI: 10.1007/s12393-020-09243-y

Smith, D. P., Oechsle, O., Rawling, M. J., Savory, E., Lacoste, A. M. B., & Richardson, P. J. (2021). Expert-Augmented Computational Drug Repurposing Identified Baricitinib as a Treatment for COVID-19. *Frontiers in Pharmacology*, *12*, 709856. DOI: 10.3389/fphar.2021.709856

Snijder, B., Kandasamy, R. K., & Superti-Furga, G. (2014). Toward effective sharing of high-dimensional immunology data. *Nature Biotechnology*, *32*(8), 755–759.

Sobhani, N., Tardiel-Cyril, D. R., Chai, D., Generali, D., Li, J. R., Vazquez-Perez, J., & Li, Y. (2024). Artificial intelligence-powered discovery of small molecules inhibiting CTLA-4 in cancer. *BJC Reports*, *2*(1), 4.

Sobral, P. S., Luz, V. C., Almeida, J. M., Videira, P. A., & Pereira, F. (2023). Computational approaches drive developments in immune-oncology therapies for PD-1/PD-L1 immune checkpoint inhibitors. *International Journal of Molecular Sciences*, *24*(6), 5908.

Sodaei, Z., Ekrami, S., & Hashemianzadeh, S. M. (2025). Machine learning analysis of molecular dynamics properties influencing drug solubility. *Scientific Reports*, *15*(1), 26955. PMID: 40707560

Son, A., Park, J., Kim, W., Lee, W., Yoon, Y., Ji, J., & Kim, H. (2024). Integrating computational design and experimental approaches for next-generation biologics. *Biomolecules*, *14*(9), 1073.

Son, A., Park, J., Kim, W., Yoon, Y., Lee, S., Ji, J., & Kim, H. (2024). Recent Advances in Omics, Computational Models, and Advanced Screening Methods for Drug Safety and Efficacy. *Toxics*, *12*(11), 822. PMID: 39591001

Song, J., Kim, L., Shin, D., Kim, J., Um, T., Cho, A., & Chae, Y. K. (2025a). AI-based models integrating serum proteomics and clinical features to predict immune-related adverse events in NSCLC patients undergoing immunotherapy. *Cancer Research*, *85*(8, Supplement_1), 3667–3667.

Song, X., Liang, H., Nan, F., Chen, W., Li, J., He, L., & Zhang, D. (2025b). Autoimmune Diseases: Molecular Pathogenesis and Therapeutic Targets. *MedComm*, *6*(7), e70262.

Soni, K., & Hasija, Y. (2022). Artificial intelligence assisted drug research and development. 2022 IEEE Delhi Section Conference (DELCON), Srivastava, D., Korsakova, A., Wang, Q., Ruiz, L., Yuan, H., & Kelley, D. R. (2025). Borzoi-informed fine mapping improves causal variant prioritization in complex trait GWAS. bioRxiv, 2025.2007. 2009.663936.

Soremekun, O., Dib, M.-J., Rajasundaram, S., Fatumo, S., & Gill, D. (2023). Genetic heterogeneity in cardiovascular disease across ancestries: Insights for mechanisms and therapeutic intervention. *Cambridge Prisms. Precision Medicine*, *1*, e8. DOI: 10.1017/pcm.2022.13

Spero, D. (2006). *Diabetes: Sugar-coated crisis: Who gets it, who profits, and how to stop it*. New Society Publishers.

Srinivas, S. S., & Runkana, V. (2024). Cross-modal learning for chemistry property prediction: large language models meet graph machine learning. *arXiv preprint arXiv:2408.14964*.

Stokes, J. M., Yang, K., Swanson, K., Jin, W., Cubillos-Ruiz, A., Donghia, N. M., MacNair, C. R., French, S., Carfrae, L. A., & Bloom-Ackermann, Z. (2020). A deep learning approach to antibiotic discovery. *Cell, 180*(4), 688-702. e613.

Stokes, J. M., Yang, K., Swanson, K., Jin, W., Cubillos-Ruiz, A., Donghia, N. M., MacNair, C. R., French, S., Carfrae, L. A., Bloom-Ackerman, Z., Tran, V. M., Chiappino-Pepe, A., Badran, A. H., Andrews, I. W., Chory, E. J., Church, G. M., Brown, E. D., Jaakkola, T. S., Barzilay, R., & Collins, J. J. (2020). A Deep Learning Approach to Antibiotic Discovery. *Cell*, *180*(4), 688–702.e13. DOI: 10.1016/j.cell.2020.01.021 PMID: 32084340

Strauss, B., Short, S., & Lotfian, P. (2023, March 31). The evolution of personalised nutrition: Executive summary. *The Evolution of Personalised Nutrition*.

Strickland, E. (2019). IBM Watson, heal thyself: How IBM overpromised and underdelivered on AI health care. *IEEE Spectrum*, *56*(4), 24–31. https://spectrum.ieee.org/ibm-watson

Subbiah, V. (2023). The next generation of evidence-based medicine. *Nature Medicine*, *29*(1), 49–58. DOI: 10.1038/s41591-022-02160-z PMID: 36646803

Subramanian, N., Torabi-Parizi, P., Gottschalk, R. A., Germain, R. N., & Dutta, B. (2015). Network representations of immune system complexity. *Wiley Interdisciplinary Reviews. Systems Biology and Medicine*, *7*(1), 13–38.

Su, J., Yang, L., Sun, Z., & Zhan, X. (2024). Personalized Drug Therapy: Innovative Concept Guided With Proteoformics. *Molecular & Cellular Proteomics*, *23*(3), 100737. DOI: 10.1016/j.mcpro.2024.100737

Sumit, M., & Dhara, V. G. (2025). Use of systems biology approaches toward target discovery, validation, and drug development. In *Biopharmaceutical Informatics* (pp. 281–305). CRC Press.

Sun, D., Gao, W., Hu, H., & Zhou, S. (2022). Why 90% of clinical drug development fails and how to improve it? In *Acta Pharmaceutica Sinica B* (Vol. 12, Issue 7, pp. 3049–3062). Chinese Academy of Medical Sciences. https://doi.org/DOI: 10.1016/j.apsb.2022.02.002

Sun, Z. Y., Yuan, J., Jaiswal, D., Ge, J., Liang, T., Wei, J., & Feng, Z. (2025). AntiB-MPNN: Structure-guided graph neural networks for precision antibody engineering. *Advancement of Science*, •••, 04278.

Su, Q., Cheng, G., & Huang, J. (2023). A review of research on eligibility criteria for clinical trials. *Clinical and Experimental Medicine*, *23*(6), 1867–1879. DOI: 10.1007/s10238-022-00975-1

Suri, G. S., Kaur, G., & Shinde, D. (2024). Beyond boundaries: Exploring the transformative power of AI in pharmaceuticals. *Discover Artificial Intelligence*, *4*(1), 82.

Suriyaamporn, P., Pamornpathomkul, B., Patrojanasophon, P., Ngawhirunpat, T., Rojanarata, T., & Opanasopit, P. (2024). The artificial intelligence-powered new era in pharmaceutical research and development: A review. *AAPS PharmSciTech*, *25*(6), 188. PMID: 39147952

Suttithumsatid, W., Shah, M. A., Bibi, S., & Panichayupakaranant, P. (2022). alpha-Glucosidase inhibitory activity of cannabidiol, tetrahydrocannabinol and standardized cannabinoid extracts from Cannabis sativa. *Current Research in Food Science*, *5*, 1091–1097. DOI: 10.1016/j.crfs.2022.07.002 PMID: 35856057

Su, X., Xu, Y., Tan, Z., Wang, X., Yang, P., Su, Y., Jiang, Y., Qin, S., & Shang, L. (2020). Prediction for cardiovascular diseases based on laboratory data: An analysis of random forest model. *Journal of Clinical Laboratory Analysis*, *34*(9), e23421. DOI: 10.1002/jcla.23421 PMID: 32725839

Su, Y., Zeng, X., Zhang, L., Bian, Y., Wang, Y., & Ma, B. (2025). ABTrans: A transformer-based model for predicting interaction between anti-Aβ antibodies and peptides. *Interdisciplinary Sciences, Computational Life Sciences*, *17*(1), 140–152.

Swanson, K., Walther, P., Leitz, J., Mukherjee, S., Wu, J. C., Shivnaraine, R. V., & Zou, J. (2024). ADMET-AI: A machine learning ADMET platform for evaluation of large-scale chemical libraries. *Bioinformatics (Oxford, England)*, *40*(7), btae416.

Swartz, M. A., Hirosue, S., & Hubbell, J. A. (2012). Engineering approaches to immunotherapy. *Science translational medicine, 4*(148), 148rv9-148rv9.

Taherdoost, H., & Ghofrani, A. (2024). AI's role in revolutionizing personalized medicine by reshaping pharmacogenomics and drug therapy. In *Intelligent Pharmacy* (Vol. 2, Issue 5, pp. 643–650). KeAi Publishing Communications Ltd. https://doi .org/DOI: 10.1016/j.ipha.2024.08.005

Talebi, N., & Azimi, M. (2025). Federated learning for multi-institutional AI in healthcare via digital pathology. *Preprints*. https://doi.org/DOI: 10.20944/preprints202509.1352.v1

Talevi, A., Morales, J. F., Hather, G., Podichetty, J. T., Kim, S., Bloomingdale, P. C., Kim, S., Burton, J., Brown, J. D., & Winterstein, A. G. (2020). Machine learning in drug discovery and development part 1: A primer. *CPT: Pharmacometrics & Systems Pharmacology*, *9*(3), 129–142. PMID: 31905263

Tan, R. K., Liu, Y., & Xie, L. (2022). Reinforcement learning for personalized drug discovery and design for complex diseases: a systems pharmacology perspective. *arXiv preprint arXiv:2201.08894*.

Tangari, G., Ikram, M., Sentana, I. W. B., Ijaz, K., Kaafar, M. A., & Berkovsky, S. (2021). Analyzing security issues of Android mobile health and medical applications. *Journal of the American Medical Informatics Association : JAMIA*, *28*(10), 2074–2084. DOI: 10.1093/jamia/ocab131

Tang, S. W., Tang, W. H., & Leonard, B. E. (2020). Safety of traditional medicine and natural product supplements in psychiatry. *International Clinical Psychopharmacology*, *35*(1), 1–7. DOI: 10.1097/YIC.0000000000000279 PMID: 31361653

Tang, Y., Kim, J. Y., Carman, K. M., Bahmani, A., Chen, Q., Rosenberger, M. G., & Ferguson, A. L. (2023). Data-driven discovery of innate immunomodulators via machine learning-guided high throughput screening. *Chemical Science (Cambridge)*, *14*(44), 12747–12766.

Tariq, M. U. (2025). AI in the Classroom: Revolutionizing Instruction and Student Engagement. In M. Kessinger, G. Nelson, L. Lennex, & K. Nettleton (Eds.), *Enhancing Classroom Instruction and Student Skills With AI* (pp. 35-62). IGI Global Scientific Publishing. https://doi.org/DOI: 10.4018/979-8-3373-4576-5.ch002

Tariq, M. U. (2025). Decolonizing Education Systems Through Action Research and Action Learning. In Mapotse, T., Tetteh, E., & Matsekoleng, T. (Eds.), *Enabling Indigenous Knowledge Systems in Action Research and Action Learning* (pp. 107–128). IGI Global Scientific Publishing., DOI: 10.4018/979-8-3693-3542-0.ch006

Tariq, M. U. (2025). Machine Learning Techniques for Personalized Rehabilitation: Enhancing Patient Outcomes Through Predictive Algorithms. In Korupalli, V., Ranasinghe, P., & Feldman, D. (Eds.), *Predictive Algorithms for Rehabilitation and Assistive Systems* (pp. 221–252). IGI Global Scientific Publishing., DOI: 10.4018/979-8-3373-0194-5.ch009

Tariq, M. U. (2025). The Challenge of Artificial Intelligence in Environmental Sustainability: Opportunities, Risks, and Policy Implications. In Ahmadi, A., & Mna, A. (Eds.), *Nexus of Environmental Quality and Technology Innovation* (pp. 267–292). IGI Global Scientific Publishing., DOI: 10.4018/979-8-3373-1822-6.ch012

Taroni, J. N., Grayson, P. C., Hu, Q., Eddy, S., Kretzler, M., Merkel, P. A., & Greene, C. S. (2018). MultiPLIER: a transfer learning framework reveals systemic features of rare autoimmune disease. *bioRxiv*.

Teachey, D. T., Lacey, S. F., Shaw, P. A., Melenhorst, J. J., Maude, S. L., Frey, N., & Grupp, S. A. (2016). Identification of predictive biomarkers for cytokine release syndrome after chimeric antigen receptor T-cell therapy for acute lymphoblastic leukemia. *Cancer Discovery*, *6*(6), 664–679.

Teodoro, D., Naderi, N., Yazdani, A., Zhang, B., & Bornet, A. (2025). A scoping review of artificial intelligence applications in clinical trial risk assessment. *npj. Digital Medicine*, *8*(1), 486. DOI: 10.1038/s41746-025-01886-7

Tetko, I. V., & Clevert, D. A. (2025). Advanced machine learning for innovative drug discovery. In *Journal of Cheminformatics* (Vol. 17, Issue 1). BioMed Central Ltd. https://doi.org/DOI: 10.1186/s13321-025-01061-w

Thaingtamtanha, T., Ravichandran, R., & Gentile, F. (2025). On the application of artificial intelligence in virtual screening. *Expert Opinion on Drug Discovery*, *20*. Advance online publication. DOI: 10.1080/17460441.2025.2508866 PMID: 40388244

Thakkar, R., Upreti, D., Ishiguro, S., Tamura, M., & Comer, J. (2023). Computational design of a cyclic peptide that inhibits the CTLA4 immune checkpoint. *RSC Medicinal Chemistry*, *14*(4), 658–670.

Thakkar, S., Slikker, W.Jr, Yiannas, F., Silva, P., Blais, B., Chng, K. R., Liu, Z., Adholeya, A., Pappalardo, F., & Soares, M. L. C. (2023). Artificial intelligence and real-world data for drug and food safety–A regulatory science perspective. *Regulatory Toxicology and Pharmacology*, *140*, 105388. PMID: 37061083

Théry, C., Witwer, K. W., Aikawa, E., Alcaraz, M. J., Anderson, J. D., Andriantsitohaina, R., Antoniou, A., Arab, T., Archer, F., Atkin-Smith, G. K., Ayre, D. C., Bach, J.-M., Bachurski, D., Baharvand, H., Balaj, L., Baldacchino, S., Bauer, N. N., Baxter, A. A., Bebawy, M., & Zuba-Surma, E. K. (2018). Minimal information for studies of extracellular vesicles 2018 (MISEV2018): A position statement of the International Society for Extracellular Vesicles and update of the MISEV2014 guidelines. *Journal of Extracellular Vesicles*, *7*(1), 1535750. DOI: 10.1080/20013078.2018.1535750

Tian, H., Ketkar, R., & Tao, P. (2022). Accurate admet prediction with xgboost. *arXiv preprint arXiv:2204.07532*.

Tian, W. W., Tang, B. H., Liu, L., Yu, D. M., & Hua, H. (2024). Research progress on curcumin improving chronic low-grade inflammation and related diseases. *Zhongguo Zhong yao za zhi= Zhongguo Zhongyao Zazhi=. Zhongguo Zhongyao Zazhi*, *49*(10), 2607–2618.

Tomar, P., Goel, F., Pal, A., & Garg, V. K. (2025). The Future of Drug Development: Leveraging AI for Faster and Safer Innovation. *International Journal of Advances in Scientific Research*, *16*(04), 5–11.

Tomer, R., Jain, S., Gahlot, P. S., Bajiya, N., & Raghava, G. P. S. (2025). In Silico Tool for Predicting and Scanning Rheumatoid Arthritis-Inducing Peptides in an Antigen (p. 2025.03.19.644081). *bioRxiv*. https://doi.org/DOI: 10.1101/2025.03.19.644081

Tomlinson, C., Thimma, M., Alexandrakis, S., Castillo, T., Dennis, J. L., Brooks, A., Bradley, T., Turnbull, C., Blaveri, E., Barton, G., Chiba, N., Maratou, K., Soutter, P., Aitman, T., & Game, L. (2008). MiMiR—an integrated platform for microarray data sharing, mining and analysis. *BMC Bioinformatics*, *9*, 379. DOI: 10.1186/1471-2105-9-379

Topol, E. J. (2019). High-performance medicine: The convergence of human and artificial intelligence. *Nature Medicine*, *25*(1), 44–56. PMID: 30617339

Trares, K., Ackermann, J., & Koch, I. (2022). The canonical and non-canonical NF-κB pathways and their crosstalk: A comparative study based on Petri nets. *Bio Systems*, *211*, 104564.

Tripathi, M. K., Nath, A., Singh, T. P., Ethayathulla, A. S., & Kaur, P. (2021). Evolving scenario of big data and Artificial Intelligence (AI) in drug discovery. *Molecular Diversity*, *25*(3), 1439–1460. DOI: 10.1007/s11030-021-10256-w PMID: 34159484

Turner, M., Millar, S., Kusiak, C., Fuller, F. D., Walsh, J., & Zhuang, R. (2024). Accelerating Crohn's Disease clinical trials using generative artificial intelligence. In *journal of crohns & colitis* (Vol. 18, pp. i1002-i1002). GREAT CLARENDON ST, OXFORD OX2 6DP, ENGLAND: OXFORD UNIV PRESS.

Tu, Y., Tan, L., Tao, H., Li, Y., & Liu, H. (2023). CETSA and thermal proteome profiling strategies for target identification and drug discovery of natural products. *Phytomedicine*, *116*, 154862. DOI: 10.1016/j.phymed.2023.154862

Twala, B. (2025). AI-driven precision diagnosis and treatment in Parkinson's disease: A comprehensive review and experimental analysis. *Frontiers in Aging Neuroscience*, *17*, 1638340. DOI: 10.3389/fnagi.2025.1638340

Tyagi, E., Kumari, P., Prakash, A., & Bhuyan, R. (2025). Revolutionizing Anti-Cancer Drug Discovery: The Role of Artificial Intelligence. *International Journal of Bioinformatics and Intelligent Computing*, *4*, 1–38.

U.S. FDA. (2023). *U.S. Food & Drug Administration (FDA): Digital Health Technologies for Remote Data Acquisition in Clinical Investigations – Guidance for Industry, Investigators, and Other Stakeholders*. Retrieved 1 November 2025 from https://www.fda.gov/regulatory-information/search-fda-guidance-documents/digital-health-technologies-remote-data-acquisition-clinical-investigations

U.S. Food and Drug Administration. (2021). *Artificial intelligence/machine learning (AI/ML)-based software as a medical device (SaMD) action plan*. U.S. Department of Health and Human Services.

U.S. Food and Drug Administration. (2023). *Using AI/ML in the development of drug and biological products: Discussion paper and request for feedback*. U.S. Department of Health and Human Services.

Ueno, H. (2023). Artificial intelligence as dual-use technology. In *Fusion of Machine Learning Paradigms: Theory and Applications* (pp. 7-32). Springer.

Ugolkov, Y., Nikitich, A., Leon, C., Helmlinger, G., Peskov, K., Sokolov, V., & Volkova, A. (2024). Mathematical modelling in autoimmune diseases: From theory to clinical application. *Frontiers in Immunology*, *15*, 1371620.

Ujiie, H., Rosmarin, D., Schön, M. P., Ständer, S., Boch, K., Metz, M., & Ludwig, R. J. (2022). Unmet medical needs in chronic, non-communicable inflammatory skin diseases. *Frontiers in medicine*, *9*, 875492.

Unlu, O., Varugheese, M., Shin, J., Subramaniam, S. M., Stein, D. W. J., St Laurent, J. J., & Blood, A. J. (2025). Manual vs AI-assisted prescreening for trial eligibility using large language models - a randomized clinical trial. *Journal of the American Medical Association*, *333*(12), 1084–1087. DOI: 10.1001/jama.2024.28047

Upadhyay, J., Nandave, M., & Kumar, A. (2024). Role of artificial intelligence in pharmacovigilance. In *Pharmacovigilance Essentials: Advances, Challenges and Global Perspectives* (pp. 347–363). Springer Nature Singapore.

Urbina, F., Lentzos, F., Invernizzi, C., & Ekins, S. (2022). Dual use of artificial-intelligence-powered drug discovery. *Nature Machine Intelligence*, *4*(3), 189–191. PMID: 36211133

Vadde, R., & Gupta, M. K. (2025). Machine learning approaches for neuroblastoma risk prediction and stratification. *Critical Reviews™ in Oncogenesis, 30*.

Valcárcel, G., Lazarenkov, A., López-Rubio, A. V., Berenguer, C., Calafell-Segura, J., Rodríguez-Ubreva, J., & Sardina, J. L. (2025). Modulating immune cell fate and inflammation through CRISPR-mediated DNA methylation editing. *Science Advances, 11*(29), eadt1644.

Valenza, C., Saldanha, E. F., Gong, Y., De Placido, P., Gritsch, D., Ortiz, H., Trapani, D., Conforti, F., Cremolini, C., Peters, S., Mateo, J., Subbiah, V., Parsons, H. A., Partridge, A. H., & Curigliano, G. (2025). Circulating tumor DNA clearance as a predictive biomarker of pathologic complete response in patients with solid tumors treated with neoadjuvant immune checkpoint inhibitors: A systematic review and meta-analysis. *Annals of Oncology : Official Journal of the European Society for Medical Oncology*, *36*(7), 726–736. DOI: 10.1016/j.annonc.2025.03.019

Vall, A., Sabnis, Y., Shi, J., Class, R., Hochreiter, S., & Klambauer, G. (2021). The Promise of AI for DILI Prediction. *Frontiers in Artificial Intelligence*, *4*, 638410. DOI: 10.3389/frai.2021.638410 PMID: 33937745

Vallée, A. (2025). Digital twins for personalized Medicine require epidemiological data and mathematical modelling. *Journal of Medical Internet Research*, *27*, e72411.

Vamathevan, J., Clark, D., Czodrowski, P., Dunham, I., Ferran, E., Lee, G., Li, B., Madabhushi, A., Shah, P., Spitzer, M., & Zhao, S. (2019). Applications of machine learning in drug discovery and development. In *Nature Reviews Drug Discovery* (Vol. 18, Issue 6, pp. 463–477). Nature Publishing Group. https://doi.org/DOI: 10.1038/s41573-019-0024-5

Vamathevan, J., Apweiler, R., & Birney, E. (2019). Biomolecular data resources: Bioinformatics infrastructure for biomedical data science. *Annual Review of Biomedical Data Science*, *2*(1), 199–222.

Vamathevan, J., Clark, D., Czodrowski, P., Dunham, I., Ferran, E., Lee, G., Li, B., Madabhushi, A., Shah, P., & Spitzer, M. (2019). Applications of machine learning in drug discovery and development. *Nature Reviews. Drug Discovery*, *18*(6), 463–477. PMID: 30976107

Van Hasselt, J. C., & Iyengar, R. (2019). Systems pharmacology: Defining the interactions of drug combinations. *Annual Review of Pharmacology and Toxicology*, *59*(1), 21–40.

Vaterkowski, M., Daniel, C., La Rosa, A., Kalra, D., Jaulent, M.-C., Lame, G., & Kempf, E. (2025). Electronic health record based recruitment support systems: A scoping review to improve patient inclusion within clinical trials. *International Journal of Medical Informatics*, *201*, 105900. DOI: 10.1016/j.ijmedinf.2025.105900

Vayena, E., Blasimme, A., & Cohen, I. G. (2018). Machine learning in medicine: Addressing ethical challenges. *PLoS Medicine, 15*(11), e1002689. PMID: 30399149

Vázquez, N. G., Nada, H., Upadhyay, S., & Gabr, M. T. (2025). Phenotypic and targeted drug discovery in immune therapeutics: Challenges, opportunities, and future directions. *RSC Advances, 15*(36), 29937–29951.

Velayuthaprabhu, S., & Archunan, G. (2005). Evaluation of anticardiolipin antibodies and antiphosphatidylserine antibodies in women with recurrent abortion. *Indian Journal of Medical Sciences, 59*, 347–352.

Velayuthaprabhu, S., Archunan, G., & Balakrishnan, K. (2007). Placental thrombosis in experimental anticardiolipin antibodies-mediated intrauterine fetal death. *American Journal of Reproductive Immunology (New York, N.Y.), 57*, 270–276.

Velayuthaprabhu, S., Matsubayashi, H., & Archunan, G. (2016). Beta-2 GPI induced tissue factor and placental apoptosis for the pathophysiology of pregnancy loss in antiphospholipid syndrome. *International Journal of Research in Medical Sciences, 4*(8), 3109–3113.

Velayuthaprabhu, S., Matsubayashi, H., Sugi, T., Nakamura, M., Ohnishi, Y., Ogura, T., & Archunan, G. (2013). Expression of apoptosis in placenta of experimental antiphospholipid syndrome (APS) mouse. *American Journal of Reproductive Immunology (New York, N.Y.), 69*(5), 486–494.

Velayuthaprabhu, S., Matsubayashi, H., Sugi, T., Nakamura, M., Ohnishi, Y., Ogura, T., Tomiyama, T., & Archunan, G. (2011). A unique preliminary study on fetal resorption and placental apoptosis in mice with passive immunization of anti-phosphatidylethanolamine antibodies and anti-Factor XII antibodies. *American Journal of Reproductive Immunology (New York, N.Y.), 66*, 373–384.

Verma, J., Khedkar, V. M., & Coutinho, E. C. (2010). 3D-QSAR in drug design—A review. *Current Topics in Medicinal Chemistry, 10*(1), 95–115. DOI: 10.2174/156802610790232260

Vignesh, M. (2024). Al in Predictive. *AI-Powered Advances in Pharmacology*, 61.

Vijayan, R. S. K., Kihlberg, J., Cross, J. B., & Poongavanam, V. (2022). Enhancing preclinical drug discovery with artificial intelligence. *Drug Discovery Today, 27*(4), 967–984. DOI: 10.1016/j.drudis.2021.11.023

Vijayaragavan, V., Vijayakumar, M., Dharshini, P., Karunakaran, K., Kesavan, K., & Raj, R. D. S. (2025). AI and automation in organ-on-a-chip technology: advancing personalized medicine and disease modelling. In *2025 IEEE 6th International Conference in Robotics and Manufacturing Automation (ROMA)* (pp. 40-45). IEEE.

Vinluan, F. (2025). An AI Biotech Hauls In $600 M [*MedCity News*, NA-NA.]. *Plus More Funding Highlights to Close, 1Q*, 2025.

Visan, A. I., & Negut, I. (2024). Integrating artificial intelligence for drug discovery in the context of revolutionizing drug delivery. *Life (Chicago, Ill.), 14*(2), 233. PMID: 38398742

Vitali, F., Mulas, F., Marini, P., & Bellazzi, R. (2013). Network-based target ranking for polypharmacological therapies. *Journal of Biomedical Informatics, 46*(5), 876–881.

Vitanza, N. A., Wilson, A. L., Huang, W., Seidel, K., Brown, C., Gustafson, J. A., Yokoyama, J. K., Johnson, A. J., Baxter, B. A., Koning, R. W., Reid, A. N., Meechan, M., Biery, M. C., Myers, C., Rawlings-Rhea, S. D., Albert, C. M., Browd, S. R., Hauptman, J. S., Lee, A., & Park, J. R. (2023). Intraventricular B7-H3 CAR T Cells for Diffuse Intrinsic Pontine Glioma: Preliminary First-in-Human Bioactivity and Safety. *Cancer Discovery, 13*(1), 114–131. DOI: 10.1158/2159-8290.CD-22-0750

Voigt, I., Inojosa, H., Dillenseger, A., Haase, R., Akgün, K., & Ziemssen, T. (2021). Digital twins for multiple sclerosis. *Frontiers in Immunology, 12*, 669811. DOI: 10.3389/fimmu.2021.669811

Vollstedt, E.-J., Madoev, H., Aasly, A., Ahmad-Annuar, A., Al-Mubarak, B., Alcalay, R. N., Alvarez, V., Amorin, I., Annesi, G., Arkadir, D., Bardien, S., Barker, R. A., Barkhuizen, M., Basak, A. N., Bonifati, V., Boon, A., Brighina, L., Brockmann, K., Carmine Belin, A., & Klein, C. (2023). Establishing an online resource to facilitate global collaboration and inclusion of underrepresented populations: Experience from the MJFF Global Genetic Parkinson's Disease Project. *PLoS One, 18*(10), e0292180. DOI: 10.1371/journal.pone.0292180

Vo, N. H. H., Phung, H. T. T., Chung, K. L., & Vu, T. Y. (2023). Design and evaluating the efficacy of novel antibodies enhancing binding on CTLA-4 and PD-1 immune checkpoints. *Journal of Advanced Engineering and Computation, 7*(4), 224–236.

Vora, L. K., Gholap, A. D., Jetha, K., Thakur, R. R. S., Solanki, H. K., & Chavda, V. P. (2023). Artificial intelligence in pharmaceutical technology and drug delivery design. *Pharmaceutics, 15*(7), 1916.

Vora, L. K., Gholap, A. D., Jetha, K., Thakur, R. R. S., Solanki, H. K., & Chavda, V. P. (2023). Artificial Intelligence in Pharmaceutical Technology and Drug Delivery Design. *Pharmaceutics, 15*(7). Advance online publication. DOI: 10.3390/pharmaceutics15071916 PMID: 37514102

Wagner, M., Schmidt, J., & Torres, O. (2023). Exploiting smart kitchen scales: Implications for nutrition tracking integrity. *DEF CON 31 Conference Proceedings*.

Walker, A. S., & Clardy, J. (2021). A Machine Learning Bioinformatics Method to Predict Biological Activity from Biosynthetic Gene Clusters. *Journal of Chemical Information and Modeling*, *61*(6), 2560–2571. DOI: 10.1021/acs.jcim.0c01304 PMID: 34042443

Wallach, I., Dzamba, M., & Heifets, A. (2015). AtomNet: a deep convolutional neural network for bioactivity prediction in structure-based drug discovery. *arXiv preprint arXiv:1510.02855*.

Wang, L. L., Lo, K., Chandrasekhar, Y., Reas, R., Yang, J., Burdick, D., Eide, D., Funk, K., Katsis, Y., & Kinney, R. (2020). Cord-19: The covid-19 open research dataset. *ArXiv*, arXiv: 2004.10706 v10704.

Wang, R., Wu, F., Gao, X., Wu, J., Zhao, P., & Yao, J. (2024c). Iggm: A generative model for functional antibody and nanobody design. bioRxiv, 2024-09.

Wang, T., Gao, X., Huai, Z., Gong, Z., Mao, T., Fan, X., & Huang, X. (2023). Revolutionizing antibody discovery industry with highly efficient and accurate AI-based epitope-specific antibody de novo design workflow. *Antibody Therapeutics, 6*(Suppl 1), tbad014-024.

Wang, Y., Li, Z., & Farimani, A. B. (2023). *Graph Neural Networks for Molecules*. https://doi.org/DOI: 10.1007/978-3-031-37196-7_2

Wang, Z., Gao, C., Glass, L. M., & Sun, J. (2022). Artificial intelligence for in silico clinical trials: A review. arXiv preprint arXiv:2209.09023.

Wang, Z., Gao, C., Glass, L. M., & Sun, J. (2022b). Artificial intelligence for in silico clinical trials: A review. *arXiv preprint arXiv:2209.09023*.

Wang, B., Tan, X., Guo, J., Xiao, T., Jiao, Y., Zhao, J., & Wang, Y. (2022a). Drug-induced immune thrombocytopenia toxicity prediction based on machine learning. *Pharmaceutics*, *14*(5), 943.

Wang, D., Fu, Z., Xing, Y., Tan, Y., Han, L., Yu, H., & Wang, T. (2020). Rapid identification of chemical composition and metabolites of Pingxiao Capsule in vivo using molecular networking and untargeted data-dependent tandem mass spectrometry. *Biomedical Chromatography*, *34*(9), e4882. PMID: 32396262

Wang, H., Chen, Y., Wang, L., Liu, Q., Yang, S., & Wang, C. (2023). Advancing herbal medicine: Enhancing product quality and safety through robust quality control practices. *Frontiers in Pharmacology*, *14*, 1265178. DOI: 10.3389/fphar.2023.1265178 PMID: 37818188

Wang, H., Hao, X., He, Y., & Fan, L. (2024a). AbImmPred: An immunogenicity prediction method for therapeutic antibodies using AntiBERTy-based sequence features. *PLoS One*, *19*(2), e0296737.

Wang, J. (2025). Multi-modal topology-aware graph neural network for robust chemical–protein interaction prediction. *International Journal of Molecular Sciences*, *26*(17), 8666.

Wang, J. W., Dai, M. W., Liang, P., Hou, J., & Meng, M. (2025). Correlation does not equal causation: The imperative of causal inference in machine learning models for immunotherapy. *Frontiers in Immunology*, *16*, 1630781.

Wang, L., Wang, L., Wu, P., & Ding, L. (2025). Cardiovascular Magnetic Resonance imaging analysis using neural networks. *Journal of Radiation Research and Applied Sciences*, *18*(4), 101874. DOI: 10.1016/j.jrras.2025.101874

Wang, L., Zhang, J., Shan, G., Liang, J., Jin, W., Li, Y., Su, F., Ba, Y., Tian, X., Sun, X., Zhang, D., Zhang, W., & Chen, C. L. (2021). Establishment of a Lung Cancer Discriminative Model Based on an Optimized Support Vector Machine Algorithm and Study of Key Targets of Wogonin in Lung Cancer. *Frontiers in Pharmacology*, *12*, 728937. DOI: 10.3389/fphar.2021.728937 PMID: 34630106

Wang, L., Zhou, Z., Yang, X., Shi, S., Zeng, X., & Cao, D. (2024b). The present state and challenges of active learning in drug discovery. *Drug Discovery Today*, *29*(6), 103985.

Wang, R., Jiao, Z., Yang, L., Choi, J. W., Xiong, Z., Halsey, K., Tran, T. M. L., Pan, I., Collins, S. A., Feng, X., Wu, J., Chang, K., Shi, L.-B., Yang, S., Yu, Q.-Z., Liu, J., Fu, F.-X., Jiang, X.-L., Wang, D.-C., & Bai, H. X. (2022). Artificial intelligence for prediction of COVID-19 progression using CT imaging and clinical data. *European Radiology*, *32*(1), 205–212. DOI: 10.1007/s00330-021-08049-8

Wang, W. (2024). *AI Based Drug Screening Process: From Data Mining to Candidate Drug Validation*. Bioscience Methods., DOI: 10.5376/bm.2024.15.0005

Wang, X., Xu, X., Tao, W., Li, Y., Wang, Y., & Yang, L. (2012). A systems biology approach to uncovering pharmacological synergy in herbal medicines with applications to cardiovascular disease. *Evidence-Based Complementary and Alternative Medicine : eCAM, 519031*. Advance online publication. DOI: 10.1155/2012/519031 PMID: 23243453

Wang, Y., Jafari, M., Tang, Y., & Tang, J. (2019). Predicting Meridian in Chinese traditional medicine using machine learning approaches. *PLoS Computational Biology*, *15*(11), e1007249. DOI: 10.1371/journal.pcbi.1007249 PMID: 31765369

Wang, Y., Zhao, H., Sciabola, S., & Wang, W. (2023). cMolGPT: A Conditional Generative Pre-Trained Transformer for Target-Specific De Novo Molecular Generation. *Molecules (Basel, Switzerland)*, *28*(11). Advance online publication. DOI: 10.3390/molecules28114430 PMID: 37298906

Wang, Z. (2024). Securing Bluetooth Low Energy: A literature review. *arXiv*.

Wang, Z.-Y., Cheng, J., Wang, Y., Yuan, H.-T., Bi, S.-J., Wang, S.-X., Hou, Y.-M., Zhang, X., Xu, B.-H., Wang, Z.-Y., Zhang, Y., Jiang, W.-J., Chen, Y.-G., & Zhang, M.-X. (2024). Macrophage ILF3 promotes abdominal aortic aneurysm by inducing inflammatory imbalance in male mice. *Nature Communications*, *15*(1), 7249. DOI: 10.1038/s41467-024-51030-4

Warokar, P., & Lote, S. (2024). Ethical and Regulatory Consideration in AI-Assisted Drug Development. *DMIHER Int. Conf. Artif. Intell. Healthc., Educ. Ind., IDICAIEI*. 2024 2nd DMIHER International Conference on Artificial Intelligence in Healthcare, Education and Industry, IDICAIEI 2024. Scopus. https://doi.org/DOI: 10.1109/IDICAIEI61867.2024.10842700

Wasdin, P. T., Johnson, N. V., Janke, A. K., Held, S., Marinov, T. M., Jordaan, G., & Georgiev, I. S. (2025). Generation of antigen-specific paired chain antibody sequences using large language models. bioRxiv, 2024-12.

Weerasekara, S., Darras, N., Fernandez, N., Chen, M., Ainbinder, A., & Price, C. (2025). CellClique: Dissecting tumor microenvironments at the single cell level using generative AI and spatial transcriptomics. *Cancer Research*, *85*(8, Supplement_1), 2418–2418.

Wei, F., Wang, S., & Gou, X. (2021). A review for cell-based screening methods in drug discovery. In *Biophysics Reports* (Vol. 7, Issue 6, pp. 504–516). Science Press. https://doi.org/DOI: 10.52601/bpr.2021.210042

Weissler, E. H., Naumann, T., Andersson, T., Ranganath, R., Elemento, O., Luo, Y., Freitag, D. F., Benoit, J., Hughes, M. C., Khan, F., Slater, P., Shameer, K., Roe, M., Hutchison, E., Kollins, S. H., Broedl, U., Meng, Z., Wong, J. L., Curtis, L., & Ghassemi, M. (2021). The role of machine learning in clinical research: Transforming the future of evidence generation. *Trials*, *22*(1), 537. DOI: 10.1186/s13063-021-05489-x PMID: 34399832

Weller, J. A., & Rohs, R. (2024). Structure-based drug design with a deep hierarchical generative model. *Journal of Chemical Information and Modeling*, *64*(16), 6450–6463. PMID: 39058534

WHO. (2021). Ethics and governance of artificial intelligence for health. World Health Organization. https://www.who.int/publications/i/item/9789240029200

WHO. (2024). Benefits and risks of using artificial intelligence for pharmaceutical development and delivery. World Health Organization. https://www.who.int/publications/i/item/9789240088108

Wieder, O., Kohlbacher, S., Kuenemann, M., Garon, A., Ducrot, P., Seidel, T., & Langer, T. (2020). A compact review of molecular property prediction with graph neural networks. *Drug Discovery Today. Technologies*, *37*, 1–12. DOI: 10.1016/J.DDTEC.2020.11.009 PMID: 34895648

Wiefling, S., Dürmuth, M., & Lo Iacono, L. (2021). Verify it's you: How users perceive risk-based authentication. *IEEE Security and Privacy*, *19*(6), 47–57. DOI: 10.1109/MSEC.2021.3092188

Wigh, D. S., Goodman, J. M., & Lapkin, A. A. (2022). A review of molecular representation in the age of machine learning. In *Wiley Interdisciplinary Reviews: Computational Molecular Science* (Vol. 12, Issue 5). John Wiley and Sons Inc. https://doi.org/DOI: 10.1002/wcms.1603

Wizemann, T., Nass, S. J., Andrada, A., & Amankwah, F. K. (2020). The role of NIH in drug development innovation and its impact on patient access: proceedings of a workshop.

World Health Organization. (2021). Ethics and governance of artificial intelligence for health: WHO guidance.

World Health Organization. (2023). Regulatory system strengthening for medical products: Why it matters. 93. Xu, J., Hagler, A., & Feher, M. (2021). AI in pharmaceutical research: from molecule design to clinical trial simulation. *Frontiers in Pharmacology*, *12*, 700680.

Wouters, O. J., McKee, M., & Luyten, J. (2020). Estimated Research and Development Investment Needed to Bring a New Medicine to Market, 2009-2018. *Journal of the American Medical Association*, *323*(9), 844. DOI: 10.1001/jama.2020.1166

Wouters, O. J., McKee, M., & Luyten, J. (2020). Estimated research and development investment needed to bring a new medicine to market, 2009-2018. *Journal of the American Medical Association*, *323*(9), 844–853. PMID: 32125404

Wouters, O. J., McKee, M., & Luyten, J. (2020). Research and Development Costs of New Drugs-Reply. *Journal of the American Medical Association*, *324*(5), 518. DOI: 10.1001/jama.2020.8651 PMID: 32749488

Wu, C., Chen, J., Lai-Han Leung, E., Chang, H., & Wang, X. (2022). Editorial: Artificial Intelligence in Traditional Medicine. *Frontiers in Pharmacology*, *13*, 933133. DOI: 10.3389/fphar.2022.933133 PMID: 35991902

Wu, Q., Chen, Y., Gu, Y., Fang, S., Li, W., Wang, Q., Fang, J., & Cai, C. (2020). Systems pharmacology-based approach to investigate the mechanisms of Danggui-Shaoyao-san prescription for treatment of Alzheimer's disease. *BMC Complementary Medicine and Therapies*, *20*(1), 282. DOI: 10.1186/s12906-020-03066-4 PMID: 32948180

Wuttke, M., Li, Y., Li, M., Sieber, K. B., Feitosa, M. F., Gorski, M., Tin, A., Wang, L., Chu, A. Y., Hoppmann, A., Kirsten, H., Giri, A., Chai, J.-F., Sveinbjornsson, G., Tayo, B. O., Nutile, T., Fuchsberger, C., Marten, J., Cocca, M., & Pattaro, C. (2019). A catalog of genetic loci associated with kidney function from analyses of a million individuals. *Nature Genetics*, *51*(6), 957–972. DOI: 10.1038/s41588-019-0407-x

Xiang, Y., Zhang, M., Jiang, D., Su, Q., & Shi, J. (2023). The role of inflammation in autoimmune disease: A therapeutic target. *Frontiers in Immunology*, *14*, 1267091. DOI: 10.3389/fimmu.2023.1267091

Xiao, M., Zheng, Q., Popa, P., Mi, X., Hu, J., Zou, F., & Zou, B. (2025). Drug molecular representations for drug response predictions: A comprehensive investigation via machine learning methods. *Scientific Reports*, *15*(1). Advance online publication. DOI: 10.1038/s41598-024-84711-7 PMID: 39748003

Xiaotong, C., LEUNG, Y.-L. A., & Jiangang, S. (2022). Artificial intelligence and its application for cardiovascular diseases in Chinese medicine. *Digital Chinese Medicine*, *5*(4), 367–376.

Xia, Q. D., Xun, Y., Lu, J. L., Lu, Y. C., Yang, Y. Y., Zhou, P., Hu, J., Li, C., & Wang, S. G. (2020). Network pharmacology and molecular docking analyses on Lianhua Qingwen capsule indicate Akt1 is a potential target to treat and prevent COVID-19. *Cell Proliferation*, *53*(12), e12949. DOI: 10.1111/cpr.12949 PMID: 33140889

Xia, X. (2017). Bioinformatics and drug discovery. *Current Topics in Medicinal Chemistry*, *17*(15), 1709–1726. PMID: 27848897

Xia, X., Zhu, C., Zhong, F., & Liu, L. (2023). MDTips: A multimodal-data-based drug–target interaction prediction system fusing knowledge, gene expression profile, and structural data. *Bioinformatics (Oxford, England)*, *39*(7), btad411. PMID: 37379157

Xia, Y., Wang, Y., Wang, Z., & Zhang, W. (2024). A comprehensive review of molecular optimization in artificial intelligence-based drug discovery. *Quantitative Biology*, *12*(1), 15–29. DOI: 10.1002/qub2.30

Xin, K., Wei, X., Shao, J., Chen, F., Liu, Q., & Liu, B. (2024). Establishment of a novel tumor neoantigen prediction tool for personalized vaccine design. *Human Vaccines & Immunotherapeutics*, *20*(1), 2300881.

Xu, B., Lu, Y., Li, C., Yue, L., Wang, X., Hao, N., & Chen, J. (2024). Smiles-mamba: Chemical mamba foundation models for drug admet prediction. *arXiv preprint arXiv:2408.05696*.

Xu, Y., Liu, X., Cao, X., Huang, C., Liu, E., Qian, S., Liu, X., Wu, Y., Dong, F., Qiu, C. W., Qiu, J., Hua, K., Su, W., Wu, J., Xu, H., Han, Y., Fu, C., Yin, Z., Liu, M., & Zhang, J. (2021). Artificial intelligence: A powerful paradigm for scientific research. *Innovation (Cambridge (Mass.))*, *2*(4), 100179. DOI: 10.1016/j.xinn.2021.100179 PMID: 34877560

Xu, Z., Ren, F., Wang, P., Cao, J., Tan, C., Ma, D., Zhao, L., Dai, J., Ding, Y., & Fang, H. (2025). A generative AI-discovered TNIK inhibitor for idiopathic pulmonary fibrosis: A randomized phase 2a trial. *Nature Medicine*, •••, 1–9. PMID: 40461817

Yadav, K. L., Desai, N., Prajapati, A., Narkhede, S., & Luhar, S. (2025). From bench to bedside: AI-enabled drug repurposing for innovative therapies in complex diseases. *Asian Journal of Pharmaceutical Research*, *15*(1), 72–76.

Yan, D., Zhou, Q., Wang, J., & Zhang, N. (2017). Bayesian regularisation neural network based on artificial intelligence optimisation. *International Journal of Production Research*, *55*(8), 2266–2287.

Yang, D., Peng, X., & Peng, S. (2023). Transformer-based models for phla binding affinity prediction. In *2023 IEEE 14th International Conference on Software Engineering and Service Science (ICSESS)* (pp. 297-300). IEEE.

Yang, J., Li, H., Wang, F., Xiao, F., Yan, W., & Hu, G. (2021). Network-based target prioritization and drug candidate identification for multiple sclerosis: From analyzing "Omics Data" to druggability simulations. *ACS Chemical Neuroscience*, *12*(5), 917–929.

Yang, Y., & Cheng, F. (2025). Artificial intelligence streamlines scientific discovery of drug–target interactions. *British Journal of Pharmacology*. PMID: 39843168

Yan, H., & Zou, C. (2021). [Mechanism and material basis of Lianhua Qingwen capsule for improving clinical cure rate of COVID-19: a study based on network pharmacology and molecular docking technology]. *Nan Fang Yi Ke da Xue Xue Bao = Journal of Southern Medical University*, *41*(1), 20–30. DOI: 10.12122/j.issn.1673-4254.2021.01.03 PMID: 33509749

Yaqoob, T., Abbas, H., & Atiquzzaman, M. (2019). Security vulnerabilities, attacks, countermeasures, and regulations of networked medical devices—A review. *IEEE Communications Surveys and Tutorials*, *21*(4), 3723–3768.

Yeh, H. Y., Chao, C. T., Lai, Y. P., & Chen, H. W. (2020). Predicting the Associations between Meridians and Chinese Traditional Medicine Using a Cost-Sensitive Graph Convolutional Neural Network. *International Journal of Environmental Research and Public Health*, *17*(3). Advance online publication. DOI: 10.3390/ijerph17030740 PMID: 31979314

Yenduri, L. K., Chaithra, M. H., Shahedhadeennisa, S., Annamalai, M., Rajesh, L., & Imran, S. M. (2025). Quantum computing and machine learning for transforming precision medicine and drug discovery. In *Modern SuperHyperSoft Computing Trends in Science and Technology* (pp. 339–366). IGI Global Scientific Publishing.

Yepez, D. B., Porta, D. S., Aguas, L. M., & Jattin, F. M. (2025). Optimizing treatment to control LDL cholesterol using machine learning. *Computers in Biology and Medicine*, *195*, 110599. DOI: 10.1016/j.compbiomed.2025.110599

Yeung, Y. T., Aziz, F., Guerrero-Castilla, A., & Arguelles, S. (2018). Signalling pathways in inflammation and anti-inflammatory therapies. *Current Pharmaceutical Design*, *24*(14), 1449–1484.

Ye, Y., Shen, Y., Wang, J., Li, D., Zhu, Y., Zhao, Z., & Wan, J. (2023). SIGANEO: Similarity network with GAN enhancement for immunogenic neoepitope prediction. *Computational and Structural Biotechnology Journal*, *21*, 5538–5543.

Yim, S., Hwang, W., Han, N., & Lee, D. (2022). Computational discovery of cancer immunotherapy targets by intercellular CRISPR screens. *Frontiers in Immunology*, *13*, 884561.

Yin, M., Zhou, H., Wu, J., Zhu, Y., Zhan, Y., Kong, Z., & Wu, J. (2025). S2alm: Sequence-structure pre-trained large language model for comprehensive antibody representation learning. *Research, 8*, 0721.

Yingngam, B. (2025). AI in Clinical Trial Design and Patient Recruitment. In M. Lytras & S. alajlan (Eds.), *Transforming Pharmaceutical Research With Artificial Intelligence* (pp. 27-74). DOI: DOI: 10.4018/979-8-3693-6270-9.ch002

Yingngam, B., Navabhatra, A., & Sillapapibool, P. (2024). AI-Driven Decision-Making Applications in Pharmaceutical Sciences. In *Using Traditional Design Methods to Enhance AI-Driven Decision Making* (pp. 1–63). IGI Global Scientific Publishing.

Yingngam, B., & Sethabouppha, B. (2024). Advanced AI applications for drug discovery. In Shah, I., & Sial, Q. (Eds.), *Advances in Computational Intelligence for the Healthcare Industry 4.0* (pp. 42–86)., DOI: 10.4018/979-8-3693-2333-5.ch003

Yong, L., Fangmin, D., & Renbin, X. (2007). Path synthesis of rapid mechanisms by artificial immune networks. *Journal-Huazhong University of Science and Technology Nature Science Edition*, *35*(3), 70.

You, Z., Ma, J., Li, H., Hu, Y. F., & Huang, J. D. (2025). BConformeR: a conformer based on mutual sampling for unified prediction of continuous and discontinuous antibody binding sites. *arXiv preprint arXiv:2508.12029.*

Yousif, M. G., Fatima, G., Castro, H. J., Al-Amran, F. G., & Rawaf, S. (2023). Unraveling post-COVID-19 immune dysregulation using machine learning-based immunophenotyping. *arXiv preprint arXiv:2310.01428.*

Yuan, Q., Wei, X., Xiong, X., Li, M., & Zhang, Y. (2020). A hybrid neural collaborative filtering model for drug repositioning. In *2020 IEEE International Conference on Bioinformatics and Biomedicine (BIBM)* (pp. 515-518). IEEE.

Yu, H., Jung, J., Yoon, S., Kwon, M., Bae, S., Yim, S., Lee, J., Kim, S., Kang, Y., & Lee, D. (2017). CODA: Integrating multi-level context-oriented directed associations for analysis of drug effects. *Scientific Reports*, *7*(1), 7519. DOI: 10.1038/s41598-017-07448-6 PMID: 28790372

Yu, T., & Chen, K. (2025). Enhancing cardiac disease detection via a fusion of machine learning and medical imaging. *Scientific Reports*, *15*, 26269. DOI: 10.1038/s41598-025-12030-6

Yu, W., Ma, M., Chen, X., Min, J., Li, L., Zheng, Y., Li, Y., Wang, J., & Wang, Q. (2017). Traditional Chinese Medicine and Constitutional Medicine in China, Japan and Korea: A Comparative Study. *The American Journal of Chinese Medicine*, *45*(1), 1–12. DOI: 10.1142/S0192415X1750001X PMID: 28068838

Yu, X., Zhu, X., Zhang, L., Qin, J. J., Feng, C., & Li, Q. (2022). In Silico Screening and Validation of PDGFRA Inhibitors Enhancing Radioiodine Sensitivity in Thyroid Cancer. *Frontiers in Pharmacology*, *13*, 883581. DOI: 10.3389/fphar.2022.883581 PMID: 35645805

Zand, A., Stokes, Z., Sharma, A., van Deen, W. K., & Hommes, D. (2022). Artificial intelligence for inflammatory bowel diseases (IBD); accurately predicting adverse outcomes using machine learning. *Digestive Diseases and Sciences*, *67*(10), 4874–4885.

Zech, J. R., Badgeley, M. A., Liu, M., Costa, A. B., Titano, J. J., & Oermann, E. K. (2018). Variable generalization performance of a deep learning model to detect pneumonia in chest radiographs: A cross-sectional study. *PLoS Medicine*, *15*(11), e1002683. DOI: 10.1371/journal.pmed.1002683 PMID: 30399157

Zhan, X., Liu, Y., Guo, Y., Zhou, W., Yan, Y., Zeng, H., & Feng, Y. (2025). Single cell resolved spatial immune repertoire unveils spatial heterogeneity of lymphoid aggregates in human immune disorders. bioRxiv, 2025-01.

Zhang, D., Yang, S., Yuan, X., & Zhang, P. (2021). Interpretable deep learning for automatic diagnosis of 12-lead electrocardiogram. *iScience*, *24*(4), 102373. DOI: 10.1016/j.isci.2021.102373

Zhang, G., Yan, C., Ji, X., Zhang, T., Zhang, T., & Xu, W. (2017). DolphinAttack: Inaudible voice commands. In *Proceedings of the 2017 ACM SIGSAC Conference on Computer and Communications Security* (pp. 103-117). ACM. DOI: 10.1145/3133956.3134052

Zhang, H., Ni, W., Li, J., & Zhang, J. (2020). Artificial Intelligence-Based Traditional Chinese Medicine Assistive Diagnostic System: Validation Study. *JMIR Medical Informatics*, *8*(6), e17608. DOI: 10.2196/17608 PMID: 32538797

Zhang, H., Ni, W., Li, J., & Zhang, J. (2020). Artificial intelligence–based traditional Chinese medicine assistive diagnostic system: Validation study. *JMIR Medical Informatics*, *8*(6), e17608. PMID: 32538797

Zhang, H., Zhu, T., Ren, M., He, Z., Tao, S., Li, M., & Bu, D. (2025a). Accurate immune protein structure prediction by large language model and transfer learning. https://doi.org/DOI: 10.21203/rs.3.rs-7153530/v1

Zhang, K., Yang, X., Wang, Y., Yu, Y., Huang, N., Li, G., & Yang, S. (2025). Artificial intelligence in drug development. *Nature Medicine*, •••, 1–15. PMID: 39833407

Zhang, M., Peng, Y., Wang, M., Gao, B., Zhao, L., & Li, X. (2019). The influence of compatibility of Si-Ni decoction with metabolism in intestinal bacteria on transports of toxic diterpenoid alkaloids from processed aconite root across Caco-2 monolayers. *Journal of Ethnopharmacology*, *228*, 164–178. DOI: 10.1016/j.jep.2018.09.022 PMID: 30223050

Zhang, M., Zhang, C., Sheng, V. S., & Fuhry, D. (2019). Behaviometric: A behavior biometric user authentication approach based on machine learning techniques. In *Proceedings of the 28th ACM International Conference on Information and Knowledge Management* (pp. 2357–2360).

Zhang, Q., Guo, Y., Zhang, B., Liu, H., Peng, Y., Wang, D., & Zhang, D. (2022). Identification of hub biomarkers of myocardial infarction by single-cell sequencing, bioinformatics, and machine learning. *Frontiers in Cardiovascular Medicine*, *9*, 939972. DOI: 10.3389/fcvm.2022.939972 PMID: 35958412

Zhang, Q., Wang, Y., Chen, A., Huang, X., Dong, Q., Li, Z., Gao, X., Wu, T., Li, W., Cong, P., Wan, H., Dai, D., He, M., Liang, H., Wang, S., & Xiong, L. (2021). Xiaoxuming Decoction: A Traditional Herbal Recipe for Stroke With Emerging Therapeutic Mechanisms. *Frontiers in Pharmacology*, *12*, 802381. DOI: 10.3389/fphar.2021.802381 PMID: 34970152

Zhang, T., Lin, Y., & Gao, Q. (2023a). Bispecific antibodies targeting immunomodulatory checkpoints for cancer therapy. *Cancer Biology & Medicine*, *20*(3), 181–195.

Zhang, T., Zhang, X., Wu, Z., Ren, J., Zhao, Z., Zhang, H., & Wang, T. (2025b). VGAE-CCI: Variational graph autoencoder-based construction of 3D spatial cell–cell communication network. *Briefings in Bioinformatics*, *26*(1), bbae619.

Zhang, W., Huai, Y., Miao, Z., Qian, A., & Wang, Y. (2019). Systems Pharmacology for Investigation of the Mechanisms of Action of Traditional Chinese Medicine in Drug Discovery. *Frontiers in Pharmacology*, *10*, 743. DOI: 10.3389/fphar.2019.00743 PMID: 31379563

Zhang, X., Rahnavard, A., & Crandall, K. A. (2025c). Machine learning enhances biomarker discovery: From multi-omics to functional genomics. *Medical Research Archives*, *13*(8).

Zhang, Y., Ari, S. L., Gupta, S., Zaemes, J., Shah, N. J., Alaoui, A., & Atkins, M. B. (2023b). 1317 Enhancing patient safety in melanoma treatment: Harnessing machine learning for predicting immune-related adverse events. *Journal for Immunotherapy of Cancer*, *11*(1, Supplement).

Zhang, Y., Bhosle, A., Bae, S., McIver, L. J., Pishchany, G., Accorsi, E. K., Thompson, K. N., Arze, C., Wang, Y., & Subramanian, A. (2022). Discovery of bioactive microbial gene products in inflammatory bowel disease. *Nature*, *606*(7915), 754–760. PMID: 35614211

Zhao, H. X., Qi, W., Liu, K., Zhao, J., Hu, X., & Deng, W. Q. (2025). Accelerating drug discovery for Disease X via AlphaFold2 driven drug repositioning strategy. *Physical Chemistry Chemical Physics*.

Zhao, L., He, Q., Song, H., Zhou, T., Luo, A., Wen, Z., & Lin, X. (2024). Protein A-like peptide design based on diffusion and ESM2 Models. *Molecules (Basel, Switzerland)*, *29*(20), 4965.

Zhao, Y., He, B., Xu, F., Li, C., Xu, Z., Su, X., & Yao, J. (2023). DeepAIR: A deep learning framework for effective integration of sequence and 3D structure to enable adaptive immune receptor analysis. *Science Advances*, *9*(32), eabo5128.

Zhavoronkov, A., Ivanenkov, Y. A., Aliper, A., Veselov, M. S., Aladinskiy, V. A., Aladinskaya, A. V., Terentiev, V. A., Polykovskiy, D. A., Kuznetsov, M. D., & Asadulaev, A. (2019). Deep learning enables rapid identification of potent DDR1 kinase inhibitors. *Nature Biotechnology*, *37*(9), 1038–1040. PMID: 31477924

Zhavoronkov, A., Vanhaelen, Q., & Oprea, T. I. (2020). Will Artificial Intelligence for Drug Discovery Impact Clinical Pharmacology? *Clinical Pharmacology and Therapeutics*, *107*(4), 780–785. DOI: 10.1002/cpt.1795

Zhazykbayeva, S., Pabel, S., Mügge, A., Sossalla, S., & Hamdani, N. (2020). The molecular mechanisms associated with the physiological responses to inflammation and oxidative stress in cardiovascular diseases. *Biophysical Reviews*, *12*(4), 947–968. DOI: 10.1007/s12551-020-00742-0

Zhou, J., Sturtevant, D., Biyani, N., Bhatia, K., & Dave, S. (2022). MCL-319 LP-284–A Highly Potent Small Molecule Targeting Mantle Cell Lymphoma. *Clinical Lymphoma, Myeloma & Leukemia*, *22*, S396.

Zhou, J., Sturtevant, D., Love, C., Kulkarni, A., Biyani, N., Kathad, U., Thacker, E., Dave, S., & Bhatia, K. (2023). LP-284, a small molecule acylfulvene, exerts potent antitumor activity in preclinical non-Hodgkin's lymphoma models and in cells deficient in DNA damage repair. *Oncotarget*, *14*, 597. PMID: 37306526

Zhou, M., Huang, Z., Ma, Z., Chen, J., Lin, S., Yang, X., & Zhong, J. (2025a). The next frontier in antibody-drug conjugates: Challenges and opportunities in cancer and autoimmune therapy. *Cancer Drug Resistance (Alhambra, Calif.)*, *8*, 34.

Zhou, X. J., Laouar, Y., & Tsoi, L. C. (2025b). Community series in towards precision medicine for immune-mediated disorders: Advances in using big data and artificial intelligence to understand heterogeneity in inflammatory responses, volume II. *Frontiers in Immunology*, *16*, 1553004.

Zhou, Y., & Wang, F. (2022). Explainable AI in healthcare and drug discovery: Trends and challenges. *Trends in Pharmacological Sciences*, *43*(6), 457–469. PMID: 35469690

Zhou, Z., Kearnes, S., Li, L., Zare, R. N., & Riley, P. (2019). Optimization of molecules via deep reinforcement learning. *Scientific Reports*, *9*(1), 10752.

Zhu, H. (2020). Big Data and Artificial Intelligence Modeling for Drug Discovery. *Annual Review of Pharmacology and Toxicology*, *60*, 573–589. PMID: 31518513

Zhu, I., Piraner, D. I., & Roybal, K. T. (2023). Synthesizing a smarter CAR T cell: Advanced engineering of T-cell immunotherapies. *Cancer Immunology Research*, *11*(8), 1030–1043.

Zhu, M., Zhang, H., Zhou, Q., Sheng, S., Gao, Q., Geng, Z., Chen, X., Lai, Y., Jing, Y., Xu, K., Bai, L., Wang, G., Wang, J., Jiang, Y., & Su, J. (2025). Dynamic GelMA/DNA Dual-Network Hydrogels Promote Woven Bone Organoid Formation and Enhance Bone Regeneration. *Advanced Materials (Deerfield Beach, Fla.)*, *37*(24), e2501254. DOI: 10.1002/adma.202501254

Zhu, T., Liu, B., Chen, N., Liu, Y., Wang, Z., & Tian, X. (2025). Artificial intelligence-driven innovations in pharmaceutical development and drug delivery systems. *Current Topics in Medicinal Chemistry*.

Zollinger-Read, C., & Filer, A. (2025). Therapeutics update in immune-mediated rheumatic diseases: Rheumatoid arthritis, idiopathic inflammatory myositis and ANCA-associated vasculitis. *Clinical Medicine (London, England)*, *25*(5), 100507. DOI: 10.1016/j.clinme.2025.100507

About the Contributors

Jen-Tsung Chen is a professor of cell biology at the National University of Kaohsiung in Taiwan. He teaches cell biology, genomics, proteomics, plant physiology, and plant biotechnology. Dr. Chen's research interests include bioactive compounds, chromatography techniques, plant molecular biology, plant biotechnology, bioinformatics, and systems pharmacology. He is an active editor of academic books and international journals to advance the exploration of multidisciplinary knowledge involving plant physiology, plant biotechnology, nanotechnology, materials science, ethnopharmacology, and systems biology. He serves as an associate editor, editorial board member, and guest editor in reputed journals. Dr. Chen published books in collaboration with international publishers, and he is handling book projects on diverse topics such as AI technologies, drug discovery, drug development, herbal medicine, medicinal biotechnology, nanotechnology, bioengineering, plant functional genomics, plant speed breeding, epigenetics, functional RNAs, and CRISPR-based genome editing. Dr. Chen is a productive author in academic publications and was recognized as one of the World's Top 2% Scientists 2023, 2024, and 2025 by Elsevier and Stanford University. Dr. Chen received the Springer Nature Editor of Distinction Award in 2025.

***

Akhil Arun is a gold medalist PharmD (Post Baccalaureate) graduate with an MBA in Hospital Administration and Healthcare. A Harvard-trained researcher (GCSRT Program), Dr. Akhil specializes in clinical pharmacy, pharmacoeconomics, and translational research. He is the inventor of a UK-design-patented Automated Insulin Delivery Pen and has presented his cost-effectiveness research at 11th World Congress on Health Economics,Health Policy and Healthcare Management. Dr. Akhil's core strengths lie in clinical research, scientific writing, academic mentorship, and health communication.

Yash Chandrakant Bari is an undergraduate student in the Department of Pharmacy at Saraswathi Vidya Bhavan's College of Pharmacy, University of Mumbai. His research interests focus on drug development and the applications of artificial intelligence in pharmaceutical sciences. He is currently pursuing a Bachelor of Pharmacy (B.Pharm) degree (2022–2026). For professional correspondence, he can be reached at yashbari0904@gmail.com or via LinkedIn:

Joyeta Ghosh is a dedicated faculty member and researcher with a passion for exploring diverse aspects of Nutrition and Dietetics. Her expertise spans areas including Metabolic Syndrome, Cancer Biology, Genomics, Neurophysiology, and Stress Physiology. With a Ph.D. in Nutritional Biochemistry from the University of Calcutta (DST-INSPIRE Fellow)(2021), a Masters in Applied Nutrition from AIIPH, Kolkata, and a Bachelor's in Food and Nutrition (Honors) from the University of Calcutta, Dr. Ghosh has built a strong academic foundation. She further expanded her skillset with an M.Sc. in Data Science from Liverpool John Moores University, UK. Her core skills encompass experimental design with human subjects, fieldwork, statistical data analysis, and a wide range of laboratory techniques. As a consultant and data scientist in Nutrition Artificial Intelligence, Dr. Ghosh continues to push the boundaries of innovation in the field. Her commitment to excellence in teaching and research, coupled with a relentless pursuit of knowledge, drives her contributions to the advancement of science and nutrition.

Salar Hafez-Ghoran was born and raised in Sardasht, West Azerbaijan, Iran. He holds a Ph.D. degree in Phytochemistry (Golestan University and Shiraz University of Medical Sciences, Iran). In 2022, he won a post-doctoral fellowship from the H.E.J. Research Institute of Chemistry, International Center for Chemical and Biological Sciences (ICCBS), University of Karachi, Pakistan. Currently, he is a Postdoctoral Research Associate in the Center for Excellence Post-Harvest Technologies (CEPHT) at North Carolina Agricultural and Technical State University, Kannapolis, USA. His research interests include: Whole Grains' Bioactive Compounds, Food Chemistry, Metabolism and Biotransformation, Isolation and Structure Elucidation of Secondary Metabolites, Ethnopharmacology.

M. Karpakavalli is a pharmacist, teacher and a medicinal chemist since from past two decades. Now, she is working as a Professor & Head, Dept. of Pharmaceutical Chemistry, Karpagam College of Pharmacy, Coimbatore, Tamil Nadu. now has 21 years of teaching & academic research experience. Rewarded with Ph.D guideship from The TN Dr. MGR Medical University, Chennai in 2019and Best academician award from AEDS and NABARD Govt. sectors, in 2021, Distinguished alumni Award in 2025, ¬ Rewarded with "NPTEL STAR-

Enthusiastic Award" in October 2022; "NPTEL STAR-Believer Award" in October 2023; "NPTEL STAR-Motivated Learner Award" in October 2023; "NPTEL STAR-Discipline Star Award" in October 2023; and "NPTEL STAR-Believer Award" in April 2024; "NPTEL STAR-Enthusiastic Award" in Jul-Dec 2024 and "NPTEL STAR-Evangelist Award" in Jul-Dec 2024. She has been a co-chair, poster evaluator, a lead lecturer, a moderator in national & international level seminars/workshops and has delivered scientific speeches in STTP/FDP/national level conferences. She has 40 publications in national and 14 publications in international levels with 191 citations, 07 H-index and 06 i10 index metrics. She has worked as an editor for a college souvenir, newsletters and IJHC guest editor for the issue (Vol 34 (4), 2024) and has been an author for two Pharmacy books and for three book chapters. She is a member of pharmacy professional bodies viz., TNSPC, IPA, IPGA, APTI, & AEDS. She is a recognized Inspector of PCI, New Delhi and The TN DR MGR Medical University, Chennai, Tamil Nadu; Recognized Examiner of the TN DR MGR Medical University, Chennai, Tamil Nadu and other equivalent Universities for Pharmacy Curriculum; Member of Advisor Panel of an academic excelling Dfree Novelish Association, AP ; Editorial Board Member-Journal of Ethno-pharmacology & Toxicology; Journal of Medical Surgical and Allied Sciences; Innovative Publications (P) Ltd., and Reviewer for many scientific journals

Rohan Pai is currently an assistant professor at Shobhaben Pratapbhai Patel School of Pharmacy & Technology Management. He has completed his Ph.D. (Tech.) in Pharmaceutics from the Institute of Chemical Technology, Mumbai, where he worked on the development of novel drug delivery systems for ophthalmic applications using computer-aided approaches for screening materials and systematically designing nanocarrier based drug delivery systems. Previously, he was employed in the Formulation and Development department of Rubicon Research Pvt. Ltd. as a Research Officer, where he was actively involved in the development and evaluation of a polymer and a polymeric delivery system based on their platform technology. His research interests include Nano Delivery Systems, Experimental Designs, Computer-Aided Formulation Development.

Gaurav Singh Pilkhwal is a Pharm.D intern at School of Pharmaceutical Sciences,Shri Guru Ram Rai University, Dehradun, India.With a focus on pharmaceutical reaserch and clinical practice and contribute to advancing knowledge in drug development, pharmacotherapy,and patient care.

Anika Singh is a Biotechnology major specializing in nanotechnology, cancer therapeutics, and computational drug screening. She has conducted basic research on silica-coated ZnO nanoparticles for pharmaceutical degradation, p-Tau biomarker detection using nanochips, and AI driven drug screening approaches. She has experience and interest aligns with molecular biology techniques, microbial assays, and interdisciplinary device design. Her long-term goal is to contribute to data-driven drug development and precision nanomedicine.

N.L Swathi is an esteemed academic researcher and medical writer with extensive expertise in medical technology and AI-assisted diagnostics. She has made significant contributions to the field through her research and publications, particularly focusing on integrating advanced technologies into healthcare systems to enhance diagnostic accuracy and therapeutic efficacy. She believes in the power of integrating technology in healthcare to achieve precise outcomes, which is reflected in her pioneering work and dedication to advancing medical science. Her work has been recognized for its impact on both clinical practice and healthcare innovation.

Fatemeh Taktaz was born and raised in Shiraz, Fars, Iran. She holds a Ph.D. degree in Clinical and Experimental Medical Science (University of Campania "Luigi Vanvitelli", Naples, Italy). Currently, she is a Postdoctoral Research Associate in the Center for Excellence Post-Harvest Technologies (CEPHT) at North Carolina Agricultural and Technical State University, Kannapolis, USA. Her research interests include: The role of Whole Grains on Cardiovascular Disease, Nutritional Biochemistry, Diabetes, Obesity, Human metabolism, Epigenetics, Cellular and Molecular Biology, Enzymology, Chronic Disease.

Muhammad Usman Tariq has more than 16+ year's experience in industry and academia. He is a prolific author of research articles, case studies, book chapters, and academic books, with work spanning a wide range of disciplines. His contributions also include several patents. He is founder and CEO of The Case HQ, a unique repository for courses, narrative and video case studies. Additionally, he is President of Gulf Higher Education (Gulf HE) focused on advancing academic practice. He has been working as a consultant and trainer for industries representing six sigma, quality, health and safety, environmental systems, project management, and information security standards. His work has encompassed sectors in aviation, manufacturing, food, hospitality, education, finance, research, software and transportation. He has diverse and significant experience working with accreditation agencies of ABET, ACBSP, AACSB, WASC, CAA, EFQM and NCEAC. He is a Principal Fellow of Advance HE UK, Senior Fellow of SEDA UK, and Chartered Fellow of CIPD UK other than Senior Member IEEE.

Anita Ioana Visan is a Scientific Researcher 2nd degree at the National Institute for Lasers, Plasma and Radiation Physics (INFLPR), highly specialized in the development and characterization of advanced functional coatings for biomedical and antimicrobial applications.Her primary research focuses on using laser-based deposition techniques, including Pulsed Laser Deposition (PLD) and Matrix Assisted Pulsed Laser Evaporation (MAPLE), to synthesize thin coatings from materials such as calcium phosphates, biopolymers, flavonoids, and antimicrobial peptides. Dr. Vi an's work extends to the fields of Artificial Intelligence in Materials Science & Engineering, specifically applying predictive models for drug discovery, controlled-release systems, and optimizing complex fabrication processes like laser cladding and deposition. She also has experience researching energy materials, including thermoelectric materials and gas sensors, and thin film characterization.She has authored or co-authored 36 ISI indexed articles, with 20 of those as the main or corresponding author. Her total citations are 962 (896 without self-citations), and her Hirsh index is 18 (according to Web of Science).She holds 3 patents covering innovations in composite systems for medical device functionalization, a hot probe method for Seebeck coefficient measurement, and a fluid decontamination procedure using UV-C radiation and metamaterials.Dr. Vi an was the Project Director for a PN III Exploratory Research Project (valued at 242,575 euros) and has played a key role in 11 other national research projects and 2 international grants.She was awarded the prestigious L'Oréal National Scholarship - UNESCO For Women in Science 2020 in the Life Sciences category.Her patents and inventions have earned significant recognition, including a Gold Medal (PRO INVENT 2025), a Diploma of Excellence and "Pro Invent" Medal (PRO INVENT 2023), and a Silver Medal (INFOINVENT 2023).She has won multiple Best Oral and Best Poster Presentation awards at various international conferences and workshops.

Mrudula Santosh Wani is a Biomedical Engineering student in the Department of Biomedical Engineering at Vidyalankar Institute of Technology. Her research focuses on Medical engineering based concepts, with a particular interest in AI in Healthcare, Medical Imaging Technology and Biomedical Equipment Management. She is pursuing her Bachelor's in Technology in Biomedical Engineering in same institute from year 2022 to 2026. Mrudula is the author of Ethical Considerations in AI Driven Drug Development and Pharmaceutical Industry.

Bancha Yingngam is an Associate Professor in the Faculty of Pharmacy, Ubon Ratchathani University, Thailand, specializing in Pharmaceutical Sciences and Technology. He earned both his pharmacy degree and PhD from Ubon Ratchathani University, and subsequently undertook a postdoctoral fellowship at Karl-Franzens-Universität Graz, Austria (2013–2021). Dr. Yingngam has published more than 80 scholarly works and serves as a reviewer for over 100 Scopus-indexed journals. His academic achievements include an h-index of 19 (Scopus) and recognition on Stanford University and Elsevier's World Top 2% Scientists list (2025) in the field of pharmacology and pharmacy, highlighting his substantial impact in pharmaceutical research.

Index

A

C

D

E

F

G

H

I

M

www.ingramcontent.com/pod-product-compliance
Lightning Source LLC
LaVergne TN
LVHW081317300926
849161LV00008B/1790